Blood & Circulatory Disorders Sourcebook

Basic Information about Disorders Such As Anemia, Hemorrhage, Shock, Embolism, and Thrombosis, along with Facts Concerning Rh Factor, Blood Banks, Blood Donation Programs, and Transfusions

Edited by Linda M. Ross. 600 pages. 1998. 0-7808-0203-9. $75.

Burns Sourcebook

Basic Information about Heat, Chemical, Electrical, and Sun Burns, along with Facts about Burn Treatment and Recovery, and Reports on Current Research Initiatives

Edited by Allan R. Cook. 600 pages. 1998. 0-7808-0204-7. $75.

Cancer Sourcebook

Basic Information on Cancer Types, Symptoms, Diagnostic Methods, and Treatments, Including Statistics on Cancer Occurrences Worldwide and the Risks Associated with Known Carcinogens and Activities

Edited by Frank E. Bair. 932 pages. 1990. 1-55888-888-8. $75.

"This publication's nontechnical nature and very comprehensive format make it useful for both the general public and undergraduate students."
— Choice, Oct '90

"This compact collection of reliable information, written in a positive, hopeful tone, is an invaluable tool for helping patients and patients' families and friends to take the first steps in coping with the many difficulties of cancer." — Medical Reference Services Quarterly, Winter '91

"An important resource for the general reader trying to understand the complexities of cancer."
— American Reference Books Annual, '91

Cancer Sourcebook for Women

Basic Information about Specific Forms of Cancer That Affect Women, Featuring Facts about Breast Cancer, Cervical Cancer, Ovarian Cancer, Cancer of the Uterus and Uterine Sarcoma, Cancer of the Vagina, and Cancer of the Vulva; Statistical and Demographic Da' ment Suggestions;

Edited by Allan]
pages. 1996. 0-78(

"This timely boc sumer health and libraries."

"The availability under one cover of all these pertinent publications, grouped under cohesive headings, makes this certainly a most useful sourcebook."
— Choice, Jun '96

"Laudably, the book portrays the feelings of the cancer victim, as well as her mate . . . .both benefit from the gold mine of information nestled between the two covers of this book. It is hard to conceive of any library that would not want it as part of its collection. Recommended."
— Academic Library Book Review, Summer '96

". . . written in easily understandable, non-technical language. Recommended for public libraries or hospital and academic libraries that collect patient education or consumer health materials."
— Medical Reference Services Quarterly, Spring '97

New Cancer Sourcebook

Basic Information about Major Forms and Stages of Cancer, Featuring Facts about Primary and Secondary Tumors of the Respiratory, Nervous, Lymphatic, Circulatory, Skeletal, and Gastrointestinal Systems, and Specific Organs; Statistical and Demographic Data, Treatment Options, and Strategies for Coping

Edited by Allan R. Cook. 1,313 pages. 1996. 0-7808-0041-9. $75.

"This book is an excellent resource. The dialogue is simple, direct, and comprehensive."
— Doody's Health Sciences Book Review, Nov '96

"The amount of factual and useful information is extensive. The writing is very clear, geared to general readers. Recommended for all levels."
— Choice, Jan '97

Cardiovascular Diseases & Disorders Sourcebook

Basic Information about Cardiovascular Diseases and Disorders, Featuring Facts about the Cardiovascular System, Demographic and Statistical Data, Descriptions of Pharmacological and Surgical Interventions, Lifestyle Modifications, and a Special Section Focusing on Heart Disorders in Children

Edited by Karen Bellenir and Peter D. Dresser. 683 pages. 1995. 0-7808-0032-X. $75.

". . . comprehensive format provides an extensive overview on this subject." — Choice, Jun '96

"Easily understood, complete, up-to-date resource. This well executed public health tool will make valu-
to those that need it most,
The typeface, sturdy non-
binding add a feel of quali-
ublications. Highly recom-
eneral libraries."
Book Review, Summer '96

Continues next page

Communication Disorders Sourcebook

Basic Information about Deafness and Hearing Loss, Speech and Language Disorders, Voice Disorders, Balance and Vestibular Disorders, and Disorders of Smell, Taste, and Touch

Edited by Linda M. Ross. 533 pages. 1996. 0-7808-0077-X. $75.

"This is skillfully edited and is a welcome resource for the layperson. It should be found in every public and medical library."
— Doody's Health Sciences Book Review, May '96

Congenital Disorders Sourcebook

Basic Information about Disorders Acquired during Gestation, Including Spina Bifida, Hydrocephalus, Cerebral Palsy, Heart Defects, Craniofacial Abnormalities, Fetal Alcohol Syndrome, and More, along with Current Treatment Options and Statistical Data

Edited by Karen Bellenir. 607 pages. 1997. 0-7808-0205-5. $75.

Consumer Issues in Health Care Sourcebook

Basic Information about Consumer Health Concerns, Including an Explanation of Physician Specialties, How to Choose a Doctor, How to Prepare for a Hospital Visit, Ways to Avoid Fraudulent "Miracle" Cures, How to Use Medications Safely, What to Look for when Choosing a Nursing Home, and End-of-Life Planning

Edited by Wendy Wilcox. 600 pages. 1998. 0-7808-0221-7. $75.

Contagious & Non-Contagious Infectious Diseases Sourcebook

Basic Information about Contagious Diseases like Measles, Polio, Hepatitis B, and Infectious Mononucleosis, and Non-Contagious Infectious Diseases like Tetanus and Toxic Shock Syndrome, and Diseases Occurring as Secondary Infections Such As Shingles and Reye Syndrome, along with Vaccination, Prevention, and Treatment Information, and a Section Describing Emerging Infectious Disease Threats

Edited by Karen Bellenir and Peter D. Dresser. 566 pages. 1996. 0-7808-0075-3. $75.

Diabetes Sourcebook

Basic Information about Insulin-Dependent and Noninsulin-Dependent Diabetes Mellitus, Gestational Diabetes, and Diabetic Complications, Symptoms, Treatment, and Research Results, Including Statistics on Prevalence, Morbidity, and Mortality, along with Source Listings for Further Help and Information

Edited by Karen Bellenir and Peter D. Dresser. 827 pages. 1994. 1-55888-751-2. $75.

"Very informative and understandable for the layperson without being simplistic. It provides a comprehensive overview for laypersons who want a general understanding of the disease or who want to focus on various aspects of the disease."
— Bulletin of the MLA, Jan '96

Diet & Nutrition Sourcebook

Basic Information about Nutrition, Including the Dietary Guidelines for Americans, the Food Guide Pyramid, and Their Applications in Daily Diet, Nutritional Advice for Specific Age Groups, Current Nutritional Issues and Controversies, the New Food Label and How to Use It to Promote Healthy Eating, and Recent Developments in Nutritional Research

Edited by Dan R. Harris. 662 pages. 1996. 0-7808-0084-2. $75.

"It is so refreshing to find a reliable and factual reference book. Recommended to aspiring professionals, librarians, and others seeking and giving reliable dietary advice. An excellent compilation."
— Choice, Feb '97

"Recommended for public and medical libraries that receive general information requests on nutrition. It is readable and will appeal to those interested in learning more about healthy dietary practices."
— Medical Reference Services Quarterly, Fall '97

Ear, Nose & Throat Disorders Sourcebook

Basic Information about Disorders of the Ears, Nose, Sinus Cavities, Tonsils, Adenoids, Pharynx, and Larynx, along with Statistical and Demographic Data and Reports on Current Research Initiatives

Edited by Linda M. Ross. 600 pages. 1998. 0-7808-0206-3. $75.

Endocrine & Metabolic Diseases & Disorders Sourcebook

Basic Information for the Layperson about Disorders Such As Graves' Disease, Goiter, Cushing's Syndrome, and Hormonal Imbalances, along with Reports on Current Research Initiatives

Edited by Linda M. Ross. 600 pages. 1998. 0-7808-0207-1. $75.

Continues on back end sheets

PUBLIC HEALTH
SOURCEBOOK

Health Reference Series

Volume Thirty-four

PUBLIC HEALTH SOURCEBOOK

*Basic Information about Government
Health Agencies Including National
Health Statistics and Trends, Healthy
People 2000 Program Goals and
Objectives, the Centers for Disease Control
and Prevention, the Food and Drug
Administration, and the National Institutes
of Health, Along with Full Contact
Information for Each Agency*

Edited by
Wendy Wilcox

Omnigraphics, Inc.

Public health sourcebook   'HIC NOTE

⟩wing publications produced by the National
⟩nt of Health and Human Services (DHHS),
the U.S. General Accounting Office (GAO), tne U.S. Department of Agriculture (USDA),
the U.S. Public Health Service (PHS), the U.S. Food and Drug Administration (FDA), and
the U.S. Department of Education, National Institute of Disability and Rehabilitation
Research (NIDRR): NIH 96-5, NIH 96-4104; FDA 96-1092, FDA 96-1228, FDA 96-1254;
FDA Consumer magazine (6/95, 12/96, 7-8/96); HRSA-M-DSEA-96-5, B0033-1994; PHS 95-
1237, PHS 96-1120, PHS 96-1785, PHS 96-1857; USDA AIB-711; GAO-PEMD-95-14, GAO/
PEMD-95-21, GAO/PEMD-95-22, GAO/PEMD-96-6; and NIDRR: No. 16, No. 9, No. 3. Full
citation information is given on the first page of each chapter.

Edited by Wendy Wilcox
Peter D. Dresser, Managing Editor, *Health Reference Series*
Karen Bellenir, Series Editor, *Health Reference Series*

Omnigraphics, Inc.
Matthew P. Barbour, *Manager, Production and Fulfillment*
Laurie Lanzen Harris, *Vice President, Editorial Director*
Peter E. Ruffner, *Vice President, Administration*
James A. Sellgren, *Vice President, Operations and Finance*
Jane J. Steele, *Marketing Consultant*

Frederick G. Ruffner, Jr., Publisher
©1998, Omnigraphics, Inc.
Library of Congress Cataloging-in-Publication Data

Public health sourcebook ; basic information about government
   health agencies . . . / edited by Wendy Wilcox.
      p. cn. — (Health reference series ; v. 34)
   Includes bibliographical references and index.
   ISBN 0-7808-0220-9 (lib. bdg. ; alk. paper)
      1. Public health—United States. 2. Public health—United
   States—Statistics. 3. Public health administration—United
   States—Directories. 4. Public health—United States—
   Information services. I. Wilcox, Wendy. II. Series
RA445.P835 1998   98-15705
362, 1'0973—dc21   CIP

∞

Printed in the United States

Table of Contents

v

Part II—Healthy People 2000

Part III—Centers for Disease Control and Prevention

Part IV—Food and Drug Administration

Part V—National Institutes of Health

Part VI—Appendices

Preface

About this Book

According to 1994 statistics from the Centers for Disease Control and Prevention, the average American can expect to live 75.7 years from birth, an increase of .2 years from 1993. This increase is attributed to a decline in the mortality rate from heart disease, cancer, pneumonia and influenza. With a longer life expectancy, however, Americans also have greater probability of experiencing disease and disabilities.

This volume contains basic information on how to obtain disease trends and statistics, health-related data and literature from federal and state government agencies, along with contact information for federal and state health agencies. Persons suffering from disease or disability, family members, friends and the general public will benefit from contacting the various agencies listed for materials and information.

How to Use this Book

This book is divided into parts and chapters. Parts focus on broad areas of interest. Chapters are devoted to single topics within a part.

Part I: United States Health Statistics and Trends provides an overview of health conditions and disabilities in the United States, including birth and death statistics, chronic disease statistics, leading causes of death and ethnic disease trends.

Part II: Healthy People 2000 presents the program goals and objectives of the Healthy People 2000 program, offers a look at how Americans are faring with the objectives, and includes ideas for healthy worksites.

Part III: Centers for Disease Control and Prevention offers an overview of the agency's centers and institute, information about vaccination for adults and children, and notifiable and infectious disease data.

Part IV: Food and Drug Administration explains the FDA's role in monitoring the quality of prescription and over-the-counter drugs, medical devices and the nation's food supply. It includes information on how policies are established, how citizens can become involved in the process or report problems, and how to obtain documents and other materials.

Part V: National Institutes of Health offers a complete listing of subagencies within the NIH, including major programs and research effort. It also provides contact information for each institute.

Part VI: Appendices includes a comprehensive list of health information resourses available from the federal government and an alphabetical listing of State Health Departments, including addresses and available telephone and facsimile numbers. A list of selected public health agency internet web sites is also included.

Note from the Editor

This book is part of Omnigraphics' Health Reference Series. The series provides basic information about a broad range of medical concerns. It is not intended to serve as a tool for diagnosing illnesses, in prescribing treatments, or as a substitute for the physician/patient relationship. All persons concerned about medical symptoms or the possibility of disease are encouraged to seek professional care from an appropriate health care provider.

Part One

United States Health
Statistics and Trends

Chapter 1

Health Status, Medical Care Use, and Number of Disabling Conditions in the United States

Approximately 37.7 million people, or 15 percent of the noninstitutionalized United States population, have disabilities, defined here as a limitation in activity caused by a chronic condition or impairment. More than one-third of this group has two or more disabling conditions. People with multiple disabling conditions have poorer health and use more medical services than those with only one condition.

All estimates presented in this report are based on the 1992 National Health Interview Survey (NHIS).

Age and Number of Disabling Conditions

The overall rate of disability increases with age, from 6 percent of children and youth to 45 percent of adults aged 75 and older (Table 1.1). The proportion of individuals with activity limitation who have multiple disabling conditions also rises sharply with age. One in six children and youth with disabilities has more than one condition, compared to half of those aged 65 and over.

Restricted Activity

Individuals with disabilities have, on average, two months of restricted activity days per year, spending 25 days of that time in bed. For those with two or more conditions, the number of restricted activity days climbs to an average of three months per year, with nearly

NIDRR Disability Statistics Abstract, No. 9, June 1995.

Table 1.1. Health Status and Medical Care Use of Persons With Chronic Conditions Causing Limitation in Activity, by Age and Number of Conditions, 1992.

	Total	Under 18	18-44	Age 45-64	65-74	75 +
Limited in activity (in thousands)*	37,733	4,047	10,681	11,064	6,362	5,578
One condition	23,583	3,354	7,905	6,325	3,254	2,744
Two or more conditions	14,150	693	2,776	4,738	3,108	2,834
Limited in activity (Percentage of total population)	15.0	6.1	10.1	22.8	34.4	45.3
One condition	9.4	5.0	7.5	13.0	17.6	22.3
Two or more conditions	5.6	1.0	2.6	9.8	16.8	23.0
Restricted activity days (per person)	62.6	26.8	58.1	69.1	66.7	79.8
One condition	45.1	24.5	47.6	48.0	46.0	55.0
Two or more conditions	91.9	38.2	88.0	97.3	88.2	103.9
Bed-disability days (per person)	24.8	12.0	20.9	26.3	26.5	36.5
One condition	15.8	10.6	15.4	15.8	13.9	25.8
Two or more conditions	39.7	19.0	36.4	40.3	39.7	46.8
Physician visits (per person)	14.0	9.6	13.5	14.6	14.5	16.5
One condition	11.2	8.4	11.7	11.4	12.2	11.3
Two or more conditions	18.8	15.3	18.7	18.9	16.9	21.6
Hospital discharges (per 100 persons)	30.5	20.5	22.7	31.5	38.5	41.9
One condition	24.4	18.8	19.3	24.5	33.0	35.9
Two or more conditions	40.7	28.6	32.4	40.9	44.2	47.7
Feeling poor or fair (percent)	43.8	18.2	34.2	52.2	53.3	53.0
One condition	32.2	15.8	27.4	37.9	40.8	42.1
Two or more conditions	63.2	29.7	53.7	71.3	66.3	63.6

* Totals may not add due to rounding
Source: 1992 National Health Interview Survey

six weeks spent in bed. Restricted activity and bed-disability days increase with age. Persons 75 years old and over with one condition have 8 weeks of restricted activity days compared with 15 weeks for those with multiple disabling conditions.

Medical Services Use

Individuals with disabilities see a doctor an average of 14 times in a year; this also increases with age, rising from 10 visits for children and youth under 18 to 17 visits for those aged 75 and over. Those with two or more disabling conditions have almost twice as many visits as those with one condition (19 vs. 11 visits).

People with disabilities have 31 hospital discharges per 100 persons per year. As with physician visits, there is a steady rise in frequency of hospitalization with age and number of conditions. People aged 75 or over with multiple disabling conditions have nearly 50 hospital discharges per 100 persons per year. However, the average length of hospital stay is fairly constant, between seven and nine days, across both age and condition groups (data not shown).

Self-Reported Health Status

Overall, more than two out of five people with disabling conditions rate their health as fair or poor. While the frequency of fair or poor health increases with both age and number of conditions, the disparity between those with one condition and those with multiple conditions narrows with age.

Comparisons by Gender and Race

Women have slightly higher rates of disability and multiple disabling conditions than men (Table 1.2). Women with disabilities have more restricted activity days and more bed-disability days than men, but the differences due to number of conditions are greater than the differences associated with gender. This distinction is particularly apparent in adults aged 18 and over (Figure 1.1). Women have more physician visits than men, but are hospitalized somewhat less frequently (Table 1.2).

Blacks have a higher rate of multiple disabling conditions, a greater likelihood of rating their health fair or poor, and a higher average number of bed disability days than whites. However, in all measures of health status and medical services use the differences

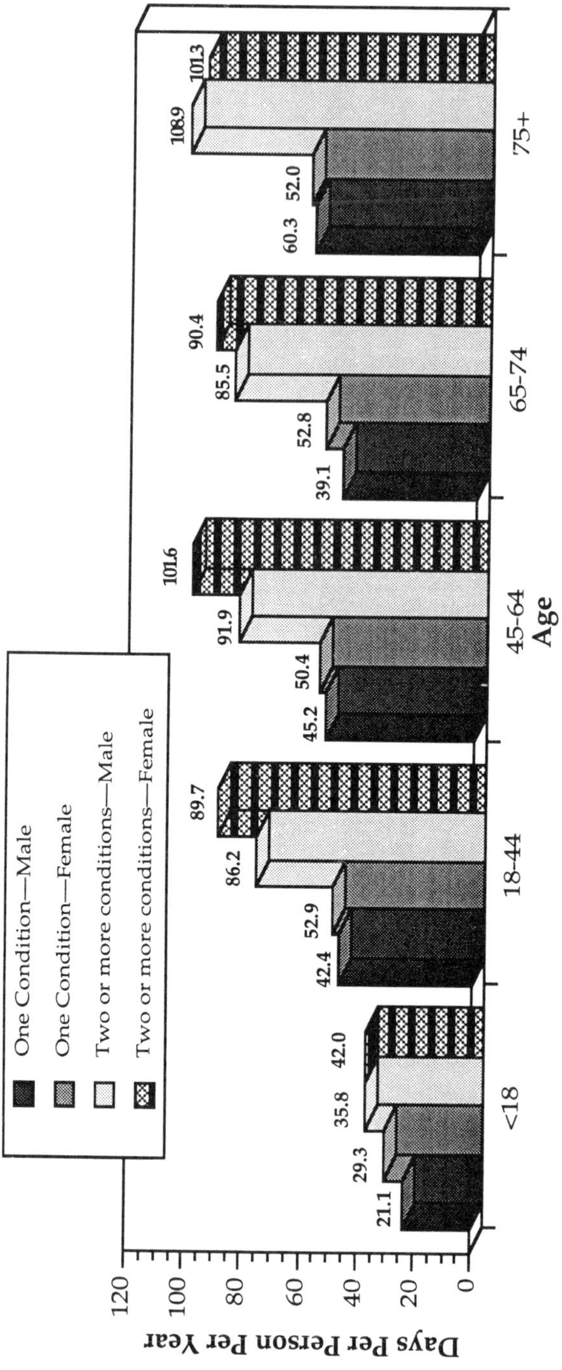

Figure 1.1. Restricted Activity Days for Persons with Chronic Conditions Causing Limitation.

Legend:
- One Condition—Male
- One Condition—Female
- Two or more conditions—Male
- Two or more conditions—Female

<18
21.1, 29.3, 35.8, 42.0

18-44
42.4, 52.9, 86.2, 89.7

45-64
45.2, 50.4, 91.9, 101.6

65-74
39.1, 52.8, 85.5, 90.4

75+
60.3, 52.0, 108.9, 101.3

Age

Days Per Person Per Year: 0, 20, 40, 60, 80, 100, 120

Table 1.2.
Health Status and Medical Care Use of Persons with Chronic Conditions Causing Limitation in Activity, by Gender, Race and Number of Conditions, 1992.

	Gender		Race ‡	
	Male	Female	White	Black
Limited in activity (in thousands)*	17,783	19,950	31,693	5,008
One condition	11,543	12,039	20,082	2,862
Two or more conditions	6,240	7,910	11,611	2,146
Limited in activity (Percentage of total population)	14.6	15.4	15.1	15.9
One condition	9.4	9.3	9.6	9.1
Two or more conditions	5.1	6.1	5.5	6.8
Restricted activity days (per person)	57.2	67.4	61.2	71.8
One condition	40.5	49.4	44.9	48.2
Two or more conditions	88.1	94.9	89.4	103.2
Bed-disability days (per person)	22.4	26.9	23.6	31.4
One condition	14.0	17.6	15.1	20.8
Two or more conditions	37.9	41.1	38.4	45.5
Physician visits (per person)	12.7	15.2	13.8	15.0
One condition	10.1	12.1	11.3	11.1
Two or more conditions	17.5	19.8	18.2	20.2
Hospital discharges (per 100 persons)	31.9	29.4	30.6	30.3
One condition	25.3	23.6	24.6	23.7
Two or more conditions	44.0	38.1	40.9	39.1
Feeling poor or fair (percent)	42.6	44.9	41.8	55.8
One condition	31.6	32.7	30.7	42.1
Two or more conditions	62.8	63.5	61.0	74.1

* Totals may not add due to rounding
‡ Excludes races other than white and black

Source: 1992 National Health Interview Survey

associated with number of disabling conditions exceed those associated with race.

In summary, persons with chronic conditions or impairments that limit activity have high medical care usage. Within this group, those with multiple disabling conditions are even higher users of the health care system. These data underscore the need for health care providers and researchers to focus on the prevention of secondary or multiple conditions.

— by Laura Trupin and Dorothy P. Rice

Chapter 2

Health Conditions and Impairments Causing Disability

Approximately 38 million Americans with disabilities report a total of 61 million disabling conditions—any chronic health disorder, injury, or impairment that contributes to a person's being limited in social or other activities. This figure comprises 42 million chronic conditions classified as physical health disorders, 16 million as impairments (such as orthopedic and sensory impairments, paralysis, learning disabilities, and mental retardation), two million as mental health disorders, and about one million injuries that are not classified as impairments.

This abstract presents data on the prevalence of disabling conditions among the civilian noninstitutionalized population of the United States. The data are obtained from the National Health Interview Survey (NHIS), a continuing national household survey consisting of 49,401 household interviews with 128,412 people in 1992. In the NHIS, disability is defined as a limitation in social or other activity that is caused by a chronic mental or physical disorder, injury, or impairment.

Impairments are deficits of bodily structure or function, either congenital in origin or acquired from a past or ongoing disorder or injury. Impairments include deficits of senses (vision, hearing, and sensation) or speech, absence of limbs or other anatomy, learning disabilities, deformities, paralysis, and other orthopedic impairments. In the NHIS, impairments are coded according to a classification

NIDRR Disability Statistics Abstract, No. 16, September 1996.

scheme developed by the National Center for Health Statistics. Health disorders (including diseases) and injuries, however, are coded to the World Health Organization's International Classification of Diseases, Ninth Revision (ICD-9).

The classification method presents several complications. First, since many impairments are caused by ongoing disorders, both the impairment and the disorder may be coded as disabling conditions. For example, for a person who has had a leg amputated due to a bone

Table 2.1. *Conditions Causing Disability by Broad ICD and Impairment Categories.*

ICD Chapter		Number (1,000s)	Percent of all Conditions
	ALL CONDITIONS	61,047	100.0
	DISORDERS AND INJURIES	44,721	73.3
13	Diseases of the musculoskeletal system and connective tissue (710-739)	10,530	17.2
7	Diseases of the circulatory system (390-459)	10,170	16.7
8	Diseases of the respiratory system (460-519)	4,774	7.8
6	Diseases of the nervous system and sense organs (320-389)	4,373	7.2
3	Endocrine, nutritional and metabolic diseases and immunity disorders (240-279)	3,409	5.6
15-16	Certain conditions originating in the perinatal period (760-799) and symptoms, signs, ill-defined conditions (780-779)	2,843	4.7
5	Mental disorders (290-316), excluding mental retardation	2,035	3.3
9	Diseases of the digestive system (520-579)	1,728	2.8
2	Neoplasms (140-239)	1,628	2.7
17	Injury and poisoning (800-999), not involving impairment	1,205	2.0
10	Diseases of the genitourinary system (580-629)	778	1.3
1	Infectious and parasitic diseases (001-139)	378	0.6
12	Diseases of the skin and subcutaneous tissue (680-709)	362	0.6
14	Congenital anomalies (740-759)	287	0.5
4	Diseases of the blood and blood-forming organs (280-289)	217	0.4
	IMPAIRMENTS	16,326	26.7
	Orthopedic impairments	8,608	14.1
	Learning disability and mental retardation	1,575	2.6
	Visual impairments	1,294	2.1
	Hearing impairments	1,175	1.9
	Paralysis	1,071	1.8
	Deformities	900	1.5
	Absence or loss of limb/other body part	788	1.3
	Speech impairments	545	0.9
	Other and ill-defined impairments	371	0.6

Note: Conditions in ICD Chapter 11, complications of pregnancy, childbirth, and the puerperium (630-676), are not used.

Source: United States National Health Interview Survey, 1992

cancer still active at the time of the interview, both the impairment (absence of limb) and the disorder (cancer) will be coded separately. A further complication results from a somewhat arbitrary distinction, in certain instances, between disorders and impairments, depending on how the condition is described. If a respondent reports "back trouble," it will be coded as an impairment, while an answer of "slipped disc" will be classified as a disorder. Thus, only by combining back-related impairments and disorders can the true number of disabling back problems be estimated.

Finally, injuries are handled in a special way. When an injury has caused an impairment, only the impairment is coded. Injuries that have not caused impairments are coded to the injuries chapter of the ICD. For example, if a person mentions last year's automobile accident as a cause of activity limitation, without specifying a particular impairment, the person's condition is coded as an injury, not an impairment.

The 37.7 million people with activity limitations report an average of 1.6 conditions per person, for a total of 61 million limiting conditions (see Table 2.1. Some 73.3 percent of these are classified as disorders and injuries, with the remainder as impairments. Among the disorders and injuries, the most prevalent are musculoskeletal disorders, which represent 17.2 percent of all limiting conditions, followed by circulatory disorders, at 16.7 percent. Respiratory conditions rank third at 7.8 percent, with nervous and sensory disorders at 7.2 percent and endocrine, nutritional, metabolic, and immunity disorders at 5.6 percent of all disabling conditions. These top five categories, each representing a chapter of the ICD, account three-quarters (74.4 percent) of all diseases and disorders reported as causing limitation in activity, or more than half (54.3 percent) of all activity-limiting conditions.

The 16.3 million impairments reported to cause activity limitation constitute about one-quarter (26.7 percent) of all disabling conditions. More than half of these are orthopedic impairments, representing 14.1 percent of disabling conditions. A distant second is the category of learning disabilities and mental retardation, accounting for 2.6 percent. Visual impairments rank third, at 2.1 percent, followed by hearing impairments, at 1.9 percent and paralysis, at 1.8 percent of all disabling conditions reported.

The remaining impairments—1.3 percent of all conditions causing activity limitation—include deformities, absence or loss (e.g., of a limb), and speech impairments.

Table 2.2 lists the most common specific health conditions and impairments that cause activity limitation in the U.S. Heart disease is the most prevalent, at 7.9 million cases—13 percent of all conditions mentioned. Back problems (including those classified as impairments or disorders) are a close second at 7.7 million conditions, or 12.6 percent of all disabling conditions. Arthritis (rheumatoid arthritis plus osteoarthrosis and allied disorders) ranks third at 5.7 million, followed by orthopedic impairments of lower extremity (2.8 million), asthma (2.6 million), and diabetes (2.6 million). Mental disorders, which are mainly the mental illnesses (since learning disability and mental retardation are classified separately), rank seventh at 2.0 million conditions, followed by disorders of the eyes (1.6 million, not including

Table 2.2. *Most Common Conditions Causing Activity Limitation.*

Rank		Number (1,000s)	Percent of all Conditions
	ALL CONDITIONS	61,047	100.0
1	Heart disease (390-429)	7,932	13.0
2	Deformities, orthopedic impairments and disorders of the spine or back	7,672	12.6
3	Osteoarthrosis and allied disorders (715-716)	5,048	8.3
4	Orthopedic impairment of lower extremity	2,817	4.6
5	Asthma (493)	2,592	4.2
6	Diabetes (250)	2,569	4.2
7	Mental disorders (290-316), excluding learning disability and mental retardation	2,035	3.3
8	Disorders of the eye (360-379)	1,577	2.6
9	Learning disability and mental retardation	1,575	2.6
10	Cancer (140-208)	1,342	2.2
11	Visual impairments	1,294	2.1
12	Orthopedic impairment of shoulder and/or upper extremities	1,196	2.0
13	Other unknown and unspecified causes	1,188	1.9
14	Hearing impairments	1,175	1.9
15	Cerebrovascular disease (430-438)	1,174	1.9

Source: United States National Health Interview Survey, 1992

visual impairments), and then by learning disability and mental retardation (1.6 million). If the latter is combined with mental illnesses, the total for all mental disorders is 3.6 million, placing the category fourth overall.

Cancer ranks in tenth place (1.3 million), followed by visual impairments (1.3 million), and then orthopedic impairments of shoulder and/or upper extremity (1.2 million). The residual category of unknown and unspecified causes ranks thirteenth (1.2 million) at 1.9 percent of all conditions, followed by hearing impairments (1.2 million), also at 1.9 percent of all conditions. Cerebrovascular disease completes the list at fifteenth with slightly under 1.2 million conditions.

These data also highlight the substantial role that injury plays in causing disability. In addition to the 1.2 million injuries (occurring more than 3 months ago) that limit activity but are not classified as impairments, another 7.2 million impairments have injury coded as a cause. Thus, injuries make up 13.4 percent of all disabling conditions. However, disorders clearly play the largest role as causes of disability.

— by Mitchell P. LaPlante

Chapter 3

Child Health USA

Preface

Child Health USA '95 is the seventh annual report on the health status and service needs of America's children. This book is a compilation of secondary data for 50 health status indicators. It provides both a graphical and textual summary of the data and addresses long-term trends where applicable.

Child Health USA is published to provide reliable and current data for public health professionals and other individuals in the private and public sectors. The succinct format of the book is intended to facilitate the use of the information as a snapshot of measures of the health of children in the United States.

Data are presented for infants, children, adolescents, and women of childbearing age. In addition to health status, health services utilization and population characteristics are addressed. This information provides the reader with a multi-dimensional perspective of the health of children in the United States, in accordance with the World Health Organization's definition of health: "A state of complete physical, mental, and social well-being, and not merely the absence of disease or infirmity."

Some statistics in Child Health USA reveal the extent of progress toward Healthy People 2000 goals or a reduction in the prevalence of unhealthful behaviors, while others reveal burgeoning or escalating

DHHS Publication No. HRSA-M-DSEA-96-5, September 1996.

health problems of women, children, and youth. We hope the information provided in this book will be helpful to policy and decision-makers responsible for implementing or expanding programs that affect the health of children in the United States.

Introduction

While the statistical trends presented in this document reveal areas of progress, they also illustrate the extent to which some heath risks continue to plague the lives of children and families as they prepare to enter the next millennium. In the United States today, the leading health risk for both children and adults is neither a disease nor a medical condition. It is poverty, which can affect nutrition, access to health care, and living conditions that are conducive to health. Poverty has steadily risen among children during the last three decades. Although children under age 18 represent just 26.2 percent of the total U.S. population, they constitute 38.4 percent of the nation's poor. In the United States, a child is born into poverty every 32 seconds. And then there's the tragedy of violence, both at home and in society. In 1994, state child protective services in 48 states determined that 1,012,000 children were victims of child abuse and neglect. It is likely that, above and beyond these figures, large numbers of cases of abuse and neglect go undetected and unreported. More than half of all reports of child maltreatment come from professionals: educators, law enforcement and justice officials, health and social service professionals, and child care providers, while less than 20 percent are reported by the victim's family. These statistics underscore how critically important it is for all professionals who work with children, indeed for all adults, to take responsibility for the health and well-being of the nation's most vulnerable citizens.

Firearms are the second leading cause of death due to injury among adolescents 15 to 19. It is estimated that fifteen children are killed by firearms each day. In the last ten years, the proportion of adolescent deaths due to homicide has increased by 50 percent. In 1993, 65 percent of all firearm deaths in 15 to 19 year olds were linked to homicide, an additional 27 percent involved suicide and 7 percent were unintentional.

AIDS is also taking a terrible toll on children, who are increasingly both affected and infected by HIV/AIDS. Advances in the knowledge, screening and therapy for reducing the transmission of the HIV virus from pregnant women to their infants show some promise for stemming the rates of pediatric AIDS.

16

Among teenagers, the proportion of AIDS cases in teen girls compared to boys jumped by 25 percent just in the past two years (1993-1995). Girls now comprise 35 percent of all teen AIDS cases, and girls are acquiring AIDS primarily through heterosexual contact.

AIDS has become one of the leading killers of women of reproductive age in the U.S. (many of whom were infected as teenagers), and women comprise the fastest growing group to become infected with HIV. Thus, it is critical that AIDS education and prevention efforts target both girls and boys.

Researchers estimate that every day approximately 3,000 young people become regular smokers. Many smokers start their habit as teenagers, and a large portion of them continue to smoke throughout the rest of their lives. Sixty-nine percent of adult daily smokers report having tried their first cigarette by age 18. Every year, more than 400,000 people die from diseases caused by tobacco use.

Teen smoking rates decreased in the late 1970s, remained relatively stable during the 1980s, and have resumed a steady increase among 8th, 10th, and 12th graders throughout the 1990s. In 1995, one in three high school seniors said that they had smoked cigarettes in the last 30 days, and 91 percent of 10th graders reported that cigarettes were easy to obtain. The Clinton Administration responded in 1995 by proposing a major tobacco initiative to reduce the access and appeal of tobacco products to youth.

Yet another area in which tobacco use has proven negative effects is during pregnancy. Along with the consequences for the mother's long-term health, smoking in pregnancy, particularly during the first trimester, is one of the scientifically documented risk factors for low birth weight and infant mortality. Thus Title V programs, in conjunction with other government-sponsored activities, have continued to promote smoking-cessation activities for pregnant women and women of reproductive age.

The U.S. has made great progress in improving maternal and child health, yet it still has many objectives to meet. The road to making children a national priority in this country is long, and the way uphill. But it is the direction we must continue to take.

Maternal Mortality

From 1935 to 1993, the maternal mortality rate dropped from 582 maternal deaths per 100,000 live births to 7.5. Though all causes of maternal mortality declined dramatically over that period, the overall decline was largely due to marked decreases in maternal deaths from infection, toxemia, and hemorrhage.

17

Significant improvements in the care of women during labor, delivery, and the postpartum period have been made over the last 60 years. Technical improvements (including sterile techniques) in the management of vaginal and cesarean deliveries and the advent of effective antibiotics probably accounted for much of the decrease in maternal mortality. It is also likely that the development of widely used prenatal care protocols contributed to the decline in mortality from chronic or pregnancy-induced conditions

Although maternal mortality has decreased significantly over the past 60 years, it is still a serious problem. Many of these deaths might be preventable if the health care system worked more effectively.

Chart 3.1. *Maternal Mortality: 1935-1993. Source (I.1): National Center for Health Statistics.*

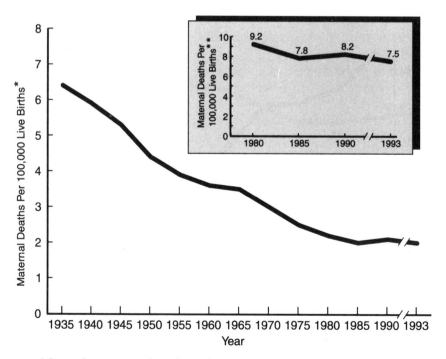

* *Data values represented on a log scale.*
** *Actual data values.*

Late Fetal Deaths

The rate of fetal deaths decreased from 14.9 per 1,000 live births plus late fetal deaths in 1950 to 3.8 in 1993. Part of the decline in the 1950s and 1960s was due to improvements in obstetric technique. There is some evidence that late fetal deaths are likely related to maternal nutrition. Smoking during pregnancy also increases the risk of late fetal death. Prenatal care that promotes good nutrition may have a role in preventing late fetal deaths.

Low Birth Weight

The prevalence of low birth weight in the total population increased from 7.0% in 1950 to 8.3% in 1965. The increase in low birth weight prevalence between 1950 and 1965 was partially attributable to improved reporting, especially for the poorer segments of the population. It decreased to a low of 6.8% in 1985. However, 7.2 the percentage of low birth weight births has been slowly increasing.

Infant Mortality

The survival of infants in the U.S. has markedly improved over the past 60 years. In 1935, there were 55.7 infant deaths per 1,000 live births; while in 1993, the U.S. infant mortality rate was 8.4. Advances in public health and medical practices—improvements in sanitation, the initiation of childhood immunizations, better medical treatment of infectious and other illnesses, and improvements in maternity and newborn care—all have contributed to the infant mortality decrease.

Although the U.S. infant mortality rate continues to improve and is at an all-time low, the U.S. ranks only 22nd among industrialized nations.

Neonatal and Postneonatal Mortality

Though there have been substantial decreases in both neonatal and postneonatal mortality in the U.S. over the past 60 years, the relationship between neonatal and postneonatal mortality has not remained constant. Postneonatal mortality declined more rapidly than neonatal mortality from the 1940s through the mid 1960s due to improvements in living conditions and in pediatric care. The gap between neonatal and postneonatal mortality has diminished from the 1970s because of dramatic improvements in perinatal intensive care. In the collection and presentation of data socio-demographic characteristics are used to develop a comprehensive and accurate picture of the country's diverse maternal and child population. These characteristics include race and ethnicity, age, and poverty status.

At the national, state, and local levels, policy makers use population information to systematically address health-related issues of mothers and children. By carefully analyzing and comparing data, health workers can often isolate high-risk populations that require specific interventions. Policy makers can then develop effective programs that meet the needs of those populations.

The following section presents data on a number of population characteristics that have an impact on maternal and child health program development and evaluation. These include data on the population distribution by age, poverty status, and living arrangements.

Chart 3.2. *U.S. Resident Population by Age Group: 1995. Source (II.1): U.S. Bureau of the Census.*

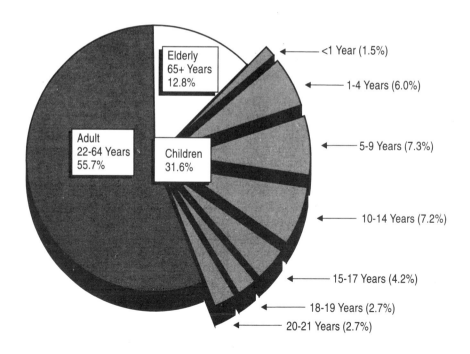

Data on school dropout rates and working mothers and child care trends are also included.

Population of Children

In 1995, there were almost 83 million children through the age of 21 in the United States, representing 31.6% of the total population.

Between 1980 and 1995, there was a 19.1 % increase in the number of children under 5 years of age.

Although there were approximately 27 million more children age 21 or younger in 1995 than in 1950, this age group is declining relative to other age groups in the population.

Chart 3.3. Related Children Under 18 Years of Age Living in Families Below 100% of Poverty: 1994. Source (II.2): U.S. Department of Commerce.

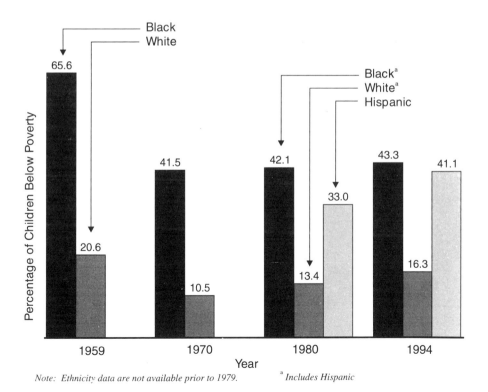

Note: Ethnicity data are not available prior to 1979.   [a] Includes Hispanic

In 1995, persons aged 65 and over represented 12.8% of the total population. By the year 2000, this group is expected to decrease by 12.6%. The child population is expected to remain at 31.5%.

Children in Poverty

In 1994, there were 14.6 million related children under 18 years of age living in families with income below the federal poverty level. This age group contains 38.4% of all the nation's poor.

Black or Hispanic children are more likely to live in poverty than are white children.

Between 1980 and 1994, the number of children living in poverty increased by almost 3.5 million. In contrast, the number of persons 65 years of age and over living in poverty decreased by 0.2 million.

In 1994, a family of four was considered to be living in poverty if its annual income was below $15,141.

Chart 3.4. *Living Arrangements of Children Under 18 Years of Age: 1970-1994. Source (II.3): U.S. Bureau of the Census.*

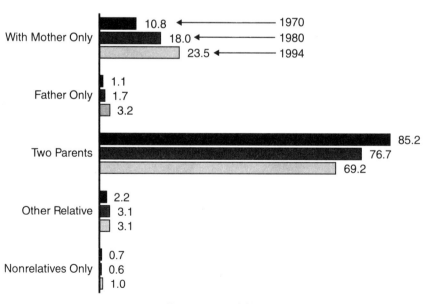

Percentage of Children

Family Composition

In 1994, 18.6 million children lived in families with only one parent. This group represented 26.7% of children younger than 18 years of age.

Since 1970, the percentage of children living with single parents has more than doubled, from 11.9% to 26.7%. A rise in the divorce rate and the number of never-married parents have contributed to this increase.

In 1994, the vast majority of single-parent families consisted of children living with their mothers. Of children living with only one parent, the proportion living with a single father increased from 9.1 % in 1970 to 12.1 % in 1994.

White children are less likely to be living with one parent than are black or Hispanic children. The proportions living with one parent in 1994 were 20.9% for white children, 31.8% for Hispanic children, and 57.1 % for black children.

Approximately two-thirds of both black children and Hispanic children who live with a single mother are below the federal poverty level. Note: A parent may be a stepparent or parent by adoption.

Health Status

The systematic assessment of the health status of children enables health workers to determine the impact of past and current health intervention and prevention programs. Program planners and policy makers identify trends by examining and comparing data from one year to the next.

In the following section, health status indicators are presented by age group: infant, child, and adolescent. Trend data for the preceding 20 years are presented for selected indicators.

The health status indicators in this section are based on vital statistics and national surveys. Population-based samples are designed to yield data that are representative of the maternal and child population affected by, or in need of, specific health services.

Comparison of National Infant Mortality Rates

Differences in the infant mortality rates among industrialized nations reflect differences in the health status of women before and during pregnancy and the quality of risk-appropriate primary health care accessible to pregnant women and their infants. Although the

United States has greatly reduced its infant mortality rate since 1965, the nation ranks lower than 21 other industrialized countries. Since 1980, Japan has had the lowest infant mortality rate in the world. In 1992, the risk of a child dying in infancy (4.5 per 1,000 live births) was 55% lower than that observed in the United States (8.5 per 1.000 live births).

Infant Mortality

In 1993, 33,466 infants died before their first birthday. The infant mortality rate was 8.4 deaths per 1,000 live births. This figure represents a decline of 1 % from the rate of 8.5 for the previous year.

The rapid decline in infant mortality, which began in the mid-1960s, slowed for both blacks and whites during the 1980s.

The 1993 infant mortality rate for black infants was 2.4 times the rate for white infants. Although the trend in infant mortality rates

Chart 3.5. Comparison of National Infant Mortality Rates: 1992. Source (III.1): National Center for Health Statistics.

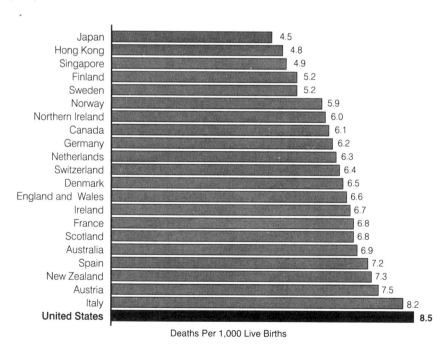

Country	Deaths Per 1,000 Live Births
Japan	4.5
Hong Kong	4.8
Singapore	4.9
Finland	5.2
Sweden	5.2
Norway	5.9
Northern Ireland	6.0
Canada	6.1
Germany	6.2
Netherlands	6.3
Switzerland	6.4
Denmark	6.5
England and Wales	6.6
Ireland	6.7
France	6.8
Scotland	6.8
Australia	6.9
Spain	7.2
New Zealand	7.3
Austria	7.5
Italy	8.2
United States	8.5

Deaths Per 1,000 Live Births

among blacks and whites has been on a continual decline throughout the 20th century, the proportional discrepancy between black and
white rates has remained unchanged.

Neonatal and Postneonatal Mortality

Neonatal

In 1993, 21,174 infants younger than 28 days died; putting the
neonatal mortality rate at 529.3 deaths per 100,000 live births. Both
the overall mortality rate and rates by leading causes of mortality
decreased from 1991 to 1993.

Blacks have the highest rates of neonatal mortality in all categories. Disorders related to short gestation and low birth weight are the
primary causes of neonatal mortality for blacks, while congenital
anomalies are the leading cause for whites.

Chart 3.6. *Leading Causes of Neonatal* Mortality: 1993. Source (III.3):
National Center for Health Statistics.*

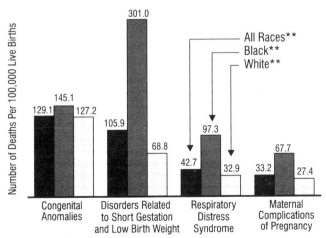

* Neonatal: less than 28 days old
** Includes Hispanic

25

Postneonatal

In 1993, 12,292 infants 28 days to 11 months old died; the post-neonatal mortality rate was 307.3 deaths per 100,000 live births, a decrease of 7.1 deaths per 100,000 live births from 1992.

The postneonatal mortality rate for blacks is at least two times that for whites in all leading causes of postneonatal mortality (three times greater when homicide is the cause), with the exception of congenital anomalies.

Chart 3.7. *Leading Causes of Postneonatal* Mortality: 1993. Source (III.3): National Center for Health Statistics.*

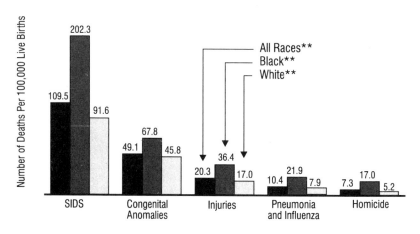

* *Postneonatal: 28 days to less than one year old*
** *Includes Hispanic*

Maternal Mortality

During the past several decades, there has been a dramatic decrease in maternal mortality in the United States. Since 1980, however, the rate of decline has slowed.

In 1993, there were 302 maternal deaths which resulted from complications during pregnancy, childbirth, or the postpartum period.

The maternal mortality rate for black women (20.5 per 100,000 live births) is more than four times the rate for white women (4.8 per 100,000 live births).

Regardless of race, the risk of maternal death increases for women over age 30; women 35-39 years old have more than twice the risk of maternal death than those aged 20-24 years. Note: 1970-1988 data based on race of child; 1989-1993 data based on race of mother.

Low Birth Weight

In 1993, 288,482 babies (7.2% of all live births) were of low birth weight, weighing less than 2,500 grams, or 5.5 pounds, at birth.

The percentage of low birth weight births among all live births rose from a low of 6.8% in 1985 to 7.2% in 1993. From 1992 to 1993, rates among blacks and Hispanics remained stable, while rates among American Indians and whites increased.

Low birth weight is the factor most closely associated with neonatal mortality. Low birth weight infants are more likely to experience long-term disabilities or to die during the first year of life than are infants of normal weight.

Factors associated with increased risk of low birth weight include poverty, low level of educational attainment, and minority status. Note: 1975-1988 data based on race of child; 1989-1993 data based on race of mother.

Child Mortality

There were 15,724 deaths of children ages 1-14 years in 1993. Injury, of any type and regardless of intent, was the primary cause of death in that age group. Among 1-4 year old children, injuries accounted for 44% of all deaths, followed by deaths due to congenital anomalies (birth defects), malignant neoplasm (tumors), diseases of the heart. and HIV or AIDS.

Injuries comprised 52% of all deaths among 5-14 year old children, followed by malignant neoplasm, congenital anomalies, diseases of the heart. and HIV or AIDS.

Childhood mortality rates have declined substantially over the past several decades. However, the decline has plateaued in recent years and, in both age groups, mortality in 1993 was slightly higher than mortality in 1992.

Childhood Deaths Due to Injury

In 1993, injuries caused the deaths of 3,093 1-4 year old children and 4,502 5-14 year old children.

Among 1-4 year old children, motor vehicle crashes, fire, and drowning were the leading causes of injury death. Motor vehicle crashes were the leading cause of injury death among 5-14 year old children, followed by firearm and drowning deaths. Almost 55% of firearm deaths among 5-14 year old children were homicides.

Hospitalization

In 1993, there were 3.4 million hospital discharges of children 1 through 21 years old, or four discharges per 100 children during the year.

Diseases of the respiratory system were the major cause of hospitalization of children 1-9 years of age and accounted for 36% of their discharges.

Hospital discharge rates decrease with age until age 9 and then increase during later adolescence.

While injuries are the leading cause of death for children older than 1 year, this category accounted for only 11% of the hospital discharges of children 1-14 years in 1993. Pregnancy and childbirth related hospitalizations accounted for 70% of discharges of young women ages 15-21.

Hospital Discharge Trends

Since 1980, there has been a 55% decrease in overall hospital discharge rates for children aged 1-14 years.

Between 1980 and 1993, there was a 54% decline in the hospital discharge rate for diseases of the respiratory system in children aged 1-14 years.

Three diagnostic categories (digestive disease, respiratory disease, and injury) accounted for 51% of the discharges of children aged 1-14 years in 1993.

Pediatric AIDS

As of December 31, 1995, 6,948 cases of AIDS in children younger than 13 years old had been reported in the U.S. This total includes 800 newly reported cases in 1995.

Pediatric cases of AIDS represent approximately 1.4% of all cases reported. The majority of pediatric AIDS cases result from transmission before or during birth, with a disproportionate number of cases occurring in black and Hispanic children. Notes: Perinatal Transmission—child's biologic mother had:

- Injecting drug use
- Sex with injecting drug user
- Sex with bisexual male
- Sex with person with hemophilia
- Sex with transfusion recipient with HIV infection
- Sex with person with HIV infection, risk not specified
- Receipt of blood transfusion, blood components, or tissue
- Has HIV infection, risk not specified

Receipt of Blood/Blood Components:

- Received clotting factor for hemophilia/coagulation disorder
- Received blood transfusion, blood components, or tissue

Child Abuse and Neglect

Investigations by state child protective services agencies in 48 states determined that 1,012,000 children were victims of substantial or indicated child abuse and neglect in 1994.

About 27% of all victims of child maltreatment were 3 years old or younger, and another 20% were between the ages of 4 and 6. Just over one-fifth of victims were youth ages 13-18.

Types of maltreatment children suffered were neglect 53%, physical abuse 26%, sexual abuse 14%, and other types of maltreatment including medical neglect and emotional maltreatment (27%). Forty-three states reported that 1,111 children died as a result of maltreatment in 1994.

In 1994, state child protective services agencies received and referred for investigation an estimated 2 million reports alleging the maltreatment of 2.9 million children. More than half of all reports alleging maltreatment (53%) came from professionals, including educators, law enforcement and justice officials, medical professionals, social service professionals and child care providers. Only one in five reports came from either the victim or a family member of the victim.

Adolescent Mortality

In 1993, there were 14,997 deaths of adolescents aged 15-19 years. In that age group, injury was the leading cause of death. The 12,047 injury deaths accounted for 80% of all deaths among 15-19 year olds in 1993. Malignant neoplasm (tumor) was the next leading cause of death, accounting for 4.8% of all deaths among 15-19 year olds. Mortality among teenagers declined substantially between 1960 and the early 1980s. There was a moderate increase in mortality among 15-19 year olds in the mid to late 1980s. The death rate among that age group has been stable since then.

Motor vehicles and firearms were the leading causes of injury mortality among 15-19 year olds in 1993. Each category accounted for approximately 40% of all injury deaths among teenagers. The next three leading causes of injury death—suffocation, drowning, and poisoning—each accounted for 2% to 3% of all injury deaths among 15-19 year olds. Motor vehicle mortality among teenagers has declined by approximately 15% over the past decade. Conversely, adolescent mortality from firearms has more than doubled over that same period.

Adolescent Deaths Due to Injury

In 1993, motor vehicle traffic crashes caused the death of 4,876 15-19 year olds. Almost 90% of those deaths were of motor vehicle occupants, either passengers or the driver. Deaths of pedestrians, motorcyclists, and pedal cyclists accounted for the remainder of motor vehicle mortality among teenagers. Data from the National Highway Traffic Safety Administration suggest that alcohol was involved in 20-25% of motor vehicle deaths among teenagers.

In 1993, 4,794 15-19 year olds were killed by firearms in the U.S. Homicide accounted for 3,118 or 65% of firearm deaths among teenagers. Approximately 27% of firearm deaths were suicide, while 7% were considered to be unintentional. Over the past decade, the proportion of firearm deaths due to homicide has increased by approximately 50%.

Teen Pregnancy and Abortion Rates

In 1991, there were 997,190 pregnancies among women less than 20 years of age. Pregnancy outcomes included 531,591 live births (53.3%) and 326,620 induced abortions (32.8%).

Although the number of abortions among females less than 20 increased sharply from 1975 to 1980, the rate has decreased steadily from 1980-1991. For the first time since 1986, there was a small but steady decline in the teen birth rate from 1991 to 1993. This trend has been documented in nearly every state.

Researchers consistently find four broad factors that predict sexual intercourse at an early age, adolescent pregnancy, and nonmarital childbearing among teenagers: early school failure, early behavior problems, poverty, and family problems/family dysfunction. Note: Data represent a woman's age at the time a pregnancy ended. More pregnancies were experienced by teenagers than were reported because most of the 19-year-olds who became pregnant had their births or abortions at age 20 and thus were not counted.

Sexual Activity

The number of students reporting ever having had sexual intercourse increased with age. Males in all grades had the highest prevalence of sexual experience.

Over 50% of students in 12th grade reported having had sexual intercourse during the preceding three months. The prevalence rate of sexual activity increased significantly from grades 9 through 12 among females, while it increased significantly from grades 10 through 12 among males.

Condom Use

More than 50% of sexually active 9th through 12th graders reported condom use during last sexual intercourse. Males were significantly more likely than females to have reported that a condom was used.

While sexual activity increased by grade for all students, condom use decreased by grade. Only 46.5% of sexually active 12th graders reported condom use, compared with 61.6% of sexually active 9th graders.

Adolescent Childbearing

In 1994, the live birth rate per 1,000 women was 1.4 for teenagers aged 10-14, 37.6 for those 15-17, and 91.5 for those 18-19 years old.

In 1994, there were 69,028 live births among black females younger than 18 years of age, which represented 10.8% of all births to black women. There were 132,366 births to white females under 18, which represented 4.2% of all births to white women.

In 1994, approximately 59 million women were of childbearing age (15-44 years) in the United States.

Adolescent and Young Adult AIDS

Adolescent AIDS

As of December 31, 1995, 2,354 cases of AIDS were reported in adolescents aged 13-19 years. This total includes 405 newly reported cases in 1995.

Whites comprised 36% of the AIDS cases among adolescents. Of these, 64% were exposed to HIV primarily through receipt of clotting factor for hemophilia/coagulation disorder or as a result of blood transfusions. Eighteen percent of whites aged 13-19 years were exposed to HIV through male-to-male sexual contact.

Forty-four percent of adolescent AIDS cases were among black, non-Hispanics. Twenty-seven percent of blacks aged 13-19 were exposed to HIV through male-to-male sexual contact.

Males comprised 65% of the 2,354 AIDS cases among adolescents aged 13-19 years. These young men were exposed to HIV primarily through receipt of clotting factor for hemophilia/coagulation disorder or as a result of blood transfusions. Thirty-eight percent of males aged 13-19 years were exposed to HIV through sexual contact with other males.

Thirty-five percent of adolescent AIDS cases were among females. Of those, 54% acquired HIV infection through heterosexual contact. Twenty-four percent had sex partners who were injecting drug users, while 16% were injecting drug users themselves.

Young Adult AIDS

As of December 31, 1995, 18,955 cases of AIDS were reported in young adults aged 20-24 years. This total includes 2,432 newly reported cases in 1995.

Across all racial/ethnic groups, men who have sex with men is the major exposure category associated with known AIDS cases in young adults. Young adult women (24% of known AIDS cases in this age group) are exposed to HIV primarily through injecting drug use (31%) or through sex with an injecting drug user (25%).

Due to the long latency period (median of 10 years to severe opportunistic infections), the majority of young adults with AIDS were most likely infected during adolescence.

Regarding Adolescent and Young Adult AIDS Statistics

- Receipt of Blood/Blood components includes received clotting factor for hemophilia/coagulation disorder and received blood transfusion, blood components, or tissue.

- The category "Men Who Have Sex with Men" includes men who have sex with men and also inject drugs.
- Heterosexual contact includes sex with: an injecting drug user, a person with hemophilia; a transfusion recipient infected with HIV; an HIV-infected person, risk not specified; a bisexual male (females only).
- On January 1, 1993, the AIDS case definition for adults and adolescents, aged 13 years and older, was expanded to include HIV-infected persons with CD4 counts of less than or equal to 200 cells/μL or a CD4 percentage of less than or equal to 14, and persons diagnosed with pulmonary tuberculosis, recurrent pneumonia and invasive cervical cancer.

Substance Abuse

Drug use among U.S. secondary school students rose again in 1995, continuing a trend that began in 1991 among 8th grade students, and in 1992, among 10th and 12th graders. Beliefs about the harmfulness of drugs have proven to be important determinants of use.

Although alcohol use rates decreased steadily from 1987 to 1993, use has increased for the past two years. Alcohol is still the most widely used substance among 12th graders. In 1995, over 51% of 12th graders reported using alcohol within the 30 days prior to the survey.

In 1995, the use of marijuana continued the strong resurgence that began in the early 1990s. The percentage of 12th graders reporting daily use increased from 1.9% to 4.6% between 1992 and 1995. The use of cocaine continued to increase slightly.

Cigarette Smoking

Trends in Thirty Day Prevalence

The University of Michigan's Institute for Social Research has found that cigarette smoking rose again in 1995 among American youth. This is the fourth year in a row that cigarette smoking increased for 8th and 10th graders, and the third year in a row for high school seniors. One in three high school seniors said that they had smoked cigarettes 30 days prior to the survey.

Increased smoking rates will have severe, lifelong consequences for this generation because a large proportion of those who initiate smoking in adolescence will continue to smoke for the rest of their lives. Hundreds of thousands of each graduating class may die prematurely as a result of cigarette smoking.

Trends in Attitudes

Among American youth, both disapproval and perceived risk of cigarette smoking have been declining over the past several years, while the prevalence of smoking has increased. Three-fourths (76%) of 8th graders say they can get cigarettes fairly easily; by 10th grade, over 90% say cigarettes are easily attainable.

Chapter 4

Births and Deaths in the United States

Abstract

Objectives

This report presents preliminary 1995 data on births and deaths in the United States from a new statistical series from the National Center for Health Statistics. U.S. data on births are shown by age, race, and Hispanic origin of mother. National and State data on marital status, prenatal care, cesarean delivery, and low birthweight are also presented. Mortality data presented include life expectancy, leading causes of death, and infant mortality.

Methods

Data in this report are based on 80-90-percent samples of 1995 births and deaths. The records are weighted to independent control counts of births, infant deaths, and total deaths registered in State vital statistics offices during 1995. Final data for 1995 may differ from the preliminary estimates.

Results

Preliminary data show that births and birth and fertility rates generally declined in 1995, especially for teenagers (3 percent); the

DHHS Publication No. (PHS) 96-1120, October 1996.

35

teen rate was 56.9 births per 1,000 women aged 15-19 years. The number, rate, and ratio of births to unmarried mothers all declined, the first time all measures have dropped simultaneously since 1940. For the sixth consecutive year, the cesarean delivery rate declined and the rate for prenatal care utilization improved. The overall low birthweight rate was unchanged at 7.3 percent.

The 1995 preliminary infant mortality rate reached a record low of 7.5 infant deaths per 1,000 live births, with record lows achieved for the white and black populations. Life expectancy matched the record high of 75.8 years attained in 1992. The largest declines in age-adjusted death rates among the leading causes of death were for homicide, Chronic liver disease and cirrhosis, and accidents. Mortality also decreased for firearm injuries, drug-induced deaths, and alcohol-induced deaths. The age-adjusted death rate for diabetes increased. For the first time, the age-adjusted death rate for Human Immunodeficiency Virus infection did not increase.

Introduction

This issue introduces a new statistical series, based on a new approach to collect and process vital statistics data and a new publication plan for the National Vital Statistics System. The new approach for vital statistics expedites the flow of data from the States to the National Center for Health Statistics (NCHS) and makes it possible to publish more detailed findings on a faster schedule.

With this publication, NCHS begins a new statistical series: Preliminary vital statistics data based on a substantial sample of records, including detailed tabulations from the natality as well as mortality files. Initially, NCHS will publish these preliminary data semiannually; however, its goal is to publish the data quarterly. This issue shows preliminary birth and death data for calendar year 1995 as well as previously published final data for 1994. The next *Monthly Vital Statistics Report (MVSR)* supplement in this series will show preliminary data for July 1995-June 1996 compared with data for July 1994-June 1995. The publication of these preliminary vital statistics is made possible by more expeditious electronic transmittal of data from the States to NCHS and by more rapid data processing at NCHS. These changes will also expedite production of final birth and death statistics.

In the past NCHS has released vital statistics data in two basic forms. Monthly provisional data based on counts of birth, marriage, divorce, and death records received in State vital registration offices have been published in the *MVSR*. Also, estimates of deaths and death rates by selected characteristics, based on a 10-percent sample of death certificates (the "Current Mortality Sample"), were published in the *MVSR*. Annual provisional data, which summarize the monthly counts and the Current Mortality Sample, have been published in *Annual Summary of Births, Marriages, Divorces, and Deaths*, an *MVSR* supplement.

Final birth and death data have been published in *MVSR* supplements entitled *Advance Report of Final Natality Statistics* and *Advance Report of Final Mortality Statistics*, respectively. These reports have been published 18-24 months after the close of the data year. Unit record data have been released on public use data tapes around the time that the final data *MVSR* supplement was published. More detailed tabulations have been published later in *Vital Statistics of the United States*.

The new series of preliminary data reports will replace the Annual Summary of provisional data, and in time, the "Current Mortality Sample," which is included in the *MVSR*. NCHS will continue to publish monthly, cumulative year-to-date, and 12-month moving average record counts in the *MVSR*. Final data will also be released in *MVSR* supplements; the publication names will be changed to *Report of Final Natality Statistics* and *Report of Final Mortality Statistics*. NCHS also plans to expand its release of vital statistics data in electronic form.

Sources and Methods

Preliminary data are based on those records received and processed by NCHS by a specified date, in this case, those 1995 births and deaths that were processed by April 30, 1996. For live births these records represent about 90 percent of the births that occurred in the United States during 1995. For deaths two files, demographic and medical (cause of death), were created. The demographic file accounted for about 90 percent of all deaths and the medical file, about 80 percent.

To produce the preliminary estimates shown in this report, the records were weighted using independent control counts of births, infant deaths, and total deaths registered in the State vital statistics offices from January through December 1995. Across tables there are some inconsistencies in the numbers of total deaths and deaths by certain demographic characteristics because the separate demographic and medical files have different sets of weights. Also, these preliminary estimates are subject to sampling variation as well as random variation.

Table 4.1. Total Births and Percent of Births with Selected Demographic and Health Characteristics, by Race and Hispanic Origin of Mother: United States, Final 1994 and Preliminary 1995.

Characteristic	All races[1]		White		Black		Hispanic[2]	
	1995	1994	1995	1994	1995	1994	1995	1994
				Number				
Births.	3,900,089	3,952,767	3,105,315	3,121,004	598,558	636,391	671,849	665,026
				Percent				
Births to mothers under								
20 years	13.2	13.1	11.5	11.3	23.2	23.2	18.0	17.8
Births to unmarried mothers.	32.0	32.6	25.3	25.4	69.5	70.4	40.8	43.1
Low birthweight[3]	7.3	7.3	6.2	6.1	13.0	13.2	6.3	6.2
Births delivered by cesarean	20.8	21.2	20.8	21.2	21.8	21.8	20.1	20.5
Prenatal care beginning in first trimester.	81.2	80.2	83.5	82.8	70.3	68.3	70.4	68.9

[1]Includes races other than white and black.
[2]Persons of Hispanic origin may be of any race.
[3]Birthweight of less than 2,500 grams (5 pounds 8 ounces).

The preliminary cause-of-death statistics have not been adjusted for the bias that occurs because cause of death is sometimes not available in the State offices when the preliminary data are sent to NCHS but is available later when copies of the final death certificates are processed. As a result estimates based on the preliminary mortality file may differ from statistics that will come from final counts. NCHS is exploring procedures to correct for biases in the number of deaths.

In addition to national and State estimates of total births and birth rates, this report includes preliminary statistics on births by age, live-birth order, marital status, race and Hispanic origin, and selected maternal and infant health characteristics, such as receipt of prenatal care, cesarean delivery, and low birthweight. Mortality data in this report are also more detailed than in the provisional data reports, with more detailed information on life expectancy, infant mortality, and causes of death.

State-specific preliminary data are shown only for those States and areas for which at least 60 percent of the records for the 12-month period have been processed. In this report all areas except Guam provided sufficient records to be included in the State-specific tabulations.

In addition, no data are shown for a particular characteristic if reporting for that item is less than 80-percent complete. Because reporting for each item in this report was at least 80 percent, no data items were suppressed.

Results

Natality Patterns

For the fifth consecutive year, births declined in the United States in 1995, to an estimated 3,900,089, 1 percent fewer than the final 1994 total, 3,952,767. The 1995 preliminary count is 6 percent lower than that for 1990 (4,158,212), the most recent high point. The crude birth rate fell 3percent between 1994 and 1995, from 15.2 to 14.8 births per 1,000 total population, reaching its lowest level in nearly two decades (14.6 in 1976). The fertility rate, which relates births to women in the childbearing ages, declined 2 percent, from 66.7 to 65.6 births per 1,000 women aged 15-44 years. The 1995 rate is lower than that for any year since 1986 (65.4).

Fertility rates in 1995 for white (64.5), American Indian (70.0), Asian or Pacific Islander (65.6), and Hispanic women (103.7) were 1 to 2 percent lower than the fertility rates in 1994. The 1995 rate for white women matched the previous low observed in 1988. Rates for

American Indian and Asian or Pacific Islander women were the lowest ever recorded. The rate for Hispanic women was at its lowest level since national data on Hispanic fertility became available. The rate for black women fell 7 percent to 71.7, an historic low level.

The birth rate for teens aged 15-19 years dropped 3 percent between 1994 and 1995, from 58.9 to 56.9 births per 1,000 women. This is the fourth consecutive year of decline in the teen rate, which has fallen 8percent since 1991 (62.1). Teen birth rates fell 3 percent or less for white, American Indian, Asian or Pacific Islander, and Hispanic teens. The rate for black teens fell substantially, from 104.5 births per 1,000 women in 1994 to 95.5 births per 1,000 women in 1995; this rate dropped 17 percent from 1991 to 1995. Despite the drop in teen birth rates, the proportion of all births occurring to women under 20 years of age increased slightly to 13.2 percent (Table 4.1). This is a reflection of the recent increases in the teenage population.

Birth rates declined 1 percent between 1994 and 1995 for women in their twenties. The rates for women aged 20-24 years (110.0 births per 1,000 women) and 25-29 years (112.4 births per 1,000 women) were each 6 percent lower than their recent high point in 1990.

Birth rates for women aged 30-34 years and 35-39 years rose 1 percent each from 1994 to 1995 to 82.5 and 34.1 per 1,000 women, respectively. The rate for women 35-39 years has risen steadily and substantially since 1978; the rate for women aged 30-34 years has increased too but at a slower pace in recent years.

The total fertility rate-an estimate of lifetime childbearing-dropped 1 percent from 1994 (2,036.0 births per 1,000 women) to 1995 (2,020.0). This hypothetical measure shows the potential impact of current fertility levels on completed family size. The rate for white women was essentially unchanged at 1,992.5 births per 1,000 women, while the rate for black women dropped 6 percent to 2,158.5. Rates for American Indian (2,061.5 births per 1,000 women), Asian or Pacific Islander (1,904.5), and Hispanic women (2,983.5) each dropped by 1 to 2 percent.

The first birth rate, a measure of family formation, was 27.3 births per 1,000 women aged 15-44 years in 1995, about 1 percent below the 1994 rate (27.5).

The preliminary number of nonmarital births declined 3 percent to 1,248,028. The proportion of all births to unmarried mothers declined 2 percent to 32.0 percent (from 32.6 percent in 1994) (Table 4.1). The proportions for white (25.3 percent) and black births (69.5 percent) were about 1 percent lower than those for 1994, while the proportion for Hispanic women, 40.8 percent, was 5 percent lower than for 1994. The birth rate for unmarried women dropped 4percent, from 46.9 to 44.9 per 1,000 unmarried women aged 1594 years, the first decline in the rate in nearly two decades. About half of the decline is due to changes in reporting procedures in California; the marital status of Hispanic mothers was more precisely determined in 1995 than in 1994. Nonetheless, even if data for California are excluded, nonmarital childbearing declined in 1995. This is the first time that all measures have dropped since 1940, when national data were first compiled. During the 5-year period 1989-94, the rate of increase in measures of nonmarital childbearing had slowed considerably compared with trends in the early to mid-1980's.

The incidence of low birthweight (birthweight of less than 2,500 grams or 5 pounds 8 ounces) was unchanged for 1995, at 7.3 percent. The percent low birthweight had risen from 6.8 percent in 1986 to 7.3 percent in 1994. Levels of low birthweight increased for white births (from 6.1 to 6.2 percent) and for Hispanic births (6.2 to 6.3 percent), while the rate for black births fell from 13.2 to 13.0 percent (Table 4.1).

The rate of cesarean delivery declined in 1995, from 21.2 to 20. 8 percent. Rates fell for white (20.8 percent) and Hispanic (20.1) women; the rate for black women was unchanged (21.8 percent). This is the sixth consecutive year of decline; the 1995 rate was 9 percent below the 1989 rate (22.8 percent).

The proportion of mothers beginning prenatal care in the first trimester continued to rise in 1995 to 81.2 percent compared with 80.2 percent in 1994. This measure has shown improvement for 6 consecutive years, rising from 75.5 percent in 1989. The proportions of white (83.5 percent), black (70.3 percent), and Hispanic (70.4) mothers receiving early care were 1 to 3 percent higher in 1995 than the comparable proportions in 1994).

Mortality Patterns

In 1995 an estimated 2,312,180 deaths occurred in the United States, 33,186 more than the previous high recorded in 1994. The crude death rate of 880.0 per 100,000 population was slightly higher than the rate of 875.4 for the previous year. The age-adjusted death rate, which eliminates the distorting effects of the aging of the population, was 503.7 per 100,000 U.S. standard million population, a record low for the United States. The comparable rate for 1994 was 507.4 per 100,000 U.S. standard million population.

The decline between 1994 and 1995 in the U.S. age-adjusted death rate continued the long-term downward trend in mortality. This trend

41

was interrupted most recently in 1993 by the high mortality associated with the influenza epidemics in 1992-93. The 1994-95 decline reflects reduced mortality for white males, black males and females, as well as Hispanic males. The mortality of white females and Hispanic females did not change significantly between the 2 years.

By age the overall reductions in mortality between 1994 and 1995 were the result of declines for most age groups under 85 years of age. Among persons 85 years old and over, mortality increased between the 2 years after declining between 1993 and 1994. Large fluctuations in mortality for persons 85 years and over are more likely to be statistical artifacts than true changes in mortality risk.

Estimated life expectancy in 1995 matched the record high of 75.8 years attained in 1992 and was slightly above the figure of 75.7 years for 1994. Record high life expectancies were reached for white and black males (73.4 years and 65.4 years, respectively) and black females (74.0 years). For white females life expectancy (79.6 years) was unchanged from the previous year, and slightly below the record high (79.8 years) reached in 1992.

The leading causes of death in 1995 were Diseases of heart (heart disease); Malignant neoplasms, including neoplasms of lymphatic and hematopoietic tissues (cancer); Cerebrovascular diseases (stroke); Chronic obstructive pulmonary disease and allied conditions (COPD); Accidents and adverse effects; Pneumonia and influenza; Diabetes mellitus (diabetes); Human immunodeficiency virus infection (HIV); Suicide; Chronic liver disease and cirrhosis; Nephritis, nephrotic syndrome, and nephrosis (kidney disease); Homicide and legal intervention (homicide); Septicemia (blood poisoning); Alzheimer's disease; and Atherosclerosis. Homicide dropped from a rank of 11th in 1994 to 12th in 1995, while kidney disease moved from 12th in 1994 to 11th in 1995.

Among the leading causes of death, reductions between 1994 and 1995 occurred in the mortality of the two leading causes of deathheart disease and cancer. For both causes of death, which combined accounted for a total of over 1.3 million deaths in 1995, the declines in age-adjusted death rates were over 1 percent (Table 4.2). While mortality in heart disease has followed a downward trend since 1950, the trend in cancer turned downward only since 1990. The 1994-95 decline in cancer mortality follows a similar reduction during 1993-94.

According to preliminary data, the largest decline between 1994 and 1995 in the age-adjusted death rates among the leading causes of death was for homicide, which decreased sharply by about 15 percent. Age-adjusted rates for chronic liver disease and cirrhosis declined by about 5 percent, continuing a 20-year downward trend. Mortality due to accidents declined by about 4 percent, continuing a general downward trend since the early 1980's. Reductions in age-adjusted death rates from accidents were shared by the two component categories—motor vehicle accidents and other types of accidents. Age-adjusted death rates for Suicide decreased by about 2 percent.

Age-adjusted death rates increased for four leading causes of death—Alzheimer's disease, Septicemia, kidney disease, and diabetes. The largest increase (8 percent), which was for Alzheimer's disease, may reflect changes in diagnostic practices rather than real increases in mortality from this cause. Diabetes mortality has been increasing for about the past 10 years.

While the number of deaths due to HIV infection increased from 42,114 in 1994 to an estimated 42,506 in 1995, the largest number reported in a single year, the age-adjusted death rate from this cause did not change between the 2 years. This marks the first time that the age-adjusted death rate for HIV infection has held steady between 2 years since 1987, when this cause of death was first uniquely classified in the morbidity and mortality statistics of the United States.

Between 1994 and 1995 the preliminary age-adjusted death rates decreased appreciably for firearm injuries (11 percent), drug-induced causes (14 percent), and alcohol-induced causes (6 percent). In addition, a marked decline occurred in the number of deaths from injuries sustained at work.

Among the major race groups, the lowest mortality was reported for Asian or Pacific Islanders. The age-adjusted death rate for this group was 39 percent below that of whites. In contrast, the rate for blacks was 59 percent higher than the age-adjusted death rate for whites. Between whites and blacks, the gap in mortality narrowed slightly between 1994 and 1995.

The preliminary infant mortality rate of 7.5 infant deaths per 1,000 live births in 1995 is a 6-percent reduction from the previous year. Declines occurred among neonates (infant deaths under 28 days of age) as well as among postneonates (aged 28 days-11 months). Between 1994 and 1995 the white infant mortality rate declined 5 percent (from 6.6 per 1,000 live births to 6.3), while the black rate declined 6 percent (from 15.8 to 14.9). The final 1995 infant mortality rate is expected to be somewhat higher than the preliminary figure, although below the 1994 rate of 8.0.

Table 4.2a. Deaths, Death Rates, and Age-adjusted Death Rates for 72 Selected Causes: United States, Final 1994 and Preliminary 1995.

[Data are based on a continuous file of records received from the States. Rates per 100,000 population; age-adjusted rates per 100,000 standard million population; see Technical notes. For explanation of asterisks preceding cause-of-death categories, see Technical notes. Figures for 1995 are based on weighted data rounded to the nearest individual, so categories may not add to totals]

Cause of death (Based on Ninth Revision, International Classification of Diseases, 1975)	1995 Number	1995 Rate	1995 Age-adjusted rate	1994 Number	1994 Rate	1994 Age-adjusted rate
All causes	2,312,203	880.0	502.9	2,278,994	875.4	507.4
Shigellosis and amebiasis (004,006)	11	*	*	15	*	*
Certain other intestinal infections (007-009)	781	0.3	0.2	746	0.3	0.2
Tuberculosis (010-018)	1,341	0.5	0.3	1,478	0.6	0.4
Tuberculosis of respiratory system (010-012)	1,064	0.4	0.3	1,129	0.4	0.3
Other tuberculosis (013-018)	277	0.1	0.1	349	0.1	0.1
Whooping cough (033)	5	*	*	8	*	*
Streptococcal sore throat, scarlatina, and erysipelas (034-035)	6	*	*	12	*	*
Meningococcal infection (036)	281	0.1	0.1	276	0.1	0.1
Septicemia (038)	21,123	8.0	4.1	20,360	7.8	4.0
Acute poliomyelitis (045)	3	*	*	-	*	*
Measles (055)	4	*	*			
Viral hepatitis (070)	3,395	1.3	1.0	3,061	1.2	0.9
Syphilis (090-097)	77	0.0	0.0	79	0.0	0.0
All other infectious and parasitic diseases[1] (001-003,005,020-032,037,039-041,*042,*044,046-054,056-066,071-088,098-139)	49,601	18.9	17.4	49,265	18.9	17.5
Malignant neoplasms, including neoplasms of lymphatic and hematopoietic tissues (140-208)	537,969	204.7	129.8	534,310	205.2	131.5
Malignant neoplasms of lip, oral cavity, and pharynx (140-149)	8,018	3.1	2.1	7,915	3.0	2.1
Malignant neoplasms of digestive organs and peritoneum (150-159)	126,404	48.1	29.0	125,353	48.1	29.3
Malignant neoplasms of respiratory and intrathoracic organs (160-165)	156,073	59.4	39.6	154,714	59.4	40.1
Malignant neoplasm of breast (174-175)	44,331	16.9	11.5	44,008	16.9	11.6
Malignant neoplasms of genital organs (179-187)	60,341	23.0	12.7	61,054	23.5	13.2
Malignant neoplasms of urinary organs (188-189)	22,492	8.6	5.0	22,432	8.6	5.1
Malignant neoplasms of all other and unspecified sites (170-173,190-199)	66,160	25.2	16.8	65,754	25.3	17.0
Leukemia (204-208)	20,021	7.6	4.8	19,669	7.6	4.9
Other malignant neoplasms of lymphatic and hematopoietic tissues (200-203)	34,128	13.0	8.2	33,411	12.8	8.2
Benign neoplasms, carcinoma in situ, and neoplasms of uncertain behavior and of unspecified nature (210-239)	7,808	3.0	1.8	7,517	2.9	1.7
Diabetes mellitus (250)	59,085	22.5	13.2	56,692	21.8	12.9
Nutritional deficiencies (260-269)	3,505	1.3	0.5	3,451	1.3	0.5
Anemias (280-285)	4,530	1.7	0.9	4,380	1.7	0.9
Meningitis (320-322)	805	0.3	0.3	770	0.3	0.3
Major cardiovascular diseases (390-448)	952,523	362.5	174.7	940,693	361.3	176.8
Diseases of heart (390-398,402,404-429)	738,781	281.2	138.2	732,409	281.3	140.4
Rheumatic fever and rheumatic heart disease (390-398)	5,225	2.0	1.2	5,415	2.1	1.2
Hypertensive heart disease (402)	24,433	9.3	4.9	23,943	9.2	5.0
Hypertensive heart and renal disease (404)	2,445	0.9	0.4	2,494	1.0	0.5
Ischemic heart disease (410-414)	482,185	183.5	89.6	481,458	184.9	91.4
Acute myocardial infarction (410)	218,579	83.2	44.0	222,399	85.4	45.6
Other acute and subacute forms of ischemic heart disease (411)	2,757	1.0	0.6	2,862	1.1	0.6
Angina pectoris (413)	843	0.3	0.1	913	0.4	0.2
Old myocardial infarction and other forms of chronic ischemic heart disease (412,414)	260,006	99.0	44.9	255,284	98.1	45.0
Other diseases of endocardium (424)	16,290	6.2	2.6	15,417	5.9	2.6
All other forms of heart disease (415-423,425-429)	208,204	79.2	39.5	203,682	78.2	39.7
Hypertension with or without renal disease (401,403)	12,479	4.7	2.3	11,765	4.5	2.2

See footnotes at end of table.

Table 4.2b. Deaths, Death Rates, and Age-adjusted Death Rates for 72 Selected Causes: United States, Final 1994 and Preliminary 1995.

[Data are based on a continuous file of records received from the States. Rates per 100,000 population; age-adjusted rates per 100,000 standard million population; see Technical notes. For explanation of asterisks preceding cause-of-death categories, see Technical notes. Figures for 1995 are based on weighted data rounded to the nearest individual, so categories may not add to totals]

Cause of death (Based on Ninth Revision, International Classification of Diseases, 1975)	1995 Number	1995 Rate	1995 Age-adjusted rate	1994 Number	1994 Rate	1994 Age-adjusted rate
Cerebrovascular diseases (430-438)	158,061	60.2	26.7	153,306	58.9	26.5
Intracerebral and other intracranial hemorrhage (431-432)	22,326	8.5	5.0	21,807	8.4	5.0
Cerebral thrombosis and unspecified occlusion of cerebral arteries (434.0,434.9)	14,075	5.4	2.3	14,629	5.6	2.4
Cerebral embolism (434.1)	635	0.2	0.1	708	0.3	0.1
All other and late effects of cerebrovascular diseases (430,433,435-438)	121,026	46.1	19.2	116,162	44.6	19.0
Atherosclerosis (440)	16,781	6.4	2.3	17,116	6.6	2.3
Other diseases of arteries, arterioles, and capillaries (441-448)	26,422	10.1	5.3	26,097	10.0	5.3
Acute bronchitis and bronchiolitis (466)	554	0.2	0.1	578	0.2	0.1
Pneumonia and influenza (480-487)	83,528	31.8	13.0	81,473	31.3	13.0
Pneumonia (480-486)	82,931	31.6	12.9	80,244	30.8	12.8
Influenza (487)	597	0.2	0.1	1,229	0.5	0.2
Chronic obstructive pulmonary diseases and allied conditions (490-496)	104,756	39.9	21.2	101,628	39.0	21.0
Bronchitis, chronic and unspecified (490-491)	3,437	1.3	0.7	3,579	1.4	0.7
Emphysema (492)	17,303	6.6	3.7	17,215	6.6	3.7
Asthma (493)	5,579	2.1	1.5	5,487	2.1	1.5
Other chronic obstructive pulmonary diseases and allied conditions (494-496)	78,437	29.9	15.3	75,347	28.9	15.1
Ulcer of stomach and duodenum (531-533)	5,433	2.1	1.0	6,088	2.3	1.2
Appendicitis (540-543)	407	0.2	0.1	380	0.1	0.1
Hernia of abdominal cavity and intestinal obstruction without mention of hernia (550-553,560)	6,214	2.4	1.1	6,142	2.4	1.1
Chronic liver disease and cirrhosis (571)	24,848	9.5	7.5	25,406	9.8	7.9
Cholelithiasis and other disorders of gallbladder (574-575)	2,686	1.0	0.5	2,855	1.1	0.5
Nephritis, nephrotic syndrome, and nephrosis (580-589)	23,845	9.1	4.4	22,976	8.8	4.3
Acute glomerulonephritis and nephrotic syndrome (580-581)	283	0.1	0.0	305	0.1	0.1*
Chronic glomerulonephritis, nephritis and nephropathy, not specified as acute or chronic, and renal sclerosis, unspecified (582-583,587)	1,510	0.6	0.3	1,546	0.6	0.3
Renal failure, disorders resulting from impaired renal function, and small kidney of unknown cause (584-586,588-589)	22,052	8.4	4.0	21,125	8.1	3.9
Infections of kidney (590)	914	0.3	0.2	973	0.4	0.2
Hyperplasia of prostate (600)	398	0.2	0.1	413	0.2	0.1
Complications of pregnancy, childbirth, and the puerperium (630-676)	247	0.1	0.1	328	0.1	0.1
Pregnancy with abortive outcome (630-638)	23	0.0	0.0	41	0.0	0.0
Other complications of pregnancy, childbirth, and the puerperium (640-676)	224	0.1	0.1	287	0.1	0.1
Congenital anomalies (740-759)	11,933	4.5	4.4	12,030	4.6	4.5
Certain conditions originating in the perinatal period (760-779)	13,222	5.0	5.2	14,487	5.6	5.7
Birth trauma, intrauterine hypoxia, birth asphyxia, and respiratory distress syndrome (767-769)	2,177	0.8	0.9	2,378	0.9	0.9
Other conditions originating in the perinatal period (760-766,770-779)	11,046	4.2	4.4	12,109	4.7	4.8
Symptoms, signs, and ill-defined conditions (780-799)	32,993	12.6	9.2	25,245	9.7	6.8
All other diseases (Residual)	212,286	80.8	40.6	203,939	78.3	40.3
Accidents and adverse effects (E800-E949)	89,703	34.1	29.2	91,437	35.1	30.3
Motor vehicle accidents (E810-E825)	41,786	15.9	15.7	42,524	16.3	16.1
All other accidents and adverse effects (E800-E807,E826-E949)	47,916	18.2	13.5	48,913	18.8	14.2
Suicide (E950-E959)	30,893	11.8	11.0	31,142	12.0	11.2
Homicide and legal intervention (E960-E978)	21,577	8.2	8.8	24,926	9.6	10.3
All other external causes (E980-E999)	2,911	1.1	1.1	3,435	1.3	1.3

See footnotes at end of table.

Table 4.2c. Deaths, Death Rates, and Age-adjusted Death Rates for 72 Selected Causes: United States, Final 1994 and Preliminary 1995.

[Data are based on a continuous file of records received from the States. Rates per 100,000 population; age-adjusted rates per 100,000 standard million population; see Technical notes. For explanation of asterisks preceding cause-of-death categories, see Technical notes. Figures for 1995 are based on weighted data rounded to the nearest individual, so categories may not add to totals]

Cause of death (Based on Ninth Revision, International Classification of Diseases, 1975)	1995			1994		
	Number	Rate	Age-adjusted rate	Number	Rate	Age-adjusted rate
Human immunodeficiency virus infection[2] (*042-*044)	42,506	16.2	15.4	42,114	16.2	15.4
Alzheimer's disease[3] (331.0)	20,415	7.8	2.7	18,584	7.1	2.5
Injury by firearms[4](E922,E955.0-E955.4,E965.0-E965.4,E970,E985.0-E985.4)	34,990	13.3	13.5	38,505	14.8	15.1
Drug-induced deaths[4] (292,304,305.2-305.9,E850-E858,E950.0-E950.5,E962.0,E980.0-E980.5)	11,933	4.5	4.3	13,923	5.3	5.0
Alcohol-induced deaths[4] (291,303,305.0,357.5,425.5,535.3,571.0-571.3,790.3,E880)	19,470	7.4	6.4	20,163	7.7	6.8
Injury at work[5]	5,543	2.1	2.0	6,008	2.3	2.2

- Quantity zero.
* Figure does not meet standards of reliability or precision (see Technical notes).
1 Includes data for deaths due to Human immunodeficiency virus infection (categories *042-*044) shown separately, see Technical notes.
2 Included in All other infectious and parasitic diseases.
3 Included in All other diseases.
4 Included in selected categories.
5 Injury at work described in Technical notes.

NOTE: Data are subject to sampling and/or random variation. For information on the relative standard errors of the data and further discussion, see Technical notes.

Table 4.3a. Life Expectancy by Age, Race, and Sex: United States, Final 1994 and Preliminary 1995.

[Data are based on a continuous file of records received from the States]

Age (in years)	All races [1]		Male		Female	
	1995	1994	1995	1994	1995	1994
0	75.8	75.7	72.6	72.4	78.9	79.0
1	75.4	75.3	72.2	72.0	78.5	78.5
5	71.5	71.4	68.3	68.1	74.6	74.6
10	66.6	66.5	63.4	63.2	69.7	69.7
15	61.6	61.6	58.5	58.3	64.7	64.8
20	56.9	56.8	53.8	53.6	59.9	59.9
25	52.2	52.1	49.2	49.1	55.0	55.1
30	47.5	47.4	44.6	44.5	50.2	50.2
35	42.8	42.8	40.1	40.0	45.4	45.4
40	38.3	38.2	35.6	35.5	40.7	40.7
45	33.7	33.7	31.3	31.2	36.0	36.0
50	29.3	29.3	27.0	26.9	31.4	31.5
55	25.1	25.1	22.9	22.8	27.0	27.1
60	21.1	21.1	19.0	18.9	22.8	22.9
65	17.4	17.4	15.6	15.5	18.9	19.0
70	14.1	14.1	12.4	12.4	15.3	15.3
75	11.0	11.0	9.7	9.6	11.9	12.0
80	8.3	8.3	7.2	7.2	8.9	9.0
85	6.0	6.1	5.2	5.2	6.3	6.4

Age (in years)	White		White male		White female	
	1995	1994	1995	1994	1995	1994
0	76.5	76.5	73.4	73.3	79.6	79.6
1	76.0	76.0	72.9	72.8	79.0	79.1
5	72.1	72.1	69.0	68.9	75.1	75.2
10	67.2	67.1	64.1	64.0	70.2	70.2
15	62.3	62.2	59.2	59.1	65.2	65.3
20	57.5	57.4	54.5	54.4	60.3	60.4
25	52.7	52.7	49.9	49.7	55.5	55.5
30	48.0	48.0	45.2	45.1	50.6	50.7
35	43.3	43.3	40.6	40.5	45.8	45.9
40	38.7	38.6	36.1	36.0	41.0	41.1
45	34.1	34.1	31.7	31.6	36.3	36.4
50	29.6	29.6	27.3	27.2	31.7	31.7
55	25.3	25.3	23.1	23.0	27.2	27.3
60	21.3	21.2	19.2	19.1	23.0	23.1
65	17.5	17.5	15.7	15.6	19.0	19.1
70	14.1	14.1	12.5	12.5	15.3	15.4
75	11.0	11.1	9.7	9.6	12.0	12.0
80	8.3	8.3	7.2	7.2	8.9	9.0
85	6.0	6.1	5.2	5.2	6.3	6.4

See footnote at end of table.

Table 4.3b. Life Expectancy by Age, Race, and Sex: United States, Final 1994 and Preliminary 1995.

[Data are based on a continuous file of records received from the States]

	Black		Black male		Black female	
	1995	1994	1995	1994	1995	1994
Age (in years)						
0	69.8	69.5	65.4	64.9	74.0	73.9
1	69.8	69.6	65.4	65.1	74.0	73.9
5	66.0	65.8	61.6	61.3	70.2	70.1
10	61.1	60.9	56.7	56.4	65.3	65.2
15	56.2	56.0	51.8	51.5	60.3	60.3
20	51.5	51.4	47.3	47.1	55.5	55.5
25	47.0	46.9	43.0	42.8	50.7	50.7
30	42.5	42.4	38.7	38.5	46.1	46.0
35	38.2	38.1	34.6	34.5	41.5	41.5
40	34.0	33.9	30.6	30.5	37.0	37.0
45	29.9	29.9	26.8	26.7	32.7	32.7
50	26.0	26.0	23.1	23.1	28.5	28.5
55	22.3	22.3	19.7	19.6	24.5	24.5
60	18.8	18.8	16.5	16.5	20.7	20.7
65	15.7	15.7	13.7	13.6	17.2	17.2
70	12.7	12.8	11.0	11.0	14.0	14.1
75	10.3	10.3	8.9	8.9	11.2	11.2
80	7.9	8.0	6.8	6.8	8.5	8.6
85	5.9	6.0	5.2	5.3	6.3	6.3

[1] Includes races other than white and black.

NOTE: Data are subject to sampling and/or random variation.

Births and Deaths in the United States

Table 4.4a. Death and Death Rates for the 10 Leading Causes of Death in Specified Age Groups: United States, Preliminary 1995.

[Data are based on a continuous file of records received from the States. Rates per 100,000 population in specified group. For explanation of asterisks preceding cause-of-death categories, see Technical notes. Figures are based on weighted data rounded to the nearest individual, so categories may not add to totals]

Rank [1]	Cause of death and age (Based on Ninth Revision, International Classification of Diseases, 1975)	Number	Rate
	All ages [2]		
. . .	All causes	2,312,203	880.0
1	Diseases of heart (390-398, 402, 404-429)	738,781	281.2
2	Malignant neoplasms, including neoplasms of lymphatic and hematopoietic tissues (140-208)	537,969	204.7
3	Cerebrovascular diseases (430-438)	156,061	60.2
4	Chronic obstructive pulmonary diseases and allied conditions (490-496)	104,756	39.9
5	Accidents and adverse effects (E800-E949)	89,703	34.1
. . .	Motor vehicle accidents (E810-E825)	41,786	15.9
. . .	All other accidents and adverse effects (E800-E807, E826-E949)	47,916	18.2
6	Pneumonia and influenza (480-487)	83,528	31.8
7	Diabetes mellitus (250)	59,085	22.5
8	Human immunodeficiency virus infection (*042-*044)	42,506	16.2
9	Suicide (E950-E959)	30,893	11.8
10	Chronic liver disease and cirrhosis (571)	24,848	9.5
. . .	All other causes (Residual)	442,073	168.2
	1-4 years		
. . .	All causes	6,355	40.4
1	Accidents and adverse effects (E800-E949)	2,277	14.5
. . .	Motor vehicle accidents (E810-E825)	814	5.2
. . .	All other accidents and adverse effects (E800-E807, E826-E949)	1,463	9.3
2	Congenital anomalies (740-759)	692	4.4
3	Malignant neoplasms, including neoplasms of lymphatic and hematopoietic tissues (140-208)	487	3.1
4	Homicide and legal intervention (E960-E978)	414	2.6
5	Diseases of heart (390-398, 402, 404-429)	256	1.6
6	Human immunodeficiency virus infection (*042-*044)	205	1.3
7	Pneumonia and influenza (480-487)	138	0.9
8	Certain conditions originating in the perinatal period (760-779)	96	0.6
9	Septicemia (038)	67	0.4
10	Benign neoplasms, carcinoma in situ, and neoplasms of uncertain behavior and of unspecified nature (210-239)	60	0.4
. . .	All other causes (Residual)	1,663	10.6
	5-14 years		
. . .	All causes	8,412	22.1
1	Accidents and adverse effects (E800-E949)	3,481	9.1
. . .	Motor vehicle accidents (E810-E825)	1,997	5.2
. . .	All other accidents and adverse effects (E800-E807, E826-E949)	1,484	3.9
2	Malignant neoplasms, including neoplasms of lymphatic and hematopoietic tissues (140-208)	999	2.6
3	Homicide and legal intervention (E960-E978)	494	1.3
4	Congenital anomalies (740-759)	457	1.2
5	Suicide (E950-E959)	329	0.9
6	Diseases of heart (390-398, 402, 404-429)	269	0.7
7	Human immunodeficiency virus infection (*042-*044)	174	0.5
8	Chronic obstructive pulmonary diseases and allied conditions (490-496)	137	0.4
9	Benign neoplasms, carcinoma in situ, and neoplasms of uncertain behavior and of unspecified nature (210-239)	120	0.3
10	Pneumonia and influenza (480-487)	115	0.3
. . .	All other causes (Residual)	1,837	4.8

See footnotes at end of table.

Table 4.4b. Death and Death Rates for the 10 Leading Causes of Death in Specified Age Groups: United States, Preliminary 1995.

[Data are based on a continuous file of records received from the States. Rates per 100,000 population in specified group. For explanation of asterisks preceding cause-of-death categories, see Technical notes. Figures are based on weighted data rounded to the nearest individual, so categories may not add to totals]

Rank [1]	Cause of death and age (Based on Ninth Revision, International Classification of Diseases, 1975)	Number	Rate
	15-24 years		
. . .	All causes	33,569	93.4
1	Accidents and adverse effects (E800-E949)	13,532	37.6
. . .	Motor vehicle accidents (E810-E825)	10,354	28.8
. . .	All other accidents and adverse effects (E800-E807, E826-E949)	3,179	8.8
2	Homicide and legal intervention (E960-E978)	6,827	19.0
3	Suicide (E950-E959)	4,789	13.3
4	Malignant neoplasms, including neoplasms of lymphatic and hematopoietic tissues (140-208)	1,599	4.4
5	Diseases of heart (390-398, 402, 404-429)	964	2.7
6	Human immunodeficiency virus infection (*042-*044)	643	1.8
7	Congenital anomalies (740-759)	425	1.2
8	Chronic obstructive pulmonary diseases and allied conditions (490-496)	220	0.6
9	Pneumonia and influenza (480-487)	193	0.5
10	Cerebrovascular diseases (430-438)	166	0.5
. . .	All other causes (Residual)	4,211	11.7
	25-44 years		
. . .	All causes	157,971	189.5
1	Human immunodeficiency virus infection (*042-*044)	30,465	36.6
2	Accidents and adverse effects (E800-E949)	25,995	31.2
. . .	Motor vehicle accidents (E810-E825)	14,087	16.9
. . .	All other accidents and adverse effects (E800-E807, E826-E949)	11,909	14.3
3	Malignant neoplasms, including neoplasms of lymphatic and hematopoietic tissues (140-208)	21,983	26.4
4	Diseases of heart (390-398, 402, 404-429)	16,719	20.1
5	Suicide (E950-E959)	12,518	15.0
6	Homicide and legal intervention (E960-E978)	9,693	11.6
7	Chronic liver disease and cirrhosis (571)	4,146	5.0
8	Cerebrovascular diseases (430-438)	3,407	4.1
9	Diabetes mellitus (250)	2,417	2.9
10	Pneumonia and influenza (480-487)	2,076	2.5
. . .	All other causes (Residual)	28,552	34.3
	45-64 years		
. . .	All causes	376,337	720.8
1	Malignant neoplasms, including neoplasms of lymphatic and hematopoietic tissues (140-208)	131,808	252.5
2	Diseases of heart (390-398, 402, 404-429)	101,975	195.3
3	Accidents and adverse effects (E800-E949)	15,021	28.8
. . .	Motor vehicle accidents (E810-E825)	7,004	13.4
. . .	All other accidents and adverse effects (E800-E807, E826-E949)	8,016	15.4
4	Cerebrovascular diseases (430-438)	15,015	28.8
5	Chronic obstructive pulmonary diseases and allied conditions (490-496)	12,889	24.7
6	Diabetes mellitus (250)	12,039	23.1
7	Chronic liver disease and cirrhosis (571)	10,310	19.7
8	Human immunodeficiency virus infection (*042-*044)	10,202	19.5
9	Suicide (E950-E959)	7,175	13.7
10	Pneumonia and influenza (480-487)	5,528	10.6
. . .	All other causes (Residual)	54,375	104.1

See footnotes at end of table.

Births and Deaths in the United States

Table 4.4c. Death and Death Rates for the 10 Leading Causes of Death in Specified Age Groups: United States, Preliminary 1995.

[Data are based on a continuous file of records received from the States. Rates per 100,000 population in specified group. For explanation of asterisks preceding cause-of-death categories, see Technical notes. Figures are based on weighted data rounded to the nearest individual, so categories may not add to totals]

Rank [1]	Cause of death and age (Based on Ninth Revision, International Classification of Diseases, 1975)	Number	Rate
	65 years and over		
. . .	All causes	1,699,752	5,069.0
1	Diseases of heart (390-398, 402, 404-429)	617,844	1,842.5
2	Malignant neoplasms, including neoplasms of lymphatic and hematopoietic tissues (140-208) ..	381,004	1,136.2
3	Cerebrovascular diseases (430-438)	139,134	414.9
4	Chronic obstructive pulmonary diseases and allied conditions (490-496)	90,299	269.3
5	Pneumonia and influenza (480-487)	74,995	223.7
6	Diabetes mellitus (250)	44,472	132.6
7	Accidents and adverse effects (E800-E949)	28,545	85.1
. . .	Motor vehicle accidents (E810-E825)	7,327	21.9
. . .	All other accidents and adverse effects (E800-E807, E826-E949)	21,218	63.3
8	Nephritis, nephrotic syndrome, and nephrosis (580-589)	20,325	60.6
9	Alzheimer's disease (331.0)	20,042	59.8
10	Septicemia (038)	17,035	50.8
. . .	All other causes (Residual)	266,057	793.4

[1] Rank based on number of deaths; see Technical notes.
[2] Includes deaths under 1 year of age.

NOTE: Data are subject to sampling and/or random variation. For information on the relative standard errors of the data and further discussion, see Technical notes.

51

Chapter 5

Reducing the Health and Economic Burden of Chronic Disease

The National Center for Chronic Disease Prevention and Health Promotion (NCCDPHP), part of the Centers for Disease Control and Prevention under the U.S. Department of Health and Human Services has among its goals reducing unnecessary illness and death related to chronic diseases such as heart disease, cancer, and diabetes. The Center has determined three national priorities that are essential to pursue if our nation is to reduce the tremendous health and economic burden of these diseases.

National Priorities for Chronic Disease Prevention

1. Strong chronic disease prevention programs should be in place in every state to target the leading causes of death and disability in our societyat a minimum, heart disease, cancer, and diabetes—and their principal risk factors: tobacco use, lack of physical activity, and poor nutrition.

2. CDC should provide the essential technical and scientific underpinnings to support these state-based programs, including:

   • Surveillance to identify populations at risk, to target program efforts, and to evaluate program effectiveness
   • Scientific and technical expertise

DHHS, Excerpts from *Unrealized Prevention Opportunities, Reducing the Health and Economic Burden of Chronic Disease*, December 1996.

- Public and professional education
- Quality assurance of screening
- Research and evaluation to develop and improve program elements
- Targeted efforts to identify prevention opportunities for other serious chronic diseases and conditions

3. Broad partnerships should be pursued and actively sustained with other governmental agencies, voluntary and professional organizations, academic institutions, and the private sector. Such partnerships have proven to be vital in developing model programs, policies, and guidelines; conducting useful prevention research; developing effective public and professional education; ensuring quality assurance for early detection practices; and extending program outreach to communities and individuals.

Reducing the Health and Economic Burden of Chronic Disease

As we enter the closing years of the 20th century, the profile of diseases contributing most heavily to death and illness among Americans is dramatically different than at its dawn. Today, chronic diseases—such as heart disease, cancer, and diabetes—are among the most prevalent, costly, and preventable of all health problems. Seven of every 10 Americans who die each year, or one and a half million people, die from a chronic disease. Heart disease and cancer account for almost two-thirds of all deaths.

Although older Americans are particularly at risk, chronic diseases also target men and women in the prime of life. Among men aged 50-64, chronic diseases account for the seven leading causes of death; among women in this age group, the 10 leading causes of death. Among younger men and women (aged 35-49), chronic diseases take a heavy toll. Moreover, most premature death among minority groups and the disadvantaged are due to chronic illness. These conditions account for the largest part of the health gap between black and white Americans.

A consideration of deaths alone severely understates the burden of chronic disease. The prolonged course of illness and disability from such chronic diseases as diabetes results in extended pain and suffering as well as in decreased quality of life for millions of Americans. Chronic disabling conditions cause major limitations in activity for more than one of every 10 Americans, or 25 million people.

54

Reducing the Health and Economic Burden of Chronic Disease

Almost every American family is in some way adversely affected by chronic diseases through the deaths of loved ones; through family members living with long-term illness, disability, and diminished quality of life; and, in many cases, through the enormous financial burden wrought by these diseases.

The vast number of Americans who are affected by chronic diseases and thus amass enormous health-care costs will escalate rapidly as our population ages. In 1995, 17% of the population was over 60 years of age; by 2020, the proportion will have increased to 25%. This aging of the population will greatly accelerate the growth in health-care costs.

The economic toll experienced by individuals and families as a result of these diseases is magnified greatly in the national toll. Chronic diseases now account for over 60% of the nation's total medical-care costs. Today, Medicare accounts for 12% of national spending on health care; by the year 2000, it will have increased by 50% and will account for 18% of health-care costs. The recent health debates surrounding health-care reform and the Medicare and Medicaid programs have at their roots our inability to pay the costs of chronic illness.

Our country cannot reduce its enormous health-care costs, much less its priority health problems, without addressing in a fundamentally more aggressive manner the prevention of chronic disease.

Prevention Opportunities in Chronic Disease

Chronic diseases rarely resolve spontaneously; they are not generally amenable to "cure" through medication or vaccines. Basic scientific research is being conducted to identify clinical and pharmacological measures to address these diseases. At the same time, effective measures exist today to prevent much of the chronic disease burden and to curtail its devastating consequences. Another generation of Americans need not suffer unnecessarily or die prematurely when so much is already known about how to prevent deaths from chronic disease.

These known prevention measures, the fruits of both behavioral and clinical research, are most effectively promoted and applied at the community level through the nation's public health framework. As the nation's prevention agency, CDC provides leadership to state and local health agencies to ensure that effective measures are widely implemented in communities throughout the country. CDC's role is to develop and disseminate surveillance mechanisms to identify populations at high risk for disease, and then to work with state and local health agencies in those communities to translate promising research findings into effective interventions that benefit individuals.

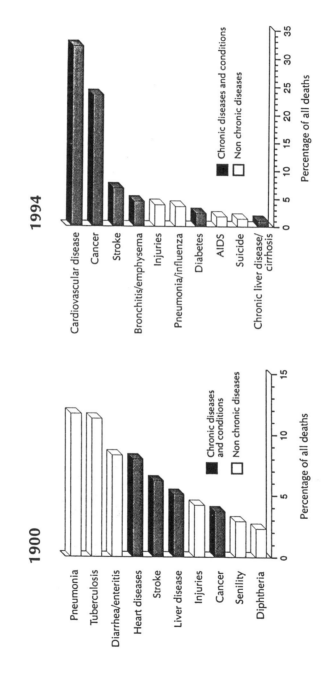

Figure 5.1. Leading Causes of Death in the United States, 1990 and 1994.

Source: Provisional data, NCHS, CDC, 1994.

Effective Framework for Prevention

The framework for efforts by CDC to prevent chronic diseases incorporates measures that have been shown to be effective and, in many cases, cost-effective in reducing the chronic disease burden. These measures include the following:

Promoting Healthy Behaviors

Several factors can increase a person's risk of chronic disease. A limited number of risk behaviors, alone or in concert, can bring inordinate suffering and early death to millions of Americans. Three such behaviorstobacco use, lack of physical activity, and poor nutritionare major contributors to heart disease and cancer, our nation's leading killers. These behaviors also exacerbate the devastating complications of diabetes and increase the risk for other serious chronic illnesses, such as chronic lung disease, arthritis, and osteoporosis.

Tobacco Use. Tobacco use is the single most preventable cause of death and disease in our society. It kills more Americans than motor vehicle crashes, AIDS, cocaine use, heroin use, homicide, and suicide combined. This one type of behavior is responsible for one of every five deaths—over 400,000 deaths each year, or 1,100 deaths every day. Each person who dies from tobacco-related lung cancer loses an average of 14 years of expected life. Those who live with such diseases as emphysema often endure prolonged suffering and disability, financial hardship, and frequent hospitalizations that have an adverse impact on the lives of family members as well.

Tobacco use costs this nation $50 billion annually, or almost $1 billion every week, in medical expenses alone, before taking into account loss of income caused by illness and premature death. Despite these staggering human and economic costs, over a quarter of adults, or 50 million Americans, continue to smoke. More than 3,000 young people aged 20 years or younger take up cigarette smoking every day. In recent years, the prevalence of smoking has been increasing among adolescents. In 1995, 33.5% of 12th graders reported smoking in the last month, a level not seen since the late 1970s.

Lack of Physical Activity and Poor Nutrition. Lack of physical activity and poor nutrition account for an estimated 300,000 deaths each year and increase an individual's risk for many chronic diseases, including heart disease, cancer, and diabetes. Twentieth-century innovations such as sedentary work environments and automobiles have removed the benefits of regular physical activity. Fully 60% of adults do not engage in adequate levels of physical activity to provide minimal health benefits. More than a third of the adults in the United States are obese; less than a quarter of the population report eating recommended amounts of fruits and vegetables.

Reducing the prevalence of these risk factors among Americans is essential to reducing the burden of chronic disease. Chronic diseases do not have to be an inevitable consequence of aging. In many cases, their origins are grounded in health-damaging behavior practiced by individuals every day for much of their lives. People who live healthfully and avoid such behaviors can expect to enjoy healthier, longer lives.

Expanding the Use of Early Detection Practices

For those chronic diseases that can be effectively treated in their early stages, screening should be considered an essential element in any American health-care system. Breast, cervical, and colorectal cancers; high blood pressure; and elevated cholesterol are among the diseases and conditions for which screening is known to save lives as well as money.

- Treatment costs for breast cancer diagnosed in the localized or in situ stage may be as much as 32% lower than treatment costs for breast cancer diagnosed in the regional or distant stages.

- One-time screening for cervical cancer among low-income elderly women can save as much as $5,907 for every 100 Papanicolaou tests performed.

In the United States, diabetes is the leading cause of new cases of blindness, the leading cause of non-traumatic lower-extremity amputations, and the leading cause of end-stage renal disease. These serious complications can be prevented or substantially curtailed through regular screening and appropriate long-term follow-up.

- An estimated 12,000 to 24,000 people become blind each year because of diabetic eye disease. Screening and treatment for eye disease among people with diabetes save the federal government at least $248 million annually. If all people with diabetes received recommended eye disease screening and follow-up, the annual savings to the federal budget could exceed $470 million.

- Over half of the 57,000 lower-extremity amputations associated with diabetes could be prevented. These preventable amputations currently cost over $285 million annually.

- At least half of the 19,000 new cases of diabetes-related kidney disease could be prevented. These preventable new cases cost over $350 million in their first year of treatment.

Providing Young People High-Quality Health Education in Schools and Community Settings

Because ingrained behaviors are difficult to change, the greatest return on investment lies in reaching individuals early, before unhealthy behaviors are adopted. This strategy is particularly important in targeting such issues as tobacco use and obesity. Fully 90% of people who become regular smokers begin smoking by age 20. Chronic illnesses often have their roots in lifelong health habits established in childhood. Because many risky behaviors begin early in life, it is crucial that intervention efforts be targeted toward young people.

Every school day, 46 million young people attend over 100,000 schools across our nation. Given the size and accessibility of this population, schools provide a unique opportunity to make an enormous, positive impact on the health of the nation. Health education programs in schools are designed to equip young people with the skills and knowledge needed to avoid unhealthy behaviors and choose healthy ones. Instructional messages are reinforced as students practice decision-making, communication, and peer-resistance skills to enable them to make positive health behavior choices and to serve as role models for others. To be most effective, these strategies should be reinforced in the community.

Such programs pay off in improved health as well as dollars. For example, planned, sequential health education has been shown to result in a 37% reduction in the onset of smoking among 7th-grade students. Moreover, for every $1 spent on school-based tobacco, drug and alcohol, and sexuality education, $14 are saved in avoided healthcare costs.

IV. Achieving Healthier Communities

An essential element in improving individual health is improving the health of communities. Collective community action is needed to create or modify community programs, policies, or practices to reduce the risk of chronic disease. Such action helps to establish a community climate that promotes and facilitates healthy living. Examples of activities include creating safe walking and cycling trails; providing low-fat/high-fruit and-vegetable menu selections in restaurants, schools, and employee cafeterias; and establishing health promotion programs (e.g., exercise and smoking cessation programs) where people work and congregate. We no longer tolerate spittoons adorning the walkways of public buildings, reusable cloth towels hanging in public restrooms, and automobiles manufactured without seat belts. Just as more healthful alternatives were developed and widely adopted to replace these unhealthy practices, so must communities address current threats to health.

Although antibiotics and vaccination programs have been considered essential tools in combating infectious diseases, analogous strategies for chronic diseases have not been fully or widely applied. Effective opportunities to prevent chronic disease exist today in a variety of settings-in communities, the work place, schools, and the clinical setting. Leadership at the national level is vital to focus and coordinate the efforts of the numerous and varied public and private partners engaged in efforts to prevent chronic disease.

CDC's Role

As the nation's prevention agency, CDC has as its mandate the prevention of unnecessary death, disease, and disability. Recognizing the tremendous burden wrought by chronic diseases in this country, CDC has long targeted chronic disease as a national priority. The agency's name was changed from the "Communicable Disease Center" to the "Center for Disease Control" in 1970 (and later to the "Centers for Disease Control and Prevention") to reflect this broader mission.

CDC's National Center for Chronic Disease Prevention and Health Promotion (NCCDPHP) works to ensure that advances in basic scientific and behavioral research are brought to bear for the benefit of individual Americans. Promising research findings are only valuable when they reach the people they are designed to benefit. It is not enough that such findings are published or that the health risks of specific behaviors are identified. Solving the research problem does not solve the health problem. The next crucial step is to ensure that these key advances are applied, reflected in state and local health policies, and widely adopted as community practices across the country. NCCDPHP's goal is to connect valuable research findings in chronic disease to real people in communities nationwide. Only then can the benefits of research make a difference in the health and lives of individual men, women, and children.

National Framework for Chronic Disease Prevention

Central to CDC's mission is providing support and assistance to states to develop comprehensive, sustainable state-based prevention programs to target the leading causes of death and disability in our society-at a minimum, heart disease, cancer, and diabetes and their principal risk factors: tobacco use, lack of physical activity, and poor nutrition. These state-based programs should target the following achievable objectives:

- Encourage healthy behaviors and reduce the prevalence of behaviors that put individuals at increased risk for chronic disease (e.g., tobacco use, lack of physical activity, and poor nutrition)

- Expand the use of prevention services, such as screening for early detection of diseases for which effective follow-up measures exist

- Provide young people with high-quality health education in schools and community settings

- Achieve healthier communities by creating opportunities and instituting policies that promote good health (e.g., providing safe walking and cycling paths; offering low-fat menu selections in restaurants, schools, and employee cafeterias; establishing health promotion programs where people work and congregate)

As such programs are established, CDC works to ensure that they are supported by elements critical for their success. These include:

- Surveillance to identify populations at risk, to target program efforts, and to evaluate program effectiveness

- Scientific and technical expertise in such areas as epidemiology and program design and evaluation

- Public and professional education

- Quality assurance of screening

- Research and evaluation to develop and improve program elements

- Targeted efforts to identify prevention opportunities for other serious chronic diseases and conditions (e.g., Alzheimer's disease, arthritis, epilepsy, iron overload, oral health conditions, and osteoporosis.)

As appropriate, CDC collaborates with both its governmental and nongovernmental partners to ensure that these elements are in place at the national level to serve as resources for state-based programs. For example, states have drawn on health communications tools developed by CDC to target tobacco use, used materials developed by CDC to educate people with diabetes on self-care, and relied on CDC for the design of surveillance systems and the analysis of surveillance data.

Underpinning all of CDC's efforts and those of the states is surveillancethe gathering of data necessary to define the disease burden, to determine the prevalence of behavioral risks, to monitor the progress of prevention efforts, and ultimately to make timely and effective public health decisions.

- Initiated in 1981 and developed in conjunction with states, CDC's state-based Behavioral Risk Factor Surveillance System (BRFSS) now enables all states to gather information on the prevalence of behavioral risk factors and other health-related measures in their individual jurisdictions. The design of the BRFSS allows for comparisons both between states and between individual states and the nation.

- Since 1990, CDC's school-based Youth Risk Behavior Surveillance System (YRBSS) has provided vital information on health-related practices among young people. This information enables states and school jurisdictions to better target prevention efforts directed toward youth.

- CDC's state-based National Program of Cancer Registries, mandated by Congress in 1992, is a fundamental tool used by states to assess the cancer burden in their jurisdictions and to make sound decisions regarding how best to allocate scarce prevention resources. This program forms the foundation for cancer control efforts at the state and local levels.

Active Partnerships are Essential

CDC plays a leadership role in coordinating and catalyzing the chronic disease prevention efforts of numerous public and private partners—other government agencies, professional organizations, voluntary organizations, academic institutions, community-based organizations, and the private sector. The expertise, experience, and outreach capabilities of these partners substantially extend CDC's effectiveness in reaching people at risk. Such partnerships enable CDC to leverage limited federal resources and thereby multiply prevention efforts.

State health departments and their local counterparts are vital links in disseminating the benefits of prevention research to individuals in communities nationwide. Within a national framework targeting chronic disease, states have primary responsibility for ensuring that needed preventive services, such as early detection, are provided; targeting public and professional education; and pursuing policies that promote good health. CDC also collaborates with newer partners—state education agencies—to implement health education in schools. State and local health and education agencies draw readily on CDC's scientific and epidemiologic expertise and experience in defining the burden of disease and risk factors, assessing the effectiveness of prevention strategies, and assisting states and communities in planning and implementing effective disease-prevention and health-promotion programs.

CDC has worked with a host of national organizations, including the Council of Chief State School Officers and the National Association of State Boards of Education, to develop model programs, policies, and guidelines to assist states in implementing high-quality health education in schools. Linkages with such organizations as the Student Coalition Against Tobacco and the National Medical Association have extended CDC's efforts to prevent tobacco use. Collaboration with voluntary organizations such as the American Cancer Society and the American Heart Association has significantly strengthened CDC's efforts in targeting cancer and health disease and their risk factors.

CDC supports 14 Prevention Research Centers at universities around the country to develop and evaluate promising prevention strategies and to assist communities in planning and evaluating their prevention efforts. These centers serve as a focal point around which various players in the health-care arena—academia, clinicians, managed-care organizations, and state and local health departments—can coalesce to target such issues as increasing physical activity among the elderly, reducing risk factors for heart disease among minorities, and facilitating breast and cervical cancer screening. By providing seed money for prevention research, these centers are able to draw the attention, expertise, and support of private foundations to help tackle priority health issues.

As new health care systems evolve, CDC is working with managed care organizations to ensure that effective prevention measures are incorporated into managed care plans. Among measures being promoted are screening for colorectal cancer, foot examinations for persons with diabetes to avert the need for amputation, and preventive counseling for such behavioral risks as tobacco use and inadequate physical activity.

Heart Disease and Stroke

Burden

- Heart disease is the nation's leading killer of both men and women and among all racial and ethnic groups.

- Heart disease is the leading cause of death among people over the age of 35.

- Heart disease and stroke cause more than 40% of all deaths in the United States, killing over 900,000 Americans each year.

- Although heart disease is commonly assumed to be a disease primarily of men, over half of all deaths caused by heart disease are in women.

- Heart disease costs this nation over $115 billion annually.

Opportunity

Three health-related behaviors—tobacco use, poor diet, and lack of physical activity—are the major risk factors for heart disease and stroke. CDC is working to reduce the prevalence of these risk behaviors through multiple intervention strategies:

- Providing national leadership and technical expertise to states for tobacco use prevention and control

- Providing leadership in the areas of nutrition and physical activity, including developing measures and recommendations for physical activity and developing a national health communications program to promote nutrition and physical activity

- Providing children with school-based health education designed to reduce the likelihood of their adopting health-damaging behaviors

- Supporting prevention research at academic institutions around the country to determine effective measures for preventing heart disease and stroke

- Administering the Preventive Health and Health Services Block Grant, an important source of funding in states for targeting heart disease and stroke

An integrated, comprehensive, and nationwide program needs to be in place to target heart disease and stroke. CDC has recently worked with the states to develop the blueprint for such a program, "Preventing Death and Disability from Cardiovascular Disease: A State-Based Plan for Action." Implementation of this plan is a crucial step in fighting the nation's leading killer.

Cancer

Burden

- In 1996, over 1,350,000 new cancer cases will be diagnosed. This estimate does not include over 800,000 cases of skin cancer that will be diagnosed.

- Cancer will kill over 550,000 people this yearmore than 1,500 people every day. One in four deaths in the United States is from this disease.

- Cancer costs this nation $104 billion annually.

Opportunity

Effective prevention measures exist to substantially reduce the number of new cancer cases each year and prevent many cancer deaths:

- Regular screening can detect cancers of the breast, cervix, colon, and rectum, among others, at an early stage when treatment is more likely to be successful. More than half of all new cases occur in these few sites. About 66% of all patients with these cancers currently survive for at least 5 years. With early detection, about 95%, or an additional 115,000 people, would survive for 5 years or more.

- About 90% of the 800,000 skin cancers that are expected in 1996 could have been prevented by protection from the sun's rays.

- All cancers caused by cigarette smoking could be prevented. Instead, 170,000 Americans will lose their lives to tobacco-related cancer this year.

- Diets high in fruits, vegetables, and fiber may reduce the incidence of some types of cancer.

Reducing the nation's cancer burden means reducing the prevalence of risk behaviors (e.g., tobacco use, poor nutrition, and sun exposure) and ensuring that screening services are available for early detection of cancers for which effective follow-up exists.

CDC's state-based National Breast and Cervical Cancer Early Detection Program provides lifesaving screening for low-income women. The program is supported by essential elements: public and provider education, quality assurance of the screening tests, and research and evaluation. In addition, CDC is assisting states in establishing or enhancing state-based cancer registries to collect information vital to program planning and evaluation and resource allocation. Early detection and critical supporting elements could also be put in place to prevent unnecessary deaths and illness from colorectal cancer and skin cancer.

CDC is working to reduce the prevalence of cancer's risk factors among Americans. Public information, especially education targeting children, is a key element of these efforts.

Diabetes

Burden

- Diabetes is the nation's seventh leading killer and is responsible for more than 169,000 deaths among Americans each year.

- Over 1,700 Americans are diagnosed with diabetes every day; 16 million Americans have the disease.

- People with diabetes risk debilitating and life-threatening complications including blindness, kidney disease, and lower-extremity amputations. People with diabetes are 2 to 4 times more likely to develop heart disease than people without the disease.

- Diabetes costs this nation more than $92 billion annually.

Opportunity

Preventing diabetes' devastating complications is not only possible; in many cases, prevention measures are cost-effective as well:

- An estimated 12,000 to 24,000 people become blind each year because of diabetic eye disease. Screening and treatment for eye disease among persons with diabetes save the federal government at least $248 million annually. If all persons with diabetes received recommended eye disease screening and follow-up, the annual savings to the federal budget could exceed $470 million.

- Over half of the 57,000 lower-extremity amputations associated with diabetes could be prevented. These amputations cost over $285 million annually.

- At least half of the 19,000 new cases of diabetes-related kidney disease could be prevented. These preventable new cases cost over $350 million in their first year of treatment.

With limited funding, CDC anticipates working with all states in FY 1997 to establish the framework for effective prevention measures:

- Improving access to care and routine screening for populations at high risk

- Ensuring high quality and consistent standards in diabetes care

- Educating people with diabetes on self-care

- Conducting state-based surveillance to better target program efforts.

Targeting the Actual Causes of Death

Though 7 of every 10 deaths among Americans are due to chronic disease, the actual underlying causes of death are often risk factors that could have been prevented. A relatively few modifiable risk behaviors, alone or in concert, bring inordinate suffering and early death to millions of Americans. Three such behaviors—tobacco use, poor nutrition, and lack of physical activity—are major contributors to heart disease and cancer, our nation's leading killers. These behaviors also exacerbate the devastating complications of diabetes and increase the risk for other serious chronic illnesses such as chronic lung disease, arthritis, and osteoporosis.

- Tobacco use is the single most preventable cause of death and disease in our society. This one behavior kills more Americans than motor vehicle crashes, AIDS, cocaine use, heroin use, homicide, and suicide combined. Tobacco use is responsible for one of every five deaths, or over 400,000 deaths each year—1,100 deaths every day. People who die of tobacco-related lung cancer die on average 14 years prematurely. Those who live with diseases such as emphysema often endure prolonged suffering and disability and frequent hospitalizations, hardships that affect the lives of their family members as well.

  Tobacco use costs this nation $50 billion annually, or roughly $1 billion every week, in medical expenses alone, before taking into account loss of income caused by illness and premature death. Despite these staggering human and economic costs, over one quarter of adults, or 50 million Americans, continue to smoke. Tragically, over 3,000 young people under the age of 20 take up cigarette smoking every day. In recent years, the prevalence of smoking has been increasing among adolescents. In 1995, 33.5% of 12th graders reported smoking in the last month, a level not seen since the late 1970s.

• Unhealthy diet and lack of physical activity account for at least 300,000 deaths each year and increase an individual's risk for many chronic diseases, including heart disease, cancer, and diabetes. More than a third of the nation's adults are obese; less than a quarter of the population report eating recommended amounts of fruits and vegetables. Twentieth-century innovations such as sedentary work environments and automobiles rob many individuals of the benefits of regular physical activity. Fully 60% of adults do not engage in adequate levels of physical activity to provide minimal health benefits.

Reducing the prevalence of these risk factors among Americans is essential to reducing the chronic disease burden. Chronic diseases do not have to be an inevitable consequence of aging. In many cases, their origins are grounded in health-damaging behaviors practiced by people every day for much of their lives. People who live healthfully and avoid such behaviors can expect to enjoy healthier, longer lives.

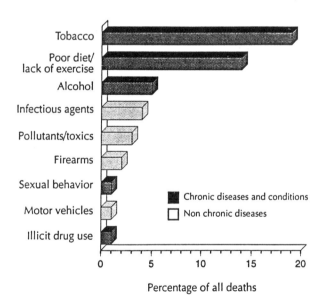

Source: McGinnis JM, Foege WH. Actual causes of death in the United States. JAMA 1992; 270:2207–12.

Figure 5.2. *Actual Causes of Death, United States, 1990.*

Figure 5.3. Leading Causes of Death Among Men and Women Aged 35-64 Years, United States, 1992.

Rank	MEN 35–49 years	MEN 50–64 years	WOMEN 35–49 years	WOMEN 50–64 years
1	Heart disease 77.4	Heart disease 396.9	Heart disease 24.9	Heart disease 155.4
2	AIDS/HIV 56.6	Lung cancer 158.2	Breast cancer 21.2	Lung cancer 81.8
3	Other unintentional injury 24.2	Cerebrovascular disease 41.9	Lung cancer 10.7	Breast cancer 64.9
4	Suicide 23.2	Chronic lung disease 37.3	Motor vehicle accident 8.4	Cerebrovascular disease 32.3
5	Motor vehicle accident 20.1	Colorectal cancer 36.6	Cerebrovascular disease 8.3	Chronic lung disease 26.0
6	Lung cancer 17.2	Chronic liver disease 35.7	Suicide 6.8	Diabetes mellitus 24.9
7	Chronic liver disease 16.8	Diabetes mellitus 28.5	AIDS/HIV 6.8	Colorectal cancer 24.8
8	Homicide 15.9	Other unintentional injury 24.6	Other unintentional injury 5.5	Ovarian cancer 18.7
9	Cerebrovascular disease 10.0	Suicide 23.4	Chronic liver disease 5.5	Chronic liver disease 14.2
10	Diabetes mellitus 7.0	AIDS/HIV 21.4	Diabetes mellitus 4.6	Pancreatic cancer 12.7

All age-adjusted death rates are per 100,000 people, standardized to the 1970 population of the United States.
Note: Dark shading denotes chronic diseases and conditions.
Source: Vital Statistics Mortality Data, National Center for Health Statistics, CDC.

Figure 5.4. Leading Causes of Death Among Men and Women 65 Years
Old and Older, United States, 1992.

Rank	MEN 65–79 years	MEN 80+ years	WOMEN 65–79 years	WOMEN 80+ years
1	Heart disease 1,422.4	Heart disease 5,056.7	Heart disease 749.5	Heart disease 3,963.1
2	Lung cancer 451.3	Cerebrovascular disease 1,030.3	Lung cancer 196.5	Cerebrovascular disease 1,010.2
3	Chronic lung disease 243.0	Pneumonia & influenza 808.2	Cerebrovascular disease 163.2	Pneumonia & influenza 521.1
4	Cerebrovascular disease 210.0	Chronic lung disease 674.1	Chronic lung disease 134.0	Chronic lung disease 267.1
5	Prostate cancer 158.8	Prostate cancer 606.1	Breast cancer 114.1	Atherosclerosis 249.2
6	Colorectal cancer 127.8	Lung cancer *563.9	Diabetes mellitus 83.9	Colorectal cancer 216.2
7	Pneumonia & influenza 107.0	Atherosclerosis 341.1	Colorectal cancer 81.0	Diabetes mellitus 197.1
8	Diabetes mellitus 91.1	Colorectal cancer 304.1	Pneumonia & influenza 57.4	Lung cancer 182.8
9	Atherosclerosis 89.5	Diabetes mellitus 216.5	Pancreatic cancer 43.1	Breast cancer 170.5
10	Urinary tract cancer 59.9	Nephritisis & nephrosis 198.1	Ovarian cancer 41.6	Other unintentional injury 126.4

All age-adjusted death rates are per 100,000 people, standardized to the 1970 population of the United States.
Note: Dark shading denotes chronic diseases and conditions.
Source: Vital Statistics Mortality Data, National Center for Health Statistics, CDC.

Figure 5.5. Death Rates* for Major Chronic Diseases Among White and Minority Groups, by Underlying Cause of Death, United States, 1990.

Disease/Condition	White American	African American	American Indian/ Alaska Native	Asian/ Pacific Islander	Hispanic American[†]
Heart disease	177.4	180.7	104.0	93.7	181.2
Stroke	48.5	76.0	33.3	45.8	47.4
Chronic obstructive pulmonary disease	32.6	24.8	21.5	15.8	22.6
Diabetes	15.9	35.7	30.3	12.4	28.3
Cirrhosis	9.4	14.5	21.2	4.7	19.0
Lung cancer	54.0	67.5	27.9	26.8	35.6
Colorectal cancer	20.6	26.6	10.1	12.6	18.2
Breast cancer	16.3	19.5	6.6	6.5	13.9
Cervical cancer	1.1	1.8	0.7	0.5	0.9
Prostate cancer	10.7	23.5	5.8	6.0	10.2
Total	**386.5**	**470.6**	**261.4**	**224.8**	**377.3**

* Age-adjusted to the 1980 U.S. standard population; rate per 100,000 persons
[†] Persons of Hispanic origin may be of any race.
Source: CDC, NCHS, National Vital Statistics Systems, 1990

Other Serious Chronic Diseases

- Alzheimer's disease is a progressive, degenerative disease that attacks the brain and results in impaired memory, thinking, and behavior. More than 3 million Americans suffer from this disease; this number is expected to more than double by 2030. This disease and related dementias are now the leading cause of long-term care needs. In 1992, costs for Alzheimer's disease exceeded $80 billion, of which the federal government bore $27 billion.

- Arthritis is a chronic and disabling condition that affected an estimated 40 million Americans in 1995; nearly 50% of individuals aged 65 and older have arthritis. Arthritis limits the activities of over 7 million people and is second only to heart disease as a cause of work disability. In 1992, direct medical costs were estimated at $15.2 billion, and total costs were estimated to be $64.8 billion.

- Chronic obstructive lung disease is nonreversible lung disease characterized by airflow impairment or obstruction, often diagnosed as emphysema or chronic bronchitis. Tobacco use is a heavy contributor to these often disabling conditions.

- Epilepsy is a chronic neurological condition affecting 2.5 million Americans. Each year, about 100,000 people are diagnosed with epilepsy, more than two-thirds of them younger than age 25.

- Iron overload, a disorder affecting 1.5 million Americans, can cause inflammation and damage to multiple body organs. Such damage can result in arthritis, cirrhosis, diabetes, impotence, heart failure, and sometimes death as vital organs fail. Iron overload is among the conditions for which screening and appropriate follow-up are indicated; screening costs $30-$100 per person compared with $50,000-$250,000 per person in medical costs for chronic disease resulting from organ failure.

- Oral health conditions will cost more than $60 billion dollars annually by the year 2000. Many oral diseases that consume large amounts of health care resources are preventable; these include dental caries, oral cancer, and periodontal disease. More than 100 million Americans lack the proven benefits provided by fluoridated water in preventing dental caries. Reducing the prevalence of tobacco use could prevent many of the 30,000 new cases of oral cancer and the 8,000 deaths that occur each year.

- Osteoporosis is a disabling condition resulting in more than 1.3 million fractures each year. Death is a common occurrence in the months immediately following hip fracture. Of individuals functionally independent and living at home at the time of the hip fracture, 15%-25% will require long-term institutional care, and 25%-35% will return home but need help with activities of daily living. In 1986, the cost of osteoporosis-related fractures was $7-$10 billion.

Opportunities to Target Other Serious Chronic Diseases

A better understanding of how some of these diseases—Alzheimer's disease, arthritis, epilepsy, iron overload, and osteoporosis—are distributed in the population and what their associated behavioral, genetic, and environmental risk factors are is greatly needed. CDC has efforts ongoing in each of these areas.

For diseases such as chronic obstructive lung disease and oral health conditions including oral cancer, certain environmental factors (e.g., lack of fluoridated water and exposure to environmental tobacco smoke) and individual behaviors clearly place one at higher risk. CDC is an active player in tobacco prevention and control efforts to combat chronic obstructive lung disease, oral cancers, and a host of other diseases and conditions.

Improving the Health of Young People: An Investment in Our Nation's Future

Burden

A limited number of behaviors contribute markedly to the leading causes of death, disease, and social problems, often including a lifetime of underachievement, in our nation. These behaviors, most often established during youth, include drug, alcohol, and tobacco use; poor nutrition; violence; sexual behaviors; lack of physical activity; and failure to use seat belts.

- Of U.S. high school students, 53% are sexually active; each year, 1 million teenagers become pregnant, and 3 million are infected with a sexually transmitted disease.

- More than 3,000 young people begin smoking each day.

- Every day, 135,000 students bring guns to school; homicide is the second leading cause of death among 15-24 year olds.

- Motor vehicle crashes account for 31% of deaths among young people aged 1-24, yet only 33% always wear seat belts.

- Only 66% of high school students report engaging in vigorous physical activity three times a week. Diets that are high in fat and contain few fruits and vegetables are the norm among many high school seniors.

Opportunity

Promoting healthy behaviors among youth and a healthful environment is an investment in our nation's future. Working with state and local health and education agencies and professional and voluntary organizations nationwide, CDC is assisting states in providing health education in schools. Such education goes beyond instruction, providing young people with opportunities to learn and practice peer-resistance and decision-making skills and thus to make positive health behavior choices.

CDC is exploring additional opportunities to promote healthy behaviors among young people, including:

- Developing and targeting health promotion programs to underserved youth

- Expanding efforts of national youth-based organizations (e.g., Boys' and Girls' Clubs of America and community and church youth groups)

- Conducting vigorous health marketing in collaboration with centers of influence for young people (e.g., athletic teams; the entertainment, clothing, and cosmetic industries; and the video market)

The Heavy Burden of Chronic Disease Among Women

To improve the health of women in the United States is in large measure to address the burden of chronic disease. The leading causes of death among women aged 65 and older include heart disease and stroke, cancer, and diabetes. These diseases do not restrict themselves to older women. Among women aged 35-64, heart disease, lung cancer, and breast cancer are the top three causes of death. Chronic health conditions such as osteoporosis, arthritis, urinary incontinence, and Alzheimer's disease are also important health issues for women.

- Although heart disease and stroke are commonly believed to primarily affect men, over half of deaths from heart disease and stroke occur in women. About 360,000 women die each year from these diseases.

- An estimated 62,000 women die each year from lung cancer, which has surpassed breast cancer as the leading cause of cancer death among women. The lung cancer death rate among women has increased by more than 400% over the last 30 years and continues to increase.

- During the 1990s, 2 million American women will be diagnosed with breast or cervical cancer, and one-half million will die from these diseases.

- Tobacco use has been shown to increase the risk of cancer, heart, and respiratory diseases and reproductive disorders among women. More than 140,000 women die each year from smoking-related illness. Even so, 22 million adult women (23% of American women) and at least 1.5 million adolescent girls currently smoke.

- More than 3.5 million women in the United States have been diagnosed with diabetes. Diabetes is the leading cause of new cases of adult blindness, end-stage kidney disease, and lower-extremity amputations. In addition, the risk for heart disease is from two to four times greater among people with diabetes than among people without diabetes.

- Osteoporosis affects 25% of women and is eight times more common in women than men. Of individuals functionally independent and living at home at the time of the hip fracture, 15%-25% will require long-term institutional care, and 25%-35% will return home but need help with the activities of daily living.

Chapter 6

Leading Causes of Death by Age, Sex, Race, and Hispanic Origin in the United States

Introduction

In recent years data users have requested leading cause-of-death data in more detailed age and race and ethnic categories than is usually available in National Center for Health Statistics (NCHS) publications. This report presents 1992 data on leading causes of death by race, sex, and Hispanic origin using three age aggregations. The report includes detailed tables illustrating the effect the different age aggregations have on the ranking of individual causes and discusses issues concerning the use of alternative age aggregations. The report also describes the cause-of-death ranking procedure used by NCHS, other agencies of the Public Health Service, and many State public health agencies.

NCHS has been publishing leading cause-of-death data since 1960 when tabulations ranking causes of death for the white and nonwhite populations and the male and female populations of the United States were introduced. In 1977 broad age categories were added to tabulations for these groups, and in 1989 NCHS began showing age, race, and sex in the same table. Although alternative groupings of the population according to race, ethnic origin, or any of a number of other demographic variables will also affect the identification and ranking of particular causes, the focus of this report is on the effect of different age aggregations.

PHS Publication No. 96-1857, June 1996.

Table 6.1. Deaths and Death Rates for the 10 Leading Causes of Death, United States, 1992.

Rank[1]	Cause of death, race, sex, and age (Ninth Revision International Classification of Diseases, 1975)		Number	Rate
. .	All causes		2,175,613	852.9
1	Diseases of heart 390–398,402,404–429		717,706	281.4
2	Malignant neoplasms, including neoplasms of lymphatic and hematopoietic tissues 140–208		520,578	204.1
3	Cerebrovascular diseases 430–438		143,769	56.4
4	Chronic obstructive pulmonary diseases and allied conditions 490–496		91,938	36.0
5	Accidents and adverse effects E800–E949		86,777	34.0
. .	Motor vehicle accidents E810–E825		40,982	16.1
. .	All other accidents and adverse effects E800–E807,E826–E949		45,795	18.0
6	Pneumonia and influenza 480–487		75,719	29.7
7	Diabetes mellitus 250		50,067	19.6
8	Human immunodeficiency virus infection *042–*044		33,566	13.2
9	Suicide E950–E959		30,484	12.0
10	Homicide and legal intervention E960–E978		25,488	10.0
. .	All other causes . . . . Residual		399,521	156.6

[1]Rank based on number of deaths.

78

NCHS publishes leading cause-of-death data annually in several publications including *Vital Statistics of the United States, Mortality, Volume II, Part A; The Advance Report of Final Mortality Statistics, Monthly Vital Statistics Report (MVSR); Annual Summary of Births, Marriages, Divorces, and Deaths (MVSR);* and *Health United States.* Rankings are typically presented for the 10 or 15 leading causes of death (Table 6.1.). Leading cause-of-death data also appear frequently in publications of many State and Federal public health agencies.

Ranking Procedures

In the 1950's, a working group made up of State and Federal representatives recommended that, to improve comparability, the various reporting agencies identifying diseases of public health importance adopt a uniform ranking procedure. This group developed the standardized procedures for ranking leading causes of death now in use by NCHS.

Causes are ranked according to the number of deaths (not rates) assigned to the 37 rankable causes from the List of 72 Selected Causes of Death, together with the category HIV infection (Human immunodeficiency virus infection, ICD-9 Nos. *042-*044). HIV infection was introduced by NCHS in 1987 data tabulations and added to the list of rankable causes. Categories on the List of 72 Selected Causes of Death excluded from ranking include the group titles Major cardiovascular diseases; Symptoms, signs, and ill-defined conditions; and category titles that begin with the words "Other" and "All Other." When a title representing a subtotal is ranked (such as tuberculosis), its component parts are not ranked (tuberculosis of the respiratory system and other tuberculosis).

NCHS introduced a separate ranking procedure for infant causes based on the number of deaths assigned to the List of 61 Selected Causes of Infant Death beginning with the 1980 data year. HIV infection was also added to this list beginning with 1987 data. NCHS publishes leading causes of neonatal and post-neonatal deaths annually. Because the data are readily available, data for infants are not presented in this report.

Mortality tabulation lists used by NCHS can be found in the NCHS Instruction Manual, Part 9 and subsequently published notices of change. Descriptions of the tabulation lists can also be found in the Technical Appendix of Vital Statistics of the United States, Volume 11, Mortality.

Effects of Age Aggregation on Ranking

The rank a cause of death receives varies according to the number of variables and the level of detail used to classify the population of interest. As with sex, race, and ethnic classifications, the age aggregation used influences both the identification of causes of death as public health problems and the relative importance of these causes once identified. For example, Chronic obstructive pulmonary disease (COPD) is not among the 10 leading causes of death for the 45 49-year-old age group but is the fifth leading cause of death for the 45-64-year-old group and the ninth leading cause of death for the 45-54-year-old group. Although each of these statements is true, each results in a different understanding of the relative importance of COPD as a public health problem. These differences can have important program implications.

The three age aggregations most widely used in NCHS presentations of general mortality data are aggregations in 5-year age groups starting with ages 5-9 and continuing through ages 80-84, with a final group 85 years and over; aggregations in 10-year age groups starting with ages 5-14 continuing through ages 75-84, with a final group 85 years and over; and aggregations in broad age groupings (1-4 years, 5-14 years, 15-24 years, 25-44 years, 45-64 years, and 65 years and over). These age categories reflect both convention and international requirements. NCHS currently uses the broadest age categories. The mortality statistics presented in this report were compiled in accordance with the World Health Organization (WHO) regulations, which specify that member nations classify causes of death by the current Manual of the International Statistical Classification of Diseases, Injuries, and Causes of Death.

Effects of Alternative Age Aggregations

Tables 6.2 and 6.3 illustrate the effect of different age aggregations on the rankings of heart disease (Diseases of heart, ICD Nos. 390-398.402,404-429) and HIV infection (Nos. *042-*044).

Heart disease was the leading cause of death for U.S. residents (all ages) in 1992. It was among the leading 10 causes in all age groups regardless of the age aggregation used. Its importance as a leading cause increases with increasing age. Using 5-year age aggregations, heart disease was the fifth or sixth leading cause of death beginning with the age group 1-4 years through the age group 25-29 yearswhen its relative importance begins to increase. It is the second leading cause by ages 40-44 years and remains at that rank through ages 65-69 years, when it becomes the leading cause of death.

Although variations in rank occur among the three age aggregations, the rankings in the broadest age grouping reflect the pattern in the more detailed 5- and 10-year age groupings. However, in the broad age grouping, the change in rank at middle age lags behind that of the more detailed groupings. Heart disease increases in importance beginning at ages 35-39 years as shown in the 5-year age groups rather than at ages 45-64 as shown in the broad age grouping. Heart disease assumes its relative importance as the leading cause at age 65 using the broadest age aggregation, at age 75 using the 10-year age aggregation, and at age 70 using the 5-year age aggregation.

In contrast to heart disease, the level of age detail used has a greater effect on the ranking of HIV infection. There are more differences and larger discrepancies in rank among the three age aggregations. HIV infection was the eighth leading cause of death in 1992 but the leading cause for 35-39-yearold age group using the 5-year age aggregation. HIV infection was never ranked first using the 10-year and the broad age aggregations but did rank second for 25-34 and 3544year-old age groups and for the 25-44-year-old age group using the 10-year and broad age aggregations. The ranking of eighth for the broad age group 45-64 years seriously understates the importance of HIV infection for the 45-49-year-old and 50-54-year-old age groups. At these ages, it ranked fourth and sixth, respectively. Although greater discrepancies in rank occurred among the different age aggregations for HIV infection than for heart disease, the 10-year and broad aggregations do reflect the ages at which HIV infection is an important cause of death.

Differences in the relative importance of the leading causes of death among different race, ethnic, and sex groups are apparent for all ages combined. Heart disease and cancer (Malignant neoplasms) are the first and second leading causes of death for the total population. Stroke (Cerebrovascular diseases), accidents, pneumonia and influenza, and diabetes are among the 10 leading causes for each group, although the ranking differs from group to group. COPD, HIV infection, and suicide are among the 10 leading causes of death for some but not all groups. Chronic liver disease and cirrhosis is not among the leading causes for the total population but is among the 10 leading causes for the Hispanic and white populations.

Certain conditions originating in the perinatal period and the puerperium is on the leading cause lists only for the Hispanic and black populations. Nephritis, nephrotic syndrome, and nephrosis; septicemia;

81

and atherosclerosis appear among the 10 leading causes only for the female population. Differences in the relative importance of the leading causes of death among different race, ethnic, and sex groups become more apparent when more detailed age aggregations are used. Cancer is the third leading cause of death for 25-44-year-olds; the fourth leading cause for males but the leading cause for females; the second leading cause for the white population, the fifth leading cause for the black population, and the fourth leading cause for the Hispanic population; and it is the fifth leading cause for white and black males and the sixth leading cause for Hispanic males 25-44 years of age.

Increased age detail provides a more accurate picture of critical age differences among these groups for different causes of death: heart disease first becomes the leading cause of death for white males 44-64 years of age and for black and Hispanic males 45-49 years of age; but it does not become the leading cause of death for black females until 65-69 years of age, for Hispanic females until 70-74 years of age, or for white females until 75-79 years of age. Compare this with the broad age groups in which heart disease becomes the leading cause for white males at 45-64 years of age and for white females at 65 years and over.

Table 6.2. *Ranking of Diseases of Heart by Alternative Age Groupings: United States 1992.*

Age	5-year age group	10-year age group	Broad age groups
All ages	1	1	1
1–4 years	5	5	5
5–9 years	5	...	...
10–14 years	6	6	6
15–19 years	5	...	...
20–24 years	5	5	5
25–29 years	6	...	...
30–34 years	6	6	...
35–39 years	4	...	4
40–44 years	2	3	...
45–49 years	2	...	...
50–54 years	2	2	2
55–59 years	2	2	...
60–64 years	2	...	...
65–69 years	2	2	...
70–74 years	1	...	1
75–79 years	1	1	...
80–84 years	1	...	...
85 years and over	1	1	...

Table 6.3. *Ranking of Human Immunodeficiency Virus Infection by Alternative Age Groupings: United States 1992.*

Age	5-year age group	10-year age group	Broad age groups
All ages	8	8	8
1–4 years	7	7	7
5–9 years	6 ⎱	7	7
10–14 years	⎰	. . .	. . .
15–19 years	10 ⎱	. . .	. . .
20–24 years	6 ⎰	6	6
25–29 years	3 ⎱	. . .	. . .
30–34 years	2 ⎰	2 ⎱	2
35–39 years	1 ⎱	2 ⎰	. . .
40–44 years	3 ⎰	. . .	. . .
45–49 years	4 ⎱	4 ⎱	. . .
50–54 years	6 ⎰	. . .	8
55–59 years	10	. . .	. . .
60–64 years	. . .	. . . ⎰	. . .
65–69 years	. . .	. . .	. . .
70–74 years	. . .	. . .	. . .
75–79 years	. . .	. . .	. . .
80–84 years	. . .	. . .	. . .
85 years and over	. . .	. . .	. . .

Chapter 7

Advance Report of Final Mortality Statistics

Abstract

Objectives

This report presents 1994 data on U.S. deaths and death rates according to such demographic and medical characteristics as age, sex, race, Hispanic origin, marital status, educational attainment, State of residence, autopsy status, and cause of death. Trends and patterns in general mortality, life expectancy, and infant and maternal mortality are also described.

Methods

Descriptive tabulations of data reported on the death certificates of 2,278,994 deaths are presented. Changes between 1993 and 1994 in numbers of deaths and death rates and differences in death rates across demographic groups in 1994 are tested for statistical significance. A decomposition procedure is used to identify causes of death accounting for changes in age-specific death rates and life expectancy.

Results

The age-adjusted death rate for the total population in 1994 decreased, and life expectancy at birth increased by 0.2 years to 75.7

DHHS Publication No. (PHS) 96-1120, September 1996.

years. The improvement in life expectancy was primarily due to a decrease in mortality from heart disease, cancer, pneumonia and influenza, and homicide, although offsetting the positive improvements were increases in mortality from Human immunodeficiency virus (HIV) infection and diabetes. The list of the 15 leading causes of death was the same as in the previous year, but the rank of some causes changed. Thus, Chronic liver disease and cirrhosis replaced homicide as the 10th leading cause of death, and Alzheimer's disease moved past atherosderosis as the 14th leading cause. Mortality declined for those under 15 years of age and those at ages 55 years and older but increased for those aged 35-44 years; causes of death contributing to this increase were HIV infection and viral hepatitis. Mortality declined for each of the major race and sex groups. Infant mortality rate declined by 4.8 percent to a record low of 8.0 infant deaths per 1,000 live births in 1994. Neonatal and postneonatal mortality rates also declined for white and black infants. The causes contributing the most to the improvement in the overall infant mortality were sudden infant death syndrome and respiratory distress syndrome.

Conclusions

The overall improvements in general mortality and life expectancy suggest a resumption of the long-term downward trend in U.S. mortality, which was briefly interrupted in 1993 by an increase in mortality associated with the influenza epidemics. The decline in U.S. infant mortality continues the steady downward trend of the past four decades.

Highlights

In 1994 a record 2,278,994 deaths were registered in the United States, 10,441 more than the previous high of 2,268,553 deaths recorded in 1993. The crude death rate for 1994 was 875.4 deaths per 100,000 population, slightly lower than the 1993 rate of 880.0. The age-adjusted death rate, which eliminates the distorting effects of the aging of the population, was 507.4 per 100,000 U.S. standard million population, 1.1 percent lower than the 1993 rate of 513.3, and 0.6percent higher than the record low of 504.5 in 1992.

The overall decline in mortality between 1993 and 1994 represents a resumption of the long-term downward mortality trend, which was interrupted by a substantial increase in mortality associated with the influenza epidemics of 1992-93. The age-adjusted rate decreased between

86

1993 and 1994 for all four major race and sex groups: White males, white females, black males, and black females.

By age death rates decreased substantially for those under 15 years of age and those at ages 55 years and older. The death rate increased by 1.4 percent between 1993 and 1994 for those aged 35-44 years. The causes of death contributing most to the increase in the death rate for those aged 35-44 years were HIV infection and viral hepatitis.

In 1994 life expectancy at birth was 75.7 years, an increase of 0.2 years compared with life expectancy in 1993, but slightly lower than the record high of 75.8 years in 1992. Women currently are expected to outlive men by an average of 6.6 years, and white persons are ex-pected to outlive black persons by an average of 7.0 years. Among the four major race-sex groups, white females continue to have the high-est life expectancy at birth (79.6 years), followed by black females (73.9 years), white males (73.3 years), and black males (64.9 years). The gain in life expectancy of 0.2 years for the total population can be explained primarily by decreasing death rates for heart disease, can-cer, pneumonia and influenza, and homicide, despite increases in death rates for HIV infection and diabetes.

The ranking of the leading causes of death for the total popula-tion in 1994 changed as follows: Chronic liver disease and cirrhosis, the 11th leading cause of death in 1993, replaced homicide as the 10th leading cause of death in 1994. Alzheimer's disease replaced athero-sclerosis as the 14th leading cause of death in 1994. However, the first nine leading causes of death in 1994-heart disease, cancer, stroke, Chronic obstructive pulmonary diseases and allied conditions (COPD), accidents, pneumonia and influenza, diabetes, HIV infection, and suicide-remained the same leading causes as those in 1993 with iden-tical rankings. These nine causes accounted for 80 percent of all deaths in 1994.

Age-adjusted death rates for eight of the leading causes of death for the total population declined between 1993 and 1994, with larg-est percentage declines occurring for nephritis, atherosclerosis, pneu-monia and influenza, homicide, and heart disease. Mortality for all other accidents, a component of the overall accidents category, de-clined by 1.4 percent between 1993 and 1994. In addition, mortality from cancer, the second leading cause of death, showed a small but significant decrease.

Age-adjusted death rates increased between 1993 and 1994 for three leading causes of death: HIV infection, diabetes, and Alzheimer's disease. The age-adjusted death rate for HIV infection increased by 11.6 percent between 1993 and 1994, higher than the rate of increase in the previous year. The age-adjusted death rate also increased by 8.7percent for Alzheimer's disease and by 4 percent for diabetes. The increase in Alzheimer's disease mortality likely reflects improvements in reporting and diagnosis of the disease rather than increases in prevalence.

Mortality from drug-induced and alcohol-induced causes increased significantly between 1993 and 1994. However, the age-adjusted death rate for firearm injuries decreased by 3 percent between 1993 and 1994.

In terms of mortality sex differentials, the age-adjusted death rate for males was 70 percent higher than that for females for all causes of death combined. For each of the 15 leading causes of death, except Alzheimer's disease, male mortality was higher than female mortality. The greatest sex differential was for HIV infection, where the age-adjusted rate for males was 5.5 times that for females. The smallest sex differential was for Alzheimer's disease, with a male-to-female ratio of about 1.0.

In 1994 mortality levels varied by race. Overall, age-adjusted death rates for the black population exceeded those of the white population by about 61 percent. Rates for the black population were also higher for most of the leading causes of death. The largest race differential continued to be for homicide, for which the age-adjusted rate for the black population was 6.6 times that of the white population. The three leading causes that had lower mortality rates for the black population were COPD, suicide, and Alzheimer's disease.

Leading causes of death differed by age. Overall, accidents were the leading cause of death for age groups 1-4, 5-14, and 15-24 years. HIV infection was the leading cause of death for those aged 25-44 years. Cancer was the leading cause of death for those aged 45-64 years, while heart disease was the leading cause for those aged 65 years and older. The leading cause of death was the same for the white and black populations for all age groups except 15-24 years and 25-44 years. For the white population, accidents were the leading cause for these two age groups. For the black population, homicide was the leading cause for those aged 15-24 years, while HIV infection was the leading cause for those aged 25-44 years.

The infant mortality rate (8.0 infant deaths per 1,000 live births) reached a record low in 1994, continuing the long-term downward trend in infant mortality.

Among the leading causes of infant death, the causes contributing the most to the improvement in the 1994 rate were sudden infant death syndrome and respiratory distress syndrome. Sudden infant death syndrome decreased from the second to the third leading cause of infant death between 1993 and 1994. Increased infant mortality from perinatal infections, pneumonia and influenza, and neonatal hemorrhage prevented the infant mortality rate from decreasing even further. Infant, neonatal, and postneonatal mortality rates declined for white and black infants between 1993 and 1994. In 1994 the infant mortality rate for black infants remained at more than twice that for white infants.

Introduction

This report, the release of national mortality statistics for 1994, presents detailed data on deaths and death rates according to a number of social, demographic, and medical characteristics. These data provide important information on mortality patterns among Americans by such variables as age, sex, race, Hispanic origin, marital status, educational attainment, State of residence, autopsy status, and cause of death. Information on these mortality patterns is critical in understanding shifts in the health and social status of the U.S. population.

The mortality data in this report can be used to monitor and evaluate the current status and long-term trends in mortality and in the health of the Nation and to identify segments of the U.S. population at greatest risk for death from specific diseases and injuries. Differences in death rates among demographic groups, including racial/ethnic groups, may reflect group differences in factors such as socioeconomic status, access to medical care, and the prevalence of specific risks.

Results and Discussion: Deaths and Death Rates

In 1994 a total of 2,278,994 deaths occurred in the United States, 10,441 more than in 1993 and 103,381 more than in 1992. Before 1994 the 1993 total of 2,268,553 deaths was the largest final number ever recorded. Although the number of deaths increased between 1993 and 1994, the crude death rate for 1994, 875.4 per 100,000 population, was 0.5 percent lower than the rate of 880.0 in 1993. In 1992 the death rate was 852.9.

Age-adjusted death rates are constructs that show what the level of mortality would be if no changes occurred in the age composition of the population from year to year. Thus, they are better indicators than unadjusted death rates for showing changes in the risk of death over a period of time when the age distribution of the population is changing. Also, they are better indicators of relative risk when comparisons of mortality are being made for sex or race subgroups of the population that have different age compositions. The age-adjusted death rate in 1994 was 507.4 deaths per 100,000 U.S. standard million population, 1.1 percent lower than the rate of 513.3 in 1993 and 12.1 percent lower than the rate of 577.0 in 1979. The 1994 rate was, however, slightly higher than the record low rate of 504.5 in 1992. Since 1979, the age-adjusted death rate has decreased every year except 1985, 1988, and 1993, years when major influenza outbreaks increased mortality in the United States.

Death Rates by Age, Sex, and Race

Between 1993 and 1994, death rates for both sexes combined declined for these age groups: Under 1 year, 1-4 years, 5-14 years, 55-64 years, 65-74 years, 75-84 years, and 85 years and over. The largest decrease (4.2 percent) occurred for the age group 1-4 years. The death rate increased for the age group 35-44 years (1.4 percent). Changes in death rates between the two years for the age groups 15-24 years, 25-34 years, and 45-54 years were not statistically significant.

The death rate for males declined between 1993 and 1994 for these age groups: Under 1 year, 1-4 years, 55-64 years, 65-74 years, 75-84 years, and 85 years and over. The largest decreases for males were for those aged under 1 year (4.9 percent) and 1-4 years (4.4 percent). The only statistically significant increase in the male death rate was for those aged 35-44 years (1.3 percent). The increase in death rates between 1993 and 1994 for males aged 35-44 years continued the increase begun between 1983 and 1984, a reversal of the downward trend for this age group since the late 1960's.

For females age-specific rates have generally been decreasing since 1950. Between 1993 and 1994, death rates declined for these age groups: Under 1 year, 5-14 years, 55-64 years, 75-84 years, and 85 years and over. The largest decrease in death rates between 1993 and 1994 occurred for females 5-14 years (6.3 percent). The only significant increase was for the age groups 35-44 years (1.7 percent). Changes in female death rates between the two years for the other age groups were not statistically significant.

The pattern of changes in age-specific death rates between 1993 and 1994 was similar for the four major race-sex groups: Death rates generally decreased for the age groups under 1 and 1-4 years and for those aged 55 years and older. For black males aged 5-14 years, however, the death rate increased by 4.2 percent. In addition, for white males and black females aged 35-44 years, the death rate increased by 1.5 and 3.2 percent, respectively.

Between 1993 and 1994, age-adjusted death rates decreased by 1.5 percent for white males and 2.1 percent for black males. The age-adjusted death rate decreased by 0.8 percent for white females and 1.2 percent for black females. Age-adjusted death rates decreased almost every year between 1980 and 1992 for white males and females but increased between 1992 and 1993. The 1994 age-adjusted rate of 617.9 was the lowest ever recorded for white males. For black males, rates decreased between 1980 and 1982, increased between 1984 and 1988, decreased between 1988 and 1992, and increased again between 1992 and 1993. Rates for black females fluctuated between 1980 and 1987, decreased each year between 1988 and 1992, and increased between 1992 and 1993.

In 1994 the age-adjusted death rate for males of all races was 1.7 times that for females. In 1950 the male-to-female ratio was 1.5. The 1970 ratio (1.7) increased to 1.8 during the late 1970's until 1987 when the ratio again declined to 1.7. For 1994 the ratio between male and female age-adjusted death rates was 1.7 for the white population and 1.8 for the black population.

In 1994 the age-adjusted death rate for the black population was 1.6 times that for the white population, the same ratio that has prevailed since 1987. For 1960-86 the race ratio was 1.5

Expectation of Life at Birth and at Specified Ages

In 1994 the average expectation of life at birth was 75.7 years, an increase of 0.2 years compared with life expectancy in 1993, but slightly lower than the record high of 75.8 years in 1992. The increase between 1993 and 1994 represents a resumption of a generally upward trend in U.S. life expectancy that has been observed throughout this century but, most recently, was interrupted by a 0.3-year decline between 1992 and 1993.

The expectation of life at birth for 1994 represents the average number of years that a group of infants would live if the infants were to experience throughout life the age-specific death rates prevailing in 1994. In 1994 life expectancy for females was 79.0 years compared with 72.4 years for males; both figures represent increases over 1993. The difference in life expectancy between the sexes was 6.6 years in 1994, the same difference as in 1993. In contrast to the widening gap from 1900 to 1972 (2.0 years in 1900, 5.5 years in 1950, and 6.5 years in 1960), the difference in life expectancy between the sexes narrowed between 1979 and 1988 (7.7 and 7.8 years throughout the period from 1972 through 1979, 7.1 years in 1984, and 6.9 years in 1988) and between 1990 and 1993.

Between 1993 and 1994, life expectancy for the white population increased from 76.3 years to 76.5 years, equaling the record high reached in 1992. Life expectancy for the black population also increased from 69.2 years in 1993 to 69.5 years in 1994; in 1992 it was 69.6 years.

The difference in life expectancy between the white and black populations was 7.0 years in 1994, slightly lower than the difference of 7.1 years in 1993. Although the white-black difference in life expectancy narrowed from 7.6 years in 1970 to 5.7 years in 1982, it increased to 7.1 years in 1989 before declining to 7.0 years in 1990 and 1991, and 6.9 years in 1992.

Among the four race-sex groups, white females continued to have the highest life expectancy at birth (79.6 years), followed by black females (73.9 years), white males (73.3 years), and black males (64.9 years). Between 1993 and 1994, life expectancy increased for black males (from 64.6 years in 1993 to 64.9 years in 1994) and for black females (from 73.7 in 1993 to 73.9 in 1994). Black males experienced an unprecedented decline in life expectancy every year for 1984-89 (3), but an annual increase in 1990, 1991, 1992, and 1994.

However, life expectancy for black males was still 0.4 years shorter than the peak life expectancy of 65.3 years attained in 1984. Before 1988 life expectancy for black females fluctuated but increased from 1988 to 1992. Overall, the largest gain in life expectancy between 1980 and 1994 was for white males (2.6 years), followed by white females (1.5 years), black females (1.4 years), and black males (1.1 years).

The 1994 life table may be used to compare life expectancies at any age from birth onward. For example, a person who has reached age 65 years may look forward to living to an older age, on the average, than one who has reached 50 years. On the basis of mortality experienced in 1994, a person aged 50 years could expect to live an average of 29.3 more years for a total of 79.3 years, and a person aged 65 years could expect to live an average of 17.4 more years for a total of 82.4 years).

Leading Causes of Death

The 15 leading causes of death in 1994 accounted for 86 percent of all deaths in the United States (Figure 7.1.). For the first time, beginning with this report, Alzheimer's disease is being treated as a rankable cause of death. The leading causes of death for 1984-94 have generally been the same, but the order has often varied. For 1994 the 1st nine and the 12th and 13th leading causes of death were the same causes and in the same order as for 1993. The only changes in the ranking were as follows: Chronic liver disease and cirrhosis, the 11th leading cause of death in 1993, became the 10th leading cause of death in 1994; Homicide and legal intervention (homicide), the 10th leading cause of death in 1993, became the 11th leading cause of death in 1994. Alzheimer's disease became the 14th leading cause of death in 1994; Atherosclerosis, the 14th leading cause of death in 1993, became the 15th leading cause of death in 1994.

For most leading causes, age-adjusted death rates are better indicators than crude death rates for showing changes in mortality risk over time. Therefore, age-adjusted rates are used to depict trends for all 15 leading causes of death. Among these causes, age-adjusted death rates were lower in 1994 than in 1993 for eight leading causes—Diseases of heart (heart disease); Malignant neoplasms, including neoplasms of lymphatic and hematopoietic tissues (cancer); Chronic obstructive pulmonary diseases and allied conditions (COPD); Pneumonia and influenza; homicide; Nephritis, nephrotic syndrome, and nephrosis (nephritis); Septicemia; and atherosclerosis (Table 7.1.) The largest declines in mortality were for nephritis (4.4 percent), atherosclerosis (4.2 percent), pneumonia and influenza (3.7 percent), homicide (3.7 percent), and heart disease (3.4 percent). Mortality from all other accidents and adverse effects, a component of accidents and adverse effects (accidents), declined by 1.4 percent between 1993 and 1994. The declines in mortality from heart disease, stroke, and atherosclerosis were consistent with the generally downward trends observed since 1950. Cancer mortality has shown a gradual but consistently downward trend since 1990. The age-adjusted death rate for homicide decreased by 3.7percent between 1993 and 1994, reversing the increase during 1992 through 1993, and resuming the downward trend observed during 1991-92.

For 1987-91 homicide mortality had risen at an average rate of more than 6 percent per year. Although the age-adjusted death rate for pneumonia and influenza decreased significantly in 1994 from that in 1993 (a year with excess influenza mortality), the rate for 1994 remained at a relatively high level—2.4 percent higher than the rate for 1992.

The age-adjusted death rate was higher in 1994 than in 1993 for three of the leading causes of death: Diabetes mellitus (diabetes), Human immunodeficiency virus (HIV) infection, and Alzheimer's disease. The age-adjusted rate for HIV infection has increased consistently since 1987, the year in which HIV infection was added to the list of rankable causes. Between 1993 and 1994, the rate for HIV infection increased by 11.6 percent, larger than the rate of increase of

93

Table 7.1. Percent of Total Deaths, Death Rates, Age-adjusted Death Rates for 1994; Percent Change in Age-adjusted Death Rates from 1993 to 1994 and 1979 to 1994, and Ratio of Age-adjusted Death Rates by Race and Sex for the 15 Leading Causes of Death for the Total Population in 1994: United States.

Rank[1]	Cause of death (Based on the Ninth Revision, International Classification of Diseases, 1975)	Percent of total deaths	Death rate	Age-adjusted death rates for 1994	Percent change from— 1993 to 1994	1979 to 1994	Ratio of— Male to Female	Black to White
...	All causes	100.0	875.4	507.4	-1.1	-12.1	1.7	1.6
1	Diseases of heart	32.1	281.3	140.4	-3.4	-29.6	1.9	1.5
2	Malignant neoplasms, including neoplasms of lymphatic and hematopoietic tissues	23.4	205.2	131.5	-0.8	0.5	1.4	1.4
3	Cerebrovascular diseases	6.7	58.9	26.5	–	-36.3	1.2	1.9
4	Chronic obstructive pulmonary diseases and allied conditions	4.5	39.0	21.0	-1.9	43.8	1.6	0.8
5	Accidents and adverse effects	4.0	35.1	30.3	–	-29.4	2.6	1.3
...	Motor vehicle accidents	1.9	16.3	16.1	0.6	-30.6	2.3	1.0
...	All other accidents and adverse effects	2.1	18.8	14.2	-1.4	-27.6	2.9	1.6
6	Pneumonia and influenza	3.6	31.3	13.0	-3.7	16.1	1.6	1.4
7	Diabetes mellitus	2.5	21.8	12.9	4.0	31.6	1.1	2.4
8	Human immunodeficiency virus infection	1.8	16.2	15.4	11.6	- - -	5.5	4.4
9	Suicide	1.4	12.0	11.2	-0.9	-4.3	4.5	0.6
10	Chronic liver disease and cirrhosis	1.1	9.8	7.9	–	-34.2	2.4	1.4
11	Homicide and legal intervention	1.1	9.6	10.3	-3.7	1.0	4.1	6.6
12	Nephritis, nephrotic syndrome, and nephrosis	1.0	8.8	4.3	-4.4	–	1.4	2.7
13	Septicemia	0.9	7.8	4.0	-2.4	73.9	1.3	2.6
14	Alzheimer's disease	0.8	7.1	2.5	8.7	1,150.0	1.0	0.7
15	Atherosclerosis	0.8	6.6	2.3	-4.2	-59.6	1.3	1.1
...	All other causes	14.3	124.9	...	...	...	...	...

... Category not applicable.
– Quantity zero.
– – Data not available.
[1]Rank based on number of deaths; see "Technical notes."

9.5 percent between 1992 and 1993. Diabetes mortality has been increasing consistently since 1986. The increase of 4.0 percent in the age-adjusted death rate for diabetes between 1993 and 1994 was similar to that for 1992-93, and larger than the rate of increase during 1990 through 1992. It was considerably smaller than the anomalous 14-percent increase during 1988-89, which has been attributed in part to the 1989 revision of the death certificate.

Between 1993 and 1994, the age-adjusted death rate for Alzheimer's disease increased by 8.7 percent. Reporting of Alzheimer's disease deaths has increased since the classification of this disease was introduced in 1979. The increase in Alzheimer's disease mortality likely reflects improvements in reporting and diagnosis of the disease rather than increases in prevalence. For three leading causes of death, including Cerebrovascular diseases (stroke), Chronic liver disease and cirrhosis, and accidents, age-adjusted death rates did not change between 1993 and 1994.

In 1994 the leading causes of death differed substantially by age. For the younger age groups—1-4,5-14, and 15-24 years—accidents were the leading cause of death. HIV infection was the leading cause of death for the age group 25-44 years. In the older age groups, chronic diseases were the leading causes: Cancer, for those aged 45-64 years, and heart disease, for those aged 65 years and over. At ages below 25 years, homicide ranked between the second and fourth leading cause of death, while for the age groups 5-14, 15-24, and 2504 years, suicide ranked between the third and sixth leading cause of death.

In 1994 the patterns in leading causes of death varied by sex. For the total male and female populations, 7 of the 10 leading causes of death were the same but differed by rank. While accidents was the third leading cause of death for males, it was the seventh leading cause for females. Similarly, while diabetes was the ninth leading cause of death for males, it was the sixth leading cause for females. Moreover, while HIV infection, suicide, and homicide were respectively the 7th, 8th, and 10th leading causes of death for males, they did not rank among the ten leading causes of death for females. The sex patterns in leading causes of death also differed according to age. Not only did the relative rankings of the leading causes of death vary by sex for a given age group, but the causes of death representing the list of top 10 causes also differed. For example, for the age group 25-44 years, HIV infection was the leading cause of death for males but was the fourth leading cause of death for females. Furthermore, while stroke was the 10th leading cause of death for males aged 15-24 years, it was not among the 10 leading causes of death for females aged 15-24 years.

In 1994 the patterns in leading causes of death also varied according to race. Within broad age groups for the white and black populations, the leading cause was the same except for the age groups 15-24 and 25-44 years. For the age group 15-24 years, the leading cause for the white population was accidents, while the leading cause for the black population was homicide. For the age group 25-44 years, the leading cause for the white population again was accidents, while the leading cause for the black population was HIV infection. For the age groups 15-24 through 65 years and over, accidents ranked higher for the white population than for the black population; while homicide and HIV infection consistently ranked higher for the black population than for the white population for all age groups under 65 years.

Age-adjusted death rates for males were higher than the rates for females for all causes of death combined and for 14 of the 15 leading causes of death (Table 7.1). Eight of the leading causes of death showed differentials in which age-adjusted death rates for males were at least 1.5 times those for females. The largest differential was for HIV infection, for which the death rate for males was 5.5 times that for females. Other large differentials were for suicide (4.5); homicide (4.1); accidents (2.6); chronic liver disease and cirrhosis (2.4); heart disease (1.9); COPD (1.6); pneumonia and influenza (1.6); nephritis (1.4); and cancer (1.4). The smallest sex difference in mortality was for Alzheimer's disease, with a male-to-female ratio of 1.04.

Mortality was higher for the black population than for the white population for most of the leading causes of death for the total population. The largest differential was for homicide, for which the age-adjusted death rate for the black population was 6.6 times that of the white population. Other causes for which the differential was large include HIV infection (4.4); nephritis (2.7); septicemia (2.6); diabetes (2.4); stroke (1.9); heart disease (1.5); cancer (1.4); and chronic liver disease and cirrhosis (1.4). Age-adjusted rates were lower for the black population than rates for the white population for three leading causes of death—COPD (18 percent), suicide (40 percent), and Alzheimer's disease (31 percent).

Causes of death can be identified that account for changes in age-specific death rates between 1993 and 1994. Thus, the 4.2-percent decrease in the death rate for those aged 1-4 years was due primarily to declines in mortality from congenital anomalies and accidents. The 3.8-percent decrease in the death rate for those aged 5-14 years was due mainly to declines in mortality from homicide, pneumonia and influenza, and COPD. Increases in mortality from HIV infection and viral hepatitis were largely responsible for a 1.4-percent increase in the death rate for those aged 35-44 years. Decreases in death rates for those in the age groups 55-64, 65-74, 75-84, and 85 years and over were due primarily to decreases in mortality from heart disease. The increase in the death rate for white males aged 35-44 years between 1993 and 1994 was due largely to an increased mortality from HIV infection and viral hepatitis. The 4.1-percent decrease in the death rate for black males aged 15-24 years was due primarily to decreases in mortality from homicide and accidents. Increases in mortality from HIV infection and stroke were largely responsible for the 3.2-percent increase in the death rate for black females aged 35-44 years.

The overall life expectancy improved from 75.5 years in 1993 to 75.7 years in 1994. despite increases in mortality from HIV infection, diabetes, and Alzheimer's disease, primarily because of decreases in mortality from heart disease, cancer, pneumonia and influenza, homicide, and perinatal conditions. Among white males, life expectancy improved by 0.2 year between 1993 and 1994 because of decreases in mortality from heart disease, cancer, COPD, pneumonia, and congenital anomalies although mortality from diabetes, viral hepatitis, suicide, and Alzheimer's disease increased. For white females, the improvement in life expectancy also reflected decreases in mortality from heart disease, pneumonia, and homicide, but was limited to a gain of 0.1 year because of increases in mortality from HIV infection, diabetes, Alzheimer's disease, accidents, and COPD. For black males, decreases in mortality from heart disease, homicide, cancer, and accidents contributed to the 0.3-year gain in life expectancy. This gain occurred despite offsetting increases in mortality from HIV infection, diabetes, stroke, hypertension, and viral hepatitis. The life expectancy for black females improved by 0.2 year, in part, because of declines in mortality from heart disease, cancer, and homicide.

Life expectancy for white males was 8.4 years higher than that for black males in 1994. Specific causes of death with much lower mortality for white males influenced this difference. The causes of death contributing the most to this difference were homicide, HIV infection, heart disease, cancer, and perinatal conditions. The life expectancy for white females was 5.7 years higher than that for black females in 1994. The causes of death contributing the most to this difference were heart disease, cancer, HIV infection, stroke, and diabetes.

Hispanic Mortality

Hispanic mortality data for 1994 are based on deaths to residents of 49 States and the District of Columbia. The crude, age-specific, and age-adjusted death rates for the Hispanic population can be compared

97

with those for the non-Hispanic white population. The crude death rate for the Hispanic population was 64 percent lower than that for the non-Hispanic white population. This difference reflects the lower age-specific mortality for the older age groups and the younger age composition of the Hispanic population compared with that of the non-Hispanic white population. The age-adjusted death rate, which controls for age-compositional differences, was 20 percent lower for the Hispanic population than for the non-Hispanic white population. The ratio of the age-adjusted death rate for the Hispanic population to that for non-Hispanic white population was 0.84 for males and 0.73 for females. Mortality of Hispanics may be somewhat understated because of net underreporting of Hispanic origin on the death certificate.

Within the Hispanic population, the age-adjusted death rate for males was 1.9 times that for females. The male-to-female ratio differed substantially by age, with Hispanic males experiencing three to four times higher death rates than Hispanic females for ages 15-44 years. The sex ratio in Hispanic mortality ranged between 1.2 and 1.6 for ages below 15 years and between 1.4 and 2.2 for ages 45 years and older.

Among specified subgroups of the Hispanic population, the age-adjusted death rate was substantially lower for Cuban Americans (358.1 deaths per 100,000 U.S. standard million population), Mexican Americans (370.4), and Central and South Americans and other and unknown Hispanics (354.0) than the age-adjusted death rate for Puerto Ricans (565.8). Among Hispanic males, Mexicans had the lowest age-adjusted death rate, while Puerto Ricans had the highest rate. Among Hispanic females, Cubans had the lowest age-adjusted death rate, while Puerto Ricans had the highest rate.

Leading causes of death for all age groups combined for the Hispanic population differed by rank and cause from those for the non-Hispanic white population in the Hispanic reporting area. Although the two leading causes of death-heart disease and cancer-were the same for both groups, they accounted for 57 percent of all deaths in 1994 for the non-Hispanic white population but for only 42 percent of the deaths for the Hispanic population.

These were the major differences in leading causes of death between the two groups: Of the 10 leading causes of death for the Hispanic population, homicide (sixth leading cause) was not among the 10 leading causes for the non-Hispanic white population. Conversely, suicide, the eighth leading cause of death for the non-Hispanic white population, was not among the 10 leading causes for the Hispanic population.

Differences in the ranking of the leading causes of death between the two population groups largely reflect differences in age composition between the two groups; that is, the Hispanic population has a greater proportion of young persons, and, accordingly, a larger proportion of deaths due to causes that are more prevalent at younger ages. Within broad age groups, leading causes were more similar between the two population groups. However, even within age categories some differences exist. Homicide and HIV infection consistently ranked higher for the Hispanic population than for the non-Hispanic white population for all age groups between 1-4 years and 45-64 years. Chronic liver disease and cirrhosis also ranked higher for the Hispanic population than for the non-Hispanic white population for those aged 45-64 years and 65 years and over.

Firearm Mortality

In 1994 a total of 38,505 persons died from firearm injuries in the United States. This number was 2.8 percent lower than the 39,595 deaths in 1993. Firearm suicide and homicide, the two major component causes, accounted for 49 and 46 percent, respectively, of all firearm injury deaths in 1994.

Of the 38,505 firearm injury deaths in 1994, 58.2 percent were for white males, 25.7 percent for black males, 10.4 percent for white females, and 3.5 percent for black females. The largest numbers of firearm deaths for males and females were for the age groups 15-24 and 25-34 years. Although the numbers of deaths were highest for white males, the age-adjusted and age-specific death rates for firearm injuries were generally highest for black males, followed by white males, black females, and white females.

In 1994 the age-adjusted death rate for firearm injuries was 15.1 deaths per 100,000 U.S. standard million population, 3 percent lower than the rate of 15.6 in 1993. The rate decreased by 14.2 percent between 1980 and 1985, increased every year between 1987 and 1991, but decreased again by 2 percent between 1991 and 1992. The 1993 age-adjusted death rate for firearm injuries was, however, 5 percent higher than the 1992 rate.

Between 1993 and 1994 the age-adjusted death rate for firearm injuries decreased by 5 percent for black males, 9 percent for black females, and 8 percent for white females; the rate did not decrease significantly for white males. In 1994 the rate for males was 6.2 times that for females, and the rate for the black population was 3.0 times that of the white population.

Between 1993 and 1994 the age-adjusted death rate decreased by 4 percent for firearm homicide and 14 percent for firearm accidents.

The rate did not decrease significantly for firearm suicide between the two years, however. In 1994 the age-specific death rates for firearm homicide were highest for the age groups 15-24 and 25-34 years, while the rates for firearm suicide peaked for those aged 75-84 years and 85 years and older.

Drug-induced Mortality

In 1994 a total of 13,923 persons died of drug-induced causes in the United States. The category drug-induced causes includes not only deaths from dependent and nondependent use of drugs (legal and illegal use), but also poisoning from medically prescribed and other drugs. It excludes accidents, homicides, and other causes indirectly related to drug use. The age-adjusted death rate for drug-induced causes in 1994 was 5.0 deaths per 100,000 U.S. standard million population, 4 percent higher than the rate of 4.8 in 1993. The rate increased by 35 percent from 1983 to 1988, then declined 14 percent between 1988 and 1990, and increased by 39 percent between 1990 and 1994. In 1994 the age-adjusted death rate for drug-induced causes for males was 2.3 times the rate for females, and the rate for the black population was 1.8 times that for the white population.

Alcohol-induced Mortality

In 1994 a total of 20,163 persons died of alcohol-induced causes in the United States. The category alcohol-induced causes includes not only deaths from dependent and nondependent use of alcohol, but also accidental poisoning by alcohol. It excludes accidents, homicides, and other causes indirectly related to alcohol use. The age-adjusted death rate for alcohol-induced causes in 1994 was 6.8 deaths per 100,000 U.S. standard million population, 1.5 percent higher than the rate of 6.7 in 1993. The rate decreased by 20 percent from 1980 to 1986, increased by 9 percent from 1986 to 1989, and then decreased by 7 percent from 1989 to 1991; since 1991 it has shown very little change. In 1994 the age-adjusted death rate for alcohol-induced causes for males was 3.5 times the rate for females, and the rate for the black population was 2.0 times the rate for the white population.

Marital Status

Eighty-nine percent of the persons 15 years of age and over who died in 1994 had been married. The proportion was larger for females

(92 percent) than for males (86 percent) and for the white population (90 percent) than for the black population (79 percent). The proportion who were widowed at the time of death was considerably greater for women (58 percent) than for men (18 percent) but fairly similar for both major race groups—38 percent of the white population and 33 percent of the black population. Some of the differences between groups can be accounted for by differences in age composition.

Educational Attainment

In an area comprised of 45 States and the District of Columbia, about 63 percent of the persons who died in 1994 had completed high school. In 1994 the percent was about the same for males (63 percent) and females (62 percent), but somewhat different for the white population (64 percent) compared with the black population (52 percent). About the same proportion of white females and white males (65 percent) who died in 1994 had completed high school. The proportion who had completed 4 years of college was smaller for white females (9.6 percent) than for white males (14.2 percent). A similar proportion of black females and black males had completed high school (about 52 percent). Slightly more black females (6.6 percent) than black males (5.8 percent) had completed 4 years of college at the time of death.

Infant Mortality

In 1994, 31,710 infant deaths were reported, 5.2 percent fewer infant deaths than the 1993 total of 33,466. The infant mortality rate of 8.0 infant deaths per 1,000 live births is the lowest final rate ever recorded for the United States. It represents a decline of 4.8 percent from the rate of 8.4 for the previous year. The mortality rate for white infants declined 2.9 percent (6.8 in 1993 compared with 6.6 in 1994); and the rate for black infants declined 4.2 percent (16.5 in 1993 compared with 15.8 in 1994).

In 1994 the infant mortality rate for black infants (15.8) was 2.4 times the rate for white infants (6.6), the same ratio as in the previous year. Historically, the black-white ratio has been increasing.

Between 1993 and 1994 the neonatal mortality rate declined by 3.8 percent, from 5.3 to 5.1 deaths for infants under 28 days per 1,000 live births. For white infants, the rate was 4.2, compared with the 1993 rate of 4.3; the change in the neonatal mortality rate between the two years was not statistically significant. For black infants the neonatal mortality rate declined by 4.7 percent, from 10.7 in 1993 to

10.2 in 1994. Neonatal mortality rates historically have declined for both races although the declines have been more rapid for the white population.

The postneonatal mortality rate—deaths to infants 28 days-11 months per 1,000 live births—declined by 6.5percent, from 3.1 in 1993 to 2.9 in 1994. For white infants the postneonatal mortality rate declined from 2.5 to 2.4 deaths per 1,000 live births. For black infants the rate was 5.6 in 1994, compared with 5.8 in 1993; the change in the postneonatal mortality rate between the two years was not statistically significant. The historical trend for postneonatal mortality was of more rapid declines in postneonatal mortality for black than for white infants.

Among the 10 leading causes of infant death, the first four—Congenital anomalies, Disorders relating to short gestation and unspecified low birthweight, and Respiratory distress syndrome—accounted for just over half (53 percent) of all infant deaths in 1994; and the remaining 6 causes accounted for only 16 percent of all infant deaths. The list of 10 leading causes of infant death was unchanged between 1993 and 1994 but the rankings of two of the leading causes of infant death changed slightly. Sudden infant death syndrome, the second leading cause in 1993, and Disorders relating to short gestation and unspecified low birthweight, the third leading cause, switched rankings in 1994.

Between 1993 and 1994 the infant mortality rate decreased for three leading causes of infant death: Respiratory distress syndrome (12.8 percent), Sudden infant death syndrome (11.7 percent), and Disorders relating to short gestation and unspecified low birthweight (0.1 percent). Infant mortality from Respiratory distress syndrome showed a rapid downward trend between 1972 and 1994. Mortality from Sudden infant death syndrome has declined since 1988. Infant mortality from Respiratory distress syndrome showed a rapid downward trend between 1972 and 1994. Mortality from Sudden infant death syndrome has declined 26.5 percent since 1988, from a rate of 140.1 to 103.0 in 1994, and between 1993 and 1994 dropped from the second leading cause of infant death to the third. For other leading causes of infant death, the infant mortality rate did not change significantly between 1993 and 1994. The causes contributing the most to the improvement in the overall infant mortality rate were Respiratory distress syndrome and Sudden infant death syndrome. The increasing rate for Infections specific to the perinatal period (perinatal infections) was the principal cause preventing the infant mortality rate from decreasing more than it did.

Differences between infant mortality rates for white and black infants by cause are reflected in differences in ranking of the leading causes of infant death as well as in differences in cause-specific infant mortality rates. Congenital anomalies was the leading cause of death for white infants, followed by Sudden infant death syndrome, Disorders relating to short gestation and unspecified low birthweight, and Respiratory distress syndrome. Combined these four causes accounted for 54.4percent of white infant deaths. In contrast, for black infants the leading cause of death was Disorders relating to short gestation and unspecified low birthweight, followed by Sudden infant death syndrome, Congenital anomalies, and Respiratory distress syndrome. These four causes accounted for 50 percent of all black infant deaths.

Although the difference between black and white infant mortality rates varied by cause, the risk was higher for black than for white infants for all the leading causes. Expressed as the ratio of the infant mortality rate for black infants to that for white infants, beginning with the highest ratio, the leading causes ranked are Disorders relating to short gestation and unspecified low birthweight; Pneumonia and influenza and Newborn affected by maternal complications of pregnancy (maternal complications) (2.7 each); Respiratory distress syndrome (2.6); perinatal infections (2.5); Sudden infant death syndrome and Newborn affected by complications of placenta, cord, and membranes (2.3 each); accidents and Intrauterine hypoxia and birth asphyxia (2.2 each); and Congenital anomalies (1.8).

Between 1993 and 1994 decreases in mortality from Sudden infant death syndrome, congenital anomalies, Respiratory distress syndrome, Other respiratory conditions of newborn, and maternal complications made the largest contributions to the 3.7 percent decrease in the white infant mortality rate. However, the white infant mortality rate would have decreased even further had it not been for increases in mortality from perinatal infections, Neonatal hemorrhage, and Pneumonia and influenza. Decreases in mortality from Sudden infant death syndrome, Respiratory distress syndrome, and Congenital anomalies made the largest contributions to the 4.2-percent decrease in the black infant mortality rate; further decrease was, however, offset by increases in mortality from short gestation and low birthweight, accidents, and Pneumonia and influenza.

Hispanic Infant Mortality

The infant mortality rate was 6.5 deaths to Hispanic infants under 1 year of age per 1,000 live births in an area comprised of 49 States and the District of Columbia. This was the same as the rate for non-Hispanic white infants. Among specified subgroups of the Hispanic population, the mortality rate for Mexican infants was 6.6 infant deaths per 1,000 live births, 8.7 for Puerto Rican infants, and 4.5 for Cuban infants. Infant mortality rates by specified Hispanic origin and race for non-Hispanic origin may be somewhat understated.

Maternal Mortality

In 1994, 328 women were reported to have died of maternal causes, compared with 302 in 1993. As in previous years, the number does not include all deaths occurring to pregnant women, but only to those deaths assigned to Complications of pregnancy, childbirth, and the puerperium (ICD 9 Nos. 630-676). The maternal mortality rate for 1994 was 8.3 deaths per 100,000 live births, compared with a rate of 7.5 in 1993. The difference in the rates between the two years was not statistically significant.

Black women have a higher risk of maternal death than white women. In 1994 the maternal mortality rate for black women was 18.5, three times the rate of 6.2 for white women. The race ratio in maternal mortality rate was 3.0 for Direct obstetric causes.

Report of Autopsy

For 1994 all States requested information on the death certificate as to whether autopsies were performed. They were reported as performed on 213,879 decedents, or 9.4 percent of the deaths that occurred in 1994, a reduction from the 9.7 percent reported for the previous year. This continues the downward trend in the percent of deaths autopsied. The percent autopsied for all causes of death combined was heavily influenced by the low rates for the three leading causes of deathheart disease (6.6 percent), cancer (2.3 percent), and stroke (2.9 percent). Among the 15 leading causes of death, the highest percents reported were for traumatic causeshomicide (97.2 percent), suicide (55.1 percent), and accidents (48.4 percent). The highest percents for non-traumatic causes were for chronic liver disease and cirrhosis (13.4percent) and Alzheimer's disease (7.1 percent).

Chapter 8

Trends in Hospital Utilization, United States

Introduction

The National Hospital Discharge Survey (NHDS) has been conducted annually since 1965. Hospital utilization statistics from the NHDS are routinely published by the National Center for Health Statistics for individual years. Because almost 30 years of data are available, there is much demand for NHDS data on trends in hospital use. Some trend data have been included in previous NHDS reports. In addition, a detailed description of trends in hospital utilization from 1965 through 1986 was presented in a previous report. The purpose of this report is to present general statistics from 1988 through 1992 on hospital utilization by patient characteristics, geographic region, and selected diagnoses and procedures.

The period beginning with 1988 was chosen for this report because that was the first year a new design was used for the NHDS. Estimates based on this new design could differ from those based on the 1965-87 design due to changes in the survey rather than actual changes in hospital utilization. Because 1988-92 data are all from the same survey design, trends for this period are not affected by design effects.

However, many users of NHDS data are interested in a longer perspective on hospital use than can be seen in 5 years of data. For historical information, estimates for 1980 and 1985 are included in most

DHHS Publication No. (PHS) 96-1785, June 1996.

of the tables in this report. Because hospital use trends during the first half of the 1980's were discussed in depth in an earlier report, they will not be discussed again here.

Data from the National Hospital Discharge Survey are used to examine a wide array of health issues. Topics such as morbidity from cerebrovascular disease, the frequency of vaginal births after previous cesarean section delivery (VBAC), and hospital use for cardiovascular disease have been studied using NHDS data. Trend analyses of NHDS data on HIV, hysterectomy, diabetes, and obstetrical procedures have been published. NHDS data are used to track objectives related to the 22 priority areas targeted in Healthy People 2000, including objectives on unintentional injuries, environmental health, maternal and infant health, diabetes and chronically disabling conditions, and sexually transmitted diseases.

Highlights

- The rate of discharges did not change significantly between 1988 and 1992, but the rate of days of care declined 10 percent.

- The average length of stay declined 6 percent for both males and females from 1988 to 1992.

- Deliveries, heart disease, and malignant neoplasms were common reasons for hospitalization and represented approximately 30 percent of first-listed diagnoses in 1988 and 1992.

- Each year from 1988 to 1992, episiotomy, aneriography and angiocardiography using contrast material, computerized axial tomography (CAT scan), diagnostic ultrasound, and fetal EKG and other fetal monitoring were each performed over 1 million times on hospital inpatients.

- In 1992, 61 percent of male newborn infants were circumcised before they were discharged from the hospital; the proportion circumcised ranged from 38 percent in the West to 78 percent in the Midwest.

- The rate for removal of coronary artery obstruction increased 57 percent for males and 96 percent for female discharges from 1988 to 1992.

- Males accounted for 67 percent of four heart-related procedures (open heart surgeries, removal of coronary obstruction, coronary artery bypass graft, and cardiac catheterizations) performed in 1988, and 65 percent in 1992.

Hospital Utilization

The focus of the report is hospital utilization from 1988 to 1992 as measured by data from the National Hospital Discharge Survey. Estimates of hospital use in 1980 and 1985 are included in the tables to provide a broader historical perspective.

A previous report on trends in hospital utilization discussed the dramatic rise of hospital discharges and days of care in the 1970's and their decline in the 1980's due to major influences from technology, an aging population, and health care policy. One of the strongest influences on hospital use in the late 1980's and 1990's was the growth of outpatient surgery. Patients who previously would have been hospitalized were undergoing surgery and returning home the same day. According to the American Hospital Association (AHA), the rise in outpatient surgery was facilitated by the development of new technologies, such as endoscopic techniques, and new anesthetic drugs that allow patients to wake up more quickly after surgery, as well as changes in reimbursement policy that promote outpatient surgery.

Outpatient or ambulatory surgeries are performed in free-standing or hospital-based ambulatory surgery centers. In 1988, 1.7 million surgical procedures were performed in approximately 980 free-standing ambulatory surgical centers (FASC's) in the United States. In 1993, this number had grown to 3.2 million surgical procedures performed in approximately 1,860 FASC's. However, the majority of outpatient surgeries occur in hospitals. Ambulatory surgeries in these hospitals increased from 10.6 million in 1988 to 12.8 million in 1992 for AHA-registered hospitals. Outpatient surgeries done in either hospitals or free-standing surgical centers are not included in the NHDS nor in this report because only hospital inpatients are within the scope of the survey. Additional information about the use of ambulatory surgery centers is being gathered in the National Survey of Ambulatory Surgery begun in 1994 by the National Center for Health Statistics.

In addition to the growth of ambulatory surgery, the aging of the U.S. population continues to influence inpatient hospital use. The median age of the civilian population was 30.1 years of age in 1980,

Table 8.1. Number and Percent Distribution of Newborn Infants Discharged from Short-stay Hospitals by Length of Stay and Average Length of Stay by Health Status: United States, 1980, 1985 and 1988-92.

Length of stay or health status	1980	1985	1988	1989	1990	1991	1992
				Number in thousands			
All newborn infants	3,824	3,794	3,733	3,884	3,869	3,880	3,689
Less than 1 day	69	84	72	89	79	81	73
1 day	270	428	531	596	693	779	873
2 days	842	1,057	1,436	1,601	1,624	1,612	1,506
3 days	1,175	1,034	704	649	636	658	632
4 days	618	528	502	485	447	385	284
5–7 days	633	497	329	298	232	198	161
8 days or more	218	167	159	166	157	167	160
				Percent distribution			
All newborn infants	100.0	100.0	100.0	100.0	100.0	100.0	100.0
Less than 1 day	1.8	2.2	1.9	2.3	2.0	2.1	2.0
1 day	7.1	11.3	14.2	15.3	17.9	20.1	23.7
2 days	22.0	27.9	38.5	41.2	42.0	41.5	40.8
3 days	30.7	27.3	18.9	16.7	16.4	17.0	17.1
4 days	16.2	13.9	13.4	12.5	11.6	9.9	7.7
5–7 days	16.6	13.1	8.8	7.7	6.0	5.1	4.4
8 days or more	5.7	4.4	4.3	4.3	4.1	4.3	4.3
				Average length of stay in days			
All newborn infants	4.3	3.8	3.5	3.4	3.3	3.2	3.1
Well[1]	3.2	2.8	2.5	2.4	2.3	2.3	2.0
Sick[2]	7.1	5.7	4.9	4.8	4.8	4.6	4.7

[1]Without any illness or risk-related diagnoses.
[2]With at least one illness or risk-related diagnosis.

32.3 years in 1988, and 33.5 years in 1992. The median age for hospital discharges was 43.9 years in 1980, 48.5 years in 1988, and 50.7 years in 1992. In 1980, persons 45 years and over accounted for 49 percent of total discharges and 64 percent of the days of care. In 1992, persons 45 years and over made up 56 percent of the discharges and 68 percent of the days of care.

Changing health care policies also affect hospital utilization. A recent example is the efforts by managed-care plans and other insurers to shorten hospital stays for women after delivery and for their newborn infants. Table 8.1 shows the trends in lengths of stay for newborn infants. In 1980, 31 percent of newborn infants stayed in the hospital 2 days or less, and 63 percent stayed 3 to 7 days. In 1988, 55 percent of newborn infants had hospital stays of 2 days or less, and 41 percent stayed 3-7 days. By 1992, 66 percent of newborn infants were hospitalized for 2 days or less and only 29 percent had stays of 3-7 days.

Utilization by Sex

The number of discharges from short-stay hospitals was approximately 31 million in both 1988 and 1992. Weighted linear regression was used to analyze trends in discharge rates, rates of days of care, and average length of stay from 1988 to 1992. The rate of discharges per 1,000 population did not change significantly during this period; it was 128.3 in 1988 and 122.1 in 1992. However, the rate of days of care per 1,000 population declined 10 percent, from 838.8 in 1988 to 751.0 in 1992. The average length of stay declined 5 percent from 1988 (6.5 days) to 1992 (6.2 days).

- Discharge rates for males and females did not change significantly from 1988 to 1992. Males had 107.5 discharges per 1,000 population in 1988 and 100.8 in 1992. For females, the discharge rates were 147.7 in 1988 and 142.2 in 1992.

- Males accounted for approximately 40 percent (12 to 13 million) of total discharges in 1988 and 1992. Females had about 19 million discharges in both these years. Over 10 percent of all discharges in 1988 and 1992 were for females with deliveries (see section on utilization by diagnosis and sex).

- Rates of days of care per 1,000 population declined significantly for males and females from 1988 to 1992. For males, the rate

109

declined 11 percent from 760.7 in 1988 to 679.7 in 1992. For females, there was a 10 percent decrease, from 912.1 in 1988 to
818.3 in 1992.

• In both 1988 and 1992, males accounted for 44 percent of days
of care and females used 56 percent of days of care.

• The average stay for males declined 6 percent from 7.1 days in
1988 to 6.7 days in 1992. For females, the average length of stay
also declined 6 percent from 6.2 days in 1988 to 5.8 days in 1992.

Utilization by Region

Weighted linear regression analysis of the rates of discharges and
days of care showed that these rates did not change significantly from
1988 to 1992 for any of the four geographic regions of the country.
Regional trends in discharge rates are shown in Figure 8.1, and average lengths of stay by region are displayed in Figure 8.2.

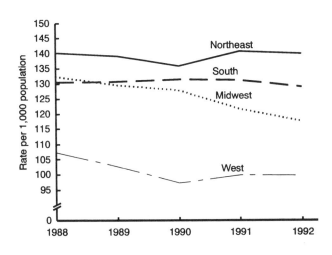

Figure 8.1. Rate of Discharges by Region: United States, 1988-92.

110

- In 1988, discharge rates per 1,000 population ranged from 107.4 per 1,000 population in the West to 140.3 in the Northeast. In 1992 the range was from 99.5 in the West to 139.9 in the Northeast.

- Rates of days of care per 1,000 population ranged from 624.3 in the West to 1,081.0 in the Northeast in 1988 and from 513.9 in the West to 1,005.1 in the Northeast in 1992.

- Average lengths of stay varied from 5.8 days in the West to 7.7 days in the Northeast in 1988 and from 5.2 days in the West to 7.2 days in the Northeast in 1992.

- In 1988, 35 percent of discharges were in the South, 25 percent were in the Midwest, 23 percent were in the Northeast, and 17 percent were in the West. The percents for 1992 were 36percent of discharges in the South, 23 percent in the Midwest, 23 percent in the Northeast, and 18 percent in the West.

- In 1988 and 1992, persons 45 years of age and over used two-thirds or more of days of care in the Northeast, Midwest, and South, but 55-62 percent of the days of care in the West.

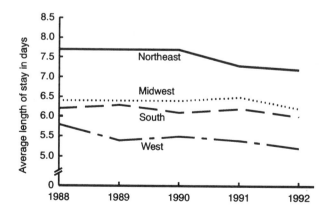

Figure 8.2. Average Length of Stay by Region: United States, 1988-92.

Table 8.2. Number of Discharges from Short-stay Hospitals, Days of Care, and Average Length of Stay, by Selected First-listed Diagnoses: United States, 1988 and 1992.

Diagnosis and ICD–9–CM codes	Discharges		Days of care		Average length of stay	
	1988	1992	1988	1992	1988	1992
	Number in thousands				Days	
All conditions[1]	31,146	30,951	203,678	190,386	6.5	6.2
Heart disease 391–392.0,393–398,402,404,410–416,420–429	3,641	3,935	25,883	26,256	7.1	6.7
Acute myocardial infarction 410	716	747	6,432	6,058	9.0	8.1
Coronary atherosclerosis 414.0	411	416	2,502	2,342	6.1	5.6
Other ischemic heart disease 411–413,414.1–414.9	921	971	4,871	4,831	5.3	5.0
Cardiac dysrhythmias 427	491	542	2,758	2,835	5.6	5.2
Congestive heart failure 428.0	634	822	5,560	6,506	8.8	7.9
Females with deliveries V27	3,781	3,910	11,029	10,040	2.9	2.6
Malignant neoplasms 140–208,230–234	1,670	1,577	15,676	13,433	9.4	8.5
Pneumonia 480–486	924	1,059	7,801	8,793	8.4	8.3
Fractures 800–829	1,014	1,016	8,558	7,842	8.4	7.7
Psychosis 290–299	781	908	11,812	11,746	15.1	12.9
Cerebrovascular disease 430–438	784	829	7,611	7,302	9.7	8.8
Arthropathies and related disorders 710–719	459	554	3,416	4,027	7.4	7.3
Cholelithiasis 574	484	512	3,162	2,236	6.5	4.4
Diabetes mellitus 250	454	476	3,734	3,274	8.2	6.9
Asthma 493	479	463	2,279	2,008	4.8	4.3
Benign neoplasms and neoplasms of uncertain behavior and unspecified nature 210–229,235–239	428	422	2,117	1,947	4.9	4.6
Intervertebral disc disorders 722	417	407	2,466	1,786	5.9	4.4
Acute respiratory infection 460–466	445	376	2,282	1,495	5.1	4.0

[1]Includes data for diagnostic conditions not shown in table.

NOTE: This table includes diagnostic categories that accounted for 400,000 or more discharges in 1988 or 1992.

Utilization by Diagnosis and Sex

Hospital use measures for selected first listed-diagnoses are shown in Table 8.2. The categories shown accounted for half or more of all discharges and days of care in 1988 and 1992. Table 8.3 lists the diagnostic categories with 200,000 or more male discharges in 1988 or 1992. These categories made up nearly half of male discharges. Diagnostic categories with 200,000 or more female discharges in 1988 or 1992 are in Table 8.4, and these categories include more than half of female discharges.

- Heart disease was the first-listed diagnosis for 12 percent (3.6 million) of discharges in 1988 and 13 percent (3.9 million) in 1992. These discharges had an average length of stay of 7.1 days in 1988 and 6.7 days in 1992. They used 13-14 percent of total days of care, and made up 23 percent of hospital deaths.

- Females hospitalized for deliveries accounted for 12 percent (3.8 million) of first-listed diagnoses in 1988 and 13 percent (3.9 million) in 1992. Because their average lengths of stay were short— 2.9 days in 1988 and 2.6 days in 1992—females with deliveries made up only 5 percent of the total days of care.

- Malignant neoplasms (cancers) were first-listed diagnoses for 5 percent of discharges in 1988 and 1992. These discharges used 7-8 percent of total days of care and had 18-18 percent of hospital deaths in 1988 and 1992. Their average length of stay was 9.4 days in 1988 and 8.5 days in 1992.

- Pneumonia, fractures, psychoses, and cerebrovascular disease each accounted for more than 700,000 discharges in 1988 and 1992. Discharges with each of these four diagnoses used more than 7 million days of care in 1988 and 1992.

- Females hospitalized for deliveries made up 20 percent of female discharges in 1988 and 21 percent in 1992.

- For males, heart disease was the first-listed diagnosis for 15 percent (2.0 million) of discharges in 1988 and 17 percent (2.1 million) in 1992. For females, 9 percent (1.7 million) of hospitalizations in 1988 and 10 percent (1.9 million) in 1992 were for heart disease.

113

Table 8.3. Number and Rate of Male Discharges from Short-stay Hospitals by Selected First-listed Diagnoses: United States, 1988 and 1992.

[Discharges of inpatients from non-Federal hospitals. Excludes newborn infants. Diagnostic categories and code numbers are based on the *International Classification of Diseases, 9th Revision, Clinical Modification* (ICD-9-CM)]

Diagnosis and ICD-9-CM codes	Number in thousands		Rate per 10,000 population	
	1988	1992	1988	1992
All conditions[1]	12,642	12,406	1,075.3	1,008.0
Heart disease 391-392.0,393-398,402,404,410-416,420-429	1,955	2,083	166.3	169.3
Acute myocardial infarction 410	451	458	38.4	37.2
Coronary atherosclerosis 414.0	278	285	23.6	23.2
Other ischemic heart disease 411-413,414.1-414.9	491	505	41.7	41.0
Cardiac dysrhythmias 427	228	256	19.4	20.8
Congestive heart failure 428.0	277	373	23.6	30.3
Malignant neoplasms 140-208,230-234	772	765	65.7	62.2
Pneumonia 480-486	472	535	40.2	43.5
Fractures 800-829	506	465	43.0	37.8
Psychosis 290-299	341	408	29.0	33.2
Cerebrovascular disease 430-438	336	375	28.5	30.5
Intervertebral disc disorders 722	247	222	21.0	18.0
Hyperplasia of prostate 600	247	221	21.0	18.0
Arthropathies and related disorders 710-719	191	212	16.3	17.2
Diabetes mellitus 250	209	207	17.7	16.8
Asthma 493	210	201	17.8	16.3
Acute respiratory infection 460-466	224	187	19.1	15.2
Inguinal hernia 550	232	98	19.7	7.9

[1] Includes data for diagnostic conditions not shown in table.

NOTE: This table includes diagnostic categories that accounted for 200,000 or more male discharges in 1988 or 1992.

- For males, malignant neoplasms made up 6 percent of first-listed diagnoses—772,000 in 1988 and 765,000 in 1992. Females had 898,000 discharges (5 percent) with a first-listed diagnosis of malignant neoplasms in 1988 and 821,000 (4 percent) in 1992.

- Only males had more than 200,000 discharges for intervertebral disc disorders in 1988 and 1992. Discharges for hyperplasia of prostate also exceeded 200,000 in both years.

- Only females had more than 200,000 discharges for cholelithiasis, benign neoplasms and neoplasms of uncertain behavior and unspecified nature, and noninfectious enteritis and colitis in 1988 and 1992.

Utilization of Selected Heart-related Procedures by Sex

Open-heart surgery, removal of coronary artery obstruction, coronary artery bypass graft, and cardiac catheterizations together accounted for 1.6 million procedures in 1988 and 2.0 million in 1992. Among these four procedures, only one significant change in rates during the 1988-92 period was found using weighted linear regression analysis. This was a 68 percent increase in the rate of removal of coronary artery obstruction. It should be noted that the data for open-heart surgery do not include coronary artery bypass graft.

- Two-thirds (67 percent) of the four heart-related procedures listed above were performed on males in 1988, and males had 65 percent of these procedures in 1992.

- In 1988, a total of 92,000 open-heart procedures were performed—53,000 on males and 39,000 on females. In 1992, there were 104,000 open-heart surgeries-57,000 on males and 48,000 on females.

- The rate per 100,000 population for removal of coronary artery obstruction increased from 93.3 in 1988 to 157.2 in 1992. The rate for males increased 57 percent (from 136.1 to 213.3 per 100,000 population) and the rate for females increased 96 percent (from 53.1 to 104.3 per 100,000 population) from 1988 to 1992.

Table 8.4. Number and Rate of Female Discharges from Short-stay Hospitals by Selected First-listed Diagnoses: United States, 1988 and 1992.

Diagnosis and ICD–9–CM codes	Number in thousands		Rate per 10,000 population	
	1988	1992	1988	1992
All conditions[1]	18,504	18,545	1,477.4	1,422.0
Females with deliveries ... V27	3,781	3,910	301.9	299.8
Heart disease ... 391–392.0,393–398,402,404,410–416,420–429	1,686	1,852	134.6	142.0
Acute myocardial infarction ... 410	265	289	21.2	22.1
Coronary atherosclerosis and other ischemic heart disease ... 411–414	565	597	45.1	45.8
Cardiac dysrhythmias ... 427	263	286	21.0	21.9
Congestive heart failure ... 428.0	357	449	28.5	34.4
Malignant neoplasms ... 140–208,230–234	898	812	71.7	62.3
Fractures ... 800–829	508	552	40.6	42.3
Fracture of neck of femur ... 820	186	205	14.9	15.7
Pneumonia ... 480–486	452	524	36.1	40.1
Psychosis ... 290–299	440	500	35.1	38.3
Cerebrovascular disease ... 430–438	448	454	35.8	34.8
Cholelithiasis ... 574	352	358	28.1	27.5
Benign neoplasms and neoplasms of uncertain behavior and unspecified nature ... 210–229,235–239	350	342	27.9	26.3
Arthropathies and related disorders ... 710–719	267	342	21.3	26.3
Diabetes mellitus ... 250	245	269	19.6	20.6
Asthma ... 493	270	263	21.5	20.1
Noninfectious enteritis and colitis ... 555–558	230	220	18.4	16.8
Acute respiratory infection ... 460–466	221	189	17.7	14.5
Abortions and ectopic and molar pregnancies ... 630–639	266	179	21.2	13.7

[1]Includes data for diagnostic conditions not shown in table.

NOTE: This table includes diagnostic categories that accounted for 200,000 or more female discharges in 1988 or 1992.

- There were 253,000 discharges with coronary artery bypass grafts in 1988 and 309,000 in 1992. Males made up 75 percent of discharges with bypass surgery (189,000) in 1988 and 72 percent (221,000) in 1992. Female discharges with bypass surgery numbered 63,000 in 1988 and 88,000 in 1992.

- An estimated 930,000 cardiac catheterizations were performed in 1988 and 1,028,000 were performed in 1992. Males underwent 598,000 catheterizations and females had 332,000 catheterizations in 1988. In 1992, the estimates were 636,000 cardiac catheterizations for males and 392,000 catheterizations for females.

Summary

After a large increase in the 1970's and an abrupt decrease in the 1980's, the discharge rates for short-stay hospitals leveled off in the 1988-92 period. However, the rate of days of care continued to decline, falling 10 percent from 1988 to 1992. Average length of stay also declined 5 percent from 1988 to 1992. Discharge rates did not change significantly in any of the four geographic regions of the country.

The major reasons for hospitalization in both 1988 and 1992 were delivery, heart disease, and malignant neoplasm. Throughout this period, the majority of procedures performed were in one of four categoriesmiscellaneous diagnostic and therapeutic procedures, obstetrical procedures, operations on the digestive system, and operations on the cardiovascular system.

Particular attention was given to commonly performed sex-specific procedures. Obstetrical procedures, such as episiotomy, fetal EKG and other fetal monitoring, and cesarean section, were among the leading procedures performed on females. Other female-specific procedures, such as hysterectomy, were also commonly done. Frequent male-specific procedures were prostatectomy and circumcision. No significant changes in rates occurred in the 1988-92 period for any of these sex-specific procedures.

The four heart-related procedures—open-heart surgery, removal of coronary artery obstruction, coronary artery bypass graft, and cardiac catheterization—were also examined by sex. Males accounted for 67 percent of these procedures in 1988 and 64 percent in 1992. The rate for one procedure, removal of coronary artery obstruction, increased significantly for both males and females during the 1988-92 period.

Chapter 9

Racial/Ethnic Patterns of Cancer in the United States

Foreword

This landmark report presents the most extensive information yet available on racial and ethnic differences in cancer experience. It cannot be overstated as to how important these data will be to our understanding of cancer. The cancer experience among ethnic and racial groups varies widely across the world as well as here in the United States. African-Americans for example, have higher incidence and mortality from many cancers compared with whites, and African American men, for instance, have the highest rate of prostate cancer in the world. Native Hawaiians also have high cancer incidence and mortality rates while Hispanics have generally lower rates, although for some cancers such as gall bladder their rates are higher than among whites. Today, with the wealth of new epidemiologic, biologic and genetic tools available, we are in a better position to capitalize on these data and find the sources of these differences. We look to these differences to help identify clues to cancer causation as well as to ways of detecting these cancers early, treating them, and ultimately, preventing them.

Differences outlined here are not necessarily the experience of each individual, of course, and it is important to understand that the racial and ethnic classifications are either self-reported, derived from medical records, or are reported in the 1990 census. Again,

NIH Publication No. NIH96-4104, April 1996.

these classifications represent guides. The differences between groups may be related to a variety of factors including biology, heredity, and perhaps most important, behavior (smoking and diet being two principal cancer-related behaviors) including behaviors related to both the public's use of the health care system and health professional practices.

Introduction

This monograph provides a concise description of the occurrence of the major cancers among several different racial/ethnic groups in the United States. Age-adjusted incidence rates are shown graphically by age group and sex for Alaska Native, American Indian (New Mexico), black, Chinese, Filipino, Hawaiian, Hispanic, Japanese, Korean, Vietnamese, white (total), white Hispanic and white non-Hispanic populations. Age adjusted mortality rates are also shown for these groups, with the exception of Koreans and Vietnamese, for whom national data are not yet available. The Alaska Native group includes persons in Alaska who identified themselves as Aleut, Eskimo or American Indian. The remaining racial/ethnic designations in this monograph correspond to those used on the 1990 decennial census form. Incidence rates are provided by the Surveillance, Epidemiology and End Results (SEER) Program of the National Cancer Institute and are based on newly diagnosed cancers between 1988 and 1992 for a subset of the United States population. Mortality rates are provided by the National Center for Health Statistics and are based on cancer deaths between 1988 and 1992 for the entire United States population.

The cancers included in this report are organized alphabetically. They are followed by a section on cancer control efforts in special population groups and an appendix. The appendix contains tables showing the number of newly diagnosed cancers, by racial/ethnic group, in specific regions of the United States during 1988-1992. It also includes estimates for the entire country of the number of newly diagnosed cancers and the number of cancer deaths in 1990. The intent of this publication is to promote a greater understanding of the cancer problem in the United States, to identify those who can benefit most by education on the potential risks and consequences of certain behaviors and exposures, and to indicate areas where more knowledge and scientific investigation are needed to understand why cancer occurs more frequently in some groups of people than others.

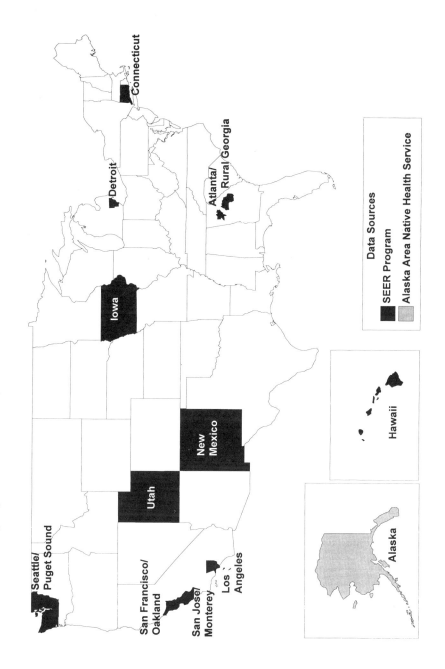

Figure 9.1. Cancer Registry Areas.

The SEER Program

The National Cancer Act of 1971 mandated the collection, analysis and dissemination of data useful in the prevention, diagnosis and treatment of cancer. This mandate led to the establishment of the Surveillance, Epidemiology and End Results (SEER) Program. As a continuing project of the National Cancer Institute, the SEER Program is responsible for monitoring the impact of cancer in the general population. Participants in the SEER Program were selected for their ability to operate and maintain a population-based cancer reporting system and for the variety and size of population subgroups within their areas (e.g., racial/ethnic, urban and rural) which are of special epidemiologic interest. Information from eleven SEER geographic areas and from the Alaska Area Native Health Service are used in this report. These areas are identified in Figure 9.1 and include: the states of Connecticut, Hawaii, Iowa, New Mexico and Utah; and the metropolitan areas of Atlanta (including 10 rural counties), Detroit, Los Angeles San Francisco/Oakland, San Jose/Monterey, and Seattle/Puget Sound. These areas cover about 14% of the total United States population. The Alaska Area Native Health Service also receives support from the National Cancer Institute and provides cancer incidence data for their Alaska Native population that is compatible with the data from the SEER areas.

Although the SEER areas cover just 14% of the total United States population, they include 78% of the Hawaiian population, 60% of the Japanese population, 49% of the Filipino population, 43% of the Chinese population, 34% of the Korean population, 31% of the Vietnamese population, 27% of the American Indian population, and 25% of the Hispanic population in the country. Since some cancers are relatively rare, the SEER areas must include large portions of these smaller racial/ethnic populations in order to calculate reliable cancer rates. Five years of cancer diagnoses and deaths, from 1988 through 1992, were accumulated to facilitate the reporting of rates in these smaller populations.

Characteristics of the SEER Population

Characteristics of the SEER population and the total United States population are compared in Figure 9.2. In 1990, the SEER population was similar to the United States population with respect to the percentage of people living below the poverty level and the percentage of adults who graduated from high school. A larger portion of the

SEER population lived in urban areas and the percentage of people in the SEER areas that were born in another country was nearly double that for the United States as a whole.

The 1990 population age distribution varies among the different racial/ethnic groups represented in the SEER Program and the Alaska Area Native Health Service. Those heavily weighted in the younger age groups include Alaska Natives, American Indians in New Mexico and Hawaiians. Japanese and non-Hispanic whites are concentrated in the older age groups. Other populations are distributed between these two extremes. Unique to the Japanese population are two bulges in the age distribution at ages 20-44 years and 60-69 years. Within the Asian groups, Vietnamese are more heavily distributed in the younger ages; Koreans, Filipinos and Chinese have slightly older distributions; and Japanese clearly have the highest percentage of persons in the older age groups. Since over 90% of the Hispanic populations represented in SEER classify themselves as white, the age distribution for the total Hispanic population and the white Hispanic population are

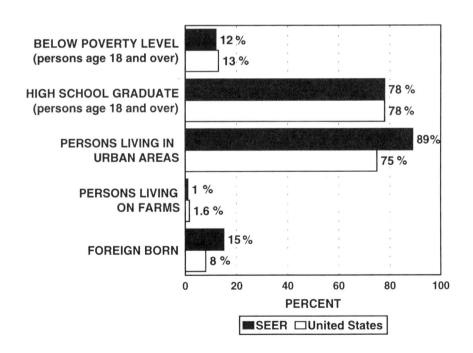

Figure 9.2. *Population Characteristics SEER areas vs. United States.*

similar. The age distribution of the total white population (which is not shown) is identical to that for the non-Hispanic white population.

Population characteristics within each of the geographic areas included in this monograph are shown in the tables at the end of this section. It is apparent that the racial/ethnic populations are not equally distributed across the SEER regions. The largest concentrations of the SEER black population are in Los Angeles (28%) and Detroit (25%), with other sizable groups in Atlanta (19%), San Francisco (12%) and Connecticut (8%). Over two-thirds of the Chinese population covered by the SEER Program is equally divided between San Francisco/Oakland (36%) and Los Angeles (35%). Smaller numbers of Chinese live in the San Jose/Monterey area (10%), Hawaii (10%), and Seattle/Puget Sound (4%). Most of the Filipino population is found in the same five areas but in different proportions (32% in Los Angeles, 24% in each of San Francisco/Oakland and Hawaii, and 11% in San Jose/Monterey, and 6% in Seattle/Puget Sound).

Most of the Hispanic population in SEER lives in Los Angeles (60%), followed by New Mexico (10%), San Francisco and San Jose/Monterey (9%), and Connecticut (4%). About 84% of the Hispanic population in San Jose/Monterey identified themselves as Mexican-American in the 1990 census (this information is not included in the tables). Mexican-Americans account for 76% of the Hispanic population in Los Angeles, 58% in San Francisco/Oakland and 57% in New Mexico. San Francisco/Oakland also has a sizable percentage of Puerto Rican Hispanics (4%). Over two-thirds of the Hispanic population in Connecticut is Puerto Rican, with smaller percentages of Mexican Americans (4%) and Cubans (3%).

One-half of the total SEER Japanese population lives in Hawaii, 25% in Los Angeles, 9% in San Francisco, and 6% in each of San Jose/Monterey and Seattle/Puget Sound. Over one-half of the Korean population (54%) is found in Los Angeles, and smaller numbers live in Seattle/Puget Sound (10%), Hawaii and San Francisco (9% in each), San Jose/Monterey (7%), Atlanta (4%), and Detroit and Connecticut (2% in each). Nearly two-thirds of the Vietnamese population is divided between Los Angeles (33%) and San Jose/Monterey (30%), 16% resides in San Francisco, 9% in Seattle/Puget Sound and 3% in each of Atlanta and Hawaii. The white population is more evenly distributed among the SEER areas with 25% in Los Angeles (which also has the largest total population of the SEER areas); 11% in each of Seattle/Puget Sound, Connecticut, and Detroit; 10% in each of Iowa and San Francisco/Oakland; and smaller percentages in the remaining areas.

Among the populations included in this monograph, Asian groups have the highest percentage of foreign born persons. This category does not include persons born in a foreign country and having at least one American parent. Of the Asian groups, Vietnamese have the largest percentage of foreign born persons in every SEER area, ranging from 71% in New Mexico to 88% in Atlanta. There are too few Vietnamese in Detroit to calculate the percentage foreign born. In Los Angeles, the high percentage of foreign born Vietnamese was matched by the percent of foreign born Koreans. In Iowa, the percentages of foreign born Chinese and Vietnamese were equal. Since a large proportion of the Vietnamese population are first generation immigrants, their cancer experience may reflect influences associated with their country of origin to a greater degree than with factors in the United States. In contrast, the percentage of foreign born Japanese tended to be among the lowest of the Asian groups in most of the SEER areas and, in Hawaii, was very low at only 8%. The percentage of foreign born Hispanics ranges from 10% to 20% in many of the SEER areas. There were higher proportions of foreign born Hispanics in Los Angeles (53%), Atlanta (48%), Connecticut (42%) and San Jose/Monterey (36%). The percentage of foreign born non-Hispanic whites ranged from one percent in Iowa to 12% in Los Angeles. The black population also had low percentages of foreign born persons, ranging from one percent in Detroit to 11% in Connecticut.

The percent of each racial/ethnic population living below the poverty level is based on answers to the income questions on the 1990 census. Households are classified by the Bureau of Census as below the poverty level when the total 1989 income of the family or householder is below the appropriate poverty threshold. The thresholds vary depending upon family size, number of children, and the age of the family householder for one and two-person households. Some studies have noted that persons living below the poverty level tend to have poorer health outcomes, including cancers more advanced at the time of diagnosis, poorer survival rates, and higher mortality rates than those living above the poverty level. Information on the percent below the poverty level is only available for American Indian, black, Hispanic (total), white (total) and Asian (total) populations.

The American Indian population in New Mexico clearly has the largest percentage of people living below the poverty level (43%). In six of the areas, black populations have the highest percentage of persons living below the poverty level, although the percentages are typically only half as large as that for American Indians in New

Mexico. About one-fifth (21%) of the Alaska Native population is living below the poverty level. Hispanics have the highest percentage of their population living below the poverty level in four of the areas (Connecticut, Los Angeles, San Jose/Monterey and Hawaii). The different populations in Hawaii are very homogeneous regarding poverty level status, with the exception of Hispanics, who have a somewhat higher percentage below the poverty level. The white population in each area has the smallest percentage below the poverty level, except in Hawaii, where they are comparable to the Asian and black populations.

Population Counts

County population estimates for July 1, 1990 were provided by the Bureau of the Census (BOC) and were used as the denominators when calculating cancer rates for American Indians, blacks, Hispanics (total, white), and whites (total, non-Hispanic) by five-year age group and sex. These populations included modifications made by the BOC to account for incomplete information from census forms regarding age, race and sex. Population counts for Chinese, Filipinos, Japanese, Koreans, and Vietnamese were obtained from unmodified 1990 census data tapes (STF2A). All of the census population data are available (or will soon be available) from the Statistical Information Office, Population Division, U.S. Bureau of the Census, Washington, D.C. 20233.

Population estimates for native Hawaiians and whites in Hawaii were provided by the Epidemiology Program of the Cancer Research Center of Hawaii. The estimates were developed from sample survey data collected by the Health Surveillance Program of the Hawaii Department of Health. The Hawaii Cancer Research Center estimates their own population figures because of a concern that their native Hawaiian population has been vastly undercounted in the last two decennial censuses due to the wording of the question on the census form regarding race. The Center staff believes that their estimates better represent the actual population size of these two groups and are based on a racial/ethnic classification more consistent with that of the cancer patients who comprise the numerators for the rate calculations. Since they do not develop estimates for all of the racial/ethnic populations in Hawaii, due to the limited size of their survey, population estimates for Hawaii are the result of a combination of BOC data and estimates derived from Hawaii's survey sample. The total Hispanic population and white Hispanic population numbers are used from the BOC. The white non-Hispanic population is derived by subtracting the BOC white Hispanic population count from Hawaii's estimate of the total white population. The black population in Hawaii is from the July 1 BOC estimate and the individual Asian populations in Hawaii are from the BOC STF2A data tapes, as they are in all of the other SEER regions.

Racial/Ethnic Differences in Cancer Rates

Differences between the cancer rates for various racial/ethnic groups included in this publication must be interpreted cautiously. Even with the over representation of many of the groups noted above, cancer rates in smaller populations (e.g., Alaska Native, American Indian, Hawaiian, Japanese, Korean, and Vietnamese) are less precise than rates in larger populations (e.g., black, white (total), white Hispanic, white non-Hispanic). An indicator of the amount of imprecision, or variability, associated with the cancer rates is the standard error. The standard errors for the age-adjusted cancer incidence and mortality rates are not specified in this monograph, but may be estimated from a formula for the standard error (SE) of a crude (unadjusted) rate as follows: $SE(rate) = rate / [events]^{1/2}$ where events refer to the number of cancer diagnoses or deaths associated with the rate. Additional information concerning the variability associated with the cancer rates will be included on a CD-ROM some time after the publication of this monograph.

Another difficulty when interpreting racial/ethnic differences in cancer rates arises from the fact that the designation of race/ethnicity for the cancer cases (used as numerators in the calculation of the rates) is based upon information recorded in medical records (incidence) or death certificates (mortality), whereas these designations are self-determined via the 1990 census questionnaire for the population counts used as denominators in the calculation of the cancer rates. Specific racial/ethnic surname lists were also used by all of the SEER registries to improve the identification of Hispanic, Chinese, Filipino, Japanese and Korean cancer patients. Cancer patients whose names matched with names on one of the surname lists were added to the appropriate racial/ethnic group, along with other cases previously identified from information contained in medical records. Inconsistencies between the racial/ethnic designations from these different sources, however, may lead to either overstating or understating the true cancer rate for a particular group. In summary, the cancer rates presented in this monograph are best used to identify general racial/ethnic patterns of cancer.

An Explanation of Terms

Two primary measures associated with assessing the impact of cancer in the general population are the number of new cancers diagnosed in a specified population during a year (incidence rate) and the number of deaths from cancer in a population during a year (mortality rate). Both of these rates are presented here as the number of cancer events (diagnoses or deaths) per 100,000 people. Since cancer diagnoses and deaths are accumulated over five years (1988-1992) for this monograph, the cancer incidence and mortality rates are calculated by dividing the number of cancers (new cases or deaths) by five times the 1990 population. The resulting rate is referred to here, as in other publications, as an average annual rate. Cancer is a disease that is very strongly associated with age; therefore, it is possible that two populations may have different cancer rates only because of their different age structures and not because of any difference in the underlying risk. A statistical method termed age-adjustment is used to enable cancer incidence (or mortality) rates to be compared between two populations with different age structures. In this monograph, the 1970 United States standard million population is used to calculate the age-adjusted rates.

A Note about Reading the Graphs

We have followed the race/ethnicity classification scheme used in the 1990 census. That is, persons declaring Hispanic ethnicity may be of any race. This results in an overlap between the Hispanic classification and the other specific racial/ethnic groups. To remind the reader of this point, each graph is divided into an upper portion with non-overlapping racial/ethnic classifications and a lower portion which contains three racial/ethnic groups (Hispanic, white Hispanic, white non-Hispanic) which overlap the populations in the upper portion of the graph.

Five Most Common Cancers in Each Racial/Ethnic Group

The top five cancer age-adjusted incidence rates and mortality rates are displayed for men and women in each racial/ethnic group.

Rankings for the total white population are identical to those for the non-Hispanic white population and are not shown in this set of graphs. Among men, lung and bronchus, prostate and colorectal cancer appear among the top five cancer incidence rates in every racial/ethnic group.

Prostate cancer is the highest reported cancer among American Indian, black, Filipino, Japanese, non-Hispanic white and Hispanic men. Cancer of the lung and bronchus is highest among men in the remaining racial/ethnic groups. In women, breast cancer incidence rates are highest in all groups except Vietnamese, for whom cervical cancer ranks higher than breast cancer. Cancers of the breast, lung and bronchus and colon and rectum appear among the top five cancer incidence rates for women in every racial/ethnic group except American Indians, for whom lung cancer does not appear. Unique to American Indian women in New Mexico is a high incidence rate for cancer of the gallbladder. Other studies have also documented elevated gallbladder cancer rates among American Indians. Stomach cancer appears among the top five cancers for men and women in each of the Asian populations with the exception of Filipinos and Chinese women.

Lung cancer is the leading cause of cancer death among men in all racial/ethnic groups except American Indians, who have higher mortality from cancers of the prostate, stomach and liver. Cancer of the prostate or colon and rectum is the second leading cause of cancer death among men in most other racial/ethnic groups. The exception is Chinese men, for whom liver cancer ranks second in mortality. Stomach cancer appears in the top five causes of cancer deaths among men in all groups except blacks, Filipinos and non-Hispanic whites. Cancer of the pancreas is among the top five causes of cancer deaths in men for all groups except Alaska Natives, American Indians, and Filipinos. Among women, the leading cause of cancer death in most racial/ethnic groups is lung cancer. Breast cancer is the leading cause of cancer death in Filipino and Hispanic women and cancer of the gallbladder ranks highest in American Indian women in New Mexico (based on 19 deaths). Breast cancer is in second place among the groups where lung cancer mortality is highest, except for Alaska Native women, who experience higher mortality from cancers of the colon and rectum. Colorectal cancer appears among the top five cancer mortality rates for all groups except American Indians and cancer of the pancreas is in the top five cancers for all groups.

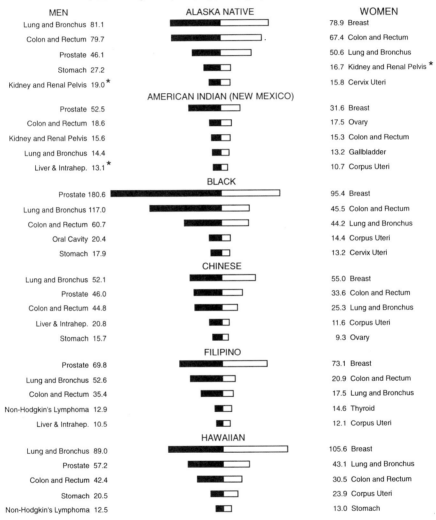

SEER INCIDENCE Rates, 1988-1992
(Rates are "average annual" per 100,000 population, age-adjusted to 1970 U.S. standard)

MEN		ALASKA NATIVE		WOMEN
Lung and Bronchus	81.1			78.9 Breast
Colon and Rectum	79.7			67.4 Colon and Rectum
Prostate	46.1			50.6 Lung and Bronchus
Stomach	27.2			16.7 Kidney and Renal Pelvis ★
Kidney and Renal Pelvis	19.0 ★			15.8 Cervix Uteri
		AMERICAN INDIAN (NEW MEXICO)		
Prostate	52.5			31.6 Breast
Colon and Rectum	18.6			17.5 Ovary
Kidney and Renal Pelvis	15.6			15.3 Colon and Rectum
Lung and Bronchus	14.4			13.2 Gallbladder
Liver & Intrahep.	13.1 ★			10.7 Corpus Uteri
		BLACK		
Prostate	180.6			95.4 Breast
Lung and Bronchus	117.0			45.5 Colon and Rectum
Colon and Rectum	60.7			44.2 Lung and Bronchus
Oral Cavity	20.4			14.4 Corpus Uteri
Stomach	17.9			13.2 Cervix Uteri
		CHINESE		
Lung and Bronchus	52.1			55.0 Breast
Prostate	46.0			33.6 Colon and Rectum
Colon and Rectum	44.8			25.3 Lung and Bronchus
Liver & Intrahep.	20.8			11.6 Corpus Uteri
Stomach	15.7			9.3 Ovary
		FILIPINO		
Prostate	69.8			73.1 Breast
Lung and Bronchus	52.6			20.9 Colon and Rectum
Colon and Rectum	35.4			17.5 Lung and Bronchus
Non-Hodgkin's Lymphoma	12.9			14.6 Thyroid
Liver & Intrahep.	10.5			12.1 Corpus Uteri
		HAWAIIAN		
Lung and Bronchus	89.0			105.6 Breast
Prostate	57.2			43.1 Lung and Bronchus
Colon and Rectum	42.4			30.5 Colon and Rectum
Stomach	20.5			23.9 Corpus Uteri
Non-Hodgkin's Lymphoma	12.5			13.0 Stomach

★ = Rate is based on fewer than 25 cases and may be subject to greater variability than the other rates which are based on larger numbers.

Figure 9.3a. *Five Most Frequently Diagnosed Cancers.*

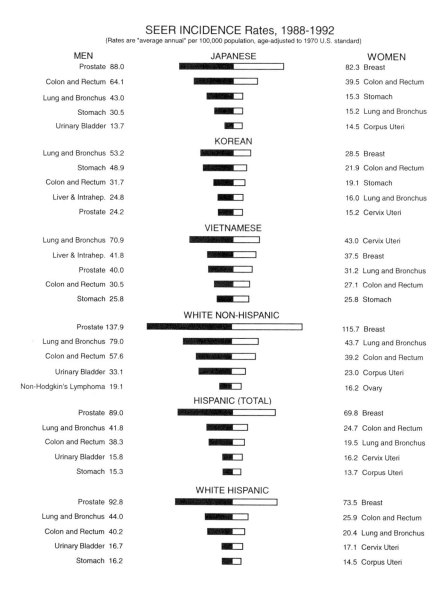

SEER INCIDENCE Rates, 1988-1992
(Rates are "average annual" per 100,000 population, age-adjusted to 1970 U.S. standard)

JAPANESE

MEN			WOMEN
Prostate	88.0	82.3	Breast
Colon and Rectum	64.1	39.5	Colon and Rectum
Lung and Bronchus	43.0	15.3	Stomach
Stomach	30.5	15.2	Lung and Bronchus
Urinary Bladder	13.7	14.5	Corpus Uteri

KOREAN

Lung and Bronchus	53.2	28.5	Breast
Stomach	48.9	21.9	Colon and Rectum
Colon and Rectum	31.7	19.1	Stomach
Liver & Intrahep.	24.8	16.0	Lung and Bronchus
Prostate	24.2	15.2	Cervix Uteri

VIETNAMESE

Lung and Bronchus	70.9	43.0	Cervix Uteri
Liver & Intrahep.	41.8	37.5	Breast
Prostate	40.0	31.2	Lung and Bronchus
Colon and Rectum	30.5	27.1	Colon and Rectum
Stomach	25.8	25.8	Stomach

WHITE NON-HISPANIC

Prostate	137.9	115.7	Breast
Lung and Bronchus	79.0	43.7	Lung and Bronchus
Colon and Rectum	57.6	39.2	Colon and Rectum
Urinary Bladder	33.1	23.0	Corpus Uteri
Non-Hodgkin's Lymphoma	19.1	16.2	Ovary

HISPANIC (TOTAL)

Prostate	89.0	69.8	Breast
Lung and Bronchus	41.8	24.7	Colon and Rectum
Colon and Rectum	38.3	19.5	Lung and Bronchus
Urinary Bladder	15.8	16.2	Cervix Uteri
Stomach	15.3	13.7	Corpus Uteri

WHITE HISPANIC

Prostate	92.8	73.5	Breast
Lung and Bronchus	44.0	25.9	Colon and Rectum
Colon and Rectum	40.2	20.4	Lung and Bronchus
Urinary Bladder	16.7	17.1	Cervix Uteri
Stomach	16.2	14.5	Corpus Uteri

Figure 9.3b. *Five Most Frequently Diagnosed Cancers.*

131

United States MORTALITY Rates, 1988-1992

(Rates are "average annual" per 100,000 population, age-adjusted to 1970 U.S. standard)

MEN	ALASKA NATIVE	WOMEN
Lung and Bronchus 69.4		45.3 Lung and Bronchus
Colon and Rectum 27.2		24.0 Colon and Rectum
Stomach 18.9*		16.0 Breast*
Kidney and Renal Pelvis 13.4*		15.5 Pancreas*
Nasopharynx 11.6*		7.4 Kidney and Renal Pelvis*

	AMERICAN INDIAN (NEW MEXICO)	
Prostate 16.2		8.9 Gallbladder*
Stomach 11.2*		8.7 Breast*
Liver & Intrahep. 11.2*		8.0 Cervix Uteri*
Lung and Bronchus 10.4*		7.4 Pancreas*
Colon and Rectum 8.5*		7.3 Ovary*

	BLACK	
Lung and Bronchus 105.6		31.5 Lung and Bronchus
Prostate 53.7		31.4 Breast
Colon and Rectum 28.2		20.4 Colon and Rectum
Esophagus 14.8		10.4 Pancreas
Pancreas 14.4		6.7 Cervix Uteri

	CHINESE	
Lung and Bronchus 40.1		18.5 Lung and Bronchus
Liver & Intrahep. 17.7		11.2 Breast
Colon and Rectum 15.7		10.5 Colon and Rectum
Stomach 10.5		5.1 Pancreas
Pancreas 6.7		4.8 Stomach

	FILIPINO	
Lung and Bronchus 29.8		11.9 Breast
Prostate 13.5		10.0 Lung and Bronchus
Colon and Rectum 11.4		5.8 Colon and Rectum
Liver & Intrahep. 7.8		3.5 Pancreas
Leukemia 5.7		3.4 Ovary

★ = Rate is based on fewer than 25 deaths and may be subject to greater variability than the other rates which are based on larger numbers.

Figure 9.3c. *Five Most Frequently Diagnosed Cancers.*

United States MORTALITY Rates, 1988-1992
(Rates are "average annual" per 100,000 population, age-adjusted to 1970 U.S. standard)

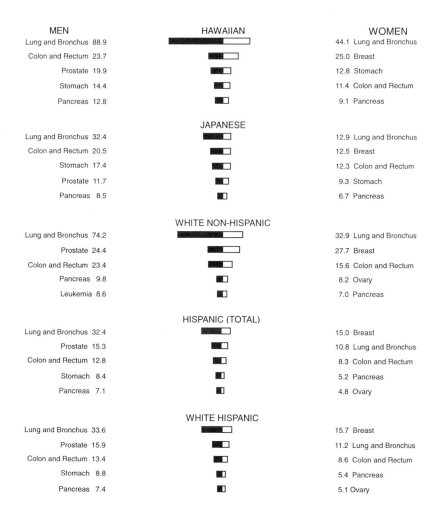

MEN	HAWAIIAN	WOMEN
Lung and Bronchus 88.9		44.1 Lung and Bronchus
Colon and Rectum 23.7		25.0 Breast
Prostate 19.9		12.8 Stomach
Stomach 14.4		11.4 Colon and Rectum
Pancreas 12.8		9.1 Pancreas
	JAPANESE	
Lung and Bronchus 32.4		12.9 Lung and Bronchus
Colon and Rectum 20.5		12.5 Breast
Stomach 17.4		12.3 Colon and Rectum
Prostate 11.7		9.3 Stomach
Pancreas 8.5		6.7 Pancreas
	WHITE NON-HISPANIC	
Lung and Bronchus 74.2		32.9 Lung and Bronchus
Prostate 24.4		27.7 Breast
Colon and Rectum 23.4		15.6 Colon and Rectum
Pancreas 9.8		8.2 Ovary
Leukemia 8.6		7.0 Pancreas
	HISPANIC (TOTAL)	
Lung and Bronchus 32.4		15.0 Breast
Prostate 15.3		10.8 Lung and Bronchus
Colon and Rectum 12.8		8.3 Colon and Rectum
Stomach 8.4		5.2 Pancreas
Pancreas 7.1		4.8 Ovary
	WHITE HISPANIC	
Lung and Bronchus 33.6		15.7 Breast
Prostate 15.9		11.2 Lung and Bronchus
Colon and Rectum 13.4		8.6 Colon and Rectum
Stomach 8.8		5.4 Pancreas
Pancreas 7.4		5.1 Ovary

Figure 9.3d. *Five Most Frequently Diagnosed Cancers.*

All Cancers Combined

Overall cancer incidence rates in the SEER regions are higher in men than women. Black men have the highest incidence rate of cancer. Non-Hispanic white men have the next highest rate which is 14% lower than that of black men. Rates for Alaska Native men and Hawaiian men follow those for whites and are over one-third lower than the rate for black men. The rate in white Hispanic men is similar to that for Hawaiian men. American Indians in New Mexico have the lowest overall cancer incidence rate among men, nearly two-thirds lower than the rate for black men. Among the Asian subgroups, Vietnamese men have the highest incidence rate, followed by Japanese, Chinese, Filipino and Korean men. The incidence rate for Korean men is more than 18% lower than that for Vietnamese men. The racial/ethnic pattern is similar when incidence rates are calculated for each of the three age groups.

Among women, the racial/ethnic differences in the incidence rates for all cancers are not as extreme as they are for men. The rate is highest for non-Hispanic white women, followed by Alaska Native (<2% lower), white (2% lower), black (8% lower) and Hawaiian (9% lower) women. The lowest rates occur in American Indian women in New Mexico and Korean women. Similar to the pattern in men, rates among women are low for Koreans, Chinese and Filipinos. The incidence rate for all cancers in Vietnamese women is the highest among Asian women, and is higher than that for white Hispanic women. Alaska Natives have the highest rate among women 30-54 years and 70 years and older. Non-Hispanic white rates are highest among women in the 55-69 year old age group.

The male-to-female ratio of age-adjusted cancer incidence rates ranges from a low of 1.1 for Alaska Natives, Hawaiians, and American Indians in New Mexico to a high of 1.7 for blacks. For Koreans, the ratio is also relatively high, at 1.5. Among the remaining racial/ethnic groups, the male-to-female rate ratio ranges from 1.2 (Filipinos and Vietnamese) to 1.4 (non-Hispanic whites). Women have higher incidence rates than men in the age group 30-54 years for every racial/ethnic group. This is due to the high rates of female breast cancer and cancers of the female genital system (ovary, corpus uteri and cervix) in this age group. In the age group 55-69 years, men have higher incidence rates than women in all groups except American Indians in New Mexico.

Similar to the SEER area incidence rates, United States mortality rates are highest for blacks, non-Hispanic whites, Alaska Natives and Hawaiians, although the relative rankings among these four groups differ somewhat from the incidence rate rankings. Among men, blacks have the greatest risk of dying from cancer, whereas for women, the highest mortality rate occurs in Alaska Natives. Mortality rates are not currently available for Koreans and Vietnamese. Among groups with relatively low mortality rates, Filipino men and women rank substantially below American Indians, Japanese, Chinese and white Hispanics.

Overall cancer mortality rates shown for American Indians in New Mexico are comparable to those for all American Indians in the U.S. (125 per 100,000 in men and 88 per 100,000 in women, not shown). The New Mexico American Indian rates for specific cancers, however, are not necessarily representative of those for American Indians living in other regions of the country. Researchers have noted that rates for cancers of the lung and bronchus, colon and rectum, and female breast are substantially lower among southwestern tribes than among northern and eastern tribes (NIH Publication No. 93-3603, 1993). Regional variations in cancer rates also occur for the other racial/ethnic groups. Differences in the rates between the racial/ ethnic groups remain important, however, and are the focus of this report.

Mortality rates by age show patterns similar to the incidence rates with a few exceptions. In contrast to the incidence patterns by age, cancer mortality rates among men in the age groups 55-69 years and 70 years and older are higher in Alaska Native men than in white men. In women aged 55-69 years, mortality among Alaska Natives exceeds that for whites, unlike the incidence pattern. Otherwise, the racial/ethnic mortality patterns by age group are generally similar to those for incidence.

The incidence-to-mortality rate ratios for Filipinos are 2.6 for men and 3.6 for women, higher than those for any other group studied. High incidence-to-mortality ratios may reflect high survival of cancer patients. Conversely, low incidence-to-mortality ratios may reflect high case fatality. High incidence-to-mortality ratios may also result when death certificates are never located through long-term follow-up of persons diagnosed with cancer (e.g., if persons diagnosed with cancer leave the country). Another possibility is that deaths within a particular racial/ethnic group may be under ascertained due to misclassification of race/ethnicity information on the death certificate. The low incidence-to-mortality rate ratios in Hawaiian men (1.4), American Indian men (1.6) and women (1.8), Alaska Native men (1.7), and black men (1.8) likely reflect higher case fatality rates in these groups.

SEER INCIDENCE Rates, 1988-1992

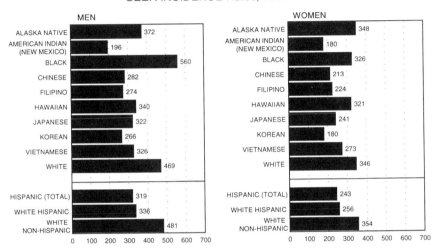

MEN

ALASKA NATIVE	372
AMERICAN INDIAN (NEW MEXICO)	196
BLACK	560
CHINESE	282
FILIPINO	274
HAWAIIAN	340
JAPANESE	322
KOREAN	266
VIETNAMESE	326
WHITE	469
HISPANIC (TOTAL)	319
WHITE HISPANIC	336
WHITE NON-HISPANIC	481

0 100 200 300 400 500 600 700

WOMEN

ALASKA NATIVE	348
AMERICAN INDIAN (NEW MEXICO)	180
BLACK	326
CHINESE	213
FILIPINO	224
HAWAIIAN	321
JAPANESE	241
KOREAN	180
VIETNAMESE	273
WHITE	346
HISPANIC (TOTAL)	243
WHITE HISPANIC	256
WHITE NON-HISPANIC	354

0 100 200 300 400 500 600 700

United States MORTALITY Rates, 1988-1992

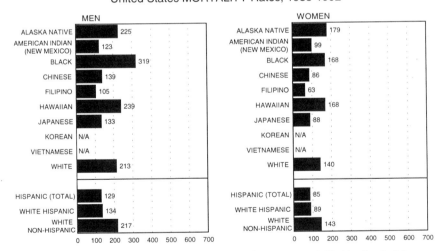

MEN

ALASKA NATIVE	225
AMERICAN INDIAN (NEW MEXICO)	123
BLACK	319
CHINESE	139
FILIPINO	105
HAWAIIAN	239
JAPANESE	133
KOREAN	N/A
VIETNAMESE	N/A
WHITE	213
HISPANIC (TOTAL)	129
WHITE HISPANIC	134
WHITE NON-HISPANIC	217

0 100 200 300 400 500 600 700

WOMEN

ALASKA NATIVE	179
AMERICAN INDIAN (NEW MEXICO)	99
BLACK	168
CHINESE	86
FILIPINO	63
HAWAIIAN	168
JAPANESE	88
KOREAN	N/A
VIETNAMESE	N/A
WHITE	140
HISPANIC (TOTAL)	85
WHITE HISPANIC	89
WHITE NON-HISPANIC	143

0 100 200 300 400 500 600 700

NOTE: Rates are "average annual" per 100,000 population, age-adjusted to 1970 U.S. standard; N/A = information not available;
★ = rate not calculated when fewer than 25 cases.

Figure 9.4a. *All Cancers Combined.*

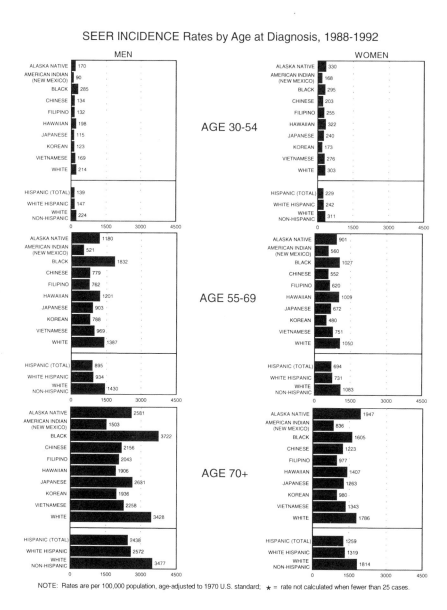

SEER INCIDENCE Rates by Age at Diagnosis, 1988-1992

MEN

	AGE 30-54
ALASKA NATIVE	170
AMERICAN INDIAN (NEW MEXICO)	90
BLACK	285
CHINESE	134
FILIPINO	132
HAWAIIAN	198
JAPANESE	115
KOREAN	123
VIETNAMESE	169
WHITE	214
HISPANIC (TOTAL)	139
WHITE HISPANIC	147
WHITE NON-HISPANIC	224

WOMEN

	AGE 30-54
ALASKA NATIVE	330
AMERICAN INDIAN (NEW MEXICO)	168
BLACK	295
CHINESE	203
FILIPINO	255
HAWAIIAN	322
JAPANESE	240
KOREAN	173
VIETNAMESE	276
WHITE	303
HISPANIC (TOTAL)	229
WHITE HISPANIC	242
WHITE NON-HISPANIC	311

MEN — AGE 55-69

ALASKA NATIVE	1180
AMERICAN INDIAN (NEW MEXICO)	521
BLACK	1832
CHINESE	779
FILIPINO	762
HAWAIIAN	1201
JAPANESE	903
KOREAN	788
VIETNAMESE	969
WHITE	1387
HISPANIC (TOTAL)	895
WHITE HISPANIC	934
WHITE NON-HISPANIC	1430

WOMEN — AGE 55-69

ALASKA NATIVE	901
AMERICAN INDIAN (NEW MEXICO)	560
BLACK	1027
CHINESE	552
FILIPINO	620
HAWAIIAN	1009
JAPANESE	672
KOREAN	480
VIETNAMESE	751
WHITE	1050
HISPANIC (TOTAL)	694
WHITE HISPANIC	731
WHITE NON-HISPANIC	1083

MEN — AGE 70+

ALASKA NATIVE	2581
AMERICAN INDIAN (NEW MEXICO)	1503
BLACK	3722
CHINESE	2156
FILIPINO	2043
HAWAIIAN	1906
JAPANESE	2631
KOREAN	1936
VIETNAMESE	2258
WHITE	3428
HISPANIC (TOTAL)	2438
WHITE HISPANIC	2572
WHITE NON-HISPANIC	3477

WOMEN — AGE 70+

ALASKA NATIVE	1947
AMERICAN INDIAN (NEW MEXICO)	836
BLACK	1605
CHINESE	1223
FILIPINO	977
HAWAIIAN	1407
JAPANESE	1263
KOREAN	980
VIETNAMESE	1343
WHITE	1786
HISPANIC (TOTAL)	1259
WHITE HISPANIC	1319
WHITE NON-HISPANIC	1814

NOTE: Rates are per 100,000 population, age-adjusted to 1970 U.S. standard; ★ = rate not calculated when fewer than 25 cases.

Figure 9.4b. *All Cancers Combined.*

United States MORTALITY Rates by Age at Death, 1988-1992

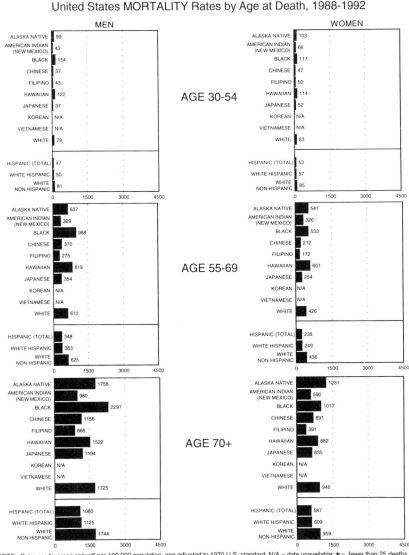

NOTE: Rates are "average annual" per 100,000 population, age-adjusted to 1970 U.S. standard; N/A = data unavailable; ★ = fewer than 25 deaths.

Figure 9.4c. All Cancers Combined.

Breast

Breast cancer is the most common form of cancer among women in the United States. The incidence of breast cancer has been rising for the past two decades, while mortality has remained relatively stable since the 1950s. Much of the increase in incidence over the past 15 years is associated with increased screening by physical examination and mammography. However, screening alone does not seem to explain all of this increase. Breast cancer occurs among both women and men, but is quite rare among men. Since the incidence rates among men are so low, there are too few cases to explore ethnic diversity. This description is limited to breast cancer among women.

The age-adjusted incidence of invasive breast cancer reveals that white, Hawaiian, and black women have the highest rates in the SEER regions. The lowest rates occur among Korean, American Indian, and Vietnamese women. The incidence rate for white non-Hispanic women is four times as high as that for the lowest group (Korean women).

In situ breast cancer occurs at much lower rates than invasive breast cancer, but has a similar racial/ethnic pattern to that for the invasive cancers. White non-Hispanic women have the highest rates, over twice the rate for Hispanic women. Rates could not be calculated for Alaska Native, American Indian, Korean, and Vietnamese women due to the small numbers of cases.

Age-specific incidence rates for invasive breast cancer present similar ethnic patterns. Among women aged 30-54 years, however, the rates among Hawaiian women are comparable to those for the white non-Hispanic women. Among women aged 55-69 years and 70 years and older, rates are highest for white, Hawaiian, and black women. In situ breast cancer incidence among women aged 30-54 years and 70 years and older is highest among white non-Hispanic women, followed by Japanese women, and white (total) women. At ages 55-69 years, in situ breast cancer is highest among white women, followed by Japanese women and black women.

Mortality rates are much lower than incidence rates for breast cancer, ranging from just 15% of the incidence rate for Japanese women to 33% of the incidence rate for black women. Racial/ethnic patterns of mortality differ slightly from those observed for incidence. The highest age adjusted mortality occurs among black women, followed by white, and Hawaiian women. The higher breast cancer mortality among black women is related to the fact that, relative to white women, a larger percentage of their breast cancers are

139

diagnosed at a later, less treatable stage. In the age groups 30-54 years and 55-69 years, black women have the highest rates, followed by Hawaiian, and white non-Hispanic women. In the 70 year and older age group, the mortality rate for white women exceeds that for black women.

Important risk factors for female breast cancer include early age at onset of menarche, late age at onset of menopause, first full-term pregnancy after age 30, a history of pre-menopausal breast cancer for mother and a sister, and a personal history of breast cancer or of benign proliferative breast disease. Obesity, nulliparity, and urban residence also have been shown to be associated with increased risk of breast cancer.

Although there are no proven methods of preventing breast cancer, randomized trials are currently underway to assess the effectiveness of tamoxifen in preventing breast cancer among high risk women and to determine whether reducing the percentage of dietary fat will reduce the incidence of breast cancer. Recent studies suggest that physical activity may have preventive potential, as well.

Cervix Uteri

Until the early 1970s, approximately 75% to 80% of cervical cancer in the United States was invasive at the time of diagnosis. Today, about 78% of cervical cancer cases are diagnosed in the in situ stage. Furthermore, both incidence and mortality for invasive cervical cancer have declined about 40% since the early 1970s. Mortality began declining just before the Papanicolaou screening test became widely utilized, however, leaving a dilemma as to the relationship between the Pap test and reductions in cervical cancer mortality. Around the world, cervical cancer is often the most common type of cancer among women.

The ethnic patterns of this disease are quite different from those of any of the other female reproductive system cancers. The highest age-adjusted incidence rate in the SEER areas occurs among Vietnamese women (43 per 100,000). Their rate is 7.4 times the lowest incidence rate, 5.8 per 100,000 in Japanese women. Incidence rates of 15 per 100,000 or higher also occur among Alaska Native, Korean, and Hispanic women.

The incidence of invasive cervical cancer exhibits different ethnic patterns by age group. Among women aged 30-54 years, Vietnamese women have the highest rate, followed by Hispanic women, and black women. The rate among Vietnamese women is nearly twice as high as that of Hispanic women, and five times as high as the rate for the group with the lowest rate, Chinese women. Vietnamese women continue to have the highest incidence of invasive cervical cancer in the age group 55-69 years, with a rate that is more than three times higher than the second ranked group, Korean women. Hispanic women have the third highest incidence in this age group, and are followed by black women. There are too few cases in the 70 and older age group to assess many of the ethnic patterns.

United States mortality rates are about 50% to 80% lower than the incidence rates. The ethnic patterns in mortality differ somewhat from those seen in incidence. Black women have the highest age-adjusted mortality rate from cervical cancer, and are followed by Hispanic women. Mortality rates are not available for comparison, however, for Vietnamese, Korean, Alaska Native or American Indian (New Mexico) women. The lowest mortality from this disease occurs among Japanese women, whose rates are less than one-fourth as high as the rates among black women. Mortality patterns by age are similar, with black women having the highest mortality in each age group. Hispanic women have the second highest mortality in the two youngest age groups, while Chinese women aged 70 years and older rank second.

The major risk factors for cervical cancer include early age at initiation of sexual activity, multiple sexual partners, infection with human papilloma virus 16, and cigarette smoking. Therefore, primary prevention is focused mainly on modification of sexual behavior and eradication of cigarette smoking. Secondary prevention occurs through screening, using the Papanicolaou test.

Colon and Rectum

Cancers of the colon and rectum are the fourth most commonly diagnosed cancers and rank second among cancer deaths in the United States. The incidence rates show wide divergence by racial/ethnic group, with rates in the Alaska Native population that are over four times as high as rates in the American Indian population (New Mexico) for both men and women. There are only minor differences, between men and women, in the order of incidence rates by racial/ethnic group. After Alaska Natives, the next highest rates in men are among Japanese, black and non-Hispanic white populations. These are followed by Chinese, Hawaiians and white Hispanics; and then Filipinos, Koreans and Vietnamese. In women, Alaska Natives are followed by black, Japanese and white non-Hispanic Americans. Next

141

are Chinese, Hawaiians, and Vietnamese; and finally white Hispanics, Koreans, and Filipinos. Incidence rates for both men and women are substantially lower among American Indians in New Mexico (18.6 per 100,000 in men, 15.3 per 100,000 in women).

In each racial/ethnic group, incidence rates for cancers of the colon and rectum among women are lower than those among men. Although the pattern of incidence rates by race/ethnicity is similar for each sex, the ratio of male-to-female rates varies. Among Filipinos and Japanese, men experience an excess of greater than 60%, while among American Indians, Alaska Natives and Vietnamese the male excess is much lower at only 13-22%. It is interesting that, although the Alaska Natives have the highest colorectal cancer incidence rates of all groups and the American Indians experience the lowest, the gender ratios of these two native American groups are similar.

Mortality patterns by race/ethnicity for cancers of the colon and rectum are similar to those for incidence, with several notable exceptions. Black, Alaska Native, and white non-Hispanic men and women, as well as Hawaiian and Japanese men, have comparatively high mortality rates. The high mortality rates among Alaska Natives and Japanese men are consistent with the high incidence rates in these groups. However, the mortality rates among white non-Hispanic and black men and women, and among Hawaiian men, appear disproportionately high.

Colon cancer accounts for 59% (Korean men) to 81% (Alaska Native men) of the combined colon and rectum cancer incidence rates. This is reflected in an racial/ethnic pattern for colon cancer incidence rates that is quite similar to the pattern for both sites combined. Incidence and mortality rates for cancers of the colon and rectum increase with age. Interestingly, the incidence rate for Hawaiian men is highest in the 55-69 year age group, and their mortality rate is second only to black men in this age group.

Migrant and other studies have provided very strong evidence that colorectal cancer risk is modifiable, and that differences in population rates may therefore be explained by lifestyle or environmental factors. Dietary factors and exercise appear to be very important. Migrants to the United States (from Japan and other countries where rates of colon and rectal cancer are lower than in the U.S.) have higher rates than do those who remain in their native country. Studies have shown that first and second generation American offspring from these migrant groups develop these cancers at rates reaching or exceeding those of the United States white population.

SEER INCIDENCE Rates, 1988-1992

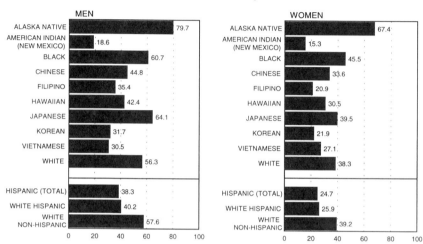

MEN | WOMEN

	MEN		WOMEN
ALASKA NATIVE	79.7	ALASKA NATIVE	67.4
AMERICAN INDIAN (NEW MEXICO)	18.6	AMERICAN INDIAN (NEW MEXICO)	15.3
BLACK	60.7	BLACK	45.5
CHINESE	44.8	CHINESE	33.6
FILIPINO	35.4	FILIPINO	20.9
HAWAIIAN	42.4	HAWAIIAN	30.5
JAPANESE	64.1	JAPANESE	39.5
KOREAN	31.7	KOREAN	21.9
VIETNAMESE	30.5	VIETNAMESE	27.1
WHITE	56.3	WHITE	38.3
HISPANIC (TOTAL)	38.3	HISPANIC (TOTAL)	24.7
WHITE HISPANIC	40.2	WHITE HISPANIC	25.9
WHITE NON-HISPANIC	57.6	WHITE NON-HISPANIC	39.2

United States MORTALITY Rates, 1988-1992

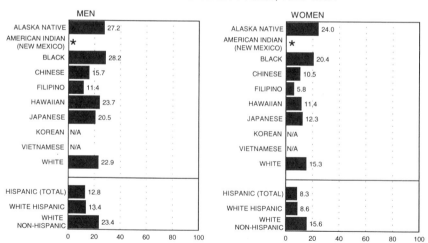

MEN | WOMEN

	MEN		WOMEN
ALASKA NATIVE	27.2	ALASKA NATIVE	24.0
AMERICAN INDIAN (NEW MEXICO)	★	AMERICAN INDIAN (NEW MEXICO)	★
BLACK	28.2	BLACK	20.4
CHINESE	15.7	CHINESE	10.5
FILIPINO	11.4	FILIPINO	5.8
HAWAIIAN	23.7	HAWAIIAN	11.4
JAPANESE	20.5	JAPANESE	12.3
KOREAN	N/A	KOREAN	N/A
VIETNAMESE	N/A	VIETNAMESE	N/A
WHITE	22.9	WHITE	15.3
HISPANIC (TOTAL)	12.8	HISPANIC (TOTAL)	8.3
WHITE HISPANIC	13.4	WHITE HISPANIC	8.6
WHITE NON-HISPANIC	23.4	WHITE NON-HISPANIC	15.6

NOTE: Rates are "average annual" per 100,000 population, age-adjusted to 1970 U.S. standard; N/A = information not available; ★ = rate not calculated when fewer than 25 cases.

Figure 9.5. Colon and Rectum Cancer Rates.

Corpus Uteri

Cancer of the corpus uteri, or endometrium, is the fourth most common cancer among women in the United States. The racial and ethnic diversity of endometrial cancer follows a pattern similar to that of breast cancer. Women with the highest age-adjusted incidence of endometrial cancer in the SEER areas include Hawaiians, whites, Japanese and blacks. The lowest rates occur among Korean, Vietnamese, and American Indian women.

Endometrial cancer increases with advancing age in most, but not all, racial/ethnic groups. Exceptions to this general pattern are Chinese and Filipino women, among whom the highest rates occur at ages 55-69 years. In younger women, ages 30-54 at diagnosis, endometrial cancer is most common among Hawaiians, Japanese, and whites. At ages 55-69 years, endometrial cancer rates are highest for white, Hawaiian, and black women. At ages 70 years and older, rates are highest among white, black, and Japanese women. There were too few cases in Hawaiian women ages 70 years and older to calculate a rate.

Age-adjusted mortality rates in the United States are highest among Hawaiian women, followed by black women. Mortality among white, Hispanic, Chinese, Japanese and Filipino women is less than one-half the rate for Hawaiian women. Age specific mortality is highest among black women in each of the three age groups (there were too few deaths among Hawaiian women to calculate rates by age). The ratio of incidence to mortality for black women is slightly over two and for Hawaiian women it is nearly three. Chinese women have incidence rates about five times higher than mortality, for white women the ratio is seven, for Japanese women it is nearly eight, and for Filipino women it is about nine. The smaller incidence-to-mortality ratios among black and Hawaiian women suggest that access to care may be a more acute problem for them.

Endometrial cancer is associated with obesity and, possibly, with abnormal glucose tolerance and diabetes. The predominant risk factor for this cancer is the use of exogenous menopausal estrogens. When menopausal estrogens are taken with progesterone, the elevation in risk is greatly reduced. Tamoxifen, a drug that is widely used to treat breast cancer, appears to have estrogen-like effects on the uterus, and may also be associated with increased risk of endometrial cancer. Excepting these risk factors, the epidemiology of endometrial cancer is not well defined.

Esophagus

Cancer of the esophagus is a common cancer in developing areas of the world (Asia, Africa and Latin America), but is less common in the United States. Historically, most esophaqeal cancers were squamous cell tumors. Recently, however, there has been a marked increase in adenocarcinoma of the esophagus, primarily among white men in developed countries of the world, including the United States. In fact, among white men, rates of adenocarcinoma of the esophagus nearly equal those of squamous cell tumors.

There is a five-fold range in the age-adjusted incidence rates for esophageal cancer among the racial/ethnic groups in the SEER regions. Men are three to five times more likely than women to be diagnosed with esophageal cancer. Among men, blacks have the highest rate (15.0 per 100,000) and Filipinos have the lowest (2.9 per 100,000). The incidence rate for black men is 60% higher than that for Hawaiians and more than 2.7 times greater than the rate for non-Hispanic white men. The rates for Chinese, Japanese and non-Hispanic white men are similar to each other (within the range of 5.3 to 5.6 per 100,000 men) and are modestly higher than the rate for white Hispanic men. Limited data are available for women. Hispanic and non-Hispanic white women have lower rates than black women. Incidence rates generally increase with age in all racial/ethnic groups. In black men, however, the incidence rate for the 55-69 year age group is close to the rate for the 70 and over age group. In black women aged 55-69 years, the incidence rate is slightly higher than for the 70 years and older age group.

United States mortality rates for esophageal cancer are nearly as high as incidence rates in the SEER regions, reflecting the generally poor survival for patients with this cancer. Among black and Hawaiian populations, the incidence-to-mortality rate ratio is less than 1.1. It is 1.1 for non-Hispanic whites, Japanese and Filipinos and 1.3 for Chinese and white Hispanics. Mortality patterns by age are similar to those seen in the incidence rates.

Heavy alcohol consumption, cigarette smoking, and, possibly, other types of tobacco use each substantially increase the risk of esophageal cancer among persons in developed countries. The use of tobacco and alcohol, in combination, results in even larger elevations in risk. In developing countries, nutritional deficiencies related to lack of fresh fruit and vegetables, drinking hot beverages, and a range of chewing and smoking habits are also important risk factors.

Kaposi's Sarcoma

Kaposi's sarcoma is a soft tissue sarcoma that was rarely diagnosed in the United States before the AIDS epidemic. It occurs primarily on the skin but may also be found in other parts of the body such as the oral cavity, esophagus, and anal canal. A small number of cases occur in organs such as the lung and stomach. Rates reported here are for all cases of Kaposi's sarcoma, regardless of the site or organ in which the disease arose. Patients with multiple skin lesions are reported only once. Mortality data for this cancer are not separately identifiable through current conventional mortality coding practices.

Age-adjusted incidence rates are calculated only for white, black, and Hispanic populations and for Filipino men due to small numbers of cases in other groups. Rates among white, black and Hispanic men are essentially equal, 5.7 to 5.9 per 100,000, while the rate among Filipino men is lower, at 1.8. Rates among women are negligible, 0.3 or less, and are not shown. Incidence rates for Kaposi's sarcoma are highest in the youngest age group (20-54 years), are considerably lower in 55-69 year age group and remain low in the 70 year and older age group.

In the age group 20-54 years, Kaposi's sarcoma is most frequently diagnosed among persons who test positive for the human immunovirus (HIV). In fact, Kaposi's sarcoma is currently such a widely recognized part of the AIDS sequelae that the incidence may be under reported because skin lesions are easily recognizable to the naked eye, may not be biopsied for pathologic confirmation, and therefore, may not be reported to a cancer registry. Before the AIDS epidemic, Kaposi's sarcoma was most commonly diagnosed in older white men of eastern European and middle eastern origin.

Kidney and Pelvis

Historically, incidence rates for kidney cancer have included cancers of the renal cells (in the main part of the kidney) and the renal pelvis (the lower part of the kidney where urine collects before entering the ureter and continuing to the bladder), although there is evidence that these cancers have different characteristics. They are presented together here for continuity. About one of five kidney cancers occur in the renal pelvis. Internationally, the highest incidence rates occur in the United States, Canada, Northern Europe, Australia, and New Zealand. The lowest rates are in Thailand, China, and the Philippines. Rates in these countries are about one-third the rates in the high risk countries.

During the years 1988 to 1992, in the SEER regions, the incidence rates for kidney cancers are about twice as high in men as in women. The highest rates in the SEER regions are in American Indian men in New Mexico. Rates are somewhat lower in blacks, Hispanics and white non-Hispanics (ranging from 10 to 13 per 100,000 for men and about six per 100,000 for women). The lowest incidence rates occur in the Asian populations. There were too few cases among Alaska Native and Vietnamese populations to calculate rates. Age-specific incidence rates for kidney cancer demonstrate a small, temporary peak in early childhood due to Wilm's tumor, an uncommon tumor of the kidney with a good prognosis. Rates then decline with age and remain low until they finally surpass the early peak at around age 40. The racial/ethnic patterns for ages 55-69 years and 70 years and over are similar to those for all ages combined. In the 30-54 year old age group, racial/ethnic differences are slight.

Kidney cancer has a relatively high mortality rate in all racial/ethnic populations. Following the incidence pattern, mortality rates are about twice as high in men as in women, regardless of age. There are too few deaths among American Indian (New Mexico), Alaska Native and Hawaiian populations to calculate reliable rates. Mortality rates for blacks are comparable to those for white non-Hispanics. Rates for the other races are lower. In all racial/ethnic groups the mortality rates increase with age.

Cancers of the kidney and renal pelvis share many risk factors although the strengths of the associations differ. For both types of cancer the only well-established risk factor is cigarette smoking. Compared to nonsmokers, smokers have about twice the risk for renal cell cancer and about four times the risk for renal pelvis cancer than nonsmokers. Other probable risk factors include obesity and, especially for cancer of the renal pelvis, heavy long-term use of analgesics (medications used to relieve pain). Cessation of cigarette smoking is the best single step in preventing these cancers. It is estimated that this measure alone would reduce by one-half the number of renal pelvis cancers and by one-third the number of renal cell cancers.

Larynx

Laryngeal cancer is relatively rare in the United States. Age-adjusted incidence rates for laryngeal cancer are not calculated for all population groups in the SEER regions due to the small number of cases in several categories, especially among women. Rates (per 100,000) among men range from a low of 2.4 among Filipinos, 2.5 in

Japanese and 2 8 in Chinese to a high of 12.7 in blacks. Rates for whites and Hispanics are intermediate. Laryngeal cancer is much less common in women, with rates ranging from a low of 0.7 among Hispanics to a high of 2.5 among blacks. Rates for white women fall between these two extremes at 1.5. The male-to-female ratio of the incidence rates is approximately five to one for blacks and whites and seven to one for Hispanics. Laryngeal cancer is uncommon in the youngest age group. Incidence rates are similar in the two older age groups, 55-69 years and 70 years and older. Within each broad age group, the incidence rate for blacks exceeds the rates for whites and Hispanics.

Age-adjusted laryngeal cancer mortality rates follow the same racial/ethnic patterns as those for incidence. Mortality rates are calculated for only a few groups, however, because of small numbers of deaths. As seen in the incidence rates, mortality rates by age group tend to be highest in black populations. An exception is the comparable mortality rate for both white women and black women aged 70 years and older.

Fortunately, the symptoms of laryngeal cancer are usually recognized early in the course of the disease leading to early treatment. Among men, incidence-to-mortality rate ratios are approximately three for whites and Hispanics, and are slightly lower for blacks at 2.3. Among women there is more consistency with each group having ratios of approximately three.

Smoking is the most important cause of laryngeal cancer, and risk is compounded with alcohol use. Risk is the highest among heavy smokers who are also heavy users of alcohol. Occupational exposures to asbestos and to some chemicals and dusts have been reported to increase the risk of cancer of the larynx, although these relationships have not been found consistently in all studies and are likely to account for only a small fraction of all laryngeal cancer cases.

Leukemias

Leukemias are cancers of the blood-forming tissues. They may be subdivided according to the particular cell type involved, the major types being lymphocytic and myelocytic (granulocytic) leukemias. Leukemias are also classified by their behavior, as either "acute" or "chronic." Childhood leukemias are mostly acute, with the lymphocytic form predominating. Both acute and chronic leukemias occur among adults; most lymphocytic leukemias among adults are chronic.

In both men and women, leukemia incidence is highest among whites and lowest among Chinese, Japanese, and Koreans. Incidence rates are shown for all leukemia types combined, but it can be noted that the ethnic patterns are generally similar to those seen when incidence is calculated separately for the lymphocytic and non-lymphocytic forms of the disease. The incidence in men is about 50% higher than in women for all racial/ethnic groups except Vietnamese, among whom the male rates are only slightly higher. Ethnic differences in the incidence rates are small in the youngest adult age group (30-54 years), but become more evident in each of the older age groups. Data for childhood leukemia (0-14 years) are not shown separately in the figures. However, we found that childhood leukemia rates are highest among Filipinos, followed by white Hispanics, non-Hispanic whites and blacks. Reliable rates could not be computed for children in the remaining racial/ethnic groups.

United States mortality rates are shown for all leukemia types combined. The mortality rates for men are generally 50% to 100% higher than those for women for all ages combined, ages 55-69 years and ages 70 years and older. Leukemia mortality rates are highest in white and black populations and in Hawaiian men. Rates among Asian populations are noticeably lower. The ratio of mortality-to-incidence rates is higher for adult leukemias than for childhood leukemias. Because treatment for childhood leukemias is quite successful, mortality from this cancer is comparatively low among children.

Established causes of leukemia include ionizing radiation (such as occurs from x-irradiation), certain drugs used in the treatment of cancer, and some chemicals (most notably benzene) used largely in industrial settings. Ionizing radiation has been associated with all forms of leukemia except the chronic lymphocytic form. It is suspected that many childhood leukemias may result from parental exposures before the time of conception or during early fetal development. cancers of the liver.

Liver and Intrahepatic Bile Duct

Primary and intrahepatic bile ducts are far more common in regions of Africa and Asia than in the United States, where they only account for about 1.5% of all cancer cases. Five-year survival rates are very low in the United States, usually less than 10%. Reported statistics for these cancers often include mortality rates that equal or exceed the incidence rates. This discrepancy (more deaths than cases) occurs when the cause of death is misclassified as "liver cancer" for some patients whose cancer originated as a primary cancer in another organ and spread (metastasized) to become a "secondary" cancer in the liver.

Non-Hispanic white men and women have the lowest age-adjusted incidence rates (SEER areas) and mortality rates (United States) for primary liver cancer. Rates in the black populations and Hispanic populations are roughly twice as high as the rates in whites. The highest incidence rate is in Vietnamese men (41.8 per 100,000), probably reflecting risks associated with the high prevalence of viral hepatitis infections in their homeland. Other Asian-American groups also have liver cancer incidence and mortality rates several times higher than the white population. Age-adjusted mortality rates among Chinese populations are the highest of all groups for which there are sufficient numbers to calculate rates. There were too few cases among Alaska Native and American Indian populations to calculate incidence or mortality rates. Most cases of liver cancer occur in the two older age groups, but younger adults are often affected in the high risk racial/ethnic groups.

About two-thirds of liver cancers are hepatocellular carcinomas (HCC), which is the cancer type most clearly associated with hepatitis B and hepatitis C viral infections and cirrhosis. Certain molds that grow on stored foods are recognized risk factors in parts of Africa and Asia. HCC occurs more frequently in men than in women by a ratio of two-to-one. About one-in-five liver cancers are cholangiocarcinomas, arising from branches of the bile ducts that are located within the liver. Certain liver parasites are recognized risk factors for this type of liver cancer, especially in parts of southeast Asia. Angiosarcomas are rare cancers that can arise from blood vessels, including the blood vessels within the liver. They account for about 1% of primary liver cancers and some of them have been associated with industrial exposures to vinyl chloride.

Lung and Bronchus

Cancer of the lung and bronchus (hereafter, lung cancer) is the second most common cancer among both men and women and is the leading cause of cancer death in both sexes. Among men age-adjusted lung cancer incidence rates (per 100,000) range from a low of about 14 among American Indians to a high of 117 among blacks, an eightfold difference. Between these two extremes, rates fall into two groups ranging from 42 to 53 for Hispanics, Japanese, Chinese, Filipinos, and Koreans and from 71 to 89 for Vietnamese, whites, Alaska Natives and Hawaiians. The range among women is much narrower, from a rate of about 15 among Japanese to nearly 51 among Alaska Natives, only a three-fold difference. Rates for the remaining female populations fall roughly into two groups with low rates of 16 to 25 for Korean, Filipino, Hispanic and Chinese women, and rates of 31 to 44 among Vietnamese, white, Hawaiian and black women. The rates among men are about two to three times greater than the rates among women in each of the racial/ethnic groups.

In the 30-54 year age group, incidence rates among men are double those among women in most of the racial/ethnic groups. In white non-Hispanics and white Hispanics, however incidence rates for women are closer to those for men. This suggests that smoking cessation and prevention programs may have been especially successful among white men and/or that such programs have not been as effective among white women.

Age-adjusted mortality rates follow similar racial/ethnic patterns to those for the incidence rates. Among men, the incidence and mortality rates are very similar. Filipino men are an exception, with an incidence rate nearly twice as large as their mortality rate. Incidence rates are also similar to mortality rates among women, with the exception of Filipinos and Hispanics. In these two groups, incidence rates are nearly twice as large as mortality rates. Among Hawaiian women, the mortality rate actually exceeds the incidence rate. This may be due to differences in the accuracy of race classification on medical records versus death certificates.

Racial/ethnic patterns are generally consistent within each age group for both incidence and mortality. An exception is the high incidence and mortality rate in Chinese women aged 70 years and older. This group tends to have low incidence and mortality rates in the younger age groups.

Cigarette smoking accounts for nearly 90% of all lung cancers. Passive smoking also contributes to the development of lung cancer among nonsmokers. Certain occupational exposures such as asbestos exposure are also known to cause lung cancer. Air pollution is a probable cause, but makes a relatively small contribution to incidence and mortality rates. In certain geographic areas of the United States, indoor exposure to radon may also make a small contribution to the total incidence of lung cancer.

Lymphomas

Lymphomas, which include Hodgkin's disease and non-Hodgkin's lymphoma, are the fifth most common type of cancer diagnosed and the sixth most common cancer cause of death in the United States.

Of the two basic lymphoma types, non-Hodgkin's lymphoma is the more common and will be discussed first.

Non-Hodgkin's Lymphoma

The age-adjusted incidence rates for non-Hodgkin's lymphoma are higher among men than women in every racial/ethnic group except Koreans, in which there is a slight preponderance among women. In both men and women, non-Hodgkin's lymphoma incidence rates are highest among non-Hispanic whites (19.1 and 12.0 per 100,000 men and women, respectively) and lowest among Koreans (5.8 and 6.0 per 100,000). This corresponds to a high to low ratio of the rates (white non-Hispanic to Korean) of 3.3 for men, and 2.0 for women. Vietnamese men have the second highest rates (after whites), followed by white Hispanic, black, Filipino, Hawaiian, Chinese and Japanese men. There were too few cases diagnosed in Alaska Native and American Indian (New Mexico) men to calculate reliable rates. Among women, white Hispanics accounted for the second highest rates, followed by Filipino, Japanese, black and Chinese women. There are insufficient numbers of lymphoma cases diagnosed in Alaska Native, American Indian (New Mexico), Hawaiian and Vietnamese women to estimate their rates reliably.

Age-adjusted mortality rates of non-Hodgkin's lymphoma are consistent with the incidence rates with one exception: the mortality rate for Hawaiian men (8.8 per 100,000) exceeds that of any other group, even though the corresponding incidence rate is considerably lower than that of white non-Hispanics. There are an insufficient number of deaths from non-Hodgkin's lymphoma among Hawaiian women to reliably asses the mortality rate for that group.

In every group, incidence rates increase with age, however the magnitude of this increase varies by racial/ethnic group. For example, from ages 30-54 years to ages 70 years and older, the incidence of non-Hodgkin's lymphoma increases about fivefold among white non-Hispanic men, but 11-fold among Filipino men. Among women, the comparable rates increase eight-fold among white non-Hispanics, but 16-fold among Filipinos. These differences reflect high incidence rates among older Filipinos, similar to those of white non-Hispanics. These high rates are not reflected, however, in the mortality data for Filipinos. Among those aged 30-54 years rates among black men and women are close to those among white non-Hispanics. Rates among black men and women aged 70 years and older, however, are only about one-half those of white non-Hispanics.

Hodgkin's Disease

Hodgkin's disease is considerably less common than non-Hodgkin's lymphoma. As a result, reliable incidence and mortality rates are available only for black, Hispanic and white populations. In both men and women, overall age-adjusted incidence rates are highest among white non-Hispanics, and considerably lower in black and Hispanic populations. Incidence rates are higher in men, compared to women, in each racial/ethnic group.

Among women 30-54 years of age, Hodgkin's disease rates are highest in the white non-Hispanic population, slightly lower in the black population, and considerably lower among Hispanics. Only in the white population are reliable rates available in the other age groups. Rates among white non-Hispanic women aged 70 years and older are about 50% greater than in the two younger groups. The rates among black men and white non-Hispanic men are similar in both the 30-54 and 55-69 year age groups. The rate in white Hispanic men aged 55-69 years (5.1 per 100,000), however, is almost double that of the younger white Hispanics (2.7 per 100,000) Rates for men over age 70 years are available only for the white population and are about one-third higher than those for the younger age groups.

Risk factors for both Hodgkin's disease and non-Hodgkin's lymphomas are largely unknown. Altered immune function, whether due to exposure to specific viruses (such as HIV and HTLV-I), or due to other causes, clearly puts people at higher risk. Herbicides and other chemicals may also increase the risk of these diseases.

Melanoma

Malignant melanoma incidence rates show substantial international variation. This variation is related to racial composition and the intensity of sunlight exposure in different geographic areas. Rates are low in races with the most skin pigmentation, such as blacks and Asians, and are high in whites. Among whites, rates are lowest in England and Scotland, about twice as high in the United States, Canada, Norway, Switzerland, and Israel and about four times higher in Australia and New Zealand. In almost every white population, but especially in Australia and the United States, malignant melanoma incidence rates have been increasing faster than nearly every other cancer. In the SEER regions, the incidence of this cancer increased rapidly during the 1970's and less so in the late 1980's. This suggests that rates may become more stable in the future.

During 1988 to 1992, there are very few cases of malignant melanoma among nonwhites, so incidence rates are very low and for many races the rates could not be calculated. Among whites, age-adjusted incidence rates are over five times higher in non-Hispanic compared to Hispanic men and over three times higher in non-Hispanic women compared to Hispanics.

The incidence rates among whites increase with age in both men and women. The size of this increase is over three-fold in men and only 62% in women. In the 30-54 year age group the difference in the rates between men and women is small. Incidence rates are nearly twice as high in men aged 55-69 years, however, and 2.3 times higher in men 70 years of age or older. Mortality rates are about 20% of the incidence rates and show a similar pattern by race (where rates can be calculated), sex, and age.

The anatomic distribution of malignant melanoma differs for men and women. Men are more likely to have melanoma on the head, neck and trunk and women are more likely to have melanoma on the lower limbs. Among white populations, the risk for malignant melanoma is highest for fair-skinned people, especially those who lack the ability to tan when exposed to sun. Risk is also higher for individuals with the highest concentration of moles on the body. The process by which sunlight is associated with the development of the disease is not well understood. However, the increasing incidence of the disease seems related to increases in voluntary sun exposure and the use of tanning devices. There is also some indication that severe burning or strong intermittent exposure, especially in childhood, may be especially high risk patterns for the disease. An excess of this cancer has been reported in family members of cases, but it is not clear if this is due to inherited genes or due to common skin type or sun exposure patterns. Currently the most established method to prevent the disease is to avoid sun exposure through use of sun screens or protective clothing when in the sun.

Ovary

Among women in the United States, cancer of the ovary ranks fifth in incidence. There are no proven methods of prevention and it often is a rapidly fatal disease.

Age-adjusted incidence rates in the SEER areas are highest among American Indian women, followed by white, Vietnamese, white Hispanic, and Hawaiian women. Rates are lowest among Korean and Chinese women. There are too few cases among Alaska Native women to calculate an incidence rate. Among women for whom there are sufficient numbers of cases to calculate rates by age, incidence in the age group 30-54 years is highest in whites, followed by Japanese, Hispanics, and Filipinos. For ages 55-69 years, the highest rates occur in whites, then Hispanics, and Japanese. Among women 70 and older, the highest rate occurs among white women followed by black and Hispanic women.

The ovarian cancer mortality patterns by racial/ethnic group differ from the incidence patterns. The age-adjusted mortality rate is highest among white women, followed by Hawaiian women, and black women. White women have the highest age-specific ovarian cancer mortality rate in each of the three age groups. The ratio of incidence to mortality rates ranges from 1.5 among black women to 3.0 among Filipino women.

Although the epidemiology of ovarian cancer is not well understood, hormonal and reproductive risk factors are implicated in the etiology of this disease. There is an inverse relationship between parity and the occurrence of ovarian cancer, with parous women having the lowest risk of this disease. The risk of cancer of the ovary also decreases with increasing length of use of oral contraceptives and there is some suggestion of a protective effect of hysterectomy.

Pancreas

Cancer of the pancreas stands out as a highly lethal disease with the poorest likelihood of survival among all of the major malignancies. It accounts for only 2% of all newly diagnosed cancers in the United States each year but 5% of all cancer deaths. Most pancreatic cancers are adenocarcinomas arising from the pancreatic ductal system. The disease is often far advanced by the time symptoms occur and the diagnosis is established. As indicated by five-year survival rates of less than 5%, successful treatment is rare. Islet cell carcinomas have a better prognosis, but account for less than 2% of all pancreatic cancers. Relatively few cancers arise from the enzyme-producing acinar (glandular) cells that form the bulk of the pancreas.

Men have higher incidence and mortality rates for pancreatic cancer than women in each racial/ethnic group. Black men and women have incidence and mortality rates that are about 50% higher than the rates for whites. Rates for native Hawaiians are somewhat higher than the rates for whites, whereas rates for Hispanics and the Asian-American groups are generally lower. There were too few cases among Alaska Native and American Indian populations to calculate rates.

Pancreatic cancer is rare in the 30-54 years age group. In the 55-69 years age group, incidence rates in the black populations exceed those for whites by about 60%. This difference diminishes somewhat among persons aged 70 years and older. Incidence rates for Japanese men and women exceed those for the white population in the oldest age group. Racial/ethnic patterns in mortality rates by age group closely follow those seen in the incidence rates.

Cigarette smoking has been identified consistently as an important risk factor for cancer of the pancreas. Other risk factors which have been suggested, but not confirmed include coffee drinking, high fat diets, diabetes mellitus and some occupations.

Prostate

Prostate cancer is the leading cancer diagnosed among men in the United States. However, racial/ethnic variations in the SEER data are striking: the incidence rate among black men (180.6 per 100,000) is more than seven times that among Koreans (24.2). Indeed, blacks in the U.S. have the highest rates of this cancer in the world. Although the incidence among whites is quite high, it is distinctly lower than among blacks. Asian and native American men have the lowest rates. The very low rate in Korean men probably reflects the fact that most of the Koreans in the SEER areas are recent immigrants from Asia, where rates are lower than in the United States.

Age-specific incidence rates show dramatic increases between age categories. The remarkably sharp increase in incidence with age is a hallmark of this cancer. Sixty percent of all newly diagnosed prostate cancer cases and almost 80% of all deaths occur in men 70 years of age and older. Mortality rates for prostate cancer are much lower than the incidence rates, because survival for men with this cancer is generally quite high.

Prostate cancer incidence has been increasing rapidly in recent years. Most of this increase has been attributed to the greater use of screening modalities, and especially the widespread introduction of the prostate-specific antigen (PSA) test. The causes of prostate cancer are not known. Men with a family history of prostate cancer are at increased risk, but whether this is genetic or due to shared environmental influences, or both, is not known. It is thought that whatever the causal factors are, they act by altering the balance of male hormones in the body. Some research has suggested that diets high in fat and red meats increase risk, while a high intake of fruits and vegetables may offer some protection. There is current interest in the possibility that the low risk of prostate cancer in certain Asian populations may result from their high intake of soy products.

156

SEER INCIDENCE Rates Among Men, 1988-1992

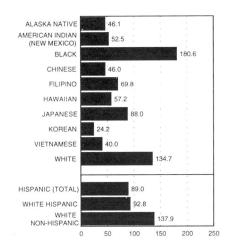

United States MORTALITY Rates Among Men, 1988-1992

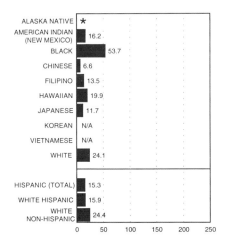

NOTE: Rates are "average annual" per 100,000 population, age-adjusted to 1970 U.S. standard; N/A = information not available;
★ = rate not calculated when fewer than 25 cases.

Figure 9.6a. *Prostate Cancer, 1988-1992.*

SEER INCIDENCE Rates Among Men by Age at Diagnosis, 1988-1992

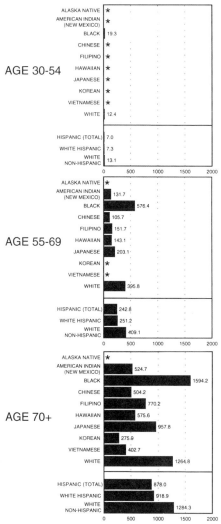

NOTE: Rates are per 100,000 population, age-adjusted to 1970 U.S. standard; ★ = rate not calculated when fewer than 25 cases.

Figure 9.6b. Prostate Cancer, 1988-1992.

United States MORTALITY Rates Among Men by Age at Death, 1988-1992

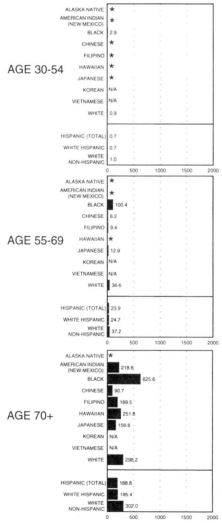

NOTE: Rates are "average annual" per 100,000 population, age-adjusted to 1970 U.S. standard; N/A = data unavailable; ★ = fewer than 25 deaths.

Figure 9.6c. *Prostate Cancer, 1988-1992.*

159

Stomach

Stomach cancer was the most common form of cancer in the world in the 1970s and early 1980s, and is probably now only surpassed by lung cancer. Stomach cancer incidence rates show substantial variation internationally. Rates are highest in Japan and eastern Asia, but other areas of the world have high stomach cancer incidence rates including eastern Europe and parts of Latin America. Incidence rates are generally lower in western Europe and the United States. Stomach cancer incidence and mortality rates have been declining for several decades in most areas of the world. For one subsite of the stomach, the cardia, incidence rates appear to be increasing, particularly among white men.

Stomach cancer incidence rates for the racial/ethnic populations in the SEER regions can be grouped broadly into three levels. Those with high age-adjusted incidence rates are Koreans, Vietnamese, Japanese, Alaska Natives and Hawaiians. Those with intermediate incidence rates are white Hispanic, Chinese, and black populations. Filipinos and non-Hispanic whites have substantially lower incidence rates than the other groups. These patterns hold for both men and women when rates are available for both sexes.

The incidence rate for Korean men is 1.6 times the rate in Japanese men, the group with the second highest rate, and is 2.4 times the rate in Hawaiians. The range in incidence rates is narrower among the groups in the intermediate level. The incidence rate for Korean men is nearly 5.8 times greater than the rate in Filipino men, the group with the lowest incidence rate. Among women, the highest incidence rate is in the Vietnamese population and is nearly 6.6 times greater than the rate in non-Hispanic whites. The male-to-female ratio of age-adjusted incidence rates is highest for Koreans (2.6) and followed closely by non-Hispanic whites and blacks (2.5 and 2.4, respectively). The ratio is less than two for other racial-ethnic groups. Notably, the incidence rates for Vietnamese men and women are the same.

The racial/ethnic patterns of stomach cancer mortality in the United States are similar to those for incidence. These patterns remain when incidence and mortality rates are calculated for the three age groups. There are some differences in the ratios of incidence rates to mortality rates. Filipinos show relatively high ratios of incidence to mortality (greater than 2); Japanese, Alaska Natives, white Hispanics. Chinese, and non-Hispanic whites show intermediate ratios (1.5-1.9); blacks and Hawaiians show low ratios of incidence to mortality rates (1.0-1.4).

Better techniques for food preservation and storage are often cited as reasons for the decline in stomach cancer incidence worldwide. Refrigeration has resulted in lower intake of salted, smoked and pickled foods and greater availability of fresh fruits and vegetables. Evidence is strong that salt intake is a major determinant of stomach cancer risk. Cigarette smoking may also play a role. Infection with helicobacter pylori, the major cause of chronic active gastritis, also appears to be important in the development of stomach cancer.

Cancer Control in Minority and Underserved Populations

Cancer affects various population subgroups in the United States in distinct ways. The statistics in this monograph show that black men have the highest incidence rate of cancer, due to excesses of prostate and lung and bronchus cancers, while American Indian men in New Mexico have the lowest rate. Among women, non-Hispanic white women have the highest incidence rate, due mainly to their excess of breast cancer, while American Indian women in New Mexico and Korean women have the lowest rates. Interestingly, the five most commonly diagnosed cancers among men in every racial/ethnic group include lung and bronchus, prostate and colorectal cancers. Oral cancers, however, are among the five most frequently diagnosed cancers only in black men and cancers of the kidney and renal pelvis are uniquely among the top five cancers in Alaska Native and American Indian (New Mexico) men. In women, cancer of the breast, lung and bronchus, and colon and rectum are among the top five cancers in every racial/ethnic group except American Indians (New Mexico). The high incidence of cervical cancer in Vietnamese women is a matter for concern and suggests a need to focus prevention and control efforts on this group. Cancers of the kidney and renal pelvis are uniquely high in Alaska Native women, mirroring the high rates seen in Alaska Native men.

Achieving better cancer control within minority and underserved populations in the United States is an important goal of the National Cancer Institute (NCI). Cancer control has been defined as the reduction of cancer incidence, mortality, and morbidity through an ordered sequence of research and interventions designed to alter cancer rates. Knowledge gained through research on specific interventions to improve cancer rates must be applied toward reducing the burden of cancer among minority populations. Specific activities supported by the NCI, include: 1) cancer surveillance, including special tracking of cancer rates among minority populations; 2) recruiting members of minority populations into clinical trials; 3) increasing and improving research targeting minority populations and increasing the participation of members of minority populations in the fields of biomedical research and medical practice; and 4) instituting community-based national education and outreach initiatives which target specific minority and underserved populations.

Cancer Surveillance

Cancer surveillance encompasses the collection, analysis and dissemination of data useful in the prevention, diagnosis, and treatment of cancer. As described in the introduction to this monograph, the SEER Program collects and reports statistics on the impact of cancer on major racial/ethnic populations in the United States. Since the composition of the United States population has changed over time, the SEER Program has adjusted its coverage of specific population subgroups to meet new needs. In 1992, to increase its coverage of minority populations, especially Hispanics, the SEER Program expanded to include Los Angeles County and the San Jose/Monterey area in California. The need for increased coverage of Hispanics arose from the tremendous influx of Hispanics into the United States during the last decade.

Recruitment to Clinical Trials

Applicants for clinical research grants and cooperative agreements from the NCI are required to include minority group representation in their study populations. Each proposal must address racial, ethnic and gender issues in the overall research design, in the rationale for the selection of the proposed study population, and in sample size calculations. Applicants are urged to carefully assess the feasibility of including the broadest possible representation of minority groups. In accordance with this policy, the representation of black, Hispanic and white populations in NCI-sponsored cancer treatment trials has closely paralleled the incident burden of disease in these groups. In some instances, minority population accrual to treatment trials has exceeded proportionality. Although there has also been a small increase in the participation of minority populations in cancer prevention trials due to outreach efforts by the NCI, these groups remain largely underrepresented in such studies. Additional efforts are needed to improve minority group participation in cancer prevention trials with the goal of reaching levels seen in treatment trials.

Research and Education

It is particularly important to direct the benefits from cancer prevention, early detection, and treatment toward minority and/or underserved populations that traditionally experience a heavy burden of cancer. The Special Populations Studies Branch of the Division of Cancer Prevention and Control, NCI currently funds four programs whose objectives are to increase research addressing the etiology, prevention, control and treatment of cancer in minority populations in the United States and to increase the pool of minority researchers. The long term goal of these programs is to reduce cancer rates in minority populations. The four programs are: the National Cancer Control Research Network; the National Hispanic Cancer Control Research Network; the Network for Cancer Control Research Among American Indian and Alaska Native Populations; and the Native Hawaiian and American Samoan Cancer Control Network. The Science Enrichment Program, an educational program aimed at encouraging minority high school students to pursue biomedical careers, is an example of a successful NCI-supported program to increase the potential pool of minority investigators.

Community-Based Outreach Initiatives

The Special Populations Studies Branch supports two outreach programs which use lay and professional leaders and coalitions to help reduce the risks of cancer among specific groups of Americans in their respective communities. These are: 1) The National Black Leadership Initiative on Cancer; and 2) The National Hispanic Leadership Initiative on Cancer. The Appalachian Leadership Initiative on Cancer is an outreach program sponsored by the Public Health Applications Research Branch, NCI. This project targets a specific geographic area, namely rural, low-income residents of the Appalachian region, rather than a racial/ethnic group.

Chapter 10

Health Status Indicators: Differentials by Race and Hispanic Origin

Introduction

The Centers for Disease Control and Prevention introduced a set of health status indicators in 1990 in response to a need for health status measures that present a broad overview of health and can be used by various levels of government. The indicators include 18 measures of health status and/or factors that put individuals at increased risk of disease or premature mortality. The development and definition of the indicators and the national data used to measure them are described in previous Statistical Notes.

One of the three broad goals of Healthy People 2000 is to reduce health disparities among Americans, including disparities between race and ethnic groups. In 1994, Committee 22.1, a group of health professionals who established the Health Status Indicators, recommended that, when possible, States and localities should analyze the indicators for each of the major population groups in their jurisdictions. Production of State and local reports by race and ethnicity is encouraged. The first part of this Statistical Note presents updates for previously published trends for the Health Status Indicators for the total population. The second part presents comparisons by race and Hispanic origin using the most recent national data. The final section provides a discussion of data issues relating to race and ethnicity.

Statistical Notes, DHHS Publication No. (PHS) 95-1237, September 1995.

Table 10.1. Health Status Indicators by Race and Hispanic Origin: United States, 1992.

Health status indicators	Total[1]	Race				
		White	Black	American Indian/ Alaska native	Asian/ Pacific islander	Hispanic origin[2]
1 Race/ethnicity-specific infant mortality as measured by the rate (per 1,000 live births) of deaths among infants under one year of age	8.5	6.9	16.8	---	---	---
Linked birth and infant death data[3]	8.6	7.1	16.6	11.3	5.8	[7]7.1
2 Total deaths per 100,000 population. (ICD-9 nos. 0-E999)[5]	504.5	477.5	767.5	453.1	285.8	[8]380.6
3 Motor vehicle crash deaths per 100,000 population. (ICD-9 nos. E810-E825)[5]	15.8	15.9	16.3	32.0	9.9	[8]16.3
4 Work-related injury deaths per 100,000 population.[7,8]	3.2	3.1	2.9	3.2	2.9	3.5
5 Suicides per 100,000 population. (ICD-9 nos. E950-E959)[5]	11.1	11.8	6.9	11.0	6.0	[8]7.2
6 Homicides per 100,000 population. (ICD-9 nos. E960-E978)[5]	10.5	6.1	39.4	10.5	5.7	[8]17.6
7 Lung cancer deaths per 100,000 population. (ICD-9 no. 162)[5]	39.3	38.8	49.8	22.2	17.9	[8]14.5
8 Female breast cancer deaths per 100,000 women. (ICD-9 no. 174)[5]	21.9	21.7	27.0	11.0	9.3	[8]13.0
9 Cardiovascular disease deaths per 100,000 population. (ICD-9 nos. 390-448)[5]	180.4	172.8	265.3	132.8	107.4	[8]120.5
Heart disease deaths per 100,000 population. (ICD-9 nos. 390-398, 402, 404-429)[5]	144.3	139.2	205.4	107.1	77.8	[8]94.8
Stroke deaths per 100,000 population. (ICD-9 nos. 430-438)[5]	26.2	24.2	45.0	19.1	23.5	[8]19.3
10 Reported incidence (per 100,000 population) of acquired immunodeficiency syndrome[7,9]	31.2	[10]17.9	[10]104.2	[10]11.9	[10]7.4	[9]52.6
11 Reported incidence (per 100,000 population) of measles[7]	0.1	0.1	---	---	---	---
12 Reported incidence (per 100,000 population) of tuberculosis[7]	9.8	[10]3.6	[10]29.1	[10]14.6	[10]44.5	20.6
13 Reported incidence (per 100,000 population) of primary and secondary syphilis[7]	10.4	[10]1.2	[10]76.5	[10]1.7	[10]1.0	6.0
14 Prevalence of low birth weight as measured by the percentage of live born infants weighing under 2,500 grams at birth	7.1	5.8	13.3	6.2	6.6	[8]6.1
15 Births to adolescents (ages 10-17 years) as a percentage of total live births	4.9	3.9	10.3	8.0	2.0	[8]7.1
16 Prenatal care as measured by the percentage of mothers delivering live infants who did not receive care during the first trimester of pregnancy	22.3	19.2	36.1	37.9	23.4	35.8
17 Childhood poverty, as measured by the proportion of children under 15 years of age living in families at or below the poverty level[7]						
Under 18 years	22.7	17.8	46.1	---	---	40.9
Under 15 years	23.4	---	---	---	---	---
5-17 years[11]	20.8	---	---	---	---	---
18 Proportion of persons living in counties exceeding U.S. Environmental Protection Agency standards for air quality during the previous year[12]	23.5	23.1	24.8	17.6	37.2	42.3

[1] Includes racial and ethnic groups not shown separately.
[2] Hispanic origin can be of any race.
[3] 1991 data.
[4] Data are for 49 States and the District of Columbia.
[5] Age adjusted to the 1940 standard population.
[6] Data are for 48 States and the District of Columbia.

[7] 1993 data.
[8] Data are for people 16 years of age and older.
[9] By date of diagnosis. Adjusted for delays in reporting; not adjusted for under reporting. Based on cases reported to CDC through September 1993.
[10] Data are for the non-Hispanic population.
[11] Related children in families.
[12] 1993 data based on 1990 county population estimates.

SOURCES:
1-3, 5-9, 14-16 - National Vital Statistics System, CDC, NCHS.
4 - Census of Fatal Occupational Injuries, Department of Labor, Bureau of Labor Statistics.
10 - AIDS Surveillance System CDC, NCID. Data are AIDS cases reported by year of diagnosis, adjusted for reporting delays. Based on cases reported to CDC through September 1993.
11 - National Notifiable Disease Surveillance System, CDC, EPO.
12 - Tuberculosis Morbidity Data, CDC, NCPS.
13 - Sexually Transmitted Disease Surveillance System, CDC, NCPS.
17 - Current Population Survey, U.S. Bureau of the Census.
18 - National Air Quality and Emission Trends Report, Office of Air and Radiation, U.S. Environmental Protection Agency.

Recent Trends for the Total Population

National data for the Health Status Indicators for the total population have been published elsewhere. Trend data are generally available for most of the indicators for the total population at the national level. The majority of the rates are declining, indicating that the total population is improving or remaining stable for most of the indicators.

The 1992 infant mortality rate of 8.5 infant deaths per 1,000 live births was the lowest rate ever recorded for the United States. Similarly, the all-cause death rate reached a record low in 1992. The age-adjusted death rate of 504.5 deaths per 100,000 population was about 3 percent below the rate of 520.2 for 1990 and 14 percent below the rate of 585.8 for 1980.

The 1992 age-adjusted death rate for motor vehicle crash deaths was 15.8 in 1992, a 16-percent decline from the 1989 rate. For homicide (including "legal intervention"), the age-adjusted death rate declined about 4 percent to 10.5 deaths per 100,000 population between 1991 and 1992, after increasing an average of nearly 5 percent per year between 1985 and 1991. For cardiovascular disease deaths, the 1992 age-adjusted death rate was 180.4 deaths per 100,000 population. Mortality from this cause, which accounts for nearly half of all deaths in the U.S., has been generally declining for decades. The 1992 age-adjusted death rates for the two major components of cardiovascular disease—heart disease and stroke—were 144.3 and 26.2, respectively. Mortality from heart disease has been declining since about 1950, while stroke mortality has been dropping steadily since U.S. mortality statistics were first published in 1900.

The age-adjusted lung cancer death rate was 39.3 per 100,000 population in 1992, slightly lower than previous years (39.9 in 1990 and 39.6 in 1991). Lung cancer mortality for the total population had been steadily increasing since at least 1950, however, the rate of increase in lung cancer mortality for men began to slow during the early 1980's and since 1990, the rates for men have declined. In contrast, the lung cancer death rate for women continues to increase. By 1986, lung cancer surpassed breast cancer as the second leading cause of cancer death in women. The female breast cancer age-adjusted death rate was 21.9 deaths per 100,000 women in 1992 (compared to 26.4 deaths per 100,000 for lung cancer) and shows a decline from previous years (23.1 in 1990 and 22.7 in 1991).

Infectious disease indicators showing improvement are the incidence of measles, tuberculosis, and syphilis. Measles incidence has

167

decreased to 0.1 per 100,000 in 1993 after increasing during the 1980's. Tuberculosis incidence decreased 7 percent to 9.8 cases per 100,000 in 1993. Tuberculosis had been increasing since 1989, due to many factors including the HIV epidemic, deterioration in the health-care system, and increases in the number of cases among foreign-born persons. For syphilis, the total population incidence was 10.4 per 100,000 in 1993, a decrease of nearly 50 percent since 1990. From 1986 through 1990, an epidemic of syphilis occurred with more than 50,000 cases reported in 1990, the highest number since 1948.

Two other indicators showing improvement are prenatal care and air quality. In 1992, 22.3 percent of mothers did not receive prenatal care during the first trimester of pregnancy, a 2-percent decrease from 1991 and the first notable improvement in more than a decade. For air quality, even though the proportion of people living in counties exceeding U.S. Environmental Protection Agency (EPA) standards for air quality has fluctuated from 1988 to 1993, there has been a general decline. In 1993, 23.5 percent of people lived in counties exceeding the EPA requirements, compared to 50.3 percent in 1988.

Health Status Indicators which are not showing improvement for the total population include work-related injury deaths, AIDS incidence, and childhood poverty. Beginning with 1992 data, work-related injury deaths are being tracked by the Census of Fatal Occupational Injuries, Department of Labor, Bureau of Labor Statistics. Previously, the National Traumatic Occupational Fatalities, National Institute for Occupational Safety and Health was used. Therefore, pre-1992 data shown in other reports are not strictly comparable to the data shown here. From 1992 to 1993 there was an increase in work-related injury deaths from 2.4 to 3.2 per 100,000 population. For AIDS incidence the national rates are by date of diagnosis corrected for delays in reporting. The 1993 incidence of acquired immunodeficiency syndrome was 31.2 cases per 100,000, up from 30.3 in 1992. Some of this increase may be due to the change in the AIDS case definition implemented in 1993. For childhood poverty, the proportion of children under age 15 living in families below the poverty level in 1993 was 23.4 percent compared to the 1990 rate of 21.4 percent.

Three indicators have remained relatively stable for the total population: suicide, births to adolescents, and low birth weight. In 1992 the age-adjusted suicide rate was 11.1 per 100,000 population. Suicide mortality has generally fluctuated within a rather narrow range since the late 1970's Adolescent births comprised 4.9 percent of total live births in 1992, a rate that has been relatively constant since 1983.

In 1991 and 1992 the overall percent of live-born infants weighing less than 2500 grams (low birth weight) was 7.1 percent, up only slightly from previous years (7.0 in 1989 and 1990).

The following sections discuss the indicators for the major race groups (white, black, American Indian and Alaska Native, and Asian and Pacific Islander) and for persons of Hispanic origin. Table 10.1 shows the most recent data by race and Hispanic origin.

White Population

Rates for the majority of the Health Status Indicators for the white population are lower than those for the total population. The 1992 rates for low birth weight, lack of early prenatal care, and tuberculosis incidence are the lowest of all the race/ethnic groups (Figures 10.1 and 10.2). The prevalence of low birth weight (5.8 percent in 1992) has remained stable at 5.6 to 5.8 percent since 1980. In 1992, about one-fifth of white mothers did not receive early prenatal care. In 1993, the tuberculosis incidence rate for non-Hispanic whites was 3.6 per 100,000, less than half the total population rate of 9.8 per 100,000. One indicator for the white population, suicide, is higher than that for the total population. Although the age-adjusted suicide rate decreased for whites from 12.1 deaths per 100,000 in 1991 to 11.8 in 1992, this rate is still the highest among all the race/ethnic groups (Figure 10.3).

Black Population

The black population has lower rates than the total population for two indicators—work-related injury deaths and suicides. For the other indicators, the rates for the black population are greater than those for the total population and are often the highest of any of the race/ethnic groups discussed. For work-related injury deaths, the 1992 black population rate of 2.9 deaths per 100,000 population is the lowest rate of any of the race/ethnic groups. For suicide, the age-adjusted rate of 6.9 deaths per 100,000 population is almost 40 percent less than the total population rate and second only to Asians and Pacific Islanders as the lowest among the major race/ethnic groups (Figure 10.3). In contrast, the black population had the highest age-adjusted total death rate in 1992 compared to the other race/ethnic groups. For five of the other eight mortality Health Status Indicators in 1992, blacks also had the highest rates. Infant mortality rates were almost twice as high for blacks (16.8 per 1,000 live births in 1992) as those for the total population (8.5 per 1,000). Despite a 6 percent decline in 1992, the age-adjusted homicide rate for blacks (39.4 deaths per 100,000 population) was almost four times that of the total population rate of 10.5 (Figure 10.3). Homicide rates for blacks have risen dramatically since the mid-1980's. For cardiovascular disease, the 1992 age-adjusted rate of 265.3 deaths per 100,000 is considerably higher than the rate of 180.4 for the total population. Similarly, lung cancer and female breast cancer age-adjusted death rates for blacks are over 20 percent greater than the total population rates (Figure 10.3).

For several infectious diseases, blacks have the highest incidence rates for any race/ethnic group (Figure 10.2). AIDS incidence for non-Hispanic blacks was 104.2 per 100,000 population in 1993, over three times that of the total population. The 1993 incidence of primary and secondary syphilis for non-Hispanic blacks (76.5 per 100,000 population) was more than seven times that of the total population incidence (10.4 per 100,000).

Low birth weight prevalence and proportion of births to adolescents were also markedly higher for blacks than for any other race/ethnic group (Figure 10.1). Between 1980 and 1992, the low birth weight prevalence among infants of black mothers rose from 12.7 percent to 13.3 percent and remained nearly twice that of the total population. The percent of births to black adolescents (10.3 percent of live births in 1992) was more than double that for the total population (4.9 percent). For childhood poverty, blacks also rank the highest of all reporting race/ethnic groups with 46.1 percent of children under age 18 living in families at or below the poverty level in 1993. This proportion is more than twice that of the total population (22.7 percent). Late or no prenatal care was also high among black mothers (36.1 percent), compared to the total population (22.3 percent).

American Indians and Alaska Natives

The American Indian and Alaska Native population have lower rates than the total population for eight indicators. Because many American Indians and Alaska Natives live in rural areas far removed from the major sources of pollution, their rates are lowest for the proportion of people living in counties exceeding EPA standards for air quality (17.6 percent in 1993). The other seven indicators that are lower than the total population estimates are: total deaths, lung cancer deaths, female breast cancer deaths, cardiovascular disease

170

deaths, AIDS incidence, syphilis incidence, and low birth weight prevalence. Stroke deaths, a component of cardiovascular disease deaths, are lower for American Indians and Alaska Natives than any other race/ethnic group with an age-adjusted rate of 19.1 deaths per 100,000 population.

The American Indians and Alaska Natives have higher rates than the total population for five indicators: infant mortality, motor vehicle crash deaths, tuberculosis incidence, percent of births to adolescents, and lack of early prenatal care. For two indicators, motor vehicle crash deaths and lack of early prenatal care, the American Indians and Alaska Natives have the highest rates of all the race/ethnic groups. The age-adjusted motor vehicle crash death rate for the American Indian and Alaska Native population was 32.0 deaths per 100,000, more than twice that of the total population rate of 15.8 deaths per 100,000 (Figure 10.3). The percentage of American Indian and Alaska Native mothers receiving late or no prenatal care was 37.9 percent, only slightly higher than the proportion for black mothers or mothers of Hispanic origin, but 70 percent higher than the total population (Figure 10.1).

It should be noted that death rates for American Indians and Alaska Natives (as well as for Asians and Pacific Islanders and persons of Hispanic origin) may be considerably underestimated and comparisons with other groups should be made with caution.

Asians and Pacific Islanders

Among the race/ethnic groups, the Asians and Pacific Islanders have the lowest overall rates for most of the Health Status Indicators. For thirteen of the indicators the Asians and Pacific Islanders are lower than the total population; for ten of these, the Asians and Pacific Islanders rank the lowest of any race/ethnic group. For 1992, Asians and Pacific Islanders had the lowest rates for total deaths, motor vehicle crash deaths, work-related injury deaths (along with blacks), suicides, homicides, female breast cancer deaths, and cardiovascular disease deaths (including heart disease) (Figure 10.3). Asians and Pacific Islanders also had the lowest infant mortality rate for 1991 at 5.8 deaths per 1,000 live births (compared with 8.6 for the total population from the Linked Birth and Infant Death File.). They also have the lowest rates for AIDS incidence, primary and secondary syphilis incidence, and percent of births to adolescents (Figures 10.1 and 10.2).

171

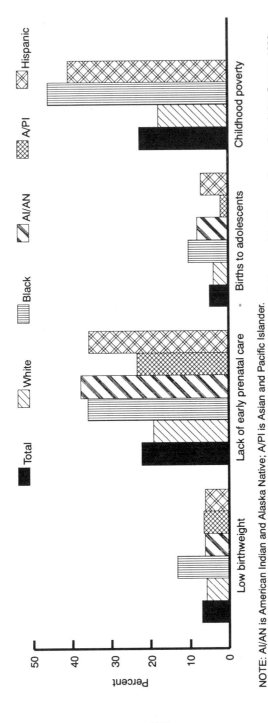

NOTE: AI/AN is American Indian and Alaska Native; A/PI is Asian and Pacific Islander.
SOURCE: CDC/NCHS, National Vital Statistics System, 1992. For childhood poverty, U.S. Bureau of the Census, Current Population Survey, 1993.

Figure 10.1. Maternal, infant and child Health Status indicators by race and Hispanic origin: United States, 1992.

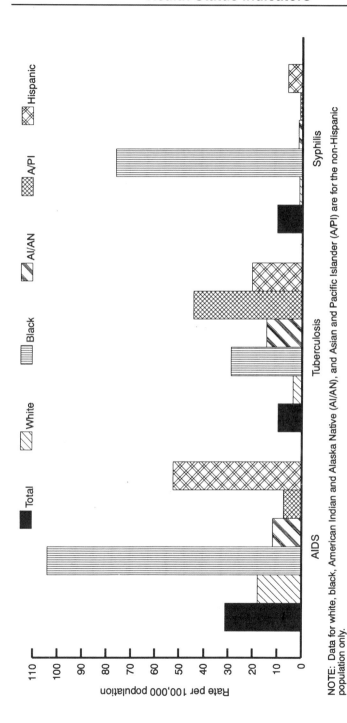

Figure 10.2. Incidence of selected infectious disease Health Status indicators by race and Hispanic origin: United States, 1993.

NOTE: Data for white, black, American Indian and Alaska Native (AI/AN), and Asian and Pacific Islander (A/PI) are for the non-Hispanic population only.

SOURCE: CDC/NCID, AIDS Surveillance System, 1993. CDC/NCPS, Tuberculosis Morbibity Data, 1993. CDC/NCPS, Sexually Transmitted Disease Surveillance System, 1993.

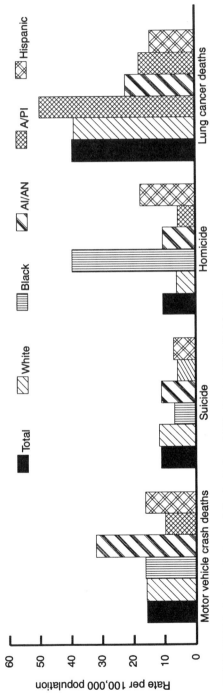

NOTE: AI/AN is American Indian and Alaska Native; A/PI is Asian and Pacific Islander.
SOURCE: CDC/NCHS, National Vital Statistics System, 1992.

Figure 10.3. Age-adjusted death rates for selected mortality Health Status indicators by race and Hispanic origin: United States, 1992.

The Asians and Pacific Islanders have higher rates than the total population for only three indicators: tuberculosis incidence, residence in poor air quality counties, and lack of early prenatal care. For tuberculosis incidence, the extremely high rate of 44.5 cases per 100,000 in 1993 was nearly five times that of the total population (9.8 per 100,000) and higher than any other race/ethnic group (Figure 10.2). This high rate of tuberculosis reflects the fact that a large proportion of immigrants, many of which are from countries with high rates of tuberculosis.

In addition, the proportion of people living in counties exceeding EPA standards in 1993 was also high for Asians and Pacific Islanders at 37.2 percent, second only to persons of Hispanic origin. In 1992, 23.4 percent of Asians and Pacific Islanders did not receive early prenatal care, slightly higher than the proportion for the total population (22.3 percent).

Hispanic Origin

For eight of the Health Status Indicators, persons of Hispanic origin have lower rates than the total population. These include infant mortality, total deaths, suicides, lung cancer deaths, female breast cancer deaths, cardiovascular disease deaths, syphilis incidence, and low birth weight prevalence. For lung cancer deaths the Hispanic origin group had the lowest rate of any of the race/ethnic groups (Figure 10.3). The 1992 age-adjusted rate for this indicator was 14.5 deaths per 100,000, more than 60 percent below the total population rate of 39.3.

For the rest of the indicators for which data are available, the rates for the Hispanic population are higher than those for the total population. For four of these indicators, Hispanics have among the highest rates when compared to the other race/ethnic groups. Work-related injury deaths are highest among workers of Hispanic origin (3.5 per 100,000 in 1993). For AIDS incidence, Hispanics have a 1993 rate of 52.6 per 100,000 (compared to the total population rate of 31.2 per 100,000) (Figure 10.2). Hispanic mothers were also less likely than all mothers to receive early prenatal care (35.8 and 22.3 percent, respectively in 1992) (Figure 10.1). Hispanics had the highest proportion of people living in counties exceeding EPA standards for air quality of any race/ethnic group in 1993 with 42.3 percent of Hispanics living in counties exceeding the requirements. This reflects the large number of Hispanics living in southern California and other places that often exceed EPA requirements.

Mortality

Studies indicate that deaths for minorities other than blacks (American Indians and Alaska Natives, Asians and Pacific Islanders, and Hispanics) from annual vital statistics files based on death certificates have been seriously underestimated. The race and Hispanic origin items on the death certificate are generally completed by the funeral director from information supplied by the next-of-kin. Underreporting comes from incorrectly reported race and also from imputing race variables where the race code was left blank. Because of this underreporting, death rates may be overestimated for whites and blacks and underestimated for other racial subgroups.

Infant mortality data for American Indians and Alaska Natives, Asians and Pacific Islanders, and Hispanics are obtained from the Linked Birth and Infant Death Files. Data from the linked files are based on the race of the mother as self-reported on the birth certificate and, therefore, do not have the problem of underestimation for minorities noted above for data based on the death certificate.

For Hispanics, an additional concern with mortality data is that not all States are included. More States have been added to the reporting area in recent years and in 1992 Oklahoma and New Hampshire were the only two States not reporting Hispanic mortality data. The mortality reporting area in 1992 encompassed 99.6 percent of the U.S. Hispanic population. In 1991 the Linked Birth and Infant Death file reporting area for infant mortality for Hispanics contained 49 States and the District of Columbia (only New Hampshire was excluded).

All death rates, except infant mortality and work-related injury deaths, are age-adjusted to the 1940 U.S. standard population. Age-adjusting is a technique that allows the user to compare rates among populations with different age distributions by "adjusting" the crude rates in each population to a standard population. Thus the user can compare the rate for a State or county with the nation, compare race and sex groups with different age compositions, or can examine trends over time in populations with a changing age distribution.

For work-related injury deaths from the Census of Fatal Occupational Injuries, Department of Labor, the actual number of deaths is small for some minority groups, resulting in rates that are highly variable. The rates from the Census of Fatal Occupational Injuries have not been adjusted for age and are limited to persons 16 years of age and older.

Infectious Diseases

Reporting systems for AIDS incidence (AIDS Surveillance System, CDC), tuberculosis incidence (Tuberculosis Morbidity Data, CDC), and syphilis incidence (Sexually Transmitted Disease Surveillance System, CDC) separate non-Hispanic from Hispanic origin. Thus data for whites, blacks, American Indians and Alaska Natives, and Asians and Pacific Islanders from these data systems do not include persons of Hispanic origin.

For AIDS, the national rates are by date of diagnosis corrected for delays in reporting; hence, the numbers for each year change as the reports are compiled and organized by the appropriate year and are not stable until after several years delay. In 1993, the AIDS case definition changed which resulted in cases being diagnosed earlier and a temporary increase in the number of cases reported. The current estimates for AIDS cases are reported through September 1994.

Racial and ethnic breakdowns are not available for measles from the National Notifiable Disease Surveillance System because of high rates of non-response to the race category.

Childhood Poverty

When the indicator for childhood poverty was developed, the under-15 age group was chosen to depict the most family-dependent of children. These data are available annually at the national level from the March Current Population Survey conducted by the U.S. Bureau of the Census. However, except for data from the decennial census, the only data available at the State level for persons under 18 years are percent of related children 5-17 years in families under the poverty threshold. The only race/ethnic breakdowns are for white, black and Hispanic children under 18. Therefore, data are shown for children under 18 years by race and Hispanic origin and total population data for children under 15 years and related children 5-17 years.

Low Birth Weight, Births to Adolescents and Prenatal Care

Data for low birth weight, births to adolescents, and prenatal care are from the National Vital Statistics System and for 1992 include data for Hispanics for 49 States and the District of Columbia. New Hampshire did not report Hispanic origin on the birth certificate in 1992.

— by Christine Plepys and Richard Klein

Part Two

Healthy People 2000

Chapter 11

Introduction to
Healthy People 2000

What Is Healthy People 2000?

As the year 2000 approaches, we have learned that a fuller measure of health and a better quality of life are within our grasp. Scientific studies over the last generation have revealed much about the factors that predispose individuals to various health threats and actions that we can take, both individually and collectively, to reduce our risks for disease, disability, and premature death.

Lifestyle changes such as reduced consumption of alcohol and quitting smoking, more exercise, and a healthier diet can help prevent disease and injury; community-wide programs can help protect populations from hazards around them or extend health promotion activities to groups in diverse settings; and clinical preventive services such as immunizations, screening for early detection, and counseling can prevent disease and help us to control it or treat it before it advances. In addition, environmental and regulatory health protection strategies addressing issues such as unintentional injuries, occupational safety and health, environmental health, food and drug safety, and oral health confer protection on large population groups.

Our new knowledge of the impact of health promotion and disease prevention activities brings with it both a keen sense of potential and

Locating Resources for Healthy People 2000 Health Promotion Projects,
U.S. Dept. Health and Human Services, September 1991.

an appreciation of how far most Americans, especially those with low incomes, are from that potential. Moreover, we are already feeling the effects of momentous new issues emerging on the horizon—the aging of our society, the prohibitive costs of many of the technologies developed for diagnosing and treating disease, and the environmental consequences of industrialization and population growth.

Reflecting the Nation's concerns with these problems and the potential for achieving a better quality of life for all Americans, the U.S. Public Health Service (PHS) of the Department of Health and Human Services led the development of a national initiative, Healthy People 2000. This document offers a vision for the new century characterized by significant reductions in preventable death and disability, enhanced quality of life, and greatly reduced disparities in the health status of populations within our society.

Healthy People 2000 grew out of a health strategy initiated in 1979 with the publication of *Healthy People: The Surgeon General's Report on Health Promotion and Disease Prevention* and expanded with publication in 1980 of Promoting Health/Preventing Disease: Objectives for the Nation, which set out an agenda for the 10 years leading up to 1990.

For the next decade, Healthy People 2000 sets three broad public health goals. Those goals are to:

1. Increase the span of healthy life for Americans;

2. Reduce health disparities among Americans; and

3. Achieve access to preventive services for all Americans.

To help meet these goals, 300 specific objectives were set in 22 separate priority areas. This national prevention agenda is established in Healthy People 2000: National Health Promotion and Disease Prevention Objectives. This report is the result of a 3-year development effort involving professionals and citizens, private organizations, and public agencies from every part of the country. Work began on the report in 1987 with the convening of a consortium that has grown to include almost 300 national membership organizations and all State health departments. After extensive public review and comment, the objectives were refined and revised to produce the published report. Listed below are the 22 priority areas in Healthy People 2000 and a general overview of the objectives addressed in each area.

The Healthy People 2000 Priority Areas

1. Physical Activity and Fitness

Because coronary heart disease is the leading cause of morbidity and mortality in the United States, the role of physical activity in preventing coronary heart disease is of particular importance and is addressed in this priority area. The objectives call for increased light-to-moderate physical activity as well as activities that promote and maintain muscular strength, muscular endurance, and flexibility. Individually focused targets have been set for special populations, especially weight reduction goals for specific socioeconomic, racial, and ethnic groups and for other high risk populations.

2. Nutrition

Dietary factors are associated with five of the ten leading causes of death in the United States—coronary heart disease, some types of cancer, stroke, non-insulin dependent diabetes mellitus, and atherosclerosis. In general, once-prevalent dietary deficiencies have been replaced by excesses and imbalances of some food components in the diet, such as the disproportionate consumption of foods high in fats. The nutrition objectives cover a broad range of concerns, including dietary deficiencies and excesses, breast feeding, growth retardation, overweight, dietary fat and saturated fat, school lunch, nutrition labeling and education. and services.

3. Tobacco

Tobacco use is responsible for more than one of every six deaths in the United States and is the most important preventable cause of death and disease in our society. An estimated 390,000 deaths are directly attributable to cigarette smoking each year in the United States. Objectives in this priority area call for reduction of death and disability from specific smoking-induced illnesses; less frequent smoking initiation and increased smoking cessation, especially among pregnant women; reduced use of smokeless tobacco; and initiation of governmental, environmental, and organizational strategies aimed at reducing tobacco use.

4. Alcohol and Other Drugs

The toll exacted on society, health, and the economy by alcohol and other drug problems is staggering and widespread across various social strata. Objectives in this priority areas call for reduced alcohol-related accidents and disorders, reduced drug-related deaths and hospital visits, increased average age of first use of alcohol or drugs, increased awareness of risks and peer disapproval among adolescents, and initiation and extension of governmental and organizational services and policies to further awareness and prevention.

5. Family Planning

Objectives here call for reduced numbers of teen pregnancies and unintended pregnancies and lowered prevalence of infertility and early adolescent experience with sexual intercourse. Nonuse of contraceptives among sexually active, never married adolescents should also decrease and effectiveness of family planning methods should increase. Other objectives address human sexuality and age-appropriate preconception counseling and education from a variety of sources, including parents, pregnancy counselors, and health care and social services providers.

6. Mental Health and Mental Disorders

These objectives seek to reduce prevalence of mental disorders and suicide among all age groups. To reduce risk, the objectives seek to increase use of community support programs by patients, increase the number of depressive patients who seek treatment, and increase the number of persons who obtain support in coping with personal and emotional problems as well as stressful life conditions. Objectives call for increased attention to sources of stress and strain as well as medical screening, counseling, and appropriate intervention, including work site stress reduction programs and self-help clearinghouses at the State level.

7. Violent and Abusive Behavior

Although violent and abusive behavior have been considered the responsibility of the fields of law enforcement, social services, and mental health, public health perspectives in preventing death and disability due to violent and abusive behavior have begun to emerge across the country. These objectives have been developed within six key areas: homicide and assaultive violence; domestic violence; child abuse; sexual assault; suicide; and weapon-related injuries. Also identified as a target is an improvement in the availability and quality of data on morbidity and disability associated with violence, particularly at the local level. The objectives also call for identifying, strengthening, and expanding effective services for victims.

8. Educational and Community-Based Programs

Attainment of the Healthy People 2000 health promotion priorities will depend substantially on educational and community-based programs that take a population-based approach to health, attempting to reach and improve the health of many people outside of traditional health care settings. Objectives in this priority areas focus on a wide range of settings and address activities that focus on multiple risk factors. Specific objectives address topics in preschool and general education that influence health, school health programs, and work site health promotion activities, as well as areas of concern for older adults and racial or ethnic minorities.

9. Unintentional Injuries

Unintentional injuries constitute the fourth leading cause of death in the United States, and result in 100,000 deaths each year. These objectives seek to reduce unintentional injury mortality and morbidity overall, with specific focus on motor vehicle crashes, falls, drowning, residential fires, hip fractures, poisonings, and head and spinal cord injuries. Strategies include increased use of safety belts, cyclist helmets, sprinklers, and smoke detectors, as well as handgun safety. Increased and improved education, design engineering, counseling, and trauma services are also addressed.

10. Occupational Safety and Health

Premature deaths, diseases, and injuries resulting from occupational exposure pose important national health problems. Overall objectives in this priority area are to reduce work-related deaths, injuries, and cumulative trauma disorders, and special targets are set for specific worker populations. Reductions are called for in incidence of occupational skin disorders and hepatitis B infection from occupational exposure. Highlighted risk reduction and health protection measures include use of motor vehicle occupant protection systems, reduced exposure to excessive noise, reduced exposures leading to high blood lead concentrations, and increased immunization protection.

11. Environmental Health

This priority area targets improvements in the way the Nation responds to environmental factors that the current knowledge base identifies as having the greatest potential for damaging human health. Several objectives in this priority area focus on reducing the total burden of environmental contaminants. For example, goals are set for cleaning up toxic waste sites, increasing recycling efforts, and reducing toxic agents released into the air, water, and soil. Where the scientific evidence is clear—lead poisoning, waterborne infectious diseases, and asthma, for example—specific objectives to prevent disease are included.

12. Food and Drug Safety

This priority area focuses on maintaining and improving a part of the public health system that has already proved its effectiveness, but requires continuing vigilance and support during the coming decade. The seven objectives in this priority area set goals to reduce incidence of specific foodborne illnesses; increase consumer awareness and application of safe food handling practices; expand regulatory coverage of commercial and institutional food services; and increase physician and pharmacist activity to monitor and alert patients to potential problems relating to their use of medications.

13. Oral Health

Although oral health status has been improving, especially in children, oral diseases are among the most prevalent health problems in the United States. Objectives include reduction of dental caries and oral diseases, such as gingivitis and oral cancer; increased oral health screening and access to care; and increased appropriate use of protective dental sealants and fluorides. The objectives also include explicit special population targets.

14. Maternal and Infant Health

In 1987, more than 3,800,000 infants were born in the United States. Of these, 38,408 died before their first birthday, and black infants died at twice the rate of white infants. In addition, maternal mortality and morbidity also require attention, including the issue of cesarean delivery, which has increased dramatically over the last

20 years. Black women die from complications of childbirth at about three times the rate of white women, and many maternal deaths are preventable. These objectives seek to reduce infant, fetal, and maternal death rates and infant morbidity by reducing specific risks such as low prenatal weight gain, smoking and substance abuse, and pregnancy complications; increasing the proportion of breast feeding mothers; and increasing preconception, prenatal, and neonatal care, screening, and counseling.

15. Heart Disease and Stroke

Cardiovascular diseases (CVD)—primarily coronary heart disease and stroke—kill more Americans than all other diseases combined. Objectives in this priority area address the major risk factors for CVD and appropriate and timely detection and management. Risk reduction objectives focus on increasing control of high blood pressure and high blood cholesterol; increasing awareness of blood cholesterol levels; reducing dietary fat intake, overweight, and smoking; and increasing physical activity. Screening activities, health care provider compliance with current high blood cholesterol management guidelines, and work sites offering education and/or control activities are also targeted.

16. Cancer

Cancer accounts for about one out of every five deaths in the United States. As well as the burden of suffering, the costs to society are high: overall costs in 1985 were $72.5 billion, about 11 percent of the total cost of disease in this country. Cancer, which includes over 100 different diseases, may strike at any age. Objectives for this priority area focus on issues in cancer prevention and detection with the greatest potential for reducing cancer incidence, morbidity, and mortality, including cigarette smoking reduction, dietary change, and improvements in early detection.

17. Diabetes and Chronic Disabling Conditions

Preventing unnecessary deaths is only one item on the public health agenda for chronic disease. The preservation of physical and mental function is also essential. Chronic and disabling conditions can have profound effects on a person's ability to function, whether it be a child with mental retardation, a young adult with a spinal cord injury, or an older adult with diabetes. Quality, not merely quantity, of life has become the issue. Overall goals are to increase the years of healthy life and to reduce the number of people who suffer limited activity due to chronic conditions. Additionally, objectives focus on reducing incidence and complications of diabetes and specific chronic conditions such as asthma, chronic back conditions, hearing and vision impairments, and serious mental retardation.

18. HIV Infection

By the end of 1992, a projected total of 365,000 cases of AIDS will have been diagnosed in the United States and 260,000 people will have died of the disease. AIDS has become the seventh leading cause of years of potential life lost in the United States, and it is the leading cause of death among intravenous drug abusers and people with hemophilia. In addition to confining incidence and reducing prevalence of HIV (human immunodeficiency virus) infection, the objectives target personal behaviors that place individuals at risk for infection, including sexual behavior and drug abuse; control of the blood supply; increased screening; counseling, and education (through school, health care facility, or work site); and discrimination protection for patients with HIV infection or AIDS.

19. Sexually Transmitted Disease

Nearly 12 million cases of sexually transmitted diseases (STDs) occur annually in the United States, 86 percent of them in persons ages 15 through 29. During the last several years, the spectrum of STDs has increased dramatically in both complexity and scope. As well as the "traditional" diseases (syphilis and gonorrhea), the list of STDs now encompasses Chlamydia trachomatis infections, genital herpes and warts, human papillomavirus, chancroid, genital mycoplasmas, cytomegalovirus, hepatitis B, vaginitis, enteric infections, and ectoparasitic diseases. These objectives focus on reducing rates of specific disease incidence behaviors, and increasing services, counseling, and prevention education.

20. Immunization and Infectious Diseases

The reduction in incidence of infectious diseases is the most significant public health achievement of the past 100 years. Smallpox was globally eradicated in 1977, and diphtheria and poliomyelitis have been virtually eliminated in the United States. Despite the remarkable advances that have been made, infectious diseases remain important causes of morbidity and mortality in the United States. These objectives call for reduced incidence of vaccine-preventable diseases, including measles, bacterial meningitis, viral hepatitis, and pneumonia. Reductions are also targeted for nosocomial infections among surgical and intensive care patients. The objectives call for increased immunization levels, especially among the very young and other high-risk groups.

21. Clinical Preventive Services

Clinical preventive services refer to those disease prevention and health promotion services—immunizations, screening for early detection of disease, and patient counseling—that are delivered to individuals in a health care setting. Improved access to and increased use of clinical preventive services are considered essential for the attainment of the national goals and objectives. (Recommended age- and gender appropriate services were presented by the U.S. Preventive Services Task Force in Guide to Clinical Preventive Services, Williams and Wilkins, 1989.) Specific objectives include increased delivery of appropriate immunizations and screening services, access to ongoing primary care, and compliance by health care providers with the Task Force recommendations.

22. Surveillance and Data Systems

These objectives recognize that public health data must be accurate, timely, and available in a usable form. The objectives in this area, which support all of the other priority areas, include developing a set of appropriate health status indicators and implementing the set in at least 40 States; identifying or creating data sources to measure progress of each of the year 2000 objectives; and developing and implementing methods for improved collection, analysis, and transfer of relevant data to and among Federal, State, and local agencies.

Chapter 12

Healthy People 2000 Midcourse Review and Revisions

1995 Report on Progress

At the midpoint of the decade, the Nation and the public health community are examining the health status of all Americans. While all of the data are not in hand, many 5-year trends have been established. Overall progress has been made on the Nation's year 2000 targets, with 50 percent proceeding in the right direction, 18 percent moving away from the targets, and 3 percent showing no change from the baseline. Tracking data are not yet available for 29 percent. The priority area midcourse reviews of the 22 Healthy People 2000 priority areas that follow provide a more detailed picture of the changes.

For racial and ethnic population groups there is a similar picture of progress, with roughly the same percentage of objectives moving in the right direction for minorities as for the total population. However, for blacks there are proportionately more objectives moving away from the targets. For Asian Americans there is a considerable problem in getting the data needed to track progress.

Another summary of progress is shown in Figure 12.2 on the status of the 47 sentinel objectives in the 22 Healthy People 2000 priority areas. The picture is also one of progress—33 objectives are proceeding in the right direction, 9 are moving away from the targets, 2 show no change from the baseline, and 3 lack data to track progress.

Excerpted from *Healthy People 2000 Midcourse Review and 1995 Revisions*, DHHS (PHS), No Document Number or Date Listed.

Prevention Opportunities

Families, schools, worksites, and community programs all provide important opportunities for prevention. Midcourse assessments of Healthy People 2000 objectives point to the continuing need to deal effectively with problems experienced by families and even whole communities—problems such as poverty, insufficient education, single parenthood, and violence, that can only be addressed through those settings.

	Right Direction	Wrong Direction	No Change	No Tracking Data*
Total Population (300 targets)	50%	18%	3%	29%
Special Populations (116)	53%	27%	3%	17%
Black (48)	50%	35%	2%	13%
Hispanic (28)	54%	14%	4%	29%
Asians/Pacific Islanders (9)	56%	11%	0%	33%
American Indians/Alaska Natives (31)	56%	31%	3%	10%

* Includes objectives with no baseline (8%) and objectives with no update beyond baseline (22%)
Source: CDC/NCHS

Figure 12.1. Progress on Racial and Ethnic Minority Objectives, 1995.

192

Figure 12.2a. Progress on 47 Sentinel Objectives.

Objective	% Change Targeted	Baseline[a]	Update[g]	Year 2000 Targets	Right Direction	Wrong Direction	No Change	No Data
HEALTH PROMOTION								
1. Physical activity								
· more people exercising regularly	+36%	22%[c]	24%[j]	30%	X			
· fewer people never exercising	-38%	24%[c]	24%[j]	15%			X	
2. Nutrition								
· fewer people overweight	-23%	26%[b]	34%[h]	20%		X		
· lower fat diets	-17%	36%[b]	34%[h]	30%	X			
3. Tobacco								
· fewer people smoking cigarettes	-48%	29%	25%	15%	X			
· fewer youth beginning to smoke	-50%	30%	27%	15%	X			
4. Alcohol and other drugs								
· fewer alcohol-related automobile deaths (per 100,000)	-13%	9.8	6.8	8.5	X			
· less alcohol use among youth aged 12–17 years	-50%	25.2%[e]	18.0%	12.6%	X			
· less marijuana use among youth aged 12–17 years	-50%	6.4%[e]	4.9%	3.2%	X			
5. Family planning								
· fewer teen pregnancies (per 1,000)	-30%	71.1[c,f]	74.3[f]	50.0[f]		X		
· fewer unintended pregnancies	-46%	56%[e]	NA	30%				X
6. Mental health and mental disorders								
· fewer suicides (per 100,000)	-10%	11.7	11.2	10.5	X			
· fewer people reporting stress-related problems	-21%	44.2%[c]	39.2%	35%	X			
7. Violent and abusive behavior								
· fewer homicides (per 100,000)	-15%	8.5	10.3[k]	7.2		X		
· fewer assault injuries (per 100,000)	-10%	9.7[d]	9.9[k]	8.7		X		
8. Educational and community-based programs								
· more schools with comprehensive school health education	NA	NA	NA	75%				X
· more workplaces with health promotion programs	+31%	65%[c]	81%[k]	85%	X			

Figure 12.2b. Progress on 47 Sentinel Objectives.

Objective	% Change Targeted	Baseline[a]	Update[g]	Year 2000 Targets	Right Direction	Wrong Direction	No Change	No Data
HEALTH PROTECTION								
9. Unintentional injuries								
· fewer unintentional injury deaths (per 100,000)	-16%	34.7	29.6	29.3	X			
· more people using automobile safety restraints	+102%	42%[e]	67%[i]	85%	X			
10. Occupational safety and health								
· fewer work-related deaths (per 100,000)	-33%	6[m]	5	4	X			
· fewer work-related injuries (per 100,000)	-22%	7.7[m]	7.9	6.0		X		
11. Environmental health								
· no children with blood lead 25 µg/dl	-100%	234,000[h]	93,000[h]	0	X			
· more people with clear air in their communities	+71%	49.7%[e]	76.5%	85%	X			
· more people in radon-tested houses	+700%	5%[l]	11.4%	40%	X			
12. Food and drug safety								
· fewer *salmonella* outbreaks	-68%	77[l]	63	25	X			
13. Oral health								
· fewer children with dental caries	-34%	54%	52%	35%	X			
· fewer older people without teeth	-44%	36%[d]	30%	20%	X			
PREVENTIVE SERVICES								
14. Maternal and infant health								
· fewer newborns with low weight	-28%	6.9%	7.1%[k]	5%		X		
· more mothers with first trimester care	+18%	76.0%	77.7%[k]	90%	X			
15. Heart disease and stroke								
· fewer coronary heart disease deaths (per 100,000)	-26%	135	114[k]	100	X			
· fewer stroke deaths (per 100,000)	-34%	30.4	26.4	20.0	X			
· better control of high blood pressure	+355%	11%[b]	21%[h]	50%	X			
· lower cholesterol levels	-6%	213 mg/dl[b]	205 mg/dl[h]	200 mg/dl	X			
16. Cancer								
· decrease cancer deaths (per 100,000)	-3%	134	133	130	X			
· increase screening for breast cancer (age>50)	+140%	25%	55%	60%	X			
· increase screening for cervical cancer (age>18)	+8%	88%	95%	95%	X			
· increase fecal occult blood testing (age>50)	+85%	27%	30%[k]	50%	X			

a 1987 unless otherwise noted
b 1976-80
c 1985
d 1986
e 1988

f 1989
g 1993 unless otherwise noted
h 1988-91
i 1990
j 1991

k 1992
l 1994
m 1983-1987
n 1984
o 1979-80 through 1986-87 influenza seasons

p 1987-88 through 1989-90 influenza seasons
q Data are expressed as measles cases
r rate per 1,000

**Figure 12.2c.
Progress on 47
Sentinel Objectives.**

Objective	% Change Targeted	Baseline[a]	Update[g]	Year 2000 Targets	Right Direction	Wrong Direction	No Change	No Data
17. Diabetes and chronic disabling conditions								
· fewer people disabled by chronic conditions	-15%	9.4%	10.6%	8%		X		
· fewer diabetes-related deaths (per 100,000)	-11%	38[d]	38[k]	34			X	
18. HIV infection								
· slower increase in HIV infection (per 100,000)	0%	400[l]	NA	400				X
19. Sexually transmitted diseases								
· fewer gonorrhea infections (per 100,000)	-25%	300[l]	172	225	X			
· fewer syphilis infections (per 100,000)	-45%	18.1[l]	10.4	10.0	X			
20. Immunization and infectious diseases								
· no measles cases	-100%	3058[e,q]	312[q]	0		X		
· fewer pneumonia and influenza deaths (per 100,000)	-63%	19.9[o]	23.1[p]	7.3		X		
· higher immunization levels (ages 19–35 months)	+53%	54-64%	67%	90%	X			
21. Clinical preventive services								
· no financial barrier to recommended preventive services	-100%	16%[f]	17%	0		X		
SURVEILLANCE AND DATA SYSTEMS								
22. Surveillance and data systems								
· common and comparable health status indicators in use across States		0 States	48 States	40 States	X			
Total					33	9	2	3

[a] 1987 unless otherwise noted
[b] 1976-80
[c] 1985
[d] 1986
[e] 1988
[f] 1989
[g] 1993 unless otherwise noted
[h] 1988-91
[i] 1990
[j] 1991
[k] 1992
[l] 1994
[m] 1983-1987
[n] 1984
[o] 1979-80 through 1986-87 influenza seasons
[p] 1987-88 through 1989-90 influenza seasons
[q] Data are expressed as measles cases
[r] rate per 1,000

A condensed version of this table was first published in McGinnis, M.J. and Lee, P.R., Healthy People 2000 at Mid-Decade. JAMA 273(14):1123-29.

Families

Beginning a family should be one of the joys of life. Through family planning, parents can ensure that they are ready to assume responsibility to care for and provide for their children. Once the choice has been made to begin a new life, the mother has the responsibility of seeking prenatal care in the first trimester of pregnancy to ensure a healthy birth. Breast feeding can also help give a child a healthy start. A nutritious diet that supports physical growth and development coupled with physical activity can ensure that a child begins life with healthy habits. It is within families that behaviors are first observed and learned. Diet and activity patterns, oral hygiene, and coping skills are established at an early age and are supported by the examples set by family members. Patterns of alcohol consumption and tobacco use are similarly established within families. For adolescents and young adults, learning about physical development can foster positive awareness of their sexuality. Promoting self-esteem and reinforcing positive behaviors also builds the mental health of children. Primary care providers can support families by ensuring that they are provided scientifically sound clinical preventive services, including immunizations, screening to detect asymptomatic disease in its early stages, and appropriate counseling to foster healthy behaviors.

Schools

For the nearly 48 million children in this country, schools play an important supporting role in maintaining and promoting good health. Schools can provide health education to prepare children and teenagers to care for themselves. Children can learn about their bodies and the health effects of different behaviors and can adopt patterns for healthy life for themselves. In and through schools, children can be linked to necessary preventive services, including nutritious meals, regular physical activity, age-appropriate immunizations, screening for early diagnosis of diseases, referrals for treatment, and appropriate counseling about the many challenges to healthy maturation. Recognizing the role of schools in ensuring health for young citizens, the need for enhancing school health education and for developing school-based and school-linked health services is clearly called for.

Low educational achievement is a consistent indicator of increased risk for preventable disease and premature death. With the passage of the Goals 2000 Educate America Act, the potential exists to initiate a broad range of actions that, together with Healthy People 2000, will result in a healthier, better educated Nation. Goals 2000 challenges the Nation to ensure that all children arrive at school ready to learn; to increase the high school completion rate; to attain student competencies in core subjects; to make U.S. students first in the world in math and science achievement; to improve teacher education and professional development; to achieve universal adult literacy and lifelong learning; to ensure safe, disciplined, and alcohol and drug-free schools; and to promote parental participation. Achieving these goals can produce a generation of educated adults for whom disease prevention and health promotion is understood, practiced, and valued.

Workplaces

Nearly 110 million people go to work each day. A prevention-based orientation to health can be enhanced by employers who promote good health for their employees through supportive policies (e.g., smoking restrictions), exercise facilities, health promotion education, health insurance, and targeted preventive services. In addition, workplace programs protect employee health through standard setting and enforcement, worker training, and safety education. By encouraging safe practices and healthy behaviors, worksite programs help sustain the national effort to reduce preventable death, disease, and disability.

Communities

Each day, millions of Americans come together to pursue neighborhood improvement projects, engage in recreation, continue their education, and maintain social support and friendship. From athletics to volunteer social service, community-based activities support better health-for participants and recipients alike. For families and neighborhoods that are least able to provide healthy, safe environments, community programs can be a bridge to a better life.

Religious institutions offer spiritual support that can promote emotional and mental health. The religious community has become increasingly engaged in the lives of its members through sponsorship of child care centers, after school programs, homeless programs, and programs for older adults. Through all of these activities, churches, temples, and other places of worship promote health.

An increasing number of community-based projects that join the skills, devotion, and energy of the community with the expertise of local public health departments and health care providers promotes better health in America's communities and neighborhoods. These healthy communities projects work to build communities that support good health decisions and promote improvements in the quality of life. Healthy People 2000 provides a framework for State and local action, helping communities tailor strategies to meet the unique needs of their residents. As of June 1995, 42 States, Guam, and the District of Columbia had used Healthy People 2000 to create their own State-level prevention agendas. Equally impressive is the degree to which private and voluntary organizations have taken on the Healthy People 2000 challenge. Acceptance of a common prevention agenda has built bridges between public and private agencies at national, State, and local levels. To emphasize the importance of action at the State level, this report is arranged with maps illustrating how statistics from various jurisdictions compare on certain indicators of health.

Prevention Challenges—Special Population Priorities

Some problems are so compelling that particular attention is required to change the behaviors of individuals and community norms. These problems occur disproportionately among the most vulnerable in the society, and solutions to these problems require the mobilization of multiple social institutions.

The population of the United States continues to grow and to diversify. At the time of the 1990 census, there were nearly 250 million Americans, with a combined minority population at 24 percent. In 1990, the racial composition of the population was 75.7 percent white non-Hispanic, 11.8 percent black non-Hispanic, 2.4 percent Asians/Pacific Islanders, and 0.7 percent American Indians/Alaska Natives. Based on official Census Bureau projections, the resident population will be 276 million by the year 2000, with a combined minority population of 28.4 percent. This growth of 17.5 million minorities reflects both migration and the natural increase of the population as births exceed deaths. Some 9 percent of the population were of Hispanic origin. By 2000 the population is expected to be 71.6 percent white non-Hispanic, 12.2 percent black non-Hispanic, 4.1 percent Asians/Pacific Islanders and 0.7 percent American Indians/Alaska Natives. Some 11.3 percent of the population are expected to be people of Hispanic origin. As America's diversity increases, so does the need to ensure that broad public health messages are culturally and linguistically appropriate.

By the year 2000, there will also be 4 million more Americans over the age of 65 than there were in 1990. The average age of the population is rising, and the number of people living beyond age 85 is at record levels. The aging of America will challenge the mental health system to minimize the effects of social isolation and depression that arise from illness and from the losses of loved ones and friends. Primary care providers will be faced with identifying risks to independence and health, counseling patients to remain physically active, providing immunizations for pneumonia and influenza, and performing periodic screenings to detect cancers, heart disease, and other life-threatening conditions.

Another special population focus in Healthy People 2000 is people with disabilities. According to the Census Bureau there were 48.9 million Americans with a disability in 1992. Almost half of these people were considered to be severely disabled, while the disability for the others was considered not severe. Among the severely disabled are the frail elderly, mentally retarded/developmentally disabled people, and adults and children with disabling physical and mental illnesses. These people may be limited in their activities of daily living

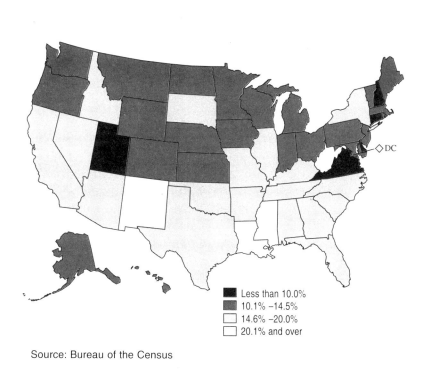

Less than 10.0%
10.1% –14.5%
14.6% –20.0%
20.1% and over

Source: Bureau of the Census

Figure 12.3. *Poverty Rates in the United States, 1992.*

such as going to work or school or in performing personal grooming, cooking or housework. Although there are no official projections of the disabled population for the year 2000, the trend data indicate that the numbers of disabled may be increasing. In part this trend reflects the aging of the population. The 1994/95 Disability Supplement to the National Health Interview Survey will provide important information on the severity, onset, and duration of disabling conditions.

For nearly every measure of health, the poor suffer more than the population as a whole. The number of people living in poverty has increased since Healthy People 2000 was published. Between 1987 and 1992, there was an increase of 4.7 million people in poverty—which brought the total population living with incomes below the official poverty level to 36.9 million Americans. Of these, 13.9 million were children under the age of 18. There are no official projections for poverty by the year 2000. As shown in Figure 12.3, poverty rates differ by State, with Mississippi having nearly three times the rate of poverty of Delaware in 1992.

These demographic trends indicate enormous challenges. To prevent premature death and disability and to thwart morbidity in a more diverse and older population in which poverty has been on the rise requires that health promotion and disease prevention messages and interventions be broadened. Resource constraints require that services be targeted to those with the greatest needs.

Conclusion

Healthy People 2000 offers goals for what can be achieved for the Nation's health by the end of this decade as well as an agenda to realize that vision. Each of the 22 priority areas is important and has substantial impact on the ability to reach the targets comprising other priority areas. Achieving the heart disease and cancer objectives also requires progress in the diet, physical activity, and tobacco use objectives. Reaching targets related to violence and unintentional injury also requires progress on the substance abuse, mental health, and educational and community based program objectives. This decade will witness profound changes in the Nation's public and personal health care system. This midcourse review reaffirms a commitment to better health in its broadest sense. Healthy People 2000 offers an important tool. Its use can ensure that efforts are focused on activities that can reduce the burden of illness and move the Nation steadily toward a higher level of health as a new century dawns.

Chapter 13

Healthy People 2000: Healthy Worksites

America's worksites can influence the health and well-being of individuals and the communities in which they live and work. From enforcing safety procedures, to mandating smoke-free workplaces, to ensuring that employee cafeterias offer healthful food choices, to making opportunities for physical fitness available, employers have many options for improving the health of their employees and their communities. Evidence continues to mount that well-designed worksite health promotion programs contribute to reductions in absenteeism; increases in productivity; health care cost containment; and improved recruitment, retention, and employee morale.

The potential of this influence is nowhere more evident than among the health promotion objectives of Healthy People 2000, the Nation's Prevention Agenda. Healthy People 2000 links health and economic policies, cultural attitudes, and democratic values to build a nationwide public health framework. The framework provides a common basis for actions to prevent unnecessary disease and disability and to achieve a better quality of life for all Americans. Employer appreciation of the benefits of worksite health promotion is essential if the Nation is to reap the rewards promised by Healthy People 2000. Fortunately, even in these times of limited resources and changing workforce demographics, both public and private sector employers are realizing the benefits of providing programs for their own employees, as well as for dependents and the communities in which they live.

DHHS Publication No. B0033-1994.

Healthy People 2000 Objectives for Worksites

The topics covered by Healthy People 2000 objectives written expressly for worksites are listed below. Divided into three categories of preventive intervention, the objectives address a full range of health promotion programming. Due to data and measurement limitations, all objectives are directed at worksites with more than 50 employees; however, health promotion activities sponsored by smaller worksites are vital to achieving significant health improvements among American adults. The complete text of the objectives is listed in Healthy People 2000: National Health Promotion and Disease Prevention Objectives.

Health Promotion Objectives

- 1.10 Worksite fitness programs
- 2.20 Worksite nutrition/weight management programs
- 3.11 Worksite smoking policies
- 4.14 Worksite alcohol and drug policies
- 6.11 Worksite stress management programs
- 8.6 Worksite health promotion activities
- 8.7 Health promotion activities for hourly workers

Health Protection Objectives

- 10.1 Work-related injury deaths
- 10.2 Nonfatal work-related injuries
- 10.3 Cumulative trauma disorders
- 10.4 Occupational skin disorders
- 10.6 Worksite occupant protection system mandates
- 10.7 Occupational noise limitations
- 10.8 Occupational lead exposure
- 10.11 Occupational lung diseases
- 10.12 Worksite health and safety programs
- 10.13 Worksite back injury prevention and rehabilitation programs

Preventive Services Objectives

- 15.16 Worksite blood pressure/cholesterol education programs
- 17.19 Employment of people with disabilities
- 18.14 Occupational exposure to HIV
- 20.11 Hepatitis B immunizations

1992 National Survey of Worksite Health Promotion Activities

In the winter and spring of 1992, the U.S. Public Health Service, through the Office of Disease Prevention and Health Promotion (ODPHP), conducted the second national survey of worksite health promotion activities. The objectives of the survey were to:

- Describe characteristics of worksite health promotion activities in the private sector;

- Measure the level of change since 1985 and track several of the national worksite objectives included in Healthy People 2000, The Nation's Prevention Agenda;

- Compare worksite activities across industries and by worksite size; and

- Describe aspects of worksite administration, evaluation, and benefits.

Demographics

The survey covered 1,507 private sector worksites with 50 or more employees in 4 size strata (50-99, 100-249, 250-749, and 750+) and 6 industry types (services; manufacturing; transportation/ communications/utilities; finance/ insurance/real estate; wholesale/ retail; agriculture/mining/construction). The worksites were diverse:

- 82 percent had no union representation;
- 7 percent reported that all employees were salaried;
- 97 percent offered health insurance plans;
- 28 percent were fully self-insured; and
- 29 percent decreased employment in the previous year.

Results

The 1992 national survey found a 25 percent increase in worksite health promotion activities since 1985. Specifically, 81 percent of worksites offered at least one health promotion activity compared with 66 percent in 1985. The HEALTHY PEOPLE 2000 target for worksite health promotion activities is 85 percent.

Improved employee health followed by improved morale and reduced health insurance costs were cited most frequently by respondents at worksites with health promotion activities.

Information and activities, including provision of resource materials, individual counseling, group classes, workshops, lectures, and special events were measured in 17 subject areas. The 1985 survey covered eight subject areas. Particularly notable were the substantial increases in offerings of worksite nutrition, weight control, physical fitness, high blood pressure, and stress management activities. Fewer worksites were offering programs in off-the-job accidents than in 1985. Programs on back care and smoking cessation have remained steady.

Progress Toward Healthy People 2000

The year 2000 worksite targets for physical activity programs, alcohol and other drug policies, and occupant protection systems have been exceeded already. The proportion of worksites with formal smoking policies increased 118 percent since 1985. In addition, the following progress has been made:

	Percent of Worksites in:		
Programs/Policies	1985	1992	2000 Target
High blood pressure/ cholesterol	17%	35%	50%
Formal smoking policy	27%	59%	75%
Nutrition/weight control	NA	37%	50%
Stress management	27%	37%	40%
Back care	29%	32%	50%

Worksite size was a strong indicator of health promotion activity. Worksites with more than 750 employees were more likely to offer activities than were smaller worksites. Size was directly related to activity level in all areas except back care and job hazard and injury prevention. There were no notable differences in activity among worksites that decreased or increased their workforce compared with those that remained the same size. No variations were noted among differing regions of the country.

The complete report is available from the National Technical Information Service (NTIS). For more information, call NTIS sales office at (703) 4874650 and request PB93-500023 (Final Report, Technical Appendix, Diskette) or PB93-100204 (Final Report and Technical Appendix only). Or write to NTIS, Springfield, VA 22161. The Summary Report (Order No. W0020) can be obtained from the National Health Information Center, P.O. Box 1133, Washington, DC 20013-1133. There is a $2 handling fee.

For More Information and Publications

Single copies of publications listed below may be ordered by writing:

National Health Information Center
P.O. Box 1133
Washington, DC 20013-1133

- *Health Promotion Goes to Work* (1993, $5)

- *Healthy People 2000: National Health Promotion and Disease Prevention Objectives*, Summary Report (1991, $4)

- *Healthy Worksites Directory of Federal Initiatives in Worksite Health Promotion* (1992, $3)

- *Locating Resources for Healthy People 2000 Health Promotion Projects* (1991, $2)

- *Summary Report, 1992 National Survey of Worksite Health Promotion Activities* (1992, $2)

- *Worksite Wellness Media Reports* (1987, $3)

Additional information and publications are available from:

Washington Business
Group on Health
777 North Capitol Street NE.
Suite 800
Washington, DC 20002

Part Three

Centers for Disease Control and Prevention

Chapter 14

About the Centers for Disease Control and Prevention

About CDC

The Centers for Disease Control and Prevention (CDC), located in Atlanta, Georgia, is an agency of the Department of Health and Human Services.

CDC Mission

To promote health and quality of life by preventing and controlling disease, injury, and disability.

CDC Pledge

CDC pledges to the American people:

* To be a diligent steward of the funds entrusted to it.
* To provide an environment for intellectual and personal growth and integrity.
* To base all public health decisions on the highest quality scientific data, openly and objectively derived.
* To place the benefits to society above the benefits to the institution.
* To treat all persons with dignity, honesty, and respect.

Centers for Disease Control Web Page.

The CDC includes 11 Centers, and Institutes, and Offices as listed below.

- Office of the Director, which include: Information Resources Management Office, Office of Health and Safety (OhASIS) and Office of Women's Health.
- National Center for Chronic Disease Prevention and Health Promotion
- National Center for Environmental Health
- National Center for Health Statistics
- National Center for HIV, STD, and TB Prevention
- National Center for Infectious Diseases
- National Center for Injury Prevention and Control
- National Institute for Occupational Safety and Health Epidemiology Program Office
- International Health Program Office
- Public Health Practice Program Office
- National Immunization Program

Centers for Disease Control and Prevention
1600 Clifton Road N.E.
Mail Stop F05
Atlanta, Georgia 30333
Toll Free (800)311-3435
(404)639-3534

Office of the Director

- Freedom of Information Act Office
- Information Resources Management Office
- Management Analysis and Services Office
- Office of Communication, Division of Media Relations
- Office of Health and Safety (OhASIS)
- Office of Women's Health

National Center for Chronic Disease Prevention and Health Promotion

Major Program Areas

- Surveillance
- Behavioral Risk Factor Surveillance System

- Youth Risk Behavior Surveillance System
- National Cancer Registries
- Modifying Risk Factors
- Tobacco
- Nutrition
- Physical Activity
- Disease Prevention and Control
- Diabetes
- Breast and Cervical Cancer
- Cardiovascular Disease
- Oral Health
- Comprehensive Approaches
- Comprehensive School Health Education
- Community Health Promotion
- Preventive Health and Health Services Block Grant
- Prevention Research Centers
- HMO-Managed Care Activity
- Clinic Management
- Maternal and Infant Health
- Maternal and Infant Health Surveillance Systems
- Maternal and Child Health Capacity Building
- Infant Mortality
- Women's Reproductive Health
- International Assistance in Reproductive Health

National Center for Environmental Health

The mission of the National Center for Environmental Health (NCEH) is to provide national leadership, through science and service, to promote health and quality of life by preventing and controlling disease, birth defects, disability, and death resulting from interactions between people and their environment.

NCEH accomplishes its mission through:

- National leadership in prevention programs.
- Public health surveillance.
- Applied research:
- Epidemiologic studies.
- Laboratory analyses.
- Statistical analyses.
- Behavioral interventions.

- Communication with the scientific community, the health community, and the public.
- Dissemination of standards, guidelines, and recommendations.
- Assistance to state and local health agencies in order to increase their capacity for preventing disability and environmental disease: technical and financial assistance.
- Training for staff.

NCEH Divisions and Programs:

- Division of Birth Defects and Developmental Disabilities (BDDD)
- Division of Environmental Hazards and Health Effects (EHHE)
- Division of Environmental Health Laboratory Sciences (EHLS)
- Programs within the Office of the Director
- Office on Disability and Health (ODH)
- Emergency Response Coordination Group (ERCG)
- International Emergency and Refugee Health Program (IERH)
- Special Programs Group (SPG)

National Center for Environmental Health (NCEH)
Centers for Disease Control and Prevention (CDC)
Mail Stop F-29
4770 Buford Highway, N.E.
Atlanta, Georgia 30341-3724
Telephone: (770) 488-7030

For State and Local Health Department Assistance:
CDC Emergency Response (24-hr assistance during emergencies): (404) 639-0615.

Toll-free telephone number for information and faxes on childhood lead poisoning, cruise ship inspection, cholesterol measurements, and list of publications: NCEH Health Line 1-888-232-6789.

National Center for Health Statistics

The mission of the National Center for Health Statistics (NCHS) is to provide statistical information that will guide actions and policies to improve the health of the American people. As the Nation's principal health statistics agency, NCHS leads the way with accurate, relevant, and timely data.

National Center for Health Statistics
internet address: nchsquery@cdc.gov
Telephone: (301) 436-8500

National Center for HIV, STD, and TB Prevention

The National Center for HIV, STD, and TB Prevention (NCHSTP) is responsible for public health surveillance, prevention research, and programs to prevent and control human immunodeficiency virus (HIV) infection and acquired immunodeficiency syndrome (AIDS), other sexually transmitted diseases (STDs), and tuberculosis (TB). Center staff work in collaboration with governmental and nongovernmental partners at community, State, national, and international levels, applying well-integrated multidisciplinary programs of research, surveillance, technical assistance, and evaluation.

NCHSTP's Prevention Approach

NCHSTP contributes to reductions in many diseases through a systematic process of (1) detecting a problem and determining the cause, (2) assessing what needs to be done by the private and public sector to control the problem, (3) developing and testing interventions to help solve the problem, (4) implementing and evaluating proven interventions through private and public efforts as nationwide prevention programs, and (5) developing prevention policies to guide further efforts.

As part of this process, NCHSTP must translate knowledge about effective methods of preventing disease and injury into nationwide strategies that reach people in communities throughout this country. The Center collects national data on HIV/AIDS, STD, and TB incidence and prevalence, and related behaviors; monitors change over time; conducts epidemiologic, laboratory, clinical, and behavioral research; and develops and evaluates prevention strategies. The translation of applied research into programs and activities that work for different groups of people at the community level is vital to all our prevention efforts. This process means field testing prevention methods for their effectiveness in real world settings and calculating their cost-effectiveness. NCHSTP works closely with its partners in State and local health agencies, national and community-based organizations, business, and academia to design and test prevention programs that work. And NCHSTP develops policies and recommendations based on this science-based process.

NCHSTP Organization

NCHSTP is organized into an Office of the Director (OD) and four divisions, with the following functions:

- The Office of the Director provides overall management, operations, communications, and policy guidance for the center. Also included in OD is an Office of Communications, which is a principal focal point for translating and disseminating science and prevention information, and a new field support unit, the Prevention Support Office (PSO), which has been created to handle grant and field staff issues across HIV, STD, and TB prevention programs.

- PSO's Program Coordination Unit is being established initially as a pilot project to facilitate program coordination and integration among the center's divisions and with State and local health department grantees for HIV, STD, and TB prevention.

- The Division of HIV/AIDS Prevention-Surveillance and Epidemiology (DHAP-SE) conducts surveillance and epidemiologic and behavioral research to monitor trends and risk behaviors and provide a basis for targeting prevention resources. In addition to work within the United States, DHAP is active in surveillance, research, prevention, evaluation, and technology transfer activities in developing countries.

- The Division of HIV/AIDS Prevention-Intervention Research and Support (DHAP-IRS) conducts behavioral intervention and operations research and evaluation and provides financial and technical assistance for HIV prevention programs conducted by State, local, and territorial health departments, national minority organizations, community-based organizations, business, labor, religious organizations, and training agencies.

- The Division of STD Prevention (DSTDP) conducts surveillance; epidemiologic, behavioral, and operations research; and program evaluation related to STDs, including syphilis, gonorrhea, chlamydia, human papillomavirus, genital herpes, and hepatitis B; assists States and selected localities in reaching those at risk for infection with STDs; works to prevent infertility and pelvic inflammatory disease and its complications, which can include ectopic pregnancy, cancer, and fetal or infant death; and collaborates with other agencies and groups, particularly community-based organizations, to enhance STD prevention awareness. DSTDP also supports programs in developing countries for surveillance, research, and prevention.

- The Division of TB Elimination (DTBE) conducts surveillance and epidemiologic, behavioral, and operations research, both in the United States and in developing countries and provides information and reducation to health care providers, persons at high risk, and the general population. It also supports State and local health department efforts in preventing and controlling TB through directly observed therapy to ensure treatment completion by patients; in following up for persons with TB, suspected of having TB, or exposed to TB; in strengthening of laboratory activities; and in TB screening among persons at high risk and preventive therapy for persons found with infection.

CDC National AIDS Hotline
(24 hours, 7 days a week)
Offers anonymous, confidential HIV/AIDS information to the American public. Provides referrals to HIV/AIDS services, and free publications and other informational materials.
(800) 342-AIDS (2437) (English)
(800) 344-7432 (Spanish)
(800) 243-7889 (TTY for hearing impaired)

CDC National STD Hotline
(Mon-Fri, 8am-11pm, EST)
Provides anonymous, confidential information on sexually transmitted diseases (STD) and how to prevent them. Also, provides referrals to clinical and other services.
(800) 227-8922

HIV/AIDS and TB Fax Information Service
(24 hours, 7 days a week)
Provides information by fax on HIV/AIDS and tuberculosis for health care professionals and others. For a list of TB documents, ask for Document #250000. For HIV/AIDS documents, follow the recorded directions.
(404) 332-4565

TB Voice Information System
24 hours, 7 days a week)
Provides recorded information on tuberculosis for health care professionals and the general public. Information can also be sent by fax or mail.
(404) 330-1231

NCHSTP Voice Information System
(24 hours, 7 days a week)
Provides information primarily for health care professionals and educators on STD and TB. Also lists state health department phone numbers.
Toll-free (888) 232-3228 (press 2,5,1 and then 1 for STD,2 for TB)

National Center for Injury Prevention and Control

Research

NCIPC conducts and monitors research on the causes, risks, and preventive measures for injuries outside the workplace, including:

- Unintentional injuries related to falls, fires and burns, drownings, poisonings, motor-vehicle crashes (including those with pedestrians), recreational activities, and play-grounds and day-care settings
- Intentional injuries related to suicide, youth violence, family and intimate violence, and firearms
- Prevention of secondary conditions among people with disabilities

NCIPC also funds research by universities and other public and private groups studying the three phases of injury control (prevention, acute care, and rehabilitation) and the two major disciplines of injury control (epidemiology and biomechanics).

National Center for Injury Prevention and Control
Office of Communication Resources
Mailstop K65
4770 Buford Highway NE
Atlanta, GA 30341-3724
Telephone (770) 488-1506
Internet address: OHCINFO@cdc.gov

National Institute for Occupational Safety and Health

NIOSH is the acronym for the National Institute for Occupational Safety and Health, a Federal agency established by the Occupational Safety and Health Act of 1970. NIOSH is part of the Centers for Disease Control and Prevention (CDC) and is responsible for conducting research and making recommendations for the prevention of work-related illness and injuries. The Institute's responsibilities include the following:

- Investigating potentially hazardous working conditions as requested by employers or employees
- Evaluating hazards in the workplace, ranging from chemicals to machinery
- Creating and disseminating methods for preventing disease, injury, and disability
- Conducting research and providing scientifically valid recommendations for protecting workers

Callers may request information about NIOSH activities, order NIOSH publications, or request information about any aspect of occupational safety and health. However, this toll-free number is NOT a hotline for medical emergencies.

Contact NIOSH toll free at: 1-800-35-NIOSH (1-800-356-4674).

Epidemiology Program Office

EPO Mission: To strengthen the public health system by coordinating public health surveillance at CDC and providing domestic and international support through scientific communications, statistical and epidemiologic consultation, and training of experts in surveillance, epidemiology, applied public health, and prevention effectiveness.

Office of the Director

- Office of Program Management and Operations
- Administrative Services Activity
- IRM Activity
- Office of Scientific Communications
- *MMWR*
- Public Health Publications Activity

Division of Prevention Research and Analytic Methods

- Prevention Effectiveness Activity
- Statistics and Epidemiology Branch
- Evaluation and Behavioral Science Methods Branch
- Community Preventive Services Guide Development Activity

Division of Applied Public Health Training

- Administrative Services Activity
- Training Development and Management Activity
- Epidemic Intelligence Service (EIS)
- Preventive Medicine Residency Program (PMR)
- Public Health Prevention Service (PHPS)
- State Branch

Division of International Health

- Program Development Activity
- Data Use and Policy Activity

Division of Public Health Surveillance and Informatics

- Systems Integration Activity
- Systems Development and Support Activity
- Systems Operations and Information Activity
- Public Health Information Systems Branch

International Health Program Office

To lead CDC's collaboration with other nations and international organizations to promote healthy lifestyles and to prevent excess disease, disability, and death. Specifically, IHPO:

- strengthens the public health capacity of other nations
- provides scientific and management expertise to the design, implementation and evaluation of integrated public health programs in developing countries
- directs CDC's response to international emergency and refugee health assistance
- facilitates all of CDC's international activities
- explores new opportunities for international collaboration in health

Associate Director for International Health
Director, **International Health Program Office**
4770 Buford Highway
Mail Stop K01
Atlanta, GA 30341-3724
Telephone: (770)488-1080

National Immunization Program

The National Immunization Program (NIP) is a part of the Centers for Disease Control and Prevention, located in Atlanta, Georgia. As a disease-prevention program, NIP provides leadership for the planning, coordination, and conduct of immunization activities nationwide. In carrying out its mission, NIP:

• Provides consultation, training, statistical, promotional, educational, epidemiological, and technical services to assist health departments in planning, developing, and implementing immunization programs.

• Supports the establishment of vaccine supply contacts for vaccine distribution to state and local immunization programs.

• Assists health departments in developing vaccine information management systems to facilitate identification of children who need vaccinations, help parents and providers ensure that all children are immunized at the appropriate age, assess vaccination levels in state and local areas, monitor the safety and efficacy of vaccines by linking vaccine administration information with adverse event reporting and disease outbreak patterns.

• Administers research and operational programs for the prevention and control of vaccine-preventable diseases.

• Supports a nationwide framework for effective surveillance of designated diseases for which effective immunizing agents are available.

• Supervises state and local assignees working on immunization activities.

Chapter 15

Emerging Infectious Diseases

Executive Summary

Thirty years ago, the threat of infectious diseases appeared to be receding. Modern scientific advances, including antibiotic drugs, vaccines against childhood diseases, and improved technology for sanitation, had facilitated the control or prevention of many infectious diseases, particularly in industrialized nations. The incidence of childhood diseases such as polio, whooping cough, and diphtheria was declining due to the use of vaccines. In addition, American physicians had fast-acting, effective antibiotics to combat often fatal bacterial diseases such as meningitis and pneumonia. Deaths from infection, commonplace at the beginning of the twentieth century, were no longer a frequent occurrence in the United States. Meanwhile, in other parts of the world, chemical pesticides like DDT were lowering the incidence of malaria, a major killer of children, by controlling populations of parasite-carrying mosquitoes.

As it turned out, our understandable euphoria was premature. It did not take into account the extraordinary resilience of infectious microbes, which have a remarkable ability to evolve, adapt, and develop resistance to drugs in an unpredictable and dynamic fashion. It also did not take into account the accelerating spread of human populations into tropical forests and overcrowded mega-cities where people are exposed to a variety of emerging infectious agents.

CISET Report Home Page

221

Today, most health professionals agree that new microbial threats are appearing in significant numbers, while well-known illnesses thought to be under control are re-emerging. Most Americans are aware of the epidemic of the acquired immunodeficiency syndrome (AIDS) and the related increase in tuberculosis (TB) cases in the United States. In fact, there has been a general resurgence of infectious diseases throughout the world, including significant outbreaks of cholera, malaria, yellow fever, and diphtheria. In addition, bacterial resistance to antibiotic drugs is an increasingly serious worldwide problem. Furthermore, the number of people infected with the human immunodeficiency virus (HIV) that causes AIDS is increasing in many countries and may reach 40 million by the year 2000. Most recently, Ebola virus, which causes an often fatal hemorrhagic illness, has appeared again in Africa, and a formerly unknown virus of the measles family that killed several horses in Australia also infected two men, one of whom died.

New diseases have also appeared within the United States, including Lyme disease, Legionnaires' disease, and most recently hantavirus pulmonary syndrome (HPS). HPS was first recognized in the southwestern United States in 1993 and has since been detected in more than 20 states and in several other countries in the Americas. Other new or re-emerging threats in the United States include multidrug-resistant TB; antibiotic-resistant bacteria causing ear infections; pneumonia; meningitis; rabies; and diarrheal diseases caused by the parasite *Cryptosporidium parvum* and by certain toxigenic strains of *Escherichia coli* bacteria.

Why Are New Infectious Diseases Emerging?

The reasons for the sharp increase in incidence of many infectious diseases—once thought to be under control—are complex and not fully understood. Population shifts and population growth; changes in human behavior; urbanization, poverty, and crowding; changes in ecology and climate; the evolution of microbes; inadequacy of public health infrastructures; and modern travel and trade have all contributed. For example, the ease of modern travel creates many opportunities for a disease outbreak in remote areas to spread to a crowded urban area. Human behavioral factors, such as dietary habits and food handling, personal hygiene, risky sexual behavior, and intravenous drug use can contribute to disease emergence. In several parts of the world, human encroachment on tropical forests has brought populations with little or no disease resistance into close proximity with insects that carry malaria and yellow fever and other, sometimes unknown, infectious diseases. In addition, local fluctuations in temperature and rainfall affect the number of microbe-carrying rodents in some areas. Finally, in many parts of the world there has been a deterioration in the local public health infrastructures that monitor and respond to disease outbreaks.

Are Infectious Disease Surveillance and Control Cost-Effective?

The costs of infectious diseases at home and abroad are staggering, and the cost-effectiveness of disease prevention has been demonstrated again and again. Every year, billions of dollars are lost in the United States in direct medical costs and lost productivity, due to intestinal infections, sexually transmitted diseases, influenza, and other viral, bacterial, or parasitic diseases. When diseases are controlled or prevented, tremendous savings can be achieved. For instance, a timely epidemiologic investigation in Washington State in 1993 led to the prompt recall of 250,000 hamburgers contaminated with *E. coli* O157, saving millions of dollars as well as preventing human suffering and death. Since smallpox was eradicated in 1977, the total investment of $32 million has been returned to the United States every 26 days. Based on the current rate of progress towards eradication of poliomyelitis, the World Health Organization predicts "global savings of half a billion dollars by the year 2000, increasing to $3 billion annually by the year 2015." Furthermore, every dollar spent on the vaccine against measles, mumps, and rubella, saves $21, while every dollar spent on the vaccine against diphtheria, tetanus, and pertussis saves $29. Clearly, public health measures that prevent or control infectious diseases are extremely cost-effective.

Today, two of the largest U.S. infectious disease health-care expenses are for the treatment of TB and AIDS. When the first cases of AIDS and drug-resistant TB were detected in the United States control measures were delayed, partly due to a lack of surveillance information. TB is an ancient disease, known throughout human history, that re-emerged in the United States in the late 1980s, sometimes in a drug-resistant or multidrug-resistant form. Government spending on infectious disease control had declined during the 1980s, and in 1986 the surveillance system for drug-resistant TB was discontinued. By 1993, multidrug-resistant TB had became a public health crisis and millions of federal dollars were necessary to control the emergency.

Unlike TB, AIDS is a newly emergent disease, unrecognized before the 1980s. AIDS might have been identified before it became established in the United States if a global surveillance system with the capacity to identify new diseases had been in place in the 1970s. As early as 1962, African doctors apparently witnessed cases of what was then known as "slim disease." Had the international community taken notice, epidemiologists might have gained a head start in learning how AIDS is transmitted and prevented, and many lives might have been saved.

Disease prevention is an investment in the young people of the world and in our collective future. Every year, an estimated four million infant and child deaths are prevented by vaccination and other preventive health measures, due to multilateral efforts. At the same time, many countries have dramatically strengthened their health-care delivery systems, even in the face of economic stagnation. On the other hand, the AIDS pandemic and the resurgence of malaria and TB are impeding economic development in many of the world's poorest countries.

Need for U.S. Leadership

The modern world is a very small place; any city in the world is only a plane ride away from any other. Infectious microbes can easily travel across borders with their human or animal hosts. In fact, diseases that arise in other parts of the world are repeatedly introduced into the United States, where they may threaten our national health and security. Thus, controlling disease outbreaks in other countries is important not only for humanitarian reasons. It also prevents those diseases from entering the United States, at great savings of U.S. lives and dollars. Moreover, U.S. support for disease investigations in other countries provides U.S. scientists with opportunities to bring U.S. capacity to focus on new pathogens like Ebola virus and consider how best to control, prevent, and treat them internationally before they arrive on our shores. Thus, U.S. interests are served while providing support to other nations.

Actively promoting the effort to develop an international partnership to address emerging infectious diseases is a natural role for the United States. American business leaders and scientists are in the forefront of the computer communications and biomedical research communities that must provide the technical and scientific underpinning for disease surveillance. The United States maintains more medical facilities and personnel abroad than any other country, in terms of both civilian and military, and public and private sector institutions. Furthermore, American scientists and public health professionals have been among the most important contributors to the international efforts to eradicate smallpox and polio. This position of leadership should be fostered.

Our earlier successes in controlling infections have bred complacency. Consequently, the component of the public health system that protects the public from infectious microbes has been neglected, both here and abroad, and its focus has narrowed. In the United States, federal, state, and local efforts to control communicable diseases are concentrated on a few targeted illnesses, with few resources allocated to address new or re-emerging diseases. This limits the ability of the U.S. medical community to detect and respond to outbreaks of newly emerging diseases, whether here or in foreign countries.

International Coordination of Infectious Disease Prevention Efforts

The challenge ahead outstrips the means available to any one country or to international organizations. The elimination of smallpox would not have been possible without a truly global effort. Similarly, multilateral leadership and resources propel the international program to eradicate polio. Both examples demonstrate the value to American citizens of resources invested in global disease prevention.

In addition, an effective global disease surveillance and response network will enable the United States to respond quickly and effectively in the event of terrorist incidents involving biological or chemical agents. The experience gained in controlling naturally occurring microbes will enhance our ability to cope with a biological warfare agent, should the need arise. The release of nerve gas in the Tokyo subway system in March 1995 has underscored our need to be well prepared to counteract deliberate attempts to undermine human health.

To address the growing threat of emerging infectious diseases the U.S. Government must not only improve its public health infrastructure, but also work in concert with other nations and international bodies, particularly WHO. The work and cost of protecting the world's people from infectious diseases must be shared by all nations. Some industrialized countries have already decided to devote substantial resources to a surveillance effort, and some less developed nations may also be ready to engage in an international effort that is so clearly in their own interests. President Clinton and the other leaders of the

G7 nations recently endorsed 11 pilot projects of the Global Information Infrastructure at the Halifax Summit, including a project entitled,
"Toward a Global Health Network." This project is designed to help
public health institutions in their fight against infectious diseases and
major health hazards. In addition, the World Health Assembly recently passed a resolution that focuses on national capacity building
related to detecting and controlling emerging infectious diseases. The
U.S. Agency for International Development (USAID), other donors,
and the WHO, are continuing to assist developing countries in establishing disease prevention and control programs and to encourage the
development of disease reporting systems.

Although international efforts must be coordinated to prevent global pandemics, disease surveillance is first of all the responsibility of
each sovereign nation. However, individual governments may not only
lack the means to respond but may also be reluctant to share national
disease surveillance information, fearing losses in trade, tourism, and
national prestige. Nevertheless, because the United States is widely
respected as the world's foremost authority on infectious disease recognition and control, we do learn about most major disease outbreaks
in other countries, although not always in an official or timely fashion. Individual doctors, laboratories, or ministries of health often seek
United States assistance when they are confronted with a disease
problem that they cannot solve. To ensure that we continue to be no-
tified when an unusual outbreak occurs, we must encourage and support other countries' efforts in national disease surveillance and
respond when asked for assistance. We must strive to develop a sense
of shared responsibility and mutual confidence in the global effort to
combat infectious diseases.

The effort to build a global surveillance and response system supports other foreign policy goals of the United States. Obviously, such
a system will help protect the health of American citizens and of people
throughout the world. In the post-Cold War period, a major objective
of U.S. foreign policy is the promotion of political stability through
sustainable economic development around the globe. Helping other
countries to help themselves to improve the lives of their citizens,
develop their economies, and find niches in the global economy is a
major goal for U.S. foreign assistance. Healthy people are more productive and better able to contribute to their country's welfare.

Building a Global Infectious Diseases Network

Surveillance

At the present time, a formal system for infectious disease surveillance does not exist on a global scale. When a cluster of cases of a new disease occurs in a remote part of Africa, Eastern Europe, Asia, or the Americas, the international community may or may not learn about it. If a new disease of unknown cause occurs in a part of the world that lacks modern communications, it may spread far and wide before it is recognized and brought under control. In most cases, however, news of a major outbreak spreads informally. When international resources are successfully mobilized, assistance in diagnosis, disease control and prevention can be made available to local health authorities. Clinical specimens can be sent to a diagnostic "reference" laboratory to rule out known disease agents. Epidemiologists can be sent into the field to help investigate the source of the new infection and determine how it is transmitted. Public health officials can use this information to implement appropriate control measures. Once the infectious agent has been identified, which is often a difficult task, experimental scientists can start to develop diagnostic tools and treatments if the disease is carried by a previously unknown agent.

The elements of a global network for disease surveillance already exist but need to be strengthened, linked, and coordinated. For instance, many U.S. Government departments and agencies maintain or support field stations and laboratories in Africa, Asia, and the Americas that may be electronically linked to provide an initial framework for a network for global infectious disease reporting. In partnership with other countries and with WHO, this skeletal surveillance network could be expanded over time to include many international resources, including national health ministries, WHO Collaborating Centers, hospitals, and laboratories operated by other nations, and American and foreign private voluntary organizations.

Information technology is revolutionizing communications worldwide; this technology needs to be applied to disease control programs, not only to effectively monitor program performance and progress, but also to detect and report emerging problems.

Response

The process of response encompasses a multitude of activities, including diagnosis of the disease; investigation to understand its source and modes of transmission; implementation of control strategies and programs; research to develop adequate means to treat it and prevent its spread; and production and dissemination of the necessary drugs and vaccines.

The international community does not always have adequate resources to respond to localized disease outbreaks and control them before they can spread across borders. If an "old" disease re-emerges, there may be a need for epidemiologic investigations and/or for emergency procurement or production of medical supplies. If the disease is new, efforts will be needed to identify the causative microbe and determine how to stop its transmission. To make the best possible use of U.S. expertise and resources, it is necessary to establish clear lines of authority and communication among U.S. Government agencies.

Response to infectious disease outbreaks, whenever and wherever they occur requires international preparation and planning. A goal of the WHO is to assist each country to develop its ability to provide laboratory diagnosis of diseases endemic to its area and to refer specimens from suspected newly emergent or re-emergent diseases to an appropriate regional reference laboratory. To reach this goal, each country must train medical workers and laboratory technicians and supply them with appropriate equipment and diagnostic resources.

In addition, several international elements must be in place to provide the wherewithal for effective and timely disease control and prevention efforts. First, regional reference laboratories must be maintained to provide diagnostic expertise and distribute diagnostic tests. Second, an international communications mechanism must be made available to receive and analyze global disease surveillance information. Third, regional procedures should be instituted to facilitate the production, procurement, and distribution of medical supplies, including vaccines for disease eradication programs. Fourth, enhanced public education in simple health measures in both industrialized and developing countries is very important.

Through programs administered by USAID and other agencies, the United States has invested in assisting developing countries to establish disease prevention and control programs, trained thousands of individuals, and strengthened scores of institutions. As a consequence, developing country researchers are better prepared to solve their own disease problems and contribute to solving global ones. Strengthening this foundation will be critical to facilitating timely and effective responses to disease outbreaks and minimizing the impact of emerging disease threats.

Research

An effective system for disease surveillance and control is critically dependent on a strong and stable research infrastructure. Scientific studies of infectious agents and the diseases they cause provide the fundamental knowledge base used to develop diagnostic tests to identify diseases, drugs to treat them, and vaccines to prevent them. Traditionally, this has been an area of U.S. strength and international leadership. To meet the new challenges represented by emerging diseases, a strong research and training effort must be sustained and strengthened. The current level of support for research and training in laboratory and field work on infectious diseases, other than AIDS and TB, is very limited. To combat new diseases for which no treatments are available, it is essential to maintain an active community of well-trained epidemiologists, laboratory scientists, clinical investigators, behavioral scientists, entomologists, and public health experts ready and able to seek new solutions for disease threats. At the present time, many of the brightest young microbiologists in the United States are leaving the field, discouraged by the lack of jobs and research funds.

USAID, National Institutes of Health (NIH), and Centers for Disease Control and Prevention (CDC) support has fostered the capacity of less developed countries to identify and solve their infectious disease problems. Applied research in these countries is aimed at preventing disease transmission through control of insect and animal vectors, environmental factors, and behavior, and at evaluating new or improved therapeutic and preventive measures. In addition, the National Oceanic and Atmospheric Administration is developing tools to predict local changes in weather that effect the incidence of vector-borne diseases.

Training

Many research programs routinely incorporate training opportunities for graduate students and postdoctoral fellows. In addition, there is an urgent need to augment specialized training programs in such areas as the handling of hazardous microbes, public health management, and field epidemiology.

Summary of Recommendations of the CISET Working Group

An interagency Government working group on emerging infectious diseases was formed in December 1994 under the auspices of the

National Science and Technology Council's Committee on International Science, Engineering, and Technology (CISET). Led by CDC, the Department of State, USAID, Food and Drug Administration, NIH, and the Department of Defense, the working group makes the following recommendations for action by the U.S. Government.

Work in partnership with other countries, with WHO, and with other international organizations to improve worldwide disease surveillance, reporting, and response by:

1. Establishing regional disease surveillance and response networks linking national health ministries, WHO regional offices, U.S. Government laboratories and field stations abroad, foreign laboratories and medical centers, and WHO Collaborating Centers.

2. Ensuring that reliable lines of communication exist between local and national medical centers and between national and regional or international reference facilities, especially in parts of the world where modern communications are lacking.

3. Developing a global alert system whereby national governments can inform appropriate worldwide health authorities of outbreaks of infectious diseases in a timely manner, and whereby individual health authorities can access regional centers.

4. Identifying regional and international resources that can provide diagnostic reagents for low incidence diseases and help identify rare and unusual diseases.

5. Assisting WHO to establish global surveillance of antibiotic resistance and drug use, as a first-step toward the development of international agreements on antibiotic usage.

6. Encouraging and assisting other countries to make infectious disease detection and control a national priority.

7. Preserving existing U.S. Government activities that enhance other countries' abilities to prevent and control emerging and re-emerging health threats.

8. Identifying and strengthening WHO Collaborating Centers that serve as unique reference centers for diseases whose re-emergence is feared.

9.   Establishing the authority of relevant U.S. Government agencies to make the most effective use of their expertise in building a worldwide disease surveillance and response network.

Strengthen the U.S. capacity to combat emerging infectious diseases by:

10. Enhancing collaborations among U.S. agencies to ensure maximum use of existing resources for domestic and international surveillance and response activities. Supporting the G7-initiated project on public health applications of the Global Information Infrastructure, entitled "Toward a Global Public Health Network."

11. Rebuilding the U.S. infectious disease surveillance public health infrastructure at the local, state, and federal levels.

12. Working with the private and public sectors to improve U.S. capacity for the emergency production of diagnostic tests, drugs, and vaccines.

13. Supporting an active community of epidemiologists, clinical investigators, laboratory scientists, health experts, and behavioral scientists ready and able to seek new solutions for new disease threats.

14. Strengthening technical training programs in disciplines related to infectious disease surveillance and response.

15. Providing accurate and timely health information to private citizens and health providers, both in the United States and abroad, when a disease outbreak occurs.

16. Strengthening infectious disease screening and quarantine efforts at ports of entry into the United States.

17. Strengthening the training of American physicians and microbiologists in the recognition of "tropical diseases" and in travel medicine in general.

18. Establishing an Interagency Task Force to coordinate the implementation of these recommendations.

19. Establishing a private sector subcommittee of the Interagency Task Force that includes representatives of the U.S. pharmaceutical industry, medical practitioners and educators, and biomedical scientists.

Chapter 16

Summary of Notifiable
Diseases in the United States

Foreward

This publication contains summary tables of the official statistics
for the reported occurrence of nationally notifiable diseases in the
United States for the year 1994. This information is collected and
compiled from reports to the National Notifiable Diseases Surveillance
System (NNDSS). Because the dates of onset and dates of diagnosis
for notifiable diseases are often unknown, these surveillance data are
presented by the week that they were reported to public health officials. These data are then finalized and published in the *MMWR Summary of Notifiable Diseases*, United States, for use by state and local
health departments; schools of medicine and public health; communications media; local, state, and federal agencies; and other agencies or persons interested in following the trends of reportable conditions in the
United States. Publication of the annual summary also ensures documentation of diseases that are considered national priorities for notification and of the annual number of cases of such diseases.

Background

As of January 1, 1994, 49 infectious diseases were designated as
notifiable at the national level. A notifiable disease is one for which
regular, frequent, and timely information on individual cases is considered necessary for the prevention and control of the disease. This

MMWR Summary of Notifiable Diseases, 1994

section briefly summarizes the history of national notifiable disease reporting in the United States.

In 1878, Congress authorized the U.S. Marine Hospital Service (the precursor to the Public Health Service, PHS) to collect morbidity reports on cholera, smallpox, plague, and yellow fever from U.S. consuls overseas; this information was to be used for instituting quarantine measures to prevent the introduction and spread of these diseases into the United States. In 1879, a specific Congressional appropriation was made for the collection and publication of reports of these notifiable diseases. The authority for weekly reporting and publication was expanded by Congress in 1893 to include data from states and municipal authorities. To increase the uniformity of the data, Congress enacted a law in 1902 directing the Surgeon General to provide forms for the collection and compilation of data and for the publication of reports at the national level. In 1912, state and territorial health authoritiesin conjunction with PHS recommended immediate telegraphic reporting of five infectious diseases and monthly reporting by letter of 10 additional diseases. The first annual summary of The Notifiable Diseases in 1912 included reports of 10 diseases from 19 states, the District of Columbia, and Hawaii. By 1928, all states, the District of Columbia, Hawaii, and Puerto Rico were participating in national reporting of nearly 30 specified conditions. At their annual meeting in 1950, the State and Territorial Health Officers authorized a conference of state and territorial epidemiologists whose purpose was to determine which diseases should be reported to PHS. CDC assumed responsibility for the collection and publication of data on nationally notifiable diseases in 1961.

The list of nationally notifiable diseases is revised periodically. For example, diseases may be added to the list as new pathogens emerge or deleted as their incidence declines. Public health officials at state health departments and CDC continue to collaborate in determining which diseases should be nationally notifiable; the Council of State and Territorial Epidemiologists (CSTE), with CDC input, makes recommendations annually for additions and deletions to the list of nationally notifiable diseases. However, reporting of nationally notifiable diseases to CDC by the states is voluntary. Reporting is currently mandated (by state legislation or regulation) only at the state level. The list of diseases that are considered notifiable, therefore, varies slightly by state. All states generally report the internationally quarantinable diseases (i.e., cholera, plague, and yellow fever) in compliance with the World Health Organization's International Health Regulations. During 1994, 49 infectious diseases were considered notifiable at the national level and were reported to CDC; 41 were reported on a weekly basis, and eight were reported monthly.

CSTE and CDC held a national surveillance conference November 30-December 2, 1994 to review the state of national infectious disease surveillance. Infectious diseases that have been approved for addition to national surveillance during 1995 are Chlamydia trachomatis (genital infections), coccidioidomycosis (for regional surveillance), cryptosporidiosis, hantavirus infection, (post-diarrheal) hemolytic uremic syndrome, pediatric infection with the human immunodeficiency virus, invasive group A streptococcal infections, streptococcal toxic-shock syndrome, and drug-resistant *Streptococcus pneumoniae*. These conditions currently are not reportable in all states, and the mechanism for reporting may not involve clinicians or consist of reports of individual cases (i.e., traditional notification methods). Reports of the number of cases of these conditions will not appear in the current year tables before 1996.

At the 1994 conference the following diseases were also proposed as deletions from the list of infectious diseases under national surveillance: amebiasis, aseptic meningitis, primary encephalitis (except for arboviral encephalitis), postinfectious encephalitis, granuloma inguinale, unspecified hepatitis, leptospirosis, lymphogranuloma venereum, rheumatic fever, and tularemia. These changes were confirmed by a vote of the full membership of CSTE in early 1995. The number of reported cases of these diseases will not appear in the current year tables after 1994.

Highlights for Selected Infectious Diseases Not Nationally Notifiable During 1994

Chlamydia

Chlamydia trachomatis infections are common among adolescents and young adults. An estimated 10% of sexually active adolescent females are infected with chlamydia. In 1994, 47 states reported 448,984 chlamydia infections. From 1984 through 1994, reported cases increased from 3.2 cases per 100,000 to 188.4. This trend may reflect increasing recognition and interest among health-care providers and public health officials.

Coccidioidomycosis

An outbreak of coccidioidomycosis occurred in Ventura County, California, following the 1994 Northridge earthquake. From January

24 through March 15, 1994, 203 infected persons were identified, compared with 52 cases that were reported through passive surveillance in the county in 1993. The National Center for Infectious Diseases (NCID/CDC) Emerging Infections Program (EIP), in collaboration with the State of California Department of Health Services, is conducting active surveillance for coccidioidomycosis in 10 California counties.

Cryptosporidiosis

In 1994, waterborne outbreaks of cryptosporidiosis were investigated in Las Vegas, Nevada, Walla Walla, Washington, and Lake Nummy, New Jersey, focusing national attention on the potential for waterborne transmission of Cryptosporidium. In September 1994, a national workshop on waterborne cryptosporidiosis was held at CDC, which resulted in guidelines and recommendations for prevention of cryptosporidiosis in severely immunosuppressed persons, appropriate public health responses to the problem, and epidemiologic and laboratory-based surveillance and research.

Hantavirus

Hantavirus Pulmonary Syndrome (HPS) is a recently recognized hantaviral illness caused by Sin Nombre virus and the newly identified Black Creek Canal and Bayou viruses. The identified rodent reservoirs for these viruses—Peromyscus maniculatus and leucopus (deer and white-footed mice) for Sin Nombre virus and its variants and Sigmodon hispidus (cotton rat) for Black Creek Canal virus—extend across the continental United States. As of July 20, 1995, national surveillance for HPS has identified 113 confirmed case-patients in 23 states (case fatality rate: 52%); 31 of these cases occurred in 1994.

Invasive Group A Streptococcal Infections

Prospective and retrospective active surveillance data for invasive group A streptococcal (GAS) infections were analyzed and several risk groups identified, including: persons who have human immunodeficiency virus (HIV) infections and acquired immunodeficiency syndrome (AIDS), injecting-drug users, persons who have cancer, diabetes mellitus, heart disease or chronic lung disease, alcohol abusers, and children who have varicella. Although different GAS strains have been identified from individual case patients, M-type 1 strains predominated.

Drug-Resistant Streptococcus Pneumoniae

In the United States, the prevalence of drug-resistant *Streptococcus pneumoniae* (DRSP) has increased since 1987 from 3.6% to 14.5%, according to limited voluntary reporting by 12 sentinel hospitals. Limited 1994 surveillance data from these hospitals indicate the proportion of invasive disease (bacteremia and meningitis) caused by penicillin-resistant pneumococci ranges from 3% to 30% and shows widespread geographic variation. Information regarding community-specific DRSP prevalence is needed to assist clinicians in choosing optimal empiric therapy. To enhance efficient and timely reporting, CDC is currently piloting an electronic laboratory-based surveillance system.

Vancomycin-Resistant Enterococci

In 1994, the percentage of nosocomial enterococci reported as resistant to vancomycin increased from 11.5% in 1993 to 13.6% among Intensive Care Unit (ICU) isolates and from 4.9% to 9.1% among non-critical care unit isolates. The increase was more dramatic among isolates from noncritical care units, suggesting that vancomycin-resistant enterococci are spreading from their focus in ICUs.

Pneumonia of Unknown Etiology

From 1979 to 1994, the overall crude death rate for pneumonia and influenza increased 59%, from 20.0 to 31.8 deaths per 100,000. Through 1992 (the most recent year for which complete data are available), pneumonia of unspecified etiology (ICD-9 code 486) accounted for most of the overall increasethe age-adjusted death rates in this diagnostic category increased 74%. Since the 1970s, several previously unrecognized infectious agents have been identified as causes of lower respiratory infections, including Legionella pneumophila, Chlamydia pneumoniae, and Sin Nombre virus. Recent prospective studies of community-acquired pneumonia indicate that an etiology cannot be identified in up to 50% of cases.

Transfusion-Associated Infectious Diseases

An Institute of Medicine committee recently released the report, "HIV and the Blood Supply: An Analysis of Crisis Decisionmaking," calling for the establishment of a surveillance system at CDC to detect, monitor, and warn of adverse effects in the recipients of blood and blood products. CDC is reviewing existing surveillance systems to highlight and address areas that need improvement. Diseases that are being examined to evaluate the level of risk associated with transfusion include HIV/AIDS, Chagas disease, babesiosis, Creutzfeld-Jakob disease, the hepatitis viruses, malaria, and transfusion-associated sepsis.

International Notes

Dengue

Although dengue fever is not endemic in the United States, its incidence is increasing in most tropical areas throughout the world. In 1994, CDC processed serum samples from 91 residents of 27 states and the District of Columbia who had traveled to countries where dengue is endemic. Among these 91 persons, 37 (40.7%) cases of dengue were diagnosed serologically or virologically.

Plague

During September and October 1994, outbreaks of bubonic and pneumonic plague were reported from sites east and north of Bombay, India, respectively. A lack of reliable epidemiologic information contributed to the ensuing international health emergency. Evidence revealed that plague did not occur in international travelers or spread beyond the original foci.

Chapter 17

Vaccines for Children: Barriers to Immunization

Section 13631 of the Omnibus Budget Reconciliation Act of 1993 created the Vaccine for Children (VFC) as an entitlement program to provide free vaccine to children 18 and younger who are eligible for Medicaid, Native American or Alaskan natives, uninsured, or under-insured (that is, whose insurance does not cover childhood vaccinations). The administration had stipulated that an increase in the cost of vaccine was a major factor in low rates of vaccination and proposed VFC to purchase and distribute vaccine supplies "to make sure that children do not become sick or die from vaccine preventable diseases." By providing free vaccines, VFC was intended to remove vaccine cost as a barrier to childhood immunization. VFC is a part of the Child-hood Immunization Initiative (CII), the goal of which is to raise immunization rates for 2-year-old children to 90 percent for most antigens. By law, VFC is to provide the states with vaccines. The schedule established by the Public Health Service's Advisory Commit-tee on Immunization Practices includes vaccines for measles, mumps, rubella, diphtheria, polio, tetanus, pertussis, hepatitis B, and hemo-philus influenza. It is expected that the recently approved hepatitis A and varicella (chicken pox) vaccines will be added.

To assess barriers to immunization and the particular significance of vaccine cost as a barrier, we talked with CDC officials and reviewed pertinent literature and agency documents, including various types of information CDC cited to address vaccine cost as a cause of delayed immunization. In addition, we reviewed four major studies sponsored

GAO/T-PEMD-95-21, May 1995.

239

by CDC in the wake of recent measles epidemics to "diagnose" and identify reasons for low immunization rates among high-risk racial and ethnic minority inner-city preschoolers in Baltimore, Los Angeles, Philadelphia, and Rochester (New York). We reviewed CDC's four studies to assess the factors associated with underimmunization. Further, we convened an expert panel of the principal investigators of these studies to help determine the extent to which the cost of vaccine for parents affects their children's vaccination status.

In our review of the available data and our discussions with the expert panel, we did not find sufficient evidence to conclude that vaccine cost has been a major barrier to children's immunization. The literature does identify many barriers, including parents' lack of awareness of their children's vaccination schedule, inadequate resources (for example, insufficient clinic staff, insufficient or inconvenient clinic hours, and inaccessible clinic locations), clinic policies that deter vaccination by requiring appointments or refusing to see walk-in patients, and various factors that cause providers to miss opportunities to immunize children at regular visits. We found that although a variety of socioeconomic and demographic variables are associated with undervaccination among inner-city children, these relationships appear to function not through cost but, rather, through other factors associated with poverty, such as family size and maternal education.

The findings from CDC's diagnostic studies indicate that most underimmunized children have access to free vaccine through Medicaid or public health clinics (that is, through private or public providers) and that they had visited their providers an average of six to eight times during a given year. During these visits, these children could have received their scheduled immunizations, but providers failed to vaccinate them. These occasions are commonly known as "missed opportunities." Specifically, a missed opportunity is defined as a health care visit during which a child eligible for vaccination on the day of the visit and with no valid contraindication for vaccination fails to receive the needed vaccine.

CDC's studies identified several factors that are associated with missed opportunities. These primarily include provider and clinic-related factors and policies, such as failure to use simultaneous vaccinations or accelerated immunization schedules for children who are behind schedule, lack of access to records of a child's immunization status, and lack of organizational support. The missed opportunities observed in the diagnostic studies occurred during both sick- and well-child care visits. In fact, incorrect beliefs regarding contraindications for immunization are a particularly important contributor to missed opportunities. For example, CDC's diagnostic study in Baltimore reported that missed opportunities occurred at approximately 25 to 30 percent of preventive visits but at more than 75 percent of sick-child visits and that a health care provider was more likely not to vaccinate a child during a sick-child visit. Table 17.1 shows immunization levels observed among children 24 months old in each of CDC's four diagnostic studies and potential levels that the investigators believed could be achieved by eliminating missed opportunities.

Table 17.1. Percentage of Actual and Potential Vaccination Coverage Among 24-Month-Old Children by Individual Vaccine Doses and Site, 1991-92[a].

City	Vaccine[b]/dose	Actual	Potential	Difference
Baltimore	DTP/DT/3	85%	93%	8%
	DTP/DT/4	58	74	16
	Polio/3	65	81	16
	MMR/1	80	89	9
Los Angeles	DTP/DT/3	54	62	8
	DTP/DT/4	26	34	8
	Polio/3	34	50	16
	MMR/1	39	48	9
Philadelphia	DTP/DT/3	82	85	3
	DTP/DT/4	57	67	10
	Polio/3	68	79	11
	MMR/1	87	94	7
Rochester	DTP/DT/3	94	99	5
	DTP/DT/4	75	96	21
	Polio/3	80	95	15
	MMR/1	90	96	6

[a]Assumes all missed opportunities to vaccinate had been eliminated.

[b]DTP/DT = diphtheria and tetanus toxoids and pertussis vaccine/diphtheria and tetanus toxoids. MMR = measles-mumps-rubella vaccine.

Source: Morbidity and Mortality Weekly Report, 43:39 (October 7, 1994), 711.

The diagnostic studies' findings regarding missed opportunities were consistent across the four studies, even though they used different methodologies. The studies concurred that 2-year-olds missed opportunities very frequently during visits to health care providers: 82 percent of children studied in Rochester missed one or more opportunities, 75 percent in Baltimore, 69 percent in Los Angeles, and 64 percent in Philadelphia. Assuming baseline coverage of 60 percent, these research projects found that eliminating all missed opportunities would alone account for a third to a half of the increase needed to reach the 90-percent goal for 1996. However, as Table 17.1 shows, eliminating missed opportunities alone would not raise immunization rates to the targeted 90 percent levels in all cases.

The results of CDC's four diagnostic studies indicate that while no single factor or category of factors accounts for undervaccination, access to health care among underimmunized children is not generally a problem. The diagnostic studies suggest that achieving and sustaining a high coverage level will require a variety of interventions aimed at changing the practices of providers that result in missed opportunities. Specifically, the findings do not provide sufficient evidence to conclude that providing free vaccines through VFC will boost coverage for most underimmunized children, for whom vaccines are already free.

In addition to the four CDC studies, we examined other studies and information cited by CDC as addressing the role of vaccine cost in delayed immunization. CDC identified six types of evidence to support the notion that vaccine cost is a barrier:

1. increases in vaccine cost over the past decade;

2. surveys of health care providers inquiring about the frequency with which they had referred patients to public health providers for immunization, their reasons for doing so, and their opinions regarding a universal vaccine purchase program;

3. reports from health departments of increased referrals from private providers;

4. surveys of parents visiting public health clinics regarding their reasons for using the clinics;

5. policy studies addressing the relationship between health insurance coverage, health care utilization, and immunization; and

6. comparisons of immunization rates between states with and without universal vaccine distribution programs.

Unlike the diagnostic studies, which examined populations at high risk of underimmunization to assess the relationship between immunization status and a variety of potential barriers, the additional research cited by CDC tended toward a more narrow investigation of particular factors, such as providers' referral patterns. We found that, for the purpose of assessing the role of vaccine cost in underimmunization, this research suffers from several conceptual and methodological problems, such as failure to distinguish vaccine costs from other fees associated with immunization, inability to determine that the factors actually measured (such as provider referrals to public health clinics) were valid indicators of eventual failure to receive immunization, and reliance on opinion data collected in surveys rather than through analysis of the immunization status of representative samples of children. For example, CDC officials acknowledged that providers' fees in the private sector would be about $40 per office visit and about $15 per dose, representing potentially about 60 percent of the total cost of full immunization, but much of the evidence they cited failed to distinguish between the cost of vaccine, which is addressed by VFC, and these fees, which are not. Comparisons of immunization rates between states operating universal distribution programs and other states do not permit accounting for the various other factors that may affect rates in these states.

To summarize, the studies we examined and the other sources of information available to us lacked sufficient evidence to conclude that the major factor addressed by VFC, vaccine cost, has been a significant barrier to immunization. It appears that efforts to address a variety of other barriers may be equally or more important in improving immunization levels. We have discussed our findings and conclusions with responsible CDC officials. They are in general agreement with our finding that there is not sufficient evidence to conclude that vaccine cost is among the most significant barriers to immunization.

Chapter 18

Vaccines for Children: Reexamination of Program Goals

Executive Summary

Purpose

More than 95 percent of the nation's children receive recommended vaccinations by the time they enter school. However, preschool children were overrepresented in the widespread measles outbreaks of 1989-91 and this was attributed to their underimmunization. In conjunction with the Children's Immunization Initiative (CII), VFC is intended to improve children's immunization coverage by reducing the cost of vaccine for their parents. At the request of Senator Dale Bumpers and Representatives Scott Nug and Ron Wyden, GAO reports on (1) the extent to which vaccine cost has prevented children from being immunized on schedule, (2) VFC'S implementation and whether VFC, as implemented, can ensure the timely vaccination of underimmunized children, and (3) promising options for improving their immunization rates.

Background

Section 13631 of the Omnibus Budget Reconciliation Act of 1993 created VFC as an entitlement program to provide free vaccine to children 18 and younger who are eligible for Medicaid or who are American Indians or uninsured. Underinsured children (those whose insurance does not cover childhood vaccinations) are also eligible for VFC vaccines but may receive them only in federally qualified health centers or rural health clinics. VFC'S fiscal year 1995 cost estimates included $412 million for vaccine purchase and $45.3 million for administrative expenses, such as vaccine distribution, vaccine ordering, and operations. The VFC legislation (signed in August 1993) mandated that the program begin operation by October 1, 1994.

The vaccines VFC currently provides to the states include antigens for measles, mumps, rubella, diphtheria, tetanus, pertussis, polio, hepatitis B, and haemophilus influenza according to a schedule set by the Advisory Committee on Immunization Practices (ACIP) of the Public Health Service. The Centers for Disease Control and Prevention (CDC) has announced that doses of influenza vaccine for high-risk children and hepatitis B vaccine for adolescents will be added in fiscal year 1996, along with speedier catch-up immunization against measles. Newly approved varicella (chicken pox) and hepatitis A vaccines will be considered. Only one of these five new additions to the vaccine schedule (the measles booster) will be covered by statutory price caps (that is, contract prices that were in effect in 1993). CDC officials estimate that VFC purchases of the new varicella vaccine could cost an additional $35 million to $560 million, depending on the extent of catch-up coverage ACIP recommends. CDC estimates that once catch-up has been completed, the annual cost of including varicella will range from $35 million to $70 million.

Results in Brief

From the available evidence, GAO concludes that the cost of vaccine for parents has not been a major barrier to children's timely immunization. Moreover, VFC'S implementation remains incomplete in six of the seven critical areas GAO reviewed. VFC'S automation, accountability, and evaluation mechanisms cannot measure its provision of vaccine to children who are at high risk of underimmunization, nor can they attribute changes in age-appropriate immunization rates to VFC. Thus, CDC cannot ensure that VFC will reach pockets of needareas or populations in which immunization rates are low and the risk of disease is consequently high. VFC'S shortcomings raise questions about its capacity to control vaccine waste and abuse.

Other options may hold better promise than VFC for improving timely vaccination among children, potentially at lower public cost, by reducing missed opportunities for immunization through Medicaid, public health clinics, and other providers with whom underimmunized children already have contact. Moreover, CDC'S analysis shows that less than 1 percent of U.S. counties reported measles cases in each year of the 1980s suggesting that specific efforts might be efficiently targeted to improving immunization in such areas.

Principal Findings

Vaccine Cost

GAO did not find sufficient evidence to conclude that the cost of vaccine for parents has been a major barrier to children's timely immunization. Immunization rates for preschool children at the outset of VFC were at or near the 90-percent national goals for 1996. Further, immunization rates among school children exceed 95 percent for all antigens in the basic series. CDC-sponsored studies clearly demonstrate that, since underimmunized children generally had access to free vaccine before VFC began, cost is less important than missed opportunities for vaccination during their regular contacts with their health care providers. The literature does identify many barriers, including parents' lack of awareness of their children's vaccination schedule, inadequate resources (for example, insufficient clinic staff, insufficient or inconvenient clinic hours, and inaccessible clinic locations), clinic policies that deter vaccination by requiring appointments or refusing to see walk-in patients, and various factors that cause providers to miss opportunities to immunize children at regular visits. The evidence CDC has cited to document that vaccine cost is a major barrier generally fails to separate vaccine costs, which VFC addresses, from the larger provider fees associated with immunization, which it generally does not. The statute does stipulate that providers may not deny vaccine to a child who is unable to pay the administration fee. However, CDC has no measures to ensure the providers' compliance with this requirement.

It is important to note that in certain population groups and areas, often referred to as pockets of need, disproportionate numbers of children are not immunized for specific diseases, creating conditions ripe for outbreak. For example, CDC's analysis of the measles outbreaks in the 1980s shows that delayed immunization led to consistently reported cases over 10 years in only 17 of 3,137 U.S. counties, suggesting that special efforts to improve immunization coverage might be targeted there.

Program Implementation

Although CDC has devoted considerable effort and resources to implementing VFC, and has made progress, implementation remains incomplete, despite assurances to the contrary following GAO's July 1994 review of VFC. In this subsequent review, as of March 1, 1995, provider enrollment, the development of provider reimbursement policy, order processing and automation arrangements, a vaccine distribution system, accountability provisions, and evaluation planning—six of VFC'S seven critical implementation tasksremained incomplete. The only completed task is contract negotiation for the purchase of vaccines.

CDC and many states cannot gauge the proportion of private immunization providers or Medicaid providers that have been enrolled. Fifteen jurisdictions cannot distribute vaccine to private providers. The physician reimbursement policy is inconsistent with the law. Order-processing software that CDC developed without analyzing its users' requirements has failed to meet their needs. CDC cannot ensure that the program reaches only entitled children or that provides will serve all entitled children. It cannot distinguish between the number of children immunized and the number of doses of vaccine distributed. The states' data on provides' vaccine needs overestimate the number of potentially eligible children and the number of doses needed to immunize them. Finally, although CDC has not released evaluation plans, it is unlikely that the program's effect can ever be assessed because important baseline data were not collected prior to its implementation and because other efforts to improve immunization were initiated concurrently. In the 12 states that already had implemented universal vaccine distribution systems, it is not clear that VFC will have any direct effect on immunization activities apart from changing the source of their financing. It is conceivable, however, that these states will add newly recommended vaccines to their programs more quickly than they would have when state funding was required.

Promising Options

CDC-funded studies have shown promise for improving immunization rates by coordinating immunization services with large public programs—such as the Special Supplemental Food Program for Women, Infants, and Children and Aid to Families with Dependent Children, which cover children who are known to be at high risk of delayed immunization. Research also links improved immunization with provider-based strategies, such as assessing clinic immunization practices and offering feedback or creating reminder and recall systems or registries to reduce missed opportunities for immunization. One CDC official has testified, based on major CDC-funded research, that immunization rates for most antigens could be improved by as much as 15 percent simply by eliminating missed opportunities.

Chapter 19

Adults Need
Tetanus Shots, Too

Kathleen Bedford had her 15 minutes of fame in a hospital lecture room full of medical students when she was 65. Because there are only about two cases of tetanus a year in the eastern part of England where she lives, the hospital held a special session for the students. For most of them, it was their first—and maybe their last—opportunity to observe someone with the infection. With her injured leg suspended in a protective frame, Bedford was the center of attention. She would have preferred celebrity in some other way.

Bedford pierced the calf of her leg with a pitchfork crusted with dirt in a freak gardening accident. She was rushed to the emergency room. Her leg was bandaged from ankle to thigh, but she received no further treatment.

When she returned to the emergency room 24 hours later, feeling quite ill, the leg was highly inflamed. After the surgeon on duty took one horrified look at her leg, he rushed her to the operating room and cut her calf open deeply across the puncture site to expose the wound to air. During the next six weeks, the wound had to remain open; hence the frame. Bedford recalls she was treated with "all kinds of pills and shots" and escaped any secondary infection, such as pneumonia.

She experienced only one tetanus symptom—transitory stiffness. But the disease could have been avoided had she been properly immunized. Like many other older adults, Bedford had neglected to keep up her immunity to tetanus with periodic booster doses of tetanus vaccine.

FDA Consumer, July-August 1996.

Lockjaw Symptoms

Tetanus is an acute, often fatal disease that occurs worldwide. It affects the central nervous system, producing both the stiffness or muscular rigidity that Bedford experienced and convulsive muscle spasm. Tetanus can be localized, with muscle contractions in the part of the body where the infection began, or it can be generalized, affecting the whole body. About 80 percent of reported tetanus cases are generalized. The incubation period ranges from 2 to 50 days, but symptoms usually occur 5 to 10 days after infection. The shorter the incubation period, the greater the chance of death.

The most frequent symptom is a stiff jaw, caused by spasm of the muscle that closes the mouth—accounting for the disease's familiar name "lockjaw." Muscle stiffness all over the body may follow. An infected person may also have other symptoms: difficulty swallowing, restlessness and irritability, stiff neck, arms or legs, fever, headache, and sore throat. As the disease progresses, the victim may develop a fixed smile and raised eyebrows due to facial muscle spasms. Spasms of the diaphragm and the muscles between the ribs may interfere with breathing, often requiring mechanical ventilation. The abdominal or back muscles may become rigid. In severe cases, patients may become so sensitive to any kind of disturbance that they suffer painful spasms all over their bodies with profuse sweating if the bed is jarred or if they feel a draft or hear a noise. Convulsions can be severe enough to break bones.

Hyperactivity of the autonomic (involuntary) nervous system may raise blood pressure dangerously or cause heart arrhythmias (irregular beats). Although tetanus victims can usually think clearly when conscious, coma may follow repeated spasms. Aspiration pneumonia is a common late complication and is found in 50 to 70 percent of autopsied cases. The mortality rate is about 25 percent in the United States and 50 percent worldwide.

Bacterial Cause

The bacteria that cause tetanus belong to the Clostridium family, also responsible for some other serious diseases. such as botulism and the type of gangrene suffered in war wounds. Clostridia bacteria are what scientists call "obligate anaerobic"—that is, they thrive only in the absence of oxygen. They also form spores, reproductive cells with thick walls that enable them to withstand unfavorable environmental conditions. Spores are tough to kill and highly resistant to heat and the usual antiseptics that treat wounds.

Tetanus bacteria may enter the body through a puncture wound or scratch. In the presence of dead tissue, tetanus spores reproduce and manufacture a poison (exotoxin) that travels through the body and causes tetanus symptoms. Though tetanus bacteria are found everywhere in the environment—in soil, street dust, and in animal intestines and feces—natural immunity to the disease is rare. This is why immunization is so important.

Vaccination with tetanus toxoid (tetanus vaccine) causes the body to respond to an inactivated form of the tetanus toxin by developing antibodies to tetanus. Tetanus toxoid is virtually 100 percent effective in preventing tetanus. It is prepared by growing tetanus bacteria (Clostridium tetani) in a special medium, and then detoxifying the resulting tetanus toxin with formaldehyde The Food and Drug Administration reviews the manufacturer's testing records for each lot of vaccine to ensure that the product is safe and effective for its intended use. FDA also sometimes tests random lots to ensure that the manufacturer's testing records are accurate.

Side effects of vaccination are few. As with the DTP shot received by children (to immunize against diphtheria, tetanus and pertussis), redness or formation of a small hard lump at the vaccination site are possible. Some individuals may have allergic reactions, such as hives, skin rash, or itching. More serious adverse reactions include the rare cases of anaphylaxis (an allergic reaction involving difficulty in breathing or swallowing and facial swelling that can be fatal) and possibly Guillain-Barre syndrome, a nerve inflammation. People who have had a severe reaction to the vaccine should not receive further doses.

Beyond Rusty Nails

The connection between a wound caused by a rusty/dirty nail and the necessity for a tetanus shot is fixed so firmly in the public mind that even the television cartoon character Homer Simpson knew he had to get a tetanus shot after stepping on a nail.

But people don't realize that tetanus can be contracted in other ways. Any puncture wound, especially one that is deep, can be infected with tetanus. Some seamstresses have contracted tetanus from sewing needles. Animal scratches and bites and other wounds contaminated by both human and animal feces and saliva are potential breeding grounds for tetanus bacteria. Infection can develop in wounds in which the flesh is torn or burned, or in wounds resulting from projectiles, such as arrows, bullets or shrapnel, or in those caused by crushing or frostbite. The disease may follow trivial wounds caused by thorns or splinters, as well as highly contaminated wounds, if oxygen is unable to reach the injured tissues. Tetanus can also develop after surgery, dental infections, and abortion. Cephalic tetanus, a rare form of the disease, is associated with chronic ear infections, in which tetanus bacteria are present in the inner ear. Tetanus has also been reported in people with no known acute injury, chronic wound, or other medical condition.

In developing countries, tetanus is a major health problem. Child birth may lake place under unsanitary conditions, causing infection in the uterus afterwards. Tetanus in newborns has emerged worldwide as the predominant form of tetanus, as the baby's umbilical stump is often sealed with mud or clay or other contaminated substances.

CDC's *Morbidity and Mortality Weekly Report* of May 6, 1994, discusses two cases of tetanus that occurred in Kansas in 1993—the first cases reported in that state since 1987—that show the importance of immunization.

The first case involved an 82-year-old man, hospitalized because of shortness of breath and weakness and difficulty chewing and swallowing. When doctors examined him, they found he had difficulty opening his jaw and noted an abrasion on his right elbow resulting from a fall two days earlier. He had never been vaccinated. Doctors administered both tetanus toxoid and tetalous immune globulin (TIG). (An injection of tetanus toxoid after the injury does not give immediate full immunity. TIG confers temporary immunity to those people who have low or no immunity to tetanus toxin by providing antitoxin directly to the body, ensuring that protective levels of antitoxin are reached quickly rather than waiting for the body's immune response.) In the next few weeks, his body was racked by spasms, followed by respiratory failure and pneumonia, which necessitated the use of a breathing machine. After treatment with antibiotics, diuretics, and neuromuscular blocking agents, he recovered and was discharged a few weeks later.

The second case involved a diabetic 57-year-old man who had stepped on a rusty nail and sought emergency treatment for tetanus that same day. Hospital personnel cleaned the wound and administered tetanus toxoid. Four days later, he returned to the emergency department complaining of severe pain in the foot, as well as chills, fever and vomiting. When he developed pain and a stiff neck, he was hospitalized immediately with a diagnosis of tetanus and received TIG. After a number of life-threatening heart and lung problems, he died following an episode of cardiac arrest. His relatives reported that he had not been previously vaccinated with tetanus toxoid.

The surviving and the deceased tetanus victims each spent about a month in the hospital and ran up medical bills of about $150,000 apiece. At that time, public health clients could have received a tetanus shot for $3.30, while vaccination with a private physician would have cost just a few dollars more.

Tetanus has become a rare disease in the United States as well as in England, with only 36 reported U.S. cases in 1994, though there may be more unreported cases. The disease has become uncommon not because tetanus bacteria have been eliminated from the environment—they're still all around us—but because immunization has provided protection.

Since adults 50 years or older account for 70 percent of tetanus infections, mature people should make certain they have received boosters within the last 10 years. If they don't know whether they were immunized as children, the primary series of shots should be completed.

—by Evelyn Zamula

Chapter 20

Vaccination Among Older Adults

Executive Summary

Purpose

Pneumococcal and influenza-associated diseases are the leading causes of vaccine-preventable death in the United States. On average, 32,800 people die from pneumococcal disease and 20,000 die from influenza each year. The elderly suffer the most from these diseases and the costs to the federal government are substantial. Annual Medicare hospital reimbursement ranges between $500 million and $1 billion for the treatment of influenza-associated illnesses alone. At the request of Senators Chafee and Gregg, GAO reviewed immunization rates among the elderly for flu and pneumococcal disease, the efforts and resources HHS has devoted to improving these rates, and the types of interventions that enhance the use of these vaccines.

Background

The PHS Advisory Committee on Immunization Practices (ACIP) and professional medical organizations recommend one-time pneumococcal vaccination and annual flu shots for all persons 65 years or older and for non-elderly persons in high-risk groups, such as persons with heart or lung disease. Safe and effective vaccines are now covered under Medicare; nonetheless, the 1993 National Health Interview

GAO/PEMD-95-14, June 1995.

Survey (NHIS) indicates that immunization rates for these diseases were below the national goals set by HHS as long ago as 1980.

Results in Brief

Although reported use of pneumococcal and influenza vaccines among the elderly has more than doubled in the past 10 years, immunization rates for both diseases remain low, and morbidity as well as mortality remain significant. Pneumococcal disease is associated with higher mortality than influenza, yet pneumococcal immunization rates are lower. Nonetheless, in the 14 years since authorization of Medicare coverage for pneumococcal vaccination, HHS has conducted few activities to enhance its use aside from providing Medicare payment. Antibiotic resistance of pneumococcal bacteria is increasing, yet reaching HHS' 60 percent vaccination goal for the year 2000 appears unlikely based on current trends.

In contrast, in the short time since Medicare began national coverage for influenza vaccination, HHS has made significant efforts to enhance the use of this vaccine. The pace of increase in influenza vaccination rates since 1989, HHS' plans to enhance its promotional strategies, and preliminary data cited by the agency are promising, suggesting that the 60 percent flu immunization goal for the year 2000 may be attained. Although immunization rates are low, CDC spends very little promoting pneumococcal and influenza vaccination. GAO believes that increasing promotion efforts would increase immunization rates and thus save lives. But HHS maintains that the appropriations report language pertaining to CDC strongly discourages the Department from spending more of its immunization funding on the elderly. GAO does not agree that the legislative history dictates CDC'S small level of spending on adult immunization. GAO reviewed the records of appropriations hearings and found that HHS has not taken a leadership role in defining pneumococcal and influenza immunization as important public health issues for the Congress and in seeking funding commensurate with their significance.

To increase vaccination rates, GAO concludes that efforts to improve health care providers' compliance with adult immunization guidelines are more promising than attempts to influence consumers' knowledge and attitudes. Physicians have a strong impact on consumers' vaccination decisions, but they often fail to recommend vaccination to those patients for whom it is indicated. Computer-based reminder systems, checklists appended to medical records, practice-based tracking systems, and issuance of standing orders for vaccination help to remedy this problem. The broad-based implementation of a hospital policy to vaccinate eligible high-risk patients before discharge shows much promise to reduce vaccine-preventable mortality among adults.

Principal Findings

Immunization Rates Are Low

HHS currently relies principally on the National Health Interview Survey to monitor rates of vaccination. The most recent available data (from the 1993 NHIS) indicate that 73 percent of older Americans had never received the pneumococcal vaccination, despite its coverage under Medicare since 1981, and 49 percent of the elderly had not been vaccinated against influenza during the 1992-93 flu season preceding Medicare coverage. Elderly blacks are between one-third and one-half as likely as older whites to get vaccinated, and persons with high-risk medical conditions or activity limitations or who describe their health as poor are generally somewhat more likely to get vaccinated. Also, elderly persons who had not visited a doctor in the last year were less than one quarter as likely to have gotten either vaccine compared with those who had three or more doctor visits. Nonetheless, even persons with five or more doctor visits were unlikely to have received pneumococcal vaccination.

HHS' Vaccination Strategies and Resource Allocations Are Inadequate

HHS officials acknowledge and agency documents reflect the significance of the public health problem presented by both illnesses. However, GAO found that HHS has taken few steps to improve pneumococcal vaccine use since Medicare coverage for the vaccine was authorized in 1981. By comparison, HHS has done more in its recent efforts to improve the use of flu vaccine. When Medicare coverage for influenza vaccination began in 1993, HCFA initiated a public information campaign through the mass media. In fiscal 1995, HCFA enhanced this effort by making data on state and county immunization rates available to health care providers and beginning limited activities through the agency's peer review organizations.

Among the HHS agencies we reviewed, HCFA makes the bulk of federal expenditures directly linked to pneumococcal and influenza immunization, primarily as Medicare payments (about $100 million in fiscal 1994). Although CDC distributed 94 percent of its $528 million fiscal 1994 immunization budget to the National Immunization Program (NIP), less than 1 percent of these funds were dedicated to adult immunization activities. The number of NIP staff positions dedicated to adult immunization activities remained constant, at five between 1987 and 1994, when it increased to seven.

Provider-Focused Strategies Show Promise for Improving Immunization

Strategies that show documented promise for enhancing pneumococcal and influenza vaccine use include physician reminder systems, the issuance of standing orders for immunizing patients, and systems for tracking patients in need of immunization. Well-designed reminders to potential vaccines were also found to be effective. Although vaccination clinics and public information campaigns have been part of successful efforts to improve vaccination rates, the independent effects of these strategies have not been rigorously evaluated.

Research suggests that a policy to vaccinate eligible patients before hospital discharge shows significant promise for reducing pneumococcal disease. Studies conducted in the United States, Canada, and the United Kingdom show that a majority of patients admitted to hospitals with pneumococcal disease had been discharged from a hospital within the previous 5 years (and had thus missed an important vaccination opportunity). ACIP has recommended that pneumococcal vaccine be offered routinely to hospitalized patients in high-risk groups before discharge to prevent future admissions for pneumococcal disease, but the data suggest that this policy has not been widely implemented.

Recommendations

GAO recommends that the Secretary of HHS take a more active leadership role in promoting pneumococcal and influenza vaccination among elderly persons by (1) seeking, in the annual appropriations process, to clarify what proportion of immunization funding should be allocated for such activities; and (2) directing HCFA and PHS to focus their efforts on promoting or supporting promising strategies, such as patient and physician reminder systems, development of standing order policies, and broad-based use of a hospital policy to vaccinate eligible patients before discharge.

Introduction

Medicare covers vaccines against two types of disease that are hazardous to the health of elderly persons—pneumonia (and other pneumococcal infections) and influenza Although these vaccines are officially recommended for all persons over 65 and for younger persons with high risk conditions, large proportions of those at risk of morbidity and mortality from these diseases do not receive inoculations against them. Consequently, Senators Chafee and Gregg asked us to assess HHS' efforts to improve these vaccination rates. Below, we describe these diseases, the safety and efficacy of the vaccines, and our approach to assessing HHS' activities to improve pneumococcal and influenza vaccination rates.

Background

Pneumococcal Disease and Influenza

Pneumonia and influenza are the sixth most common cause of death in the United States. Between 15 and 50 percent of all adult pneumonias are caused by pneumococcal bacteria and these infections are the leading cause of pneumonia requiring hospitalization. In addition to pneumonia, pneumococcal bacteria can cause serious infections of the bloodstream (bacteria) and the covering of the brain or spinal cord (meningitis).

Influenza is a highly contagious viral disease that is spread by direct contact with an infected person or through contact with the airborne virus. The public health significance of influenza vaccination derives for the rapidity with which flu epidemics evolve, the widespread morbidity associated with these epidemics, and the seriousness of complications (notably, pneumonias) that may result from the flu. Influenza viruses continually change over time; thus, people are susceptible to influenza infection throughout life.

Health Consequences

Despite antibiotic therapy, pneumococcal disease remains a leading cause of morbidity and mortality. CDC estimates that there are 268,000 cases of pneumococcal disease per year in the United States among the approximately 36 million persons 65 years old or older and that, on average, 32,800 elderly persons die each year from pneumococcal disease. People older than 65 are more likely to contract pneumococcal disease than the general population.

The incidence of influenza varies from year to year depending on the type of viral outbreak and its level of activity. The highest illness rate occurs with the A(H3N2) virus, which has caused epidemics every other year in the last decade. According to CDC, 5 to 10 percent of the elderly population become ill with influenza during A(H3N2) outbreaks. On average, type A and B viruses caused 20,000 deaths per year in the last two decades, with 80 to 90 percent of deaths occurring among the elderly.

Disease Costs

Precise annual costs for treating pneumococcal disease and influenza are not available. However, HCFA researchers have estimated that Medicare reimburses hospitals $750 million to $1 billion for the treatment of influenza-associated illness during epidemic periods and almost a half billion dollars in a non-epidemic year. The majority of cases of pneumococcal disease and influenza are treated in outpatient settings, and these estimates do not include the medical costs associated with outpatient treatment. In fiscal 1994, HHS officials reported expending approximately $100 million on Medicare coverage for pneumococcal and influenza vaccines and their administration.

Vaccine Safety and Efficacy

Pneumococcal Vaccine

Mild side effects, such as swelling and pain at the injection site, occur in about half of the people who are given the pneumococcal vaccine. However, fever, muscle pain, and more serious local reactions have been reported in less than 1 percent of recipients. The efficacy of pneumococcal vaccine has increased over the years as new vaccines were introduced to protect against a larger number of pneumococci (83 types are known). The current pneumococcal vaccine, which became available in 1983, protects against 23 types responsible for approximately 90 percent of the pneumococcal bacteremic infections found in U.S. residents.

Randomized controlled trials have demonstrated that the vaccine protected against pneumococcal infections in healthy young adults in settings outside the United States where there were high rates of pneumococcal disease. Recently, a large randomized controlled trial conducted in France found that the vaccine was 77 percent effective in reducing the incidence of pneumonia in persons living in geriatric hospitals and homes for the aged.

In contrast, three major trials with older U.S. adults in a prepaid medical plan in San Francisco, in a chronic disease hospital, and in a Department of Veterans' Affairs (VA) studyhave not demonstrated pneumococcal vaccine efficacy in preventing pneumococcal pneumonia in the absence of bacteremia. However, because the rate of pneumococcal infection is quite low, it is difficult to demonstrate vaccine efficacy in a randomized trial.

Owing to the difficulties inherent in assessing pneumococcal vaccine efficacy for older persons from randomized trials, findings from case-control studies and cohort analyses have become the standard from which CDC scientists and other experts judge vaccine efficacy. Together, these studies indicate an overall protective efficacy against invasive pneumococcal infection of 60 percent to 70 percent in elderly persons with normal immune response, regardless of such high-risk conditions as heart or lung disease.

Influenza Vaccine

Although most individuals have no side effects from influenza vaccines, some may have soreness at the injection site or may experience fever or body aches for a day or two. Unlike the 1976 "swine flu" vaccine, recent flu shots have not been linked to Guillian-Barre syndrome. According to CDC, the vaccines produced before the mid-1960s were not as purified as today's vaccines, and they sometimes produced fever, headache, muscle ache, and fatigue. These symptoms are similar to those occurring with influenza, thus some people believed that the vaccine had caused them to get the flu. Contrary to myth, it has never been possible to get the flu from influenza vaccines licensed in the United States because they have only been made from killed (inactivated) viruses, which cannot cause infection.

Influenza vaccine efficacy depends on many factors, including the age and health status of the recipient and the match between the prevalent flu strain and the strains addressed in the year's vaccine. Studies of healthy young adults have shown influenza vaccine to be 70 to 90percent effective in preventing illness. However, in the elderly, the vaccine is often more effective in reducing the severity of illness and the risk of serious complications and death than in preventing illness altogether. Studies have shown the vaccine to reduce hospitalization by about 70 percent and death by about 85 percent in noninstitutionalized elderly. Among nursing home residents, vaccine can reduce the risk of hospitalization for flu by about 50 percent, the risk of pneumonia by about 60 percent, and the risk of death by 75 to 80 percent.

Vaccination Recommendations

Both pneumococcal and influenza vaccinations are recommended for elderly persons by U.S. public health authorities. Since 1963, CDC'S Advisory Committee on Immunization Practices has recommended annual vaccination against influenza for persons age 65 and older. In 1984, ACIP began recommending a one-time pneumococcal vaccination for older persons. In 1989, ACIP also recommended revaccination of persons at highest risk of fatal pneumococcal infection and those with rapid loss of pneumococcal antibody levels for whom 6 or more years had passed since initial vaccination.

Both vaccinations are also recommended for non-elderly persons with medical conditions that make them vulnerable to severe complications from influenza infections or that put them at increased risk of pneumococcal disease. Moreover, ACIP, noting research that shows that two-thirds of persons with serious pneumococcal disease had been hospitalized in the 5-year period before the illness, recommends that pneumococcal vaccine be given to hospitalized patients in high-risk groups before discharge in order to prevent future admissions for pneumococcal disease.

Consistent with these professional recommendations, HHS has established goals for increasing these vaccination rates by the year 2000 to 60 percent of the population defined by ACIP, which includes all persons age 65 and older, and at least 80 percent of institutionalized chronically ill or older persons. The goal of immunizing 60 percent of the elderly with influenza vaccine is carried over from a 1990 target set by the Surgeon General in 1980.

Legislative Authorization for Immunization Activities

In July 1981, coverage for pneumococcal vaccine and its administration became one of the first primary preventive services added to the Medicare program. It was incorporated in title XVIU of the Social Security Act following a 1979 study by the Office of Technology Assessment that indicated pneumococcal vaccination would be cost-effective for persons age 65 and over.

OTA issued another report, in 1981, that found that influenza vaccination for persons age 65 and older would be cost-effective. In Public Law 100-203, the Congress mandated that HCFA conduct a demonstration project regarding Medicare coverage of influenza vaccination, which subsequently yielded mixed findings on the cost-effectiveness of flu coverage. According to legislative mandate, HCFA initiated Medicare coverage for the vaccine and its administration in May 1993. Consequently, today Medicare Part B covers both the cost and the administration of vaccines against pneumococcal disease and influenza for both elderly and disabled beneficiaries. Unlike most other part B services, for which beneficiaries must pay 20 percent of allowed charges, no copayment is required for these two services. Providers' claims for delivering these services are processed by a network of carriers and intermediaries contracted to HCFA, who are also responsible for educating providers about covered services.

In addition to HCFA, which administers Medicare, two other HHS units within the Public Health Service have major legislative authority for immunization activities: the National Vaccine Program Office and the Centers for Disease Control and Prevention. NVPO was established within the Office of the Assistant Secretary for Health by the National Childhood Vaccine Injury Act of 1986 (P.L. 99-660), which added title XXI to the Public Health Service Act. The office's responsibilities extend to coordination of the various federal agencies involved in immunization activities, including the CDC, and its prescribed roles include coordinating and directing federal activities relating to vaccine research, distribution, and use. As authorized by section 317 of the Public Health Service Act, CDC provides immunization assistance in the form of grants to states and other public entities and conducts research activities.

Factors That May Explain Low Immunization Rates

Awareness of Vaccine Availability

A Gallup poll conducted in the fall of 1993 found that only 25 percent of all adults 55 years old or older were aware that a safe, effective pneumococcal vaccine exists. However, a high level of vaccine awareness does not necessarily ensure high vaccination rates: a 1987 CDC study of elderly residents in two Georgia counties found that 90 percent were aware of the flu vaccine, yet only 55 percent said they had received it within the past year.

Beliefs About Susceptibility to Disease

Consumers are probably more likely to seek a particular preventive service if they believe they may be susceptible to the disease it prevents. National surveys conducted in 1977-78 by Opinion Research Corporation (ORC) indicate that adults of all ages tended to see themselves as more susceptible to influenza than to any other vaccine-preventable disease. Nonetheless, survey data from persons who did not receive immunization in the recent Medicare Influenza Demonstration revealed that the most common reason for not getting the flu vaccine was the belief that one was healthy and did not need it.

Data on beliefs about susceptibility to pneumonia are more sparse. However, almost 70 percent of elderly Hawaiians who responded to a 1988 survey recognized that pneumonia is a more common cause of illness in people over 65 than in younger people.

Beliefs About Disease Severity

Research also suggests that consumers may be more likely to seek a preventive service if they view the disease it prevents as a serious matter. With respect to flu, the ORC survey found that adults of all ages tended to perceive influenza as the least serious vaccine-preventable disease of adulthood. Survey data from the 1988 Hawaii Pneumococcal Disease Initiative indicated that 78 percent of elderly respondents viewed pneumonia as a serious disease, and 57 percent viewed influenza as a serious disease. According to CDC, influenza-attributable death is 90 percent higher than reported in current vital statistics (that is, nearly twice as high as current reports).

Beliefs About Vaccine Side Effects, Safety, and Efficacy

Concerns about vaccine side effects, safety, and efficacy were frequently cited reasons for not receiving influenza vaccination by elderly residents of the 10 communities that participated in the Medicare Influenza Demonstration. Similarly, CDC'S 1987 survey in Georgia found that 73 percent of respondents who were aware of the flu vaccine believed that it caused illness, did not protect against influenza, or was unnecessary. Of those who were aware of the pneumococcal vaccine, 36 percent believed that it would not prevent pneumonia or would make them sick. Negative attitudes lingering from the 1976 swine flu vaccine initiative may color current perceptions about flu shots in general. When respondents were asked in a 1977 ORC survey whether there are "any specific vaccinations . . . which you feel are unsafe," fully 78 percent of those who said "yes" mentioned "swine flu," whereas only 11 percent said "flu" without mentioning a specific type. Six months later, 59 percent mentioned "swine flu" and fully 30 percent mentioned "flu" without indicating a specific type.

Negative perceptions about the flu vaccine may also be related to misconceptions about its efficacy. In NIA's focus groups with elderly adults, most participants reported having had a negative experience with the flu vaccine or said they knew someone who had. Although a flu-like, winter respiratory illness may be coincident to, rather than caused by, influenza vaccination, people may conclude that the flu vaccine either failed to work or, worse, induced the illness.

Influences on Providers' Behavior

In this section, we examine potential explanations of low pneumococcal and influenza immunization rates that focus on providers' knowledge or behavior. Evidence suggests that physician recommendation is a strong motivator to accept vaccination, regardless of patient attitudes. Thus, we consider physicians' knowledge, attitudes, and practices, as well as institutional practices within hospitals, health maintenance organizations, and nursing homes. We find evidence that suggests missed opportunities to offer vaccine to elderly persons in physicians' practices and institutional contexts and failure in many cases to maintain immunization records.

Physician Knowledge and Attitudes

The available literature suggests that most primary care physicians know about the seriousness of pneumococcal and influenza disease and that half or more of these providers are familiar with the recommendations for vaccination. Moreover, most tend to have favorable attitudes about vaccine safety and efficacy, though some doubts about vaccine efficacy linger among a minority of physicians. For example, in 1980, CDC found that about 90 percent of primary care physicians were aware and supportive of flu vaccination recommendations for the elderly. Fewer physicians knew the indications for pneumococcal vaccination. However, two-thirds of general and family practitioner respondents and just over one-half of responding internists believed that elderly people should get pneumococcal vaccination. CDC also found that most primary care physicians (over 70 percent) believed that influenza vaccine is very safe, and that it is effective for at least 60 percent of patients. Fewer than 10 percent expressed concerns about pneumococcal vaccine safety or effectiveness.

These findings are consistent with more recent results from focus groups run by the National Institute on Aging in 1993 and findings from the 1988 Hawaii Pneumococcal Disease Initiative, which found that among the 35 percent of physicians responding to a survey, roughly half recognized age over 65 as an indication for flu and pneumococcal immunization. HHS officials commenting on this report noted a continuing need for provider education, but agreed with our conclusion that physicians' vaccination practices should be the major focus of attention.

Medical education in adult immunization and vaccine-preventable disease is brief but widespread. In a 1991 survey of U.S. medical schools and primary care residency programs, CDC found that almost 90 percent of medical schools reported teaching about influenza, spending an average of 30 minutes to 1 hour on the subject. In addition, about one-third of internal medicine residency programs reported teaching about vaccine-preventable disease in adults, prevention of these diseases, and vaccination indications. Although HHS officials argued that current instructional practices are insufficient, it remains unclear whether or to what extent enhancement of routine medical instruction would affect provider practices.

Physician Practices: Recommendations to Patients

The significance of a physician's vaccination recommendation has been clearly demonstrated. Its absence acts as a barrier to vaccine receipt; its presence is a motivator to get vaccinated.

Most surveyed physicians report that they recommend vaccination to their patients for whom it is indicated (i.e., elderly persons and those with high-risk conditions). Evidence shows, however, that neither physicians' knowledge nor their self-reported implementation of vaccination recommendations is a reliable predictor of their actual immunization practices. For example, although almost all primary care physicians surveyed by ORC in 1980 believed and recommended that high-risk patients should be vaccinated and reported recommending the flu vaccine to their high-risk patients, they reported vaccinating only about one-half of these patients, on average, and only about one-third of their non-high-risk elderly patients. An unknown number of patients may have refused their physician's recommendation.

Stronger evidence of a discrepancy between physicians' immunization knowledge or attitudes and their practices comes from a study conducted at a primary care clinic in Milwaukee in the mid-1980s. Of the 92 physicians practicing at this clinic, over 75 percent knew flu vaccine recommendations, contraindications, and objectives, and two-thirds believed the vaccine was between 70 and 90 percent effective. Yet when medical records were examined from 3 peak months of the 1984-85 flu season, only 41 percent of these physicians' eligible patients had been offered vaccine. Rates of offering vaccine varied widely across physicians, from zero to 90 percent, with vaccination refused by only 9 percent of those to whom it was offered.

Record-Keeping

Maintaining an immunization record is a basic aspect of providing vaccine-related care. However, only 42 percent of internists surveyed in 1987 by the American College of Physicians reported maintaining immunization data for their patients. Among the types of preventive and diagnostic data covered by the survey, immunization status was among the least frequently recorded, outranking only information on sexual activities and seat-belt use.

Interestingly, most of the internist participants in NIA's focus groups mentioned forgetting as an important reason why they had not administered the pneumococcal vaccine to more patients. Physicians explained that patients usually are in the office for other reasons, and vaccination is relatively low on their list of priorities.

Another factor that apparently contributes to suboptimal immunization practices is that, according to a 1988 CDC survey of all physicians practicing in Hawaii, most of those responding did not consider vaccination to be a part of their practice.

Institutional Practices

Hospitals

Several studies have shown that hospitals admit patients at high risk of pneumococcal and influenza disease and miss opportunities to vaccinate them before their discharge. An analysis of the medical records of 1,633 Medicare beneficiaries in the Shenandoah region of Virginia with any type of pneumonia admission to hospitals in 1983 showed that 62 percent of these beneficiaries had been discharged at least once from a hospital (often from the same hospital) in the same region in the previous 4 years. Almost 90 percent of these patients had high-risk medical conditions listed on their previous discharge summaries. Additional research, conducted in the United States and the United Kingdom, showed that approximately two-thirds of patients hospitalized with pneumococcal bacteremia during the study period had been discharged at least once in the preceding 3 to 5 years. Similarly, a Canadian study found that although only 8 percent of the elderly in Manitoba had been discharged from a hospital during the

1982-83 vaccination season, this group accounted for almost 45 percent of subsequent influenza-associated hospitalizations and fully two-thirds of all hospital deaths from influenza-associated illness. Moreover, HHS officials reported that a survey of medical/surgical hospitals completed in 1994 found that over 60 percent of responding hospitals had no policy for vaccinating inpatients or outpatients against pneumococcal disease or influenza.

Health Maintenance Organizations

The Health Maintenance Organization Act of 1973 (as amended) mandates immunizations as one of the basic services to be included in the benefits offered by federally qualified HMOs. In 1987-88, CDC commissioned a survey of HMO's with 25,000 members or more that had at least 3 years of operational experience, but received responses from less than 25 percent of them. Among those HMOs responding to the survey, fewer than 50 percent had written policies specifying use of vaccines for adults, fewer than 20 percent issued an immunization record to members, high-risk members were not consistently identified, reminder systems were generally unavailable to physicians or members, administrative encouragement was lacking, promotion of vaccine use was limited, and data management systems were not adequate to monitor immunization levels.

Nursing Homes

HHS has not routinely monitored immunization rates in nursing homes. Available data on influenza immunization in nursing homes suggest that vaccination rates may have improved between the 1980s and 1990s, but that they are still quite variable across facilities. In the early and mid-1980s, findings from CDC'S studies of 67 nursing homes in six states showed that, on average, only 55 to 65 percent of nursing home residents were vaccinated against influenza in any given year. However, when Abt Associates surveyed over 500 nursing homes as part of the Medicare Influenza Demonstration from 1990 to 1992, it found higher overall vaccination rates of about 70 percent, on average. The studies found that having a vaccination policy, not requiring a physician's order for vaccination, and not requiring patient consent were associated with slightly higher vaccination rates. CDC also found a significant difference in vaccination rates between homes requiring consent from family members, which had vaccinated an average of 57 percent of patients, and homes that did not require familial consent, which had vaccinated 90 percent.

Summary

We identified several factors that may help explain why pneumococcal and influenza immunization rates are below HHS goals. We found that consumers lack awareness of the availability of pneumococcal vaccine. In the case of influenza vaccination, public awareness is high, but elderly people tend to underestimate the seriousness of, and their susceptibility to, influenza-related disease. Moreover, recent data suggest that consumers may have exaggerated concerns about influenza vaccine side effects, safety, and efficacy. However, it is difficult to accurately predict the extent to which addressing attitudinal factors alone might increase vaccination rates above current levels.

Regardless of the patient's personal attitudes about the vaccine, a physician's recommendation appears to be a strong motivator for a patient to get vaccinated. However, evidence suggests that physicians' actual immunization practices are often inconsistent with their intentions or self-reported practices. Forgetting to offer vaccine and the perceived limits or demands of a physician's practice are more plausible explanations for this than lack of knowledge; available evidence suggests that most physicians know basic facts about pneumococcal and influenza disease and that half or more are familiar with vaccine recommendations.

With respect to the role of health care organizations, limited data from the late 1980s suggest poor immunization practices in HMOs, and data from the mid-1980s imply uneven immunization practices in nursing homes. Importantly, we found strong evidence of missed opportunities to offer vaccination to high-risk patients before their discharge from hospitals.

Part Four

Food and Drug Administration

Chapter 21

How Much Do You Know about Food and Drug Administration?

The Food and Drug Administration regulates a large number of consumer products—but not everything! How good are you at distinguishing which products FDA regulates from those it doesn't? Take this quiz and see.

Circle the one item in each of the following groups that is not under the jurisdiction of the Food and Drug Administration. Answers follow.

1. a. Spam
   b. puppy food
   c. chocolate-covered cherries
   d. frozen spinach
   e. imported caviar

2. a. aspirin
   b. anti-lice shampoo
   c. insect repellent
   d. eye shadow
   e. lipstick

3. a. pesticide residues in lettuce
   b. canned tomatoes
   c. oven cleaner
   d. spaghetti
   e. pet turtles

FDA Consumer, FDA Publication No. 96-1228, March 1996.

4. a. airport security x-ray machines
   b. laser products used in lumber mills
   c. magnetic resonance imaging (MRI) diagnostic equipment
   d. smoke detectors
   e. microwave ovens

5. a. TV sets
   b. over-the-counter antacid
   c. TV ads for aspirin
   d. diphtheria, pertussis and tetanus vaccine
   e. human plasma

6. a. baby pacifiers
   b. baby bottle nipples
   c. ceramic ware for food use
   d. coffee mugs
   e. eye chart

7. a. illegal heroin use
   b. veterinary tetracycline
   c. barbiturates
   d. medicinal oxygen
   e. methadone

8. a. kidney dialysis machine
   b. tongue depressor
   c. toothpaste
   d. fluoridated toothpaste
   e. hair dryer

9. a. label on beer
   b. ground coffee
   c. coffee beans
   d. rabbit meat
   e. canned tuna

10. a. home canning equipment
   b. food warehouse
   c. drug warehouse
   d. hearing aid dispenser (retailer)
   e. exporting of drugs

11. a. Halloween make-up
    b. theatrical make-up
    c. soap
    d. eye mascara
    e. nail polish

12. a. vaccine for horses
    b. penicillin for horses
    c. medicated feed for hogs
    d. pet parrots
    e. bird feed

13. a. tap water
    b. club soda
    c. bottled mineral water
    d. ginger ale
    e. bottled water for water cooler

14. a. tamper-resistant packaging for over-the-counter (OTC) drugs
    b. child-proof packaging for OTC drugs
    c. plastic containers for soft drinks
    d. Valentine heart containing chocolates
    e. a tube containing medical ointment

15. a. grooming cream for dogs
    b. artificial limb for dogs
    c. laser scanner at supermarket checkout
    d. mercury vapor lamps
    e. vitamin C tablets

Answers

1. Answer a: Spam is a meat product. The U.S. Department of Agriculture is responsible for regulating meat (and poultry) products. Caviar and all seafood and seafood products, whether imported or domestically produced, are regulated under the Federal Food, Drug, and Cosmetic Act (FD&C Act) as a food. So, too, are the other choices.

2. Answer c: insect repellents are regulated as pesticides by the Environmental Protection Agency. Both aspirin and shampoos that get rid of lice are drugs; eye shadow and lipstick are cosmetics; all are regulated by FDA.

3. Answer c: Oven cleaners are regulated by the Consumer Product Safety Commission (CPSC). Canned tomatoes and spaghetti are regulated as foods by FDA. Tolerances for pesticide residues in foods are established by EPA. but FDA is responsible for ensuring that these tolerances are not exceeded on foods (except for meat, poultry and certain egg products, which are under USDA's jurisdiction). A tolerance level is the maximum amount of a pesticide residue permitted in or on a food. FDA enforces a ban on the sale and distribution of turtles less than 4 inches long, the size most often sold as pets. Pet turtles frequently carry salmonella bacteria, which may cause severe diarrhea in children and adults. Baby turtles were sold as pets in the United States until 1975, when the national Centers for Disease Control and Prevention determined that the bacterial contamination could not be prevented by any known treatment.

4. Answer d: Smoke detectors—both photoelectric and ionization chamber types—are regulated by the Consumer Product Safety Commission. The radioactive source used in the ionization chamber detector is naturally occurring, not electronic and, therefore, is not a substance that would be regulated by FDA. (The level of radiation exposure to home occupants from ionization chamber detectors is much less than that received from the low level of natural background radiation.) Under the FD&C Act, FDA is responsible for protecting consumers from unnecessary exposure to radiation emitted from electronic products. (These provisions were originally separate from the FD&C Act and were referred to as the Radiation Control for Health and Safety Act. They were later incorporated into the FD&C Act when the Safe Medical Devices Act of 1990 was enacted). Airport security x-ray machines and microwave ovens must be properly shielded so that the radiation generated by these products (x-radiation and microwave radiation, respectively) does not harm anyone. MRI diagnostic equipment is regulated as a medical device under the FD&C Act. It

is also subject to enforcement as an electronic product emitting radiation because it uses radio waves and a strong magnetic field to produce its images. Laser products used in lumber mills must conform to an FDA standard that ensures their safety. This standard applies to all laser products, whether medical, industrial or consumer.

5. Answer c: The only advertisements over which FDA has direct jurisdiction are those for prescription drugs. FTC oversees advertising for other FDA-regulated products. TV sets are regulated under the radiological health provisions of the FD&C Act. All televisions must comply with a performance standard that ensures their safety. This standard also applies to video display terminals used with computers. Over-the-counter and prescription drugs, as well as human biological products (such as vaccines and blood products), are regulated by FDA.

6. Answer a: Baby pacifiers are regulated by CPSC unless they are marketed with health claims, in which case they are under FDA's jurisdiction. Food-contact articles, including baby bottle nipples, ceramic ware intended for food use and coffee mugs are regulated by FDA. So are eye charts, which, as diagnostic products, are considered to be medical devices

7. Answer a: Illegal use of heroin is the responsibility of the Drug Enforcement Administration, the key federal agency that polices illicit, or "street" drugs. (If heroin were being studied for medical uses, FDA would regulate it as an investigational drug.) Barbiturates are subject to abuse and thus may, potentially, wind up on the "street," bringing them under DEA's purview. However, barbiturates have legitimate medical uses, and FDA is responsible or ensuring they are properly manufactured and labeled. FDA regulates methadone as a drug, and methadone maintenance treatment programs are monitored under regulations promulgated by both FDA and the National Institute on Drug Abuse (NIDA). Medicinal oxygen is regulated by FDA as a drug. Animal drugs, including veterinary tetracycline, are regulated by FDA.

8. Answer e: Hair dryers are regulated by CPSC. Kidney dialysis machines and tongue depressors, as different as they are in

complexity, are both considered to be medical devices. FDA regulates nonfluoridated toothpastes as cosmetics, and fluoridated toothpastes as drugs.

9. Answer a: Labels on beer and other malt beverages, distilled spirits (liquors), and wines are regulated by the Bureau of Alcohol, Tobacco, and Firearms under the Federal Alcohol Administration Act. Ground coffee, coffee beans, rabbit meat, and canned tuna are all regulated by FDA as foods. (The Federal Meat Inspection Act, which gives USDA authority over meat products, covers cattle, sheep, swine, goats, and horses. Other meat products, including game meats such as rabbit are regulated by FDA.)

10. Answer a: Home canning equipment, under a memorandum of understanding between FDA and CPSC, is regulated by CPSC. FDA's jurisdiction includes the facilities where the products it regulates are stored, such as food and drug warehouses. Hearing aid dispensing establishments are bound by specific FDA regulations that impose conditions for the sale of hearing aids. The regulations attempt to prevent misrepresentation and ensure adherence to proper medical standards. Regarding exporting drugs, FDA continues to have authority over its regulated products even when they are exported.

11. Answer c: The FD&C Act specifically excludes soap from its definition of cosmetics. CPSC regulates this product. All of the other choices are defined as cosmetics and, therefore, are regulated by FDA.

12. Answer a: A vaccine for horses is a veterinary biological product. FDA does not have jurisdiction over veterinary biologics. The Virus, Serum, and Toxin Act gives this responsibility to USDA. The FD&C Act gives FDA authority over pet foods and drugs, which would include veterinary penicillin, medicated feeds, and bird feed. The Public Health Service Act confers on FDA the authority to regulate the interstate movement of psittacine birds (parrots, cockatoos, macaws, parakeets, and other birds in the psittacine family). These birds are potential carriers of psittacosis, a disease that can be transmitted to people. Psittacosis, which is also known as parrot fever, can

range in severity from a mild respiratory infection to a protracted illness.

13. Answer a: The safety of public drinking water (tap water) is
protected by EPA, as decided in an agreement between that
agency and FDA. FDA has jurisdiction over bottled water,
which is considered a food under the FD&C Act. The remaining choices are also defined as foods.

14. Answer b: Child-proof packaging authority, addressed under
the Poison Prevention Packaging Act, was delegated to CPSC.
Tamper-resistant packaging, which is required for certain
OTC drugs, cosmetics, and medical devices, is FDA's responsibility. Food packaging materials, such as plastic containers
and candy boxes, are subject to regulation as food additives under the FD&C Act because of the possibility that they may leach
their chemical constituents into the food products. These potential additives are referred to as indirect food additives. A container bearing a drug product is considered to be a component
of that drug, and FDA, therefore, requires that it be appropriate for that drug.

15. Answer a: The animal counterpart of a cosmetic is commonly
referred to as a "grooming aid." Cosmetics, as defined in the
FD&C Act, apply only to human use. Therefore, products intended for cleansing or promoting attractiveness of animals
are not subject to FDA control. An artificial limb for dogs is
regulated as a veterinary medical device. While such products
do not require FDA approval, they do come under the purview
of the FD&C Act. They may not bear labeling that is false or
misleading, nor may they be otherwise misbranded or adulterated. The laser scanner must comply with the standard. Mercury vapor lamps most often used to light streets, gymnasiums,
sports arenas, banks and stores must be maintained properly
to be safe. With some types of mercury vapor lamps, if the
outer envelope is broken and the lamp continues to operate,
intense, harmful ultraviolet radiation is emitted. An FDA
standard ensures that this lighting is safe. Finally, FDA regulates vitamin C tablets as food supplements.

Chapter 22

Food and Drug Administration Almanac

Agency Overview: FDA's Mission

The Food and Drug Administration is a team of dedicated professionals working to protect, promote and enhance the health of the American people. FDA is responsible for ensuring that:

* Foods are safe, wholesome and sanitary; human and veterinary drugs, biological products, and medical devices are safe and effective; cosmetics are safe; and electronic products that emit radiation are safe.

* Regulated products are honestly, accurately and informatively represented.

* These products are in compliance with the law and FDA regulations; noncompliance is identified and corrected; and any unsafe or unlawful products are removed from the marketplace.

We strive to:

* Enforce FDA laws and regulations, using all appropriate legal means.

* Base regulatory decisions on a strong scientific and analytical base and the law; and understand, conduct and apply excellent science and research.

DHHS Publication No. (FDA) 96-1254, July 1996.

281

- Be a positive force in making safe and effective products available to the consumer, and focus special attention on rare and life-threatening diseases.

- Provide clear standards of compliance to regulated industry, and advise industry on how to meet those standards.

- Identify and effectively address critical public health problems arising from use of FDA-regulated products.

- Increase FDA's effectiveness through collaboration and cooperation with state and local governments; domestic, foreign and international agencies; industry; and academia.

- Assist the media, consumer groups, and health professionals in providing accurate, current information about regulated products to the public.

- Work consistently toward effective and efficient application of resources to our responsibilities.

- Provide superior public service by developing, maintaining and supporting a high-quality, diverse work force.

- Be honest, fair and accountable in all of our actions and decisions.

FDA's Vision

FDA in the year 2000 will be ...

- A strong science-based agency—to accurately detect and assess health risks and to set appropriate standards.

- A trusted agency—to enforce the Food, Drug, and Cosmetic Act fairly, uphold safety standards, and protect consumers.

- An enabling agency—to steward needed products and to promote Public health.

- A collaborative agency—to strengthen ties to scientific, health provider, and regulatory communities both domestically and internationally.

- A high performance agency—to capitalize on state-of-the-art information and communication technologies and management systems to enhance performance.

- An employee-valued agency—to recruit, develop and advance employees equitably, and to position the agency to meet the changing work force needs of the 21st century.

FDA principally serves the general public in its health and safety mission. FDA also recognizes its responsibilities to the industries that it regulates and will work with them in shepherding new technologies to the marketplace. Thus it strives to maximize public health protection while minimizing regulatory burden.

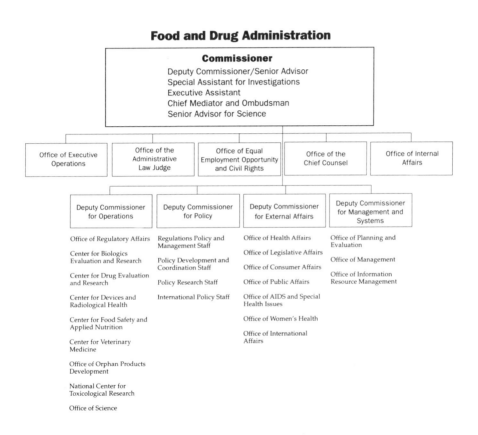

Figure 22.1. The Food and Drug Administration.

283

Major Laws Enforced by FDA

- **Food and Drugs Act of 1906** prohibits interstate commerce in misbranded and adulterated food, drinks and drugs.

- **Federal Food, Drug, and Cosmetic Act of 1938** ensures that foods are safe to eat and produced under sanitary conditions; that drugs and devices are safe and effective for their intended uses; that cosmetics are safe and made from appropriate ingredients; and that labeling and packaging is truthful, informative, and not deceptive.

- **Public Health Service Act of 1944** covers a broad spectrum of health concerns, including the regulation of biological products for human use.

- **Fair Packaging and Labeling Act of 1966** affects the contents and placement of information required on product packages.

- **Radiation Control for Health and Safety Act of 1968** protects the public from unnecessary exposure to radiation from electronic products.

- **Medical Device Amendments of 1976** assures the safety and effectiveness of medical devices.

- **Prescription Drug Marketing Act of 1987** bans the diversion of prescription drugs from legitimate commercial channels.

- **Pesticide Monitoring Improvements Act of 1988** requires the conduct of a comprehensive monitoring program for imported and domestic foods for pesticide residues.

- **Nutrition Labeling and Education Act of 1990** defines new standards for nutrition labeling, nutrient content, and health claims for foods.

- **Safe Medical Devices Act of 1990** requires the reporting of any medical device that causes or contributes to the death, serious illness, or injury of a patient.

- **Prescription Drug User Fee Act of 1992** requires drug and biologic manufacturers to pay fees for applications and supplements.

- **Mammography Quality Standards Act of 1992** requires all mammography facilities in the United States to be accredited and federally certified.

- **Dietary Supplement Health and Education Act of 1994** establishes specific labeling requirements, provides a regulatory framework, and authorizes FDA to promulgate good manufacturing practice regulations for dietary supplements.

FDA: A Record of Accomplishment

Faster Drug Approvals

- 82 new drugs approved in 16.5 months (median) in calendar year (CY) 1995, compared with 62 new drugs approved in 19 months in 1994

- 28 of the 1995 approvals were new molecular entities (NMEs)—brand new drugs as opposed to new formulations—and were approved in 15.9 months (median), compared with 22 NMEs approved in 17.5 months in 1994

- 15 of the 1995 approvals were "priority" drugs—having important therapeutic valueand were approved in 6 months (median), compared with 17 "priority" drugs approved in 15 months in 1994

- 13 of the 1995 "priority" approvals were user fee drugs approved in 5.9 months (median), compared with 12 "priority" user fee drugs approved in 10.4 months in 1994

Improved Device Reviews

- 5,594 510(k)s (which account for about 98 percent of medical devices) found substantially equivalent by FDA in 137 days (mean) in FY 1995, compared with 5,498 in 184 days in FY 1994

- 27 PMAs (premarket applications for certain class III devices) approved by FDA in 20 months (mean) in FY 1995, compared with 26 PMAs in 21.5 months in FY 1994

The Record on Reinvention

As part of Vice President Gore's National Performance Review, FDA has announced more than 30 FDA regulatory reinvention initiatives since March 1995. These initiatives will reduce regulatory burdens and streamline the regulatory process, while maintaining vital public health safeguards and speeding the marketing of safe and effective new drugs and medical devices. Following is a partial listing of these initiatives:

- Speed up approval process for cancer drugs by using tumor shrinkage as surrogate marker for accelerated approval decisions.

- Expand patient access to experimental cancer drugs approved in other countries.

- Increase patient representation on cancer drug advisory committees.

- Clarify requirements for doctors studying already approved cancer drugs.

- Eliminate Establishment License Application (ELA) for most biotech drugs.

- Eliminate lot release requirement for biotech drugs.

- Commit FDA to respond to clinical hold submissions on drugs, including biotech drugs, within 30 days.

- Harmonize application forms for drugs and biologics.

- Eliminate preapproval requirement for promotional labeling for biotech drugs.

- Allow companies to distribute certain textbooks and journal articles that discuss unapproved uses of drugs and devices.

- Allow companies to submit toxicology findings based on first analysis of studies and reduce manufacturing data needed to begin drug tests in humans.

- Develop pilot program for review of low- to moderate-risk medical devices by outside organizations.

- Collect user fees for medical device reviews.

- Expand opportunities for export of unapproved drugs and medical devices to industrialized countries.

- Exempt up to 122 categories of low-risk medical devices from premarket review, adding to 450 categories already exempted.

- Allow manufacturers of biological drugs to get licenses for pilot facilities instead of having to build full-scale manufacturing plants.

- Exclude drug and biologics manufacturers from requirements for most environmental assessments.

The International Record

- The General Accounting Office reported in October 1995 that approval times for NMEs were shorter in the United States than in the United Kingdom.

- In FY 1994, 32 NMEs were approved in the United Kingdom in a median time of 30 months.

- In CY 1994, 22 NMES were approved in the United States in a median time of 18 months.

- FDA's median approval time for new drugs approved in CY 1994 and 1995 was as fast as that in the United Kingdom and faster than those in France, Spain, Germany, Australia, Japan, Italy, and Canada, according to preliminary data from the Centre for Medicines Research (CMR), an industry-funded, not-for-profit research group in the United Kingdom. The median review time in the United States and the United Kingdom was approximately 1.3 years, according to CMR News, Spring 1996.

- The United States has had more first launches of worldwide NMEs than any single European country since 1990. In fact, analysis of worldwide NMEs launched in the United States and Europe showed the United States has had a higher percentage of first launches than the top three European countries combined, according to CMR News, Spring 1996 (United States: 33%, United Kingdom: 14%, France: 9%, Germany: 7%.)

Access to New Drugs

In *Timely Access to New Drugs in the 1990s: An International Comparison*, published in December 1995, the United States, the United Kingdom, Germany, and Japan were compared to determine whether and when new drugs introduced worldwide from 1990 through 1994 were reaching their consumers. The analysis leads to the following conclusions:

- Numerous therapies with significant public health benefits are available in the United States but have not yet been approved in these other countries. Among those of special interest are

Zerit (stavudine), to treat AIDS; Cognex (tacrine), for use in mitigating Alzheimer's disease; Cerezyme (imiglucerase), for Gaucher's disease; and Chemet (succimer), to treat lead intoxication in children.

- Virtually all of the drugs in this study that were approved in the United Kingdom, Germany, or Japan, but not in the United States, are drugs that have essentially the same therapeutic value as other drugs already on the U.S. market.

- The United States is first to approve a significant proportion of the "global" drugs—those ultimately approved in more than one of the countries under study.

Speed of approval is only one measure of performance; the quality of review and decision-making is also critical. FDA's rigorous evaluation makes its approval decision an international gold standard, automatically confirming a product's merits in many foreign marketplaces.

But it is reasonable to ask whether the time cost of that quality is excessive. The analysis presented here reveals that in 1996 FDA's tough standards do not delay consumer access to important new drugs compared with other countries. Every country has a medicine cabinet that is somewhat different, and no country stocks all the products that have been approved somewhere on the world market. But the data clearly demonstrate that the United States has available valuable drugs as soon as, and in many cases sooner than, its counterparts around the world.

The 214 new drugs in this report were introduced into the world market from January 1990 through December 1994. For purposes of this study, a new drug is defined as a new chemical entity (NCE) or a biological substance that has not been approved previously anywhere in the world.

HACCP

Eight major food companies are working with FDA in a pilot program to test a procedure to enhance food safety.

The pilot, announced Aug. 4,1994, will help FDA determine if the approach, called Hazard Analysis Critical Control Point, or HACCP, is practical for wider application in the food industry.

Under the HACCP plan, companies analyze their manufacturing processes to identify where problems are most likely to occur and where preventive measures need to be focused. The idea behind

288

HACCP is to build safety into the manufacturing process, rather than rely on inspections and sampling to identify unsafe products after they've been made.

A HACCP program is built on seven scientific principles:

1. Analyze hazards, and establish preventive measures to control identified hazards.

2. Identify critical control points.

3. Establish critical limits for each preventive measure associated with a critical control point.

4. Establish procedures to monitor the critical control points.

5. Establish corrective actions to be taken when monitoring shows that a critical limit has not been met.

6. Establish effective record keeping to document the HACCP system.

7. Establish procedures to verify the system is working consistently.

Advantages

Advocates of HACCP believe that it offers a number of advantages. Most importantly, HACCP:

- focuses on preventing hazards before they occur

- is based on sound science

- reinforces that the responsibility for ensuring food safety rests with the food manufacturer or distributor

- permits more efficient and effective government oversight, primarily because the record keeping allows government investigators to see how well a firm is complying with food safety laws over time rather than how well it is doing on any given day

- helps food companies compete more effectively in the world market.

Companies participating in the voluntary pilot program and their products are:

- Alto Dairy, Wapun, Wis.—hard cheese

- Campbell Soup Company, Camden, N.J.—refrigerated salad dressing

- Campbell-Taggart, Inc., St. Louis, Mo.—pan breads

- Con Agra, Omaha, Neb.—flour

- Ocean Spray Cranberries, Lakeville-Middleboro, Mass.—pasteurized juice

- Pillsbury, Minneapolis, Minn.—bakery products

- Hans Kissle Foods, Wilmington, Mass. (in cooperation with the Massachusetts Department of Health)—quiche

- Ralston Foods, St. Louis, Mo.—breakfast cereal.

Seafood HACCP

In December 1995, FDA published its final rule requiring mandatory HACCP systems in the seafood industry. The final rule is scheduled to take effect on Dec. 18,1997. In the interim, the agency is working with academia, the seafood industry, and others to develop and implement the training programs required to support mandatory HACCP for seafood. FDA is also writing guidelines to provide seafood processors with advice on food hazards that must be controlled through HACCP and controls that could be employed for those hazards. A draft of the guide, "Fish and Fishery Products Hazards and Controls," was published in 1994. The guide will be published annually beginning in 1996 to incorporate additional scientific data and other information.

MEDWATCH

FDA launched MEDWATCH, the agency's medical products reporting program, in June 1993 to enhance the effectiveness of post-marketing surveillance of all medical products FDA regulates. FDA is particularly interested in receiving reports of serious adverse events and important product problems. The program has four general goals:

- To increase awareness of drug- and device-induced disease.
- To clarify what should be reported.
- To make reporting easier.
- To provide feedback to the health-care community about medical product safety issues.

FDA FY 1996 Budget by Program Area

FDA's FY 1996 budget totals $918 million. This means FDA provides consumer protection over a vast array of products (worth over 1 trillion dollars) at a cost of less than $4 per American per year.

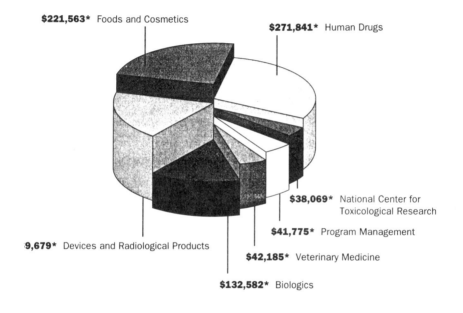

$221,563* Foods and Cosmetics

$271,841* Human Drugs

$38,069* National Center for Toxicological Research

$41,775* Program Management

9,679* Devices and Radiological Products

$42,185* Veterinary Medicine

$132,582* Biologics

*dollars in thousands

Figure 22.2. *FDA's Fiscal Year 1996 Budget by Program Area.*

Field Locations

Six regions, each responsible for a distinct part of the country, make up FDA's field operations. In addition to the six regional offices and 21 district offices shown below, there are 130 resident inspection posts located throughout the United States.

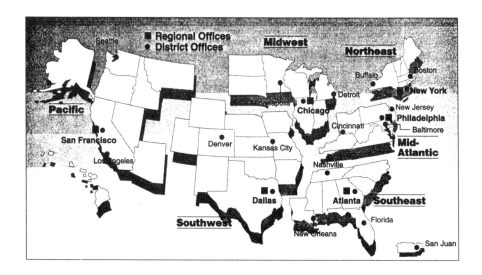

Figure 22.3. *FDA Regional Offices.*

Center for Biologics Evaluation and Research

Overview

The center's mission is to ensure the safety, efficacy, potency, and purity of biological products intended for use in the treatment, prevention or cure of diseases in humans. The primary responsibility of the center is to review the safety and efficacy of vaccines, blood products, certain diagnostic products, and other biological and biotechnology-derived human products. Center activities also include:

- evaluating the safety and effectiveness of biological products before marketing, and monitoring the preclinical and clinical testing of new biological products

- Licensing biological product and manufacturing establishments, including plasmapheresis centers, blood banks, and vaccine manufacturers

- AIDS program and policy activities, including research on AIDS therapeutic products, diagnostic tests, and vaccines

- research to establish product standards and develop improved testing methods

- compliance monitoring, lot release, and postmarket surveillance

CBER Highlights—1995

- During January 1995, FDA conducted a two-day workshop, "Licensing Blood Establishments." The workshop provided detailed guidance to the blood banking industry on registration and general licensing requirements, the managed review process, establishment license applications, product license applications, changes to be reported, special cases, preapproval programs, and how to submit licensing applications.

- In February 1995, FDA licensed the first vaccine for prevention of hepatitis A in adults and children. The vaccine is indicated for international travelers, people living in or relocating to areas where the disease is endemic, some military personnel, and certain high-risk individuals.

- In March 1995, FDA licensed the Varicella Virus Vaccine Live for the prevention of chickenpox. A single injection of the vaccine is recommended for children ages 12 months to 12 years, while two injections four to eight weeks apart are recommended for adolescents and adults (ages 13 and older) who have not contracted chickenpox. The vaccine has been shown to be safe and effective when administered at the same time as the measles, mumps, and rubella vaccines.

- In the second quarter of 1995 FDA cleared for marketing the AlaSTAT Latex-Specific IgE Allergen Test kit to measure latex antibodies in blood.

- In March 1995, FDA licensed a new anti-Rh immune globulin to prevent development of anti-Rh antibodies in Rh-negative pregnant women with an Rh-positive fetus. Anti-Rh antibodies can cause erythroblastosis fetalis, also called "blue baby syndrome") in subsequent Rh-positive fetuses.

- The Creutzfeldt-Jakob disease (CJD) ad hoc advisory committee met in June 1995 to review and evaluate data, hear opinions, and advise on the public health issues of blood product disposition associated with CJD in implicated donors. CJD is a rare, degenerative disease of the central nervous system.

- FDA conducted a workshop at NIH on Human Tissue Intended for Transplantation and Human Reproductive Tissue on June 20-21, 1995. The workshop provided an opportunity to make public and to request comments about a discussion document on screening and testing human tissue. This document, for which a notice of availability was published in the Federal Register on the first day of the conference, will be used to form the core of a guidance document on testing and screening tissue donors for high-risk behaviors and for symptoms of human immunodeficiency virus (HIV) and hepatitis.

- In June 1995, FDA issued a memorandum to blood establishments recommending the deferral of current or recent correctional facility/ institution inmates as donors of whole blood, blood components, source plasma, and source leukocytes. The recommendations were based on reports that a significant proportion of correctional institution inmates are at increased risk for infectious diseases because of their use of illicit intravenous drugs prior to incarceration.

- FDA held two biologics workshops on June 7-8, 1995. Representatives of the biologics industry and FDA district personnel discussed licensing and registration, infectious disease updates, sterile docking devices and pooled product, irradiated products, computer approach to inspections, quality assurance, recalls, and error/accident reporting.

- On Aug. 8, 1995, FDA recommended that blood establishments test donors with new HIV-1 antigen test kits as soon as the kits become available, to further reduce the risk of infecting blood recipients through contaminated transfusions.

- On Aug. 9, 1995, FDA and the National Heart, Lung, and Blood Institute met to discuss the institute's request to study the use of cord blood as bone marrow reconstitution for both children and adults with malignancies and immunodeficiencies.

- In September 1995, CBER's animal care program and facilities were reviewed by the American Association for Accreditation of Laboratory Animal Care, and full accreditation status was retained. The accreditation assures the general public that FDA biomedical research and testing is performed in a humane manner.

Center for Devices and Radiological Health

Overview

The center is responsible for ensuring the safety and effectiveness of medical devices and eliminating unnecessary human exposure to manmade radiation from medical, occupational and consumer products. The center protects the public health by:

- reviewing and evaluating medical device premarket approval applications, product development protocols, exemption requests for investigational devices, and premarket notifications (510(k)s)

- collecting information about injuries and other experiences in the use of medical devices and radiation-emitting electronic products and using this information in center activities

- developing and enforcing standards for every significant aspect of mammography, including equipment, personnel, and quality assurance programs

- developing, promulgating and enforcing performance standards for radiation-emitting electronic products and medical devices and good manufacturing practice regulations

• monitoring compliance and surveillance programs for medical devices and radiation-emitting electronic products

• providing technical and other nonfinancial assistance to small manufacturers of medical devices

CDRH Highlights—1995

Device Review

CDRH reduced the average review time for 510(k)s, devices manufacturers identify as similar to already existing products, by more than 25 percent, from 184 days in FY94 to 137 days in FY95. Half of these devices were reviewed in 90 days or less.

The backlog of 510(k)s under review for more than 90 days was reduced to nine from 498 in October 1994. The elimination of these overdue applications enables CDRH to start reviewing new 510(k) submissions soon after they come in, without relegating them to a protracted queue.

The average review time for premarket applications (PMAs) for new uses and new types of devices was reduced from 21.5 months in FY94 to 20 months in FY95.

CDRH also cut by half the number of overdue PMA supplements despite a 34 percent increase in this type of submission.

The proportion of Investigational Device Exemptions (IDEs) approved within 30 days of receipt increased from 30 percent in FY94 to 65 percent in the second half of FY95.

New Medical Device Problem Reporting Rule

On Dec. 11, 1995, FDA published a final regulation to require hospitals, nursing homes, and other health-care facilities to report deaths and serious injuries or illnesses connected with the use of medical devices. This will provide the necessary backup assurance of product safety to enable FDA to clear innovative devices for marketing more quickly. The requirements of the final regulation take effect on July 31, 1996.

Medical facilities must now report all serious device-related incidents within 10 days. Deaths must be reported directly to the agency, as well as to the manufacturer, and serious injuries or illnesses must be reported to the manufacturer, or to FDA if the firm's identity is not known. The facilities must send a summary of these reports to FDA every six months.

Manufacturers must report to FDA any device-related incident that requires immediate action to protect the public health within five days. All other reports on device-related deaths or serious injuries or illness must be made within 30 days.

In addition, manufacturers must submit an annual statement certifying the number of reports filed during the last 12 months. Device manufacturers are responsible for reporting incidents related to their products even if they are no longer being marketed.

AIDS Accomplishments from CDRH

• The center organized and co-sponsored a workshop and symposium on ultraviolet (W), HIV, and AIDS. A center study of 41 clinics found that at least 8 percent of patients undergoing therapy with UV-emitting devices are HIV-infected. This study is part of a larger research program to determine the safety of UV-emitting devices on HIV-positive patients.

• The center has developed a computer model that simulates the microscopic properties of latex condoms in relation to leakage and as a barrier to virus-sized particles.

• As part of the agency's policy to encourage condom use, the center is now allowing manufacturers to market condoms made from polyurethane and other new materials after supplying FDA with certain key test results, including data on slipping and breaking during actual use. The manufacturer must agree to conduct a postmarket contraceptive efficacy study, and the agency will reexamine the product after that study is complete. As of March 1996, FDA had cleared three such condoms.

• Results of a study of latex, polyurethane and natural membrane male condoms indicate that currently marketed latex and polyurethane are reasonably effective barriers to virus passage.

• FDA, the German Institute for Standardization, and the American Society for Testing and Materials have developed a clinical laboratory standard for the diagnosis of HIV by polymerase chain reaction. The standard will assist different diagnostic laboratories in obtaining comparable and reproducible test results.

• FDA developed new water leak tests which are now being used to detect pinholes in polyurethane female condoms.

- FDA placed an emphasis on the adequacy of current methods and developments of new methods for evaluating medical device sterilization and disinfection. Research is focusing on evaluating the effectiveness of liquid disinfectants against common contaminants.

FDA's Device Review Team

Medical devices have diverse applications, technology, and operating principles. Therefore, the technical expertise of FDA's review staff must also be diverse and tailored to the issues presented by specific devices:

- **Engineers** (including biomedical, electrical/electronics, and materials) assess information on design, specifications, and performance characteristics for a broad range of devices to ensure they are appropriate for their intended users.

- **Biologists and microbiologists** review packaging and sterilization information for many devices and are also focused on the evaluation of in vitro diagnostic products and infection control devices.

- **Physicians and other clinicians** review clinical data and other information on many devices to evaluate their intended or adverse effects and the appropriateness of proposed labeling.

- **Chemists, biochemists and toxicologists** review preclinical test data and information on device composition and manufacturing to assess the stability and toxicity of implants and other devices that come in contact with the body.

- **Medical technologists** lend their special expertise to the review of clinical laboratory devices.

- **Physicists** review imaging devices, surgical lasers, and other radiation-emitting devices.

- **Statisticians** evaluate study designs, statistical analyses, and related conclusions about safety and effectiveness.

- **Consumer safety officers** and field investigators assess the adequacy of proposed manufacturing processes and controls and the compliance status of manufacturers.

- **Human factors specialists** ensure that medical device design and labeling take user characteristics and limitations into consideration.

Center for Drug Evaluation and Research

Overview

The center promotes, protects and enhances the health of the public through the drug development and evaluation process. The center's mission is to:

- approve drugs for marketing that are effective for their labeled indications, provide benefits that outweigh their risks, are of high quality, and have directions for use that are complete and honestly communicated

- facilitate early access to promising experimental drugs being developed for serious illnesses with no adequate therapy

- promote innovation and provide scientific leadership in the drug development process

- ensure that the safety and rights of patients in drug studies are adequately protected

- ensure that product quality and safety are maintained after marketing

FDA's Drug Review Team

The members of the FDA review team simultaneously apply their special technical expertise to the review of an NDA:

- **Chemists** focus on how the drug is put together, whether the manufacturing controls and packaging are adequate to ensure the stability of the product, and whether the proposed labeling accurately reflects the effects of the drug.

- **Pharmacologists** evaluate the effects of the drug on laboratory animals in short-term and long-term studies.

- **Physicians** evaluate the results of the clinical tests-including the drug's adverse as well as therapeutic effects.

- **Statisticians** evaluate the designs for each controlled study, the validity of statistical analyses, and the conclusions of safety and effectiveness based on the study data.

- **Microbiologists** evaluate the data on anti-infectives (antibiotics, antivirals and antifungals). These drugs differ from others because they're intended to affect microbes instead of patients.

- **Other staff** evaluate the rate and extent to which the drug's active ingredient is made available to the body and the way it is distributed, metabolized and eliminated. They determine whether the evidence supports the labeling for the recommended dosing regimen.

Prescription Drug User Fee Act

Specific performance targets for application review times took effect in FY 1995. The agency monitored FY 1995 performance and found, as of Feb. 29, 1996:

New Applications

- 111 New Drug Applications
- 48 of 48 applications completed within 12-month cycle
- 63 pending action within 12-month cycle
- zero pending action and "overdue"

Effectiveness Supplements

- 76 filed
- 44 of 44 supplements completed within 12-month cycle
- 30 pending action within 12-month cycle
- 2 pending action and "overdue"

Manufacturing Supplements

- 1,248 filed
- 1,088 of 1,179 completely reviewed within six months
- 29 pending action and "overdue"

CDER reduced its user fee defined backlog of overdue original new drug applications, efficacy supplements, and manufacturing supplements to zero.

The median approval time for user fee NDA approvals was 15.9 months.

300

Center for Food Safety and Applied Nutrition

Overview

The center is responsible for the regulation of foods for human consumption and cosmetics. The mission of the center is to:

- ensure that food is microbiologically, chemically, nutritionally, and toxicologically safe

- emphasize a preventative approach to protecting public health

- promote sound nutrition

- encourage industry innovation while upholding safety standards and maintaining consumer protection

- ensure that food and cosmetic products are honestly and accurately labeled.

The center oversees a vast food industry that includes more than 30,000 U.S. food manufacturers and processors and 20,000 warehouses. The U.S. food industry contributes about 20 percent of the U.S. Gross National Product, employs about 14 million individuals, and provides an additional 4 million jobs in related industries.

FDA spent over $200 million on food safety in FY 1995. The responsibilities of the 870 people with the center include research, writing regulations, premarket safety reviews of food additives, developing educational materials, collecting and analyzing data, providing technical assistance to the states, and postmarket surveillance.

Many CFSAN employees have specialized training in physical and physiological sciences, including epidemiology and environmental health, to oversee new technologies in product handling and food transport.

Food Safety

FDA is responsible for ensuring the safety and wholesomeness of all food sold in interstate commerce, except for meat and poultry, which are under the jurisdiction of the U.S. Department of Agriculture.

The U.S. food supply is safe and wholesome—in fact, one of the safest in the world. The complexity of the food industry, and of the technologies used in food production and packaging, is increasing. The concept of food safety and quality is changing, and the volume of imported foods is on the rise.

Food is subject to natural and man-made contamination with toxins, pests, pathogenic bacteria, viruses and parasites, molds, industrial chemicals, and toxic metals. The following issues constitute FDA's current area of concern for food safety:

- biological: bacteria, viruses, parasites
- natural toxins (e.g., mycotoxins, ciguatera toxin, paralytic shellfish poison)
- pesticide residues in foods
- industrial chemicals
- toxic elements (such as lead and mercury)
- radionuclides
- tampering
- filth and decomposition
- nutrient concerns (e.g., vitamin D overdose, pediatric iron toxicity)
- dietary components (e.g., fat, cholesterol)
- allergens (e.g., sulfites)
- metabolic disorders (e.g., phenylketonuria)
- used as dietary supplements

FDA's Tools for Ensuring Food Safety

- inspection of establishments
- collection and analysis of samples
- premarket approval review (food and color additives and animal drugs)
- regulation/agreement writing
- consumer education
- laboratory studies—develop/improve analytical methods; determine health effects of food contaminants; determine effects of processing on food composition; determine health effects of dietary factors
- pilot plant food processing and packaging and biotechnology studies
- cooperative activities/technical assistance
- collection and analysis of information

Microbiological Safety

A major food safety problem confronting the nation—which every American can help prevent through safe food-handling practices—is microbial contamination of food by bacteria such as:

- *Salmonella enteritidis*
- *Campylobacter jejuni*
- *Listeria monocytogenes*
- *Vibrio vulnificus*

Salmonella is responsible for 2 million to 4 million human illnesses annually in the United States. Illnesses caused by *Campylobacter jejuni* are thought to exceed in number those caused by *Salmonella*. *Listeria monocytogenes* caused approximately 1,100 illnesses in 1993 in the United States. *Vibrio vulnificus* is a free-living marine bacterium, sometimes found in uncooked shellfish, that can cause fatal infections in those with liver disease, such as cirrhosis, or in immune-compromised individuals. It causes an average of 40 illnesses and 20 deaths a year.

Cosmetics

FDA estimates that cosmetics are being produced in more than 1,600 domestic manufacturing and repacking establishments, representing more than 40,000 product formulations. Consumer expenditures for cosmetic products exceed $20 billion annually. The cosmetics industry uses about 7,500 different cosmetic ingredients and about 4,000 fragrance ingredients.

The Center for Food Safety and Applied Nutrition is responsible for handling issues involving the safety and proper labeling of domestically manufactured and imported cosmetics, including:

- evaluation of cosmetic-related adverse reactions
- dermal tests for toxicity and absorption of colors and cosmetics
- safety research on cosmetic ingredients and contaminants
- safety research and analytical methods development for cosmetic fragrance ingredients and cosmetic preservative systems.

Current issues of concern in cosmetics include adverse reaction monitoring, drug-cosmetics enforcement, aerosol flammability (hair spray), hair dye safety, talc safety, and investigation of products containing alphahydroxy acid (AHA).

Center for Veterinary Medicine

Overview

The Center for Veterinary Medicine is a public health organization that enables the marketing of effective animal drugs, food additives, feed ingredients, and animal devices that are safe to animals, humans, and the environment. The center, in partnership with federal and state agencies and other center customers, ensures animal health and the safety of food derived from animals. The center makes timely quality decisions and takes regulatory actions to ensure that these products provide for quality health care of animals, minimize the transmission of zoonotic diseases, and increase efficiency of production of animal-derived food. To support these decisions, the center performs research and monitors product safety and efficacy.

CVM Highlights—1995

- In March 1995, CVM issued a summary of the adverse reaction reports on Posilac™ (sometribove) during the first year of marketing. Posilac, the only recombinant bovine somatotropin product approved for increasing milk production in dairy cattle, was first marketed in February 1994. CVM found that the number and severity of the reported adverse reactions during this period raised no new animal health concerns about the safety of Posilac™. In addition CVM and the states found no indication of a change in the incidence of violative drug residues in milk since Posilac™ had been in commercial use.

- In June 1995, CVM issued the ninth in a series of policy letters regarding the implementation of the generic Animal Drug and Patent Term Restoration Act, which was signed into law Nov. 16, 1988. This letter introduced a revised policy statement on the environmental review of generic animal drugs.

- In August 1995, CVM approved the first fluoroquinolone antibacterial drug for use in food-producing animals. Sarafloxacin hydrochloride was approved for use in chickens and turkeys. Fluoroquinolones are the newest class of antimicrobial drugs developed for treating infections in people and animals. This approval of a fluoroquinolone product for food animal use followed lengthy consideration about possible microbial resistance to these drugs.

- In September 1995, CVM amended the food additive regulations to allow marketing of cobalt-60 source gamma radiation to control *Salmonella* contamination in poultry feed products. Use of this technology to kill *Salmonella* in feed may help prevent the transmission of *Salmonella* from poultry products to humans.

National Center for Toxicological Research

Overview

The National Center for Toxicological Research, located in Jefferson, Ark., conducts integrated research with other FDA centers and leverages FDA resources through cooperative and collaborative agreements with other agencies, academia and industry. Research is conducted within the following research areas:

- biometry and risk assessment
- biochemical toxicology
- carcinogenesis
- chemistry
- reproductive and developmental toxicology
- genetic toxicology
- microbiology
- molecular epidemiology
- neurotoxicology
- nutritional toxicology

The focus of NCTR research is within three strategic research goals:

- **The development of knowledge bases:** Accumulation of data that have predictive values extending beyond the individual data elements and which foster the identification of data gaps and new research areas leading to the development of predictive systems in support of regulatory decision making.

- **The development of new strategies for the prediction of toxicity:** Mechanism-based assays that contribute to a profile of information that supports a regulatory decision.

- **The conduct of method-(METH), agent-(AGNT), or concept driven research:** The modification and development of better analytical and toxicological test methods, and the provision of data on specific agents of interest to FDA to facilitate current and anticipated regulatory needs.

Examples of activities under way to support these goals include:

• Research to improve the predictive value of the animal model for regulatory risk assessment and to provide essential data on the cancer risk of chloral hydrate, fumonisin B1, and malachite green.

• Investigations on the toxicity of estrogens to enhance knowledge of product safety and to develop through the use of artificial intelligence, a knowledge base for determinants of estrogenic activity.

• Design of molecular epidemiological studies on food-borne carcinogens to define biomarkers of exposure and susceptibility for humans.

• Development of analytical methods for detection of pesticides (with CFSAN) and antibiotic residues in food (with CVM); identification of microorganisms, using immunoassays and polymerase chain reaction techniques; use of pyrolysis-mass spectrometry for the rapid identification of bacteria; and development of a device to characterize gaseous components of seafood decomposition.

Deputy Commissioner/Senior Advisor to the Commissioner

The position of deputy commissioner/senior advisor to the commissioner was established in 1993. Keeping alert to developing situations in all the centers and offices, the deputy commissioner/senior advisor to the commissioner takes appropriate action to avert a crisis or defuse emergency situations. The deputy commissioner also provides an internal mechanism for reporting directly to the commissioner allegations of wrongdoing that could have a significant effect on programs or allegations of improper management action.

Office of Executive Secretariat

The Office of Executive Secretariat coordinates communication on FDA's program priorities. The core function of the Executive Secretariat is to assign, track and review for consistency, accuracy, and appropriate agency clearance correspondence and memoranda for the signature of the commissioner and deputy commissioners. This office also serves as liaison between the department and FDA and as a resource for up-to-date information on developments throughout the agency.

Office of the Chief Counsel

The Office of the Chief Counsel provides a full range of legal services to FDA in the enforcement of the Federal Food, Drug, and Cosmetic Act. The office also handles legal matters involving the Administrative Procedure Act, Federal Advisory Committee Act, Federal Tort Claim Act, and other federal statutes. The Office of the Chief Counsel:

* represents FDA in court proceedings and administrative hearings
* provides legal advice regarding agency programs
* coordinates legal matters involving FDA with the Department of Justice and other federal agencies
* drafts or reviews FDA regulations and other *Federal Register* documents
* gives legal opinions on agency regulatory issues and on petitions submitted to FDA
* reviews proposed legislation affecting FDA that originates in the Department of Health and Human Services or on which Congress requests the views of the department
* provides legal advice and assistance on matters within its expertise to the Office of the Secretary of Health and Human Services.

Office of the Chief Mediator and Ombudsman

The chief mediator and ombudsman reports directly to and acts on behalf of the commissioner in investigating and resolving issues and problems that affect products under FDA's jurisdiction. The office investigates industry complaints about FDA's regulatory processes, identifies deficiencies in those processes, responds to problems, and ensures that FDA policy is fairly and evenly applied throughout the agency. The office also mediates disputes or issues between FDA and the regulated industry that have not been resolved through conventional administrative processes.

The chief mediator and ombudsman also assigns review responsibility for combination products and other products whose jurisdiction is uncertain or in dispute, and oversees the policies and procedures governing intercenter consultations and collaborations.

Office of Special Investigations

The Office of Special Investigations investigates internal and external policy-related issues involving all areas of the agency, including inspections, congressional affairs, media relations, and scientific procedures. The office also interacts with senior-level agency administrators, center directors and their staffs, and with field employees to enhance internal communication.

Office of External Affairs

The Office of External Affairs (OEA) coordinates FDA's interactions with a variety of external audiences, through the outreach activities of the Offices of Consumer Affairs, Health Affairs, International Affairs, Legislative Affairs, Public Affairs, AIDS and Special Health Issues, Women's Health, and the Industry and Small Business Liaison Staff. OEA offices seek to inform the public regarding FDA activities and to increase public understanding of FDA and its activities, provide the agency's constituencies with opportunities to contribute to FDA decision-making, and facilitate communication between agency components and outside groups.

Office of Consumer Affairs

The Office of Consumer Affairs seeks consumer participation in agency policy-making and ensures that FDA decision makers hear consumer concerns before completing policy decisions. OCA's primary functions include public participation, consumer education, and outreach. Recent highlights include:

Public Participation

Constituents—OCA broadened its outreach to include:

- consumer advocates for international concerns in the areas of drug approvals and food safety
- environmental groups involved with FDA issues such as food safety, International Harmonization, and biotechnology.

FDA Advisory Committees—OCA recruited candidates for 10 anticipated consumer representative vacancies in 1995. Consumer representatives serve as members on 36 of the agency's 42 advisory committees and panels.

Consumer Education and Outreach

Consumer Quarterly—OCA published three issues of the newsletter. Mailed to over 1,500 consumers and *Consumer Quarterly* organizations, the newsletter provides information on public participation opportunities, developments in agency policy, and consumer information.

Breast Implants—OCA continued to operate a toll-free information service on the status of silicone and saline-filled breast implants.

Food Labeling—OCA sponsored a variety of consumer education programs that highlighted the food label and good nutrition. The most recent program, "Para Vivir Bien" is a Hispanic/Latino program developed to raise awareness about diet and health among the Hispanic/Latino population in the United States.

OCA responded to over 2,500 inquiries about the food label from consumers, schools, and health groups.

Dietary Supplements—OCA responded to over 2,600 inquiries from consumers, researchers, and health professionals interested in the safety of herbal products. The agency received over 500 comments from a national phone-in campaign from consumers protesting their right to free choice in healthcare and FDA's regulatory enforcement actions with respect to dietary supplements.

MEDWATCH Adverse Reporting Program—The Office of MEDWATCH began transferring consumer calls to OCA at the end of FY94. A total of 9,720 calls were transferred to OCA in FY95. Consumers requested safety information about FDA regulated products-in particular, dietary supplements and herbal remedies. Requests to report an adverse event targeted Rio Hair Conditioners, pedicle screws, temporomandibular joint (TMJ), and breast implants.

Office of Health Affairs

The Office of Health Affairs has lead agency responsibility for liaison with U.S. health professional organizations and the World Health Organization. The office coordinates the agency's Healthy People 2000 activities, ethical issues involving protection of human subjects and institutional review boards, the International Conference on Harmonization, patient information, and liaison with the NIH Office of Alternative Medicine. Other areas of responsibility include:

- the *FDA Medical Bulletin*
- disqualification and reinstatement of clinical investigators
- patent term extension
- appeals from decisions by the Administrative Law Judge
- international drug scheduling.

Highlights

- In October 1995, updated information sheets that help institutional review boards and clinical investigators carry out their responsibilities for the protection of human research subjects. The updates were distributed directly to institutional review boards and at related professional conferences, and are available on the FDA Internet Web site (http://www.fda.gov/oc/oha/toc.html) and via automated fax (800-993-3156).

- Began a series of regular meetings between health professional organizations and senior agency staff in October 1995 to provide an opportunity for interchange on specific topics of mutual interest.

- Briefed the assistant secretary for health, along with the Office of External Affairs and outside health professional organizations, on progress made to date regarding food and drug safety issues contained in Healthy People 2000, the national initiative to significantly improve the health of all Americans by the year 2000.

- Wrote columns for medical journals and provided exhibits at health professional organizations to enlist health professionals in the agency's campaign to inform consumers about the dangers of *Vibrio vulnificus* when eating raw oysters, mammography, patient information, and children and tobacco.

- Participated in the third International Conference on Harmonization in Yokohama, Japan, in November 1995. The conference has finalized 19 technical guidelines that harmonize scientific and technical information needed for drug registration in the European Union, Japan, and the United States. All guidelines are expected to be final by 1997.

- On Feb. 14-15, 1996, held a public patient education workshop to discuss methods and criteria for developing and evaluating prescription drug information for patients.

Office of International Affairs

The International Affairs Staff has the lead agency responsibility for liaison with foreign countries and international organizations. It also works closely with and represents the agency to the Office of the U.S. Trade Representative and the U.S. interagency staff groups dealing with international trade issues.

FDA international activities that are either coordinated, supported or implemented by the International Affairs Staff include:

- Codex Alimentarius Commission

- harmonized technical requirements for pharmaceuticals and biologicals

- international vaccine standards

- provisions for health and safety standards in the World Trade Organization Agreement and the North American Free Trade Agreement

- international agreements regarding FDA-regulated products.

Other areas of responsibility include:

- processing approvals for export of investigational drugs

- negotiating Memoranda of Understanding on regulatory matters with officials of foreign governments

- conducting international training programs and conferences.

Office of Legislative Affairs

The mission of the Office of Legislative Affairs is to manage the agency's congressional relations. OLA initiates, coordinates and provides in-depth analyses of agency legislative needs and proposed and pending legislation by preparing supporting documents, legislative proposals, and position papers for the commissioner, deputy commissioner, other agency officials, Congress, and OMB. This includes developing and coordinating testimony for the agency and the department for presentation to congressional committees; monitoring hearings; and editing transcripts of agency testimony.

OLA coordinates and prepares agency responses to congressional and legislative inquiries and other sensitive correspondence.

OLA Highlights—1995

• Responded to about 3,500 written inquiries from Congress and almost 100 priority requests from the Secretary's office and congressional committee chairmen. Subjects included safety of the blood supply, food safety and labeling, drug approvals, dietary supplements, medical devices, and veterinary drugs.

• Conducted or coordinated briefings and technical assistance sessions for members of Congress and their staffs on topics such as blood safety, sensor pads, aspirin, pedicle screw proposed rule, FDA reform, seafood, regulatory reform, food additives, and FDA laboratory and headquarters consolidation.

• Provided extensive congressional outreach on subjects such as mammography, breast cancer awareness, and women's health.

• Coordinated the development of testimony, briefing books, and preparation of witnesses for 17 congressional hearings. The hearings covered such subjects as devices, blood, drugs, food additives, pesticides, and lab consolidation.

• Ensured appropriate FDA staff involvement and awareness in 17 audits initiated by the General Accounting Office. There were 38 GAO audits in progress in 1995.

Office of Public Affairs

The Office of Public Affairs advises and assists the commissioner and other key officials on all public information programs.

The office plans, coordinates and directs all media relations for the agency. It prepares and distributes press releases and other media statements representing agency policy; coordinates research and drafting of major public statements by the commissioner and other key agency officials; compiles, publishes and distributes the weekly *FDA Enforcement Report* and the FDA Public Calendar; and manages the FDA Internet site.

It also serves as the agency focal point for developing public information programs. It designs, writes and produces consumer information material such as the official agency magazine *FDA Consumer*, the employee newsletter *FDA Today*, the *FDA Almanac*, FDA backgrounders, and brochures. It also produces public service announcements, video news releases, and other informational videos.

OPA's Freedom of Information Staff serves as the agency focal point for the receipt, control, coordination, and assignment of FOI requests to the appropriate FDA office. It ensures that the agency complies with federal laws governing the release of documents. During 1995, OPA:

- prepared and issued 19 press releases, notes to correspondents, and statements, and 69 talk papers

- handled more than 10,400 calls from the media, including about 2,000 from television and radio journalists

- conducted a public education campaign to reduce the risk of accidental childhood poisoning from iron

- published more than 60 *FDA Consumer* reprints, backgrounders, and other print and video public education materials

- received and processed 50,606 FOI requests.

Office of AIDS and Special Health Issues

The Office of AIDS and Special Health Issues is a focal point for agency coordination on AIDS, cancer, Alzheimer's disease, and other special health issues considered serious and life-threatening. The office is also a resource for the general public, including individual patients and patient advocacy groups, on policy initiatives, agency activities, and other issues related to these diseases. In addition, the office:

- serves as a resource within FDA for AIDS, cancer, Alzheimer's disease, and other special health issues

- ensures adequate and timely agency responses to individuals with questions and concerns related to AIDS, cancer, Alzheimer's disease, and other special health issues

- serves as a liaison between patients and their advocates and FDA

- serves as a channel to express patient issues and points of view to senior FDA officials

- provides consultation and policy advice to senior FDA staff

- provides FDA representation at a wide range of public and government meetings where scientific and policy matters are being discussed

- assists in the development of HHS, PHS, and national policies and practices concerning AIDS, cancer, Alzheimer's disease, and other special health issues

- coordinates meetings and workshops of interest for patient advocacy groups.

Office of Women's Health

FDA's Office of Women's Health promotes testing of FDA-regulated products in women, supports research and education to increase knowledge of women's health issues, and forms partnerships to advance women's health objectives.

1995 Highlights

- Sponsored a two-day scientific workshop on gender analysis and areas for policy development and clarification.

- Established a mammography information service, in conjunction with FDA's Center for Devices and Radiological Health, to assist women in locating an FDA-certified mammography facility. This service is available on the National Cancer Institute's (1-800)4-Cancer line.

- Funded 26 agency research and education projects in support of women's health objectives, including: Gender differences in early and long-term coronary angioplasty with the Palmaz/ Schatz stent: Expands the New Approaches to Coronary Intervention (NACI) Registry of patients treated with the Palmaz/ Schatz stent to include more women. Introduction of Mucosal Immunity to Protect Females from HIV-1: Provides the basis for using a novel carrier in vaccines designed to protect women at risk for HIV-1.

- Noninvasive Assessment of Silicone Migration from Gel-filled Breast Implants: Use of a new magnetic resonance spectroscopy method to determine the mean levels of silicone in the livers of women with silicone gel-filled breast implants.

- Hormonal Regulation of Cytokine-Producing Cells in Women with Systemic Lupus Erythematosus: Examines changes in female sex hormone levels that occur during the menstrual cycle, pregnancy and menopause to see if there is any association with the activation state of cytokine-secreting cells.

- Women's Health Internet Initiative: Provides information about women's health issues on the Internet on food safety, nutrition and cosmetics.

- Minority Women Health Empowerment Workshops.

- Pilot Tracking System for Monitoring the Participation of Women in Clinical Trials

Industry and Small Business Liaison Staff

The Industry and Small Business Liaison Staff serves as the focal point for liaison and communication activities between FDA and more than 200 trade and professional organizations representing the industries FDA regulates. The staff works closely with other offices government-wide to ensure that the special needs of small manufacturers are met in all phases of the regulatory process.

The staff also advises and assists the commissioner, deputy commissioners, and other agency officials on industry-related issues that have an impact on agency policy, direction and goals.

The staff's responsibilities include the following outreach and educational activities to regulated industry, trade and professional organizations, and educational institutions:

- mailing agency information, including meeting announcements, press releases, rule-making notices, and backgrounders

- identifying and scheduling agency speakers for annual national and international meetings and educational seminars on FDA-related matters

- assisting organizations in planning educational seminars concerning FDA issues

- initiating, arranging and coordinating agency-sponsored informational meetings—including exchange meetings, grass-roots meetings, and others—on matters of concern to regulated industry

- monitoring the positions of regulated industry on agency proposals and priorities and communicating such positions to appropriate FDA officials.

Office of Management and Systems

Office of Management

The Office of Management advises and assists the deputy commissioner for management and systems in coordinating agency management and the use of agency resources in the following areas:

- human resources
- budget, finance and accounting
- facilities management, central services, and safety
- contracts, grants and procurement
- ethics, internal controls, and financial disclosure
- management studies, organization planning, and committee management.

Highlights of Recent Activity:

- Decentralized budget decisions allowing increased management participation in and awareness of cost/benefit implications, expedited allocation of agency resources, increased incentives to reduce costs, and increased flexibility for funding priority initiatives.

- Upgraded accounts payable system allowing agency to pay 93 percent of its most paid vendors by electronic funds transfer.

- Consolidated and streamlined accounting processes for the Office of Regulatory Affairs.

- Worked with the centers to inventory existing headquarters laboratory space, develop laboratory space use standards, and develop a plan for meeting laboratory space needs through the year 2000.

- Provided position descriptions, reorganization assistance, and classification guidelines to agency managers to improve supervisory ratio, elimination of organizational layers, and reductions in headquarters and senior level positions.

- Coordinated reinvention of Performance Management Program.

- Developed Flexible Workplace Arrangement Plan and Alternative Work Schedules Plan.

- In partnership with the Office of Regulatory Affairs, transferred the full personnel authority from the Department of Health and Human Services regional personnel offices to FDA.

- Assisted the Office of Government Ethics with the first nationwide live satellite broadcast of Annual Ethics Training, saving the agency significant travel costs.

- Improved the process for formulating the agency's Annual Assurance Statement in accordance with the Federal Managers' Financial Integrity Act.

- Moved ahead with acquisition of land and design and construction of laboratory and office facilities for FDA consolidation in Montgomery County, Md., the Center for Food Safety and Applied Nutrition laboratory and office complex and Center for Veterinary Medicine office building in Prince Georges County, Md., CVM laboratory in Laurel, Md., and Office of Regulatory Affairs laboratories in Cincinnati, New York, and Los Angeles.

Office of Planning and Evaluation

The Office of Planning and Evaluation implements the agency's responsibilities associated with the Government Performance and Results Act, the Regulatory Flexibility Act, and Executive Orders pertaining to economic analysis of regulatory policies and OMB/HHS directives regarding strategic management. These responsibilities include the following:

- Design and develop strategic plans, performance management systems, and operational plans.

- Analyze management performance trends, agency cost structure, and use of program resources.

- Oversee the Prescription Drug User Fee Act performance and use of resources.

- Analyze cost and benefits of major agency regulations.

- Provide assistance to agency components in change management, program reinvention, and managing-to-cost.

- Analyze changes in domestic health-care system and changes in international and trade issues that relate to FDA responsibilities.

Office of Information Resource Management

The Office of Information Resource Management develops and implements agency information resource management policy and procedures.

The office provides leadership in the area of information technology in support of agency objectives and assists the agency in meeting increasing demands for integrating and coordinating its information resources.

Highlights of Recent Activity:

- Administrative Systems Automation Project (ASAP)—an FDA initiative to improve the efficiency and effectiveness of FDA's administrative processes through re-engineering and automation.

- Standardized Nomenclature—initiative to standardize medical terminology within the agency for scientific information contained in industry submissions.

- Information Systems Architecture—development of a common information technology infrastructure throughout the agency.

- FDA Home Page on the World Wide Web.

- Video teleconferencing.

Office of Science

The Office of Science advises and assists the senior advisor for science, the commissioner, and other key officials on scientific issues that have an impact on policy, direction, and long-range goals of the agency. The office facilitates communication among scientists inside and outside FDA, and coordinates and provides guidance on special and overall science policy in program areas that cross major agency component lines. In addition, the office:

- works with other government agencies, industry, academia, consumer organizations, Congress, and international organizations on science policy

- serves as the focal point for overall management of scientific agency research, training, contracts, and fellowship activities

- provides leadership and direction on scientific technological achievement in FDA

- evaluates the adequacy of scientific resources available to the agency and initiates action to enhance those resources

- advises the Office of Management and Systems on scientific facilities, and participates with other agency components in planning such facilities

318

- provides leadership to agency components in identifying, recruiting and retaining top-level scientists

Office of Science Highlights 1995-1996

- In November of 1995, initiated development of an agency-wide scientific information system, first to be completed in September 1996.

- Sponsored a series of agency-wide workshops on the following science topics: Immunology: May 1995, Surveillance Systems and Strategies at FDA: January 1996, and Indirect Mechanisms of Carcinogenesis: March 1996.

- Sponsored the 1995 FDA Science Symposium "Developing Alternative In Vivo Methods for Assessing Carcinogenicity."

- Planned and coordinated three Science Board meetings: May and November 1995, March 1996

Office of Policy

The Office of Policy, established in 1991, oversees the coordination of broad policy objectives directed by FDA's commissioner, manages the agency's rule-making activities, and provides policy research support to resolve policy questions involving multiple centers, differing or overlapping statutory jurisdiction, or complex and emerging developments in new science or technology. The office also coordinates policies and programs relating to international harmonization and international standard setting. Recent initiatives this office coordinated in conjunction with program officials include:

- development of proposals to reduce the use of tobacco products by children

- development of proposals for a comprehensive new food safety assurance program for both domestically produced and imported foods, based on the principles of Hazard Analysis Critical Control Points

- development of a new program to increase the dissemination of useful information about prescription drug products to patients

- coordination and development of the agency's policies on legislative proposals to reform FDA

- development of the agency's policies with respect to the regulation of food additives

- development of a new program to improve the label on over-the-counter drugs

- implementation of the Mammography Quality Standards Act

- coordination of the agency's regulatory and legislative strategy for determining how dietary supplements should be regulated

- publication of 595 *Federal Register* documents totaling approximately 1,926 pages in FY 1995

- implementation of an agency-wide electronic tracking system for *Federal Register* documents.

Office of Orphan Products Development

The term "orphan products" refers to a product that treats a rare disease affecting fewer than 200,000 Americans. The Orphan Drug Act of 1983 was enacted to stimulate the development and approval of products to treat rare diseases. Since 1983, 119 orphan drug and biological products have been approved for marketing. These products help more than 2 million Americans and millions more worldwide. Also, more than 300 grants have been awarded. Eleven products supported by the orphan products grants program have been brought to market.

FDA's Office of Orphan Products Development promotes the development of safe and effective products for the diagnosis or treatment of rare diseases or conditions, and implements the provisions of the Orphan Drug Act by:

- managing a program providing seven years of orphan drug exclusivity to sponsors of approved orphan drugs

- reviewing and evaluating sponsors' requests for orphan drug designation

- managing an extramural grants program to support clinical studies

- coordinating protocol assistance to sponsors seeking information about requirements for new drug approval

- encouraging sponsors to allow treatment use of investigational orphan drugs.

Office of Regulatory Affairs

Overview

FDA is a scientifically based law enforcement agency. The enforcement function of FDA is twofold: to safeguard the public health and to ensure honesty and fair dealing between the regulated industry and consumers.

- FDA encourages and expects compliance with the laws and regulations it enforces. To this end, the agency participates in cooperative and educational efforts designed to inform industry, health professionals, and the public of those legal requirements.

- FDA surveys and inspects regulated industry to assess compliance and discover noncompliance. Depending upon the nature of noncompliance, FDA may afford an opportunity for correction by industry. If adequate correction does not occur within a reasonable period, FDA is committed to swiftly initiating action to obtain compliance. Legal remedies include injunction, seizure and prosecution.

- FDA does not tolerate fraud, intentional violations, or gross negligence, and promptly seeks prosecution to punish and deter whenever appropriate.

ORA Highlights

In late 1995, the Customer Service Planning Team began developing a survey to discover what the agency's customers want and expect. The survey results will help the agency design a strategic plan to address concerns while continuing to focus on protecting the public health.

Meetings with regulated industry were held throughout the country during 1995 to allow open communication between agency and industry representatives at the local level.

The Compliance Accomplishments Reporting System (CARS), implemented in early FY 1996, allows field employees to report into the Field Information System database activities that resulted in corrective action, such as reconditioning or destruction.

The Public Affairs Information Reporting System (PAIRS) now allows specialists in the field to transmit data on a regular basis via the computer. With instant access to the category "topics from callers," trends in consumer interests and concerns can be identified.

FDA Public Advisory Committees

FDA enlists the aid and expertise of outstanding scientists across the country to help the agency reach decisions, particularly concerning controversial issues or new and unusual products.

- **Office of the Commissioner:** National Task Force on AIDS Drug Development; Science Board to the FDA.

- **Center for Biologics Evaluation and Research:** Allergenic Products Advisory Committee; Biological Response Modifiers Advisory Committee; Blood Products Advisory Committee; Vaccines and Related Biological Products Advisory Committee.

- **Center for Drug Evaluation and Research:** Anesthetic and Life Support Drugs Advisory Committee; Anti-Infective Drugs Advisory Committee; Antiviral Drugs Advisory Committee; Arthritis Advisory Committee; Cardiovascular and Renal Drugs Advisory Committee; Dermatologic Drugs Advisory Committee; Drug Abuse Advisory Committee; Endocrinologic and Metabolic Drugs Advisory Committee; Fertility and Maternal Health Drugs Advisory Committee; Gastrointestinal Drugs Advisory Committee; Generic Drugs Advisory Committee Medical Imaging Drugs Advisory Committee; Nonprescription Drugs Advisory Committee; Oncologic Drugs Advisory Committee; Peripheral and Central Nervous System Drugs Advisory Committee; Psychopharmacologic Drugs Advisory Committee; Pulmonary-Allergy Drugs Advisory Committee.

- **Center for Food Safety and Applied Nutrition:** Food Advisory Committee

- **Center for Devices and Radiological Health:** Device Good Manufacturing Practice Advisory Committee; Medical Devices Advisory Committee; Anesthesiology and Respiratory Therapy Devices Panel; Circulatory System Devices Panel; Clinical Chemistry and Clinical Toxicology Devices Panel; Dental Products Panel; Ear, Nose, and Throat Devices Panel; Gastroenterology and Urology Devices Panel; General and Plastic Surgery Devices Panel; General Hospital and Personal Use Devices Panel; Hematology and Pathology Devices Panel; Immunology Devices Panel; Microbiology Devices Panel; Neurological Devices Panel; Obstetrics and Gynecology Devices Panel; Ophthalmic Devices Panel; Orthopedic and Rehabilitation Devices

Panel; Radiological Devices Panel; National Mammography Quality Assurance Advisory Committee; Technical Electronic Product Radiation Safety Standards Committee.

- **Center for Veterinary Medicine:** Veterinary Medicine Advisory Committee.

- **National Center for Toxicological Research:** Ranch Hand Advisory Committee; Science Advisory Board.

Congressional Committees with FDA-Related Responsibilities

Senate

- Committee on Appropriations, Subcommittee on Agriculture, Rural Development, and Related Agencies
- Committee on Labor and Human Resources
- Committee on Agriculture, Nutrition, and Forestry
- Committee on Governmental Affairs

House of Representatives

- Committee on Appropriations, Subcommittee on Agriculture, Rural Development, Food and Drug Administration, and Related Agencies
- Committee on Agriculture
- Committee on Energy and Commerce
- Committee on Government Operations
- Committee on Merchant Marine and Fisheries
- Committee on Science, Space and Technology
- Committee on Small Business

Other Federal Agencies with FDA-Related Duties

- **U.S. Department of Agriculture**: meat and poultry; animal vaccines; grain inspection.

- **Consumer Product Safety Commission:** consumer products such as household appliances (except those that emit radiation); baby furniture; toys; child-resistant packages.

- **Environmental Protection Agency:** pesticides (sets tolerance levels for residues on feed crops and raw and processed foods); municipal water supplies.

- **Bureau of Alcohol, Tobacco, and Firearms:** alcoholic beverages; tobacco.

- **Drug Enforcement Administration:** drugs of abuse.

- **Federal Trade Commission:** nonprescription drug and cosmetic advertising.

- **National Marine Fisheries Service:** voluntary seafood inspection program.

- **Occupational Safety and Health Administration:** workplace safety standards.

- **U.S. Customs Service:** imports.

- **Federal Bureau of Investigation:** federal Anti-Tampering Act.

- **Centers for Disease Control and Prevention:** epidemiology of diseases and other health problems.

- **Nuclear Regulatory Commission:** Licensing and regulation of the nuclear industry

Getting Information from FDA

Thousands of people call or write FDA each year wanting information on a gamut of FDA-regulated items, from aspirin, tongue depressors, and canned green beans to cancer drugs, heart pacemakers, hair dyes, and infant formula.

Those people include reporters, physicians, pharmacists, members of Congress, and consumers. The following offices, all located at agency headquarters in metropolitan Washington, D.C., provide information to these different groups of people:

Office of Health Affairs
Information for and from health professionals, including questions or concerns about advertising and promotion of FDA-regulated products; telephone (1-800) 23USFDA, or (301) 443-5470; fax (1-800) 344-3332, or (301) 443-2446. Answers questions from Institutional Review Boards; telephone (301) 443-1382, fax (301) 443-0232.

Office of Legislative Affairs

Answers questions from Congress and other elected officials; telephone (301) 443-3793, fax (301) 443-2567.

Press Office

Answers questions from reporters; print media, telephone (301) 443-3285, fax (301) 443-1388; broadcast media, telephone (301) 827-3434, fax (301) 443-8512.

Office of Consumer Affairs

Answers consumers' questions. Write to FDA, Consumer Inquiries Staff, Office of Consumer Affairs (HFE-88), Room 16-63. 5600 Fishers Lane, Rockville, MD 20857; telephone (301) 443-3170

Public Affairs Specialists

More than 40 public affairs specialists throughout the country respond to consumers' questions about the agency and what it regulates. FDA's responsibilities cover:

- food (except meat and poultry, which are regulated by the U.S. Department of Agriculture)
- prescription and nonprescription drugs
- cosmetics
- vaccines, donated blood, and blood products
- medical devices
- radiation-emitting products such as microwave ovens and sun lamps
- animal feed and drugs.

Public affairs specialists have publications, posters, teachers' kits, press releases, and background papers on all kinds of FDA-related topics. They are located in the following FDA offices:

Northeast Region

One Montvale Ave.
Stoneham, MA 02180
(617) 279-1675 (ext. 184)
fax (617) 279-1687

850 Third Ave.
Brooklyn, NY 11232
(718) 965-5300 (ext. 5043)
fax (718) 965-5117

599 Delaware Ave.
Buffalo, NY 14202
(716) 551-4461 (ext. 3118)
fax (716) 551-3813

Mid-Atlantic Region

Waterview Corporate Center
10 Waterview Blvd., 3rd Floor
Parsippany, NJ 07054
(201) 331-2926
fax(201) 331-2969

2nd and Chestnut Streets
Room 900, U.S. Customhouse
Philadelphia, PA 19106
(215) 597-4390 (ext. 4202)
fax (215) 597-6649

900 Madison Ave.
Baltimore, MD 21201
(410) 962-3731
fax (410) 962-2307

Resident Inspection Post
3820 Center Road
P.O. Box 838
Brunswick, OH 44212
(330) 273-1038 (ext. 114)
fax (330) 225-7477

Southeast Region

Puerta de Tierra Station
466 Fernandez Juncos Ave.
San Juan, PR 00906-3223
(809) 729-6852
fax (809) 729-6847

60-8th St. N.E.
Atlanta, GA 30309
(404) 347-7355
fax (404) 347-1912

7200 Lake Ellenor Dr.
Suite 120
Orlando, FL 32809
(407) 648-6922 (ext. 202)
fax (407) 648-6881
6601 N.W. 25th St.

P.O. Box 59-2256
Miami, FL 33159-2256
(305) 526-2800
fax (305) 526-2693

297 Plus Park Blvd.
Nashville, TN 37217
(615) 781-5372
fax (615) 781-5383

4298 Elysian Fields Ave.
New Orleans, LA 70122
(504) 589-2420 (ext. 121)
fax (504) 589-6360

Midwest Region

300 S. Riverside Plaza
Suite 550 - South
Chicago, IL 60606
(312) 353-5863 (ext. 188)
fax (312) 886-3280

1560 East Jefferson Ave.
Detroit, MI 48207
(313) 226-6260 (ext. 149)
fax (313) 226-3076

Resident Inspection Post
101 W. Ohio St., Suite 1300
Indianapolis, IN 46204
(317) 226-6500 (ext. 13)
fax (317) 226-6506

240 Hennepin Ave.
Minneapolis, MN 55401
(612) 334-4100 (ext. 129)
fax (612) 334-4134

2675 North Mayfair Road
Suite 200
Milwaukee, WI 53226-1305
414) 771-7167
fax (414) 771-7512

Southwest Region

3310 Live Oak St.
Dallas, TX 75204
(214) 655-5315 (ext. 303)
fax (214) 655-5331

Resident Inspection Post
1445 N. Loop West
Suite 420
Houston, TX 77008
(713) 802-9095 (ext. 15)
fax (713) 802-0906

Resident Inspection Post
10127 Morocco
Suite 119
San Antonio, TX 78216
(210) 229-4531
fax (210) 229-4548

11630 West 80th St.
Lenexa, KS 66214
(913) 752-2120
fax (913) 752-2111

12 Sunnen Dr.
Suite 122
St. Louis, MO 63143
(314) 645-1167 (ext. 23)
fax (314) 645-2969

Denver Federal Center
Building 20, Room B-1121
6th Ave. and Kipling
Denver, CO 80225-0087
(303) 236-3018
fax (303) 236-3551

Pacific Region

1431 Harbor Bay Parkway	22201 23rd Dr. S.E.
Alameda, CA 94502-7070	Bothell, WA 98201-4421
(510) 337-6736	(206) 483-4953
fax (510) 337-6708	fax (206) 483-4996
19900 MacArthur Blvd.	Resident Inspection Post
Suite 300	9780 S.W. Nimbus Ave.
Irvine, CA 92715-2445	Beaverton, OR 97008-7163
(714) 798-7607	(503) 671-9332 (ext. 22)
fax (714) 798-7715	fax (503) 671-9445

Resident Inspection Post
4615 East Elwood St.
Suite 200
Phoenix, AZ 85040
(602) 379-4595 (ext. 225)
fax (602) 379-4646

Other Sources of Information about FDA

Toll-Free Numbers

* **Advisory Committee Information Hotline**—Provides current information on FDA advisory committee meetings. Call (1-800)-741-8138.

* **FDA Medical Advertising Line**—To report fraudulent or misleading advertising and promotion of FDA-regulated products. Call (1-800) 238-7332.

* **Vaccine Adverse Event Reporting System**—To report any unusual or unexpected adverse reactions associated with the administration of vaccines. Call (1-800) 822-7967.

* **Mammography Information Service**—To find a mammography facility near you that's certified by FDA. Available weekdays from 9 a.m. to 4:30 p.m. local time. Call (1-800) 422-6237; TTY (1-800) 332-8615.

* **Consumer Product Complaint Lines**—For residents in the specified areas to report problems and complaints about FDA-regulated products. In Kentucky and Ohio, call (1-800)

437-2382. In Massachusetts, Maine, Connecticut, Vermont, Rhode Island, and New Hampshire, call (1-800) 891-8295.

- **FDA's Breast Implant Information Line**—Provides up-to-date information on breast implant studies and regulatory status. Call (1-800) 532-4440; TTY (1-800) 688-6167.

- **FDA's Seafood Hotline**—Provides information on seafood safety. Public affairs specialists answer questions from noon to 4 p.m. Eastern time, Monday through Friday. At other times callers can listen to a recording on current seafood topics and leave messages to receive educational material or to report suspected seafood safety, labeling, or economic fraud problems. Call (1-800) 332-4010; (202) 205-4314 in the Washington, D.C., area.

- **AIDS Clinical Trials Information Service (ACTIS)**—Provides information about AIDS and HIV-related trials currently under way throughout the United States. ACTIS is a joint project of the Centers for Disease Control and Prevention, the National Institute of Allergy and Infectious Diseases, the National Library of Medicine, and FDA. Call (1-800) TRIALS-A between 9 a.m. and 7 p.m. Eastern time, Monday through Friday.

- **Center for Biologics Evaluation and Research Voice Information Service**—To request documents by fax or mail or to speak with knowledgeable staff, Call (1-800) 835-4709.

- **Center for Drug Evaluation and Research FAX-on-Demand**—Call (1-800) 342-2722 or (301) 827-0577.

- **MEDWATCH**—Call (1-800) 332-1088 to report adverse events, request forms, or request a copy of the FDA Desk Guide to Adverse Event and Product Problem Reporting. Modem number (1-800) 332-7737; fax (1-800) 332-0178.

Electronic Information

- **FDA on the Internet**—The FDA Internet Home Page provides up-to-date, authoritative information on food, cosmetics, human and animal drugs, biologics, medical devices, and more.

To access the FDA Home Page, use this URL (uniform resource locator): http://www.fda.gov/. From there, you can easily locate consumer education materials, press releases, industry guidance, bulletins for health professionals, and a wealth of other useful documents and data from FDA's centers and offices.

FDA's Internet site replaces the agency's electronic bulletin board, which had provided on-line information for more than a decade. The Internet site offers far more material, in a more user-friendly form, including easy-to-use full-text searches and links to other FDA documents and other government Internet sites.

You do not need an Internet connection to reach the FDA home page; you can use the same free dial-up connection that used to connect you to the FDA bulletin board:

- If Rockville, Md., is a local call, use 227-6849 or 227-6857.
- If you have FTS2000 access, use (301) 227-6849 or (301) 227-6857.
- If Rockville, Md., is not a local call and you don't have FTS2000 access, use (800) 222-0185.
- Set your terminal emulation software to: Terminal type: vtl00, vt200 - 7bit, or vt320; Characters: 8; Stop bits: 1; Parity: none; At the login prompt, type bbs. If you experience a problem, please call (301) 443-4908.

- **FDA's CD-ROM**—This subscription service is updated quarterly. Documents currently available include:

  - Center for Drug Evaluation and Research GMPs and NDA Guidelines
  - Center for Veterinary Medicine policy and procedures
  - Chemistry Review
  - Code of Federal Regulations (Title 21)
  - Compliance Policy Guides
  - Drug Study/Health Fraud Bulletins
  - FDA Import Alert Retrieval System
  - FDA Phone Book
  - Food, Drug, and Cosmetic Act and Related Laws
  - Operations Manual
  - Market Names of Fish
  - Medical Products Quality Manual
  - Preamble Medical Devices Reporting Regulations
  - Regulatory Procedures Manual, Chapters 5 and 8
  - Talk Papers/Press Releases

For more information, call FDA's Office of Information Resource Management at (301) 443-6770.

- **Periodicals**

FDA Consumer—The official magazine of FDA. Ten issues a year, each containing in-depth feature articles written for the general public on FDA-related health issues. Also includes reports from FDA's own investigators that go behind the scenes to show how the agency protects the public from unsafe or worthless products. Subscriptions available for $15 per year from the Superintendent of Documents, Government Printing Office, Washington, DC 20402-9371.

FDA Medical Bulletin—Information about FDA-related issues and activities of particular interest to health professionals. Sent to more than a million doctors and other health professionals approximately three times a year. Send requests to be placed on the mailing list to: FDA Medical Bulletin Circulation Dept. (HFI-43) 5600 Fishers Lane Rockville, MD 20857

FDA Enforcement Report—Weekly update on actions taken in connection with agency regulatory activities, including seizures, injunctions, prosecutions, and dispositions. Recalls and medical device safety alerts voluntarily conducted by firms are also included. Subscriptions are available for $78 per year from the Superintendent of Documents, Government Printing Office, Washington, DC 20402-9371.

FDA Veterinarian—Published bimonthly, this FDA publication covers current issues concerning animal drugs, food additives, and devices. Subscriptions are available for $8.50 per year from the Superintendent of Documents, Government Printing Office, Washington, DC 20402-9371.

Publications

Approved Drug Products with Therapeutic Equivalence Evaluations—Commonly called the "Orange Book," the publication is available for $55 a year from the Superintendent of Documents, Government Printing Office, Washington, DC 20402-9371. A subscription includes periodic updates of the drug listings.

Mammography Matters—A quarterly publication to help mammography facilities comply with the Mammography Quality Standards Act of 1992. Distributed to mammography facilities and other interested organizations and individuals. For information write: Editor, *Mammography Matters*, FDA (HFZ-240), Rockville, MD 20857.

User Facility Reporting Bulletin—A quarterly bulletin to assist hospitals, nursing homes, and other medical device user facilities in complying with their statutory reporting requirements under the Safe Medical Devices Act. The publication's content may be freely reproduced. For information, write: Editor, *User Facility Reporting Bulletin*, FDA (HFZ-230), Rockville, MD 20857.

Agency Files

Facts-on-Demand System-Provides companies access to the latest guidance documents on medical devices from FDA's Center for Devices and Radiological Health. Call (800) 899-0381 any time from a touch-tone phone and follow the system prompts. Up to three documents may be requested for transmission by fax. An index is available on Facts-on-Demand (document #919).

Notice of Status for Premarket Notification [510(k)] Submissions— Provides manufacturers with the status of their premarket notification submissions. After 90 days from day of receipt, a sponsor may request the status of its submission by fax on (301) 443-8818 or mail to Status Coordination, DSMA (HFZ-220), FDA, 5600 Fishers Lane, Rockville, MD 20857, USA. The status request form (document #858), which shows the required information, may be requested by phone, mail, fax, or Facts-on-Demand. An answer should be returned within three working days. Because of resource limitations, manufacturers should wait at least four weeks between requests.

Chapter 23

Food and Drug Administration Action Guide

The Federal Register: What It Is and How to Use It

The *Federal Register* is one of the most important sources for information on what FDA—or for that matter, what any government agency is doing. Published daily, Monday through Friday, the *Federal Register* carries all proposed and finalized regulations and many significant legal notices issued by the various agencies, as well as presidential proclamations and executive orders.

Subscriptions to the *Federal Register* can be purchased from the Superintendent of Documents. For price and order information, call (202) 512-1806 or (202) 512-1530 for online subscriptions. As an alternative, copies can usually be found in local libraries, county courthouses, or federal buildings.

The following are examples of how the *Federal Register* can be used to keep informed of FDA issues and activities:

- **Advance Notice**—Often, FDA will publish "Notices of Intent" in the *Federal Register* to give you the earliest possible opportunity to participate in its decisions. These notices inform you that FDA is considering an issue and that your views are welcome before a formal proposal is made.

- **Proposed Regulations**—When a formal proposal is developed, FDA publishes a "Notice of Proposed Rulemaking" in the *Federal*

DHHS Publication No. (FDA) 96-1092, Spring 1996.

Register. The notice also informs you how much time you have to submit written comments about the proposed action. If you do not feel you have enough time to study the proposal and comment on it, you can request, in writing, that Agency officials extend the comment period. If FDA extends the period, a notice of the extension will be published in the *Federal Register*. Occasionally, a second or third proposal is published in the *Federal Register* because of the nature of the comments received. Each time a proposal is substantively revised or amended, a notice is published in the *Federal Register*.

- **Final Regulations**—Ultimately, a "Final Rule" is published, and the rule specifies the date when the new regulatory requirements or regulations become effective.

- **Regulatory Agenda**—Twice a year—in April and October—FDA, along with the entire Department of Health and Human Services, publishes an agenda in the *Federal Register* that summarizes policy-significant regulations, regulations that are likely to have a significant economic impact on small entities, and other actions under development. This agenda will help you identify actions of interest early to plan your participation. Each item listed includes the name, address and telephone number of an Agency official to contact if you need more information.

- **Meetings and Hearings**—Notices are published in the *Federal Register* announcing all meetings of the Agency's advisory committees and all public meetings that provide an information exchange between FDA and industry, health professionals, consumers, and the scientific and medical communities. The notice contains the date, time and place of the meeting, as well as its agenda. The *Federal Register* also announces administrative hearings before the Agency and public hearings to gain citizen input into Agency activities. Information about meetings of advisory committees is also available by calling (1-800) 741-8138.

How to Comment on Proposed Regulations

Before you comment on regulations proposed by FDA, you may obtain more information about a proposal by contacting the person designated in the *Federal Register* statement. Whether you agree or disagree with the proposed regulations, you will want to communicate your comments in the most effective way possible. The following points will help you do this:

- Give the title, date of publication, and docket number for the proposal.

- State who you are and how the proposal affects you. (Economic costs and back-up data are more compelling than generalities.)

- Give supporting statements for your position and present new data and scientific findings, if possible.

- Whether you agree or disagree, you may suggest alternatives to the proposal or to requirements that are part of the proposal.

- The more substantive your comments, the more weight they will carry. The same thing is true for petitions. When FDA considers comments from the public, it's not a simple matter of counting up "for" or "against" options.

Comments on proposed regulations should always be forwarded to the Dockets Management Branch (HFA-306), Food and Drug Administration, Room 1-46 Park Building, 12420 Parklawn Drive, Rockville, MD 20857.

How to Obtain Agency Documents

FDA's policy is to make the fullest possible disclosure of records to the public, provided that disclosure is consistent with the rights of individuals to privacy and property (e.g., trade secret and confidential commercial information). When releasing records, the Agency must also consider the need to pursue internal policy deliberations and regulatory activities without disruption.

Under the Freedom of Information Act (FOIA), FDA is required to make available to the public all documents in its possession, with the possible exception of the following:

- documents relating solely to internal personnel rules and practices

- trade secrets and confidential commercial or financial information

- certain interagency and intraagency memoranda containing opinions and recommendations prepared to assist in Agency decision-making

335

- personnel, medical, and similar files, the disclosure of which would be a clearly unwarranted invasion of personal privacy

- investigatory records compiled for enforcement purposes when disclosure would interfere with enforcement procedures

FDA regulations specifically exempt from disclosure the following categories of information: most safety and efficacy data; manufacturing methods; production, sales or distribution data; quantitative or semiquantitative formulas; and data on design or construction of products. Address all requests for FDA records to the following:

Food and Drug Administration Freedom of Information Staff
(HFI-35) Room 12A-16 5600 Fishers Lane
Rockville, MD 20857
Phone: (301) 443-6310.
Fax: (301) 443-1726
Fax Operator (301) 443-2706

In your request, describe the information needed as accurately and fully as possible, so that it can be easily located. You need not explain why you are requesting the information.

When requesting information from FDA, keep in mind these points:

- Within 10 working days after receipt of an FOIA request, FDA must determine whether to comply with such a request. The Agency may grant itself a 10-day extension in "unusual circumstances." The Agency is required to give written notice of such an extension.

- FDA charges uniform fees for searches and copying. By law, these fees may not exceed the actual costs. FDA may waive these fees if disclosure of the information will primarily serve the general public, and not benefit an individual or business. Your letter must specifically request such a waiver and say why you believe you are entitled to it.

- If FDA denies your request for records (less than two percent of requests are denied), it must tell you the specific reason(s) for the denial and advise you of your right to appeal. Names and addresses of those responsible for the denial must be disclosed to you.

- If you receive a denial letter, you may send a letter of appeal to the Assistant Secretary for Health, Department of Health and

Human Services. File your appeal within 30 days after notification of the denial. Send the appeal letter by certified mail, return receipt requested to have proof of the timeliness of your appeal.

- The Assistant Secretary for Health has 20 working days after receipt to respond. If FDA did not take a 10-day extension the first time, the Department may do so now. Should your appeal be denied, you are entitled to judicial review.

The Freedom of Information Act pertains only to existing records. It is not a research service to compile information that cannot be readily identified. A request for specific information that is releasable to the public can be processed much more expeditiously than a request for "all information" on a particular subject. This is because "all information" may include information exempt from public disclosure, such as trade secrets, commercial or confidential information, that is not releasable and would, therefore, be subject to a denial. A full discussion of FDA's FOIA policies and procedures can be found in 21 CFR, Part 20.1-20.119.

There are a wide variety of documents that would be very helpful to you, such as FDA's Regulatory Procedures Manual or Compliance Policy Guides. If you would like a list of the available documents, write to the FOI staff listed above.

There are many FDA pamphlets and informational materials that are available without going through an FOIA request. They may be obtained by contacting an FDA Small Business Representative (SBR) or a Center small business contact person.

How to Obtain FDA Statutes and Regulations

Among the statutes enforced by FDA are: the Federal Food, Drug, and Cosmetic Act, as Amended; sections of the Public Health Service Act pertaining to biological products; the Radiation Control for Health and Education Act; the Safe Medical Devices Act; the Mammography Quality Standards Act; the Fair Packaging and Labeling Act; the Infant Formula Act; the Nutrition Labeling and Education Act; and the Dietary Supplement Health and Education Act. These are compiled in one booklet, "Federal Food, Drug, and Cosmetic Act as Amended and Related Laws," which is available from the Superintendent of Documents.

The regulations over which FDA has jurisdiction are codified under Title 21, Code of Federal Regulations (CFR). These are updated on April 1 of each year and are available for sale approximately four months later. Nine volumes are applicable to FDA and may be purchased singly or as a set from the Superintendent of Documents. The contents of each volume are listed below:

- Parts 1 to 99. General regulations for the enforcement of the Federal Food, Drug, and Cosmetic Act and the Fair Packaging and Labeling Act. Color additives.

- Parts 100 to 169. Food standards, good manufacturing practice for foods, low-acid canned foods, acidified foods, and food labeling.

- Parts 170 to 199. Food additives.

- Parts 200 to 299. General regulations for drugs.

- Parts 300 to 499. Drugs for human use.

- Parts 500 to 599. Animal drugs, feeds, and related products.

- Parts 600 to 799. Biologics and cosmetics.

- Parts 800 to 1299. Medical devices and radiological health. Regulations under the Federal Import Milk Act, the Federal Tea Importation Act, the Federal Caustic Poison Act, and for control of communicable diseases and interstate conveyance sanitation.

- Parts 1300 through end. Drug Enforcement Administration regulations and requirements.

Requirements of Laws and Regulations Enforced by the U.S. Food and Drug Administration

Requirements of Laws and Regulations Enforced by the U.S. Food and Drug Administration is an easy-to-read booklet summarizing FDA requirements. Single copies are available at no charge by writing to: Office of Consumer Affairs (HFE-88), Food and Drug Administration, 5600 Fishers Lane, Rockville. MD 20857.

How to Petition the FDA

Anyone may request or petition FDA to change or create an Agency policy or regulation under 21 CFR Part 10.30. If you believe this type of action is necessary, direct your request to FDA's Dockets Management Branch. When submitting a petition, keep these points in mind:

- Clearly state what problem you think the Agency needs to address.

- Propose specifically what the Agency's action should be. Your proposal should be based on sound, supportable facts.

- Submit the petition, an original and three copies, unless otherwise stipulated in the *Federal Register* announcement, to the Food and Drug Administration, Dockets Management Branch (HFA-305), Room 1-46 Park Building, 12420 Parklawn Drive, Rockville, MD 20857.

FDA carefully considers every petition and must respond within 180 days by either approving or denying it, or providing a tentative response indicating why FDA has been unable to reach a decision. If FDA approves the petition, it may be published in the *Federal Register*. Your petition could eventually be incorporated into Agency policy. An example showing how to prepare a citizen's petition follows.

Petition Content and Format
(Date)

Dockets Management Branch, Food and Drug Administration, Department of Health and Human Services, Room 1-46 Park Building, 12420 Parklawn Drive, Rockville, MD 20857.

Citizen Petition

The undersigned submits this petition under (relevant statutory sections, if known) of the Federal Food, Drug, and Cosmetic Act, the Public Health Service Act, or any other statutory provision for which authority has been delegated to the Commissioner of Food and Drugs (under 21 CFR, Part 5.10) to request the Commissioner of Food and Drugs to (issue, amend, or revoke a regulation or order to take or refrain from taking any other form of administrative action.

A. **Action Requested**

1. If the petition requests the Commissioner to issue, amend or revoke a regulation, give the exact wording of the existing regulation (if any) and the proposed regulation or amendment requested.

2. If the petition requests the Commissioner to issue, amend or revoke an order, include a copy of the exact wording of the citation

to the existing order (if any) and the exact wording requested for the proposed order.

3. If the petition requests the Commissioner to take or refrain from taking any other form of administrative action, state the specific action or relief requested.

B. **Statement of Grounds.** Include a well organized statement of the factual and legal grounds upon which the petition is based. Opposing views known to the petitioner should be presented.

C. **Environmental Impact Statement.** Give an environmental impact analysis report in the form specified in 21 CFR, Part 25.1(g), except for the types of actions specified in 21 CFR, Part 25.1(d).

D. **Economic Impact Statement.** The following information is to be submitted only when requested by the Commissioner following review of the petition: a statement of the effect of the requested action on 1) cost (and price) increases to industry, government, and consumers; 2) productivity of wage earners, businesses, or government; 3) competition; 4) supplies of important materials, products, or services; 5) employment; and 6) energy supply or demand. The undersigned certifies that, to the best of his/her knowledge and belief, this petition includes all information and views on which the petition relies, and that it includes representative data and information known to the petitioner which are unfavorable to the petition.

(Signature) Name of Petitioner

(Mailing Address)

(Phone)

How to Participate in Agency Decision-Making

In addition to commenting on *Federal Register* documents and petitioning the Agency, there are a number of ways that can interact with FDA to make your viewpoint known. Here are a few examples:

Public Meetings or Conferences

FDA uses public meetings and conferences to discuss significant issues with the public. The Agency may schedule public meetings, sometimes referred to as "exchange meetings," before developing a proposal, or after proposing a program change. The meetings offer a chance for you and FDA managers to discuss issues informally before the rulemaking process begins. FDA announces meetings in the *Federal Register* and trade publications.

Industry Information/Education Meetings

Many meetings and workshops are conducted in which key representatives from industry, government, academia, and professional, consumer, ethnic, and patient groups discuss subjects of vital concern to industry and the FDA.

Public Hearings

A hearing is an opportunity for you to take part in a rulemaking proceeding. FDA always announces hearings in the *Federal Register* and usually in other publications (e.g., industry newsletters) related to the topic of the hearing. Depending on the subject of the hearing, you can testify on specific issues that are included in an Agency proposal, or you can present your views about general issues on Agency programs. At all hearings, your testimony, whether it is presented orally or in writing, will become part of an official record of evidence which will help the Agency make policy decisions.

Public Advisory Committees and Panels

FDA routinely looks for qualified people to serve on a variety of public advisory committees and panels. Many of the Agency's committees and panels include two non-voting members representing consumer and industry interests. FDA requests nominations for these members through announcements in the *Federal Register*. The committees generally study current scientific work and make recommendations to the Agency on product approvals, regulations, and other actions. Membership on most committees requires a scientific background. A free copy of "FDA Public Advisory Groups," or further information about FDA advisory committees, can be obtained by contacting the Office of Committee Management (HFA-306), Food and Drug Administration, Room 310 Park Building, 12420 Parklawn Drive, Rockville, MD 20857; (301)443-2765 or fax (301) 443-8811. For current information or information updates on FDA advisory committee meetings, call the hotline by dialing (1-800) 741-8138 or (301) 443-0572, and the five digit number assigned to each advisory committee. This number will appear in each notice of meeting.

What to do When Marketing a New Product

FDA must give the manufacturer, distributor or importer permission to market certain products before they can be sold in interstate commerce. For example:

- New human and veterinary drugs and certain medical devices must be approved for safety and effectiveness, and their labeling reviewed for accuracy and thoroughness.

- Substances added to food must meet the requirements of the food additive regulations that are based on FDA's review of scientific data of safety and utility that have been submitted to FDA.

- Manufacturers of low-acid canned foods packaged in airtight bottles, plastic bags, and cans and acidified foods must register with FDA and submit detailed information about heat-treatments to destroy bacteria (and acidification, if necessary to prevent growth of bacterial spores).

- Specific premarket controls apply to biological products which have been required to be licensed under Federal law.

Marketing these kinds of products or conducting experimental investigations with them in human clinical trials, requires that one or more applications be filed with FDA and that certain procedures be followed.

In addition, although some products, such as cosmetics and some radiation-emitting items, do not need premarket approval from FDA, there are regulatory standards and regulations applicable to their manufacture and labeling that fall under FDA's jurisdiction. Therefore, to avoid unnecessary delay in bringing new products to market, it would be helpful to talk with an FDA product specialist early in your planning.

Contact Information

FDA, Northeast Region
Small Business Representative (HFR-NE17)
850 Third Ave.
Brooklyn NY 11232
Telephone: (718) 965-5300 ext. 5528
Fax: (718) 965-5759

FDA, Mid-Atlantic Region
Small Business Representative (HFR-MA17)
900 U.S. Customhouse
2nd & Chestnut St.
Philadelphia, PA 19106
Telephone: (215) 597-0537
Fax: (215) 597-6649

FDA, Southeast Region
Small Business Representative (HFR-SE17)
60 Eight St. NE
Atlanta, GA 30309
Telephone:(404) 347-4001 Ext. 5256
Fax: (404) 347-4349

FDA, Midwest Region
Small Business Representative, (HFR-MW17)
20 N. Michigan Ave., Rm. 510
Chicago, IL 60602
Telephone: (312) 353-9400 ext. 23
Fax: (312) 886-1682

FDA, Southwest Region
Small Business Representative, (HFR-SW17)
7920 Elmbrook Dr., Suite 102
Dallas, TX 75247-4982
Telephone: (214) 655-8100 ext. 128
Fax: (214) 655-8130

FDA, Pacific Region
Small Business Representative, (HFR-PA17)
Oakland Federal Building
1301 Clay Street, Suite 1180-N
Oakland, CA 94612-5217
Telephone: (510) 637-3980
Fax: (510) 637-3977

Frequently Called Numbers

Office Of External Affairs-Consumer Inquiries (301) 443-3170;
Industry and Small Business Liaison Team (301) 827-3430

343

Fax on Demand under:

Center for Biologics Evaluation and Research—FLASH-FAX (Documents via fax) (301) 827-3844 or connect to the fax system toll free at (1-800) 835-4709

Center for Devices and Radiological Health—Division of Small Manufacturers Assistance (301) 443-6597 OR toll free (1-800) 638-2041; CDRH Facts-On-Demand (Documents via fax) (1-800) 899-0381; Electronic Docket (Documents via computer modem)(1-800) 252-1366

Center For Drug Evaluation And Research—Office of Training and Communication (301) 594-1012 or Fax (301) 594-3302; Fax-on-Demand (Documents via fax) (1-800) 342-2722 or (301) 827-0577

Center for Food Safety and Applied Nutrition—Seafood hotline (1-800) FDA-4010 or (202) 205-4314

National Institutes of Health—Small Business Institutes Program (301) 599-7248 (For information about grants involving FDA regulated products)

Superintendent of Documents—Mail to: New Orders, Superintendent of Documents, P.O. Box 371954, Pittsburgh, PA 15250-7954, Telephone: (202) 512-1806, for on-line subscriptions (202) 512-1530

Access Information from the Internet—World Wide Web (WWW) FDA Home Page can be reached at the Uniform Resource Locator: http://www.fda.gov/fdahomepage.html (with hypertext links to information about various FDA responsibilities: foods, human drugs, animal drugs, biologics, cosmetics, medical devices and radiological health, toxicology, and FDA news). FDA is placing the documents that the public most frequently requests on the WWW site to give users more immediate access.

Chapter 24

Making Your Voice Heard at the Food and Drug Administration

As a regulatory agency, FDA publishes rules that establish or modify the way it regulates foods, drugs, biologics, cosmetics, radiation-emitting electronic products, and medical devices—commodities close to the daily lives of all Americans. FDA rules have considerable impact on the nation's health, industries and economy. These rules are not created arbitrarily or in a vacuum. They are formed with the public's help.

By law, anyone can participate in the rule-making process by commenting in writing on rules FDA proposes. FDA allows plenty of time for public input and carefully considers these comments when it draws up a final rule. FDA gathers public comments mainly through two channels: proposed rules and petitions.

Proposed Rules

When FDA plans to issue a new regulation or revise an existing one, it places an announcement in the *Federal Register* on the day the public comment period begins. Published every weekday, the *Federal Register* is available at many public libraries and colleges, and even on the Internet.

Issues open to public comment often are reported by the news media and may frequently be found on FDA's Internet home page.

In the *Federal Register*, the "notice of proposed rulemaking" describes the planned regulation and provides background on the issue.

FDA Backgrounder, January 19, 1996.

345

It also gives the address for submitting written comments and the name of the person to contact for more information. Also noted is the "comment period," which specifies how long the agency will accept public comments. Usually, the file—or docket— stays open for comments at least 60 days, though some comment periods have been as short as 10 days or as long as nine months. Weekends and holidays are included in the comment period.

There is no special form to fill out for comments, nor do submitters have to follow a certain style. But FDA can process comments more effectively if they are presented—either written legibly or typed—on 8-1/2-inch by 11-inch paper.

Here are some other suggestions for making sure your comment has the greatest possible impact:

- Clearly indicate if you are for or against the proposed rule or some part of it and why. FDA regulatory decisions are based largely on law and science, and agency reviewers look for reasoning, logic, and good science in comments they evaluate.

- Refer to the docket number, listed in *Federal Register* notice.

- Include a copy of articles or other references that support your comments. Only relevant material should be submitted.

- If an article or reference is in a foreign language, it must be accompanied by an English translation verified to be accurate. Translations should be accompanied by a copy of the original publication.

- To protect privacy when submitting medical information, delete names or other information that would identify patients.

- Threats, obscenities, profanities, or material defamatory to FDA or the federal government may be rejected or referred to law enforcement officials.

- Comments must be postmarked or delivered in person by the last day of the comment period.

When FDA receives a comment, it is logged in, numbered, and placed in a file for that docket. It then becomes a public record and is available for anyone to examine in FDA's reading room (Room 123, 12420 Parklawn Drive, Rockville, Md.). Under the Freedom of Information Act (FOIA), visitors to the reading room can receive free copies of comments up to 50 pages if their request is for noncommercial use. After that, each page costs 10 cents. People also can send FDA an FOIA request and have copies of comments mailed to them.

Petitions

Another way to influence the way FDA does business is to petition the agency to issue, change or cancel a regulation, or to take other action. The agency receives about 200 petitions yearly.

Petitions require careful preparation by the submitter. FDA spends considerable time and staff resources processing petitions. Individuals sometimes submit petitions, but most come from regulated industry or consumer groups. For example, a drug company might request a change in labeling for one of its products; a food company might ask that its product be exempted from some provision of a regulation; or a consumer group might petition FDA to tighten regulation of a certain product.

Petitions submitted to FDA must contain:

- **Action requested**—What rule, order, or other administrative action does the petitioner want FDA to issue, amend or revoke?

- **Statement of grounds**—The factual and legal grounds for the petition, including all supporting material, as well as information known to the petitioner that may be unfavorable to the petitioner's position.

- **Certification**—A statement that to the best of the petitioner's knowledge, the petition includes all information relevant to the petition, favorable or not. The petition must be signed and include the petitioner's address and phone number.

In addition, some petitions may require information on:

- **Environmental impact**—This information is generally required if the petition requests approval of food or color additives, drugs, biological products, animal drugs, or certain medical devices, or for a food to be categorized as GRAS (generally recognized as safe). Procedures for preparing environmental impact statements can be found in Title 21 of the Code of Federal Regulations, Sections 25.24 and 25.31. If an environmental impact statement is not required, petitions should include a statement to that effect.

- **Economic impact**—This information is required only if FDA requests it after review of the petition.

Petitions should be mailed or delivered to:

Dockets Management Branch
Food and Drug Administration
12420 Parklawn Drive, Room 1-23
Rockville, MD 20857

Ultimately, FDA management decides whether to grant a petition. But first, agency staffers evaluate it, a process that may take several weeks to more than a year, depending on the issue's complexity. After FDA grants or denies the petition, the agency will notify the petitioner directly. If not satisfied, the petitioner can take the matter to court.

For more information on submitting petitions, consult Title 21 of the Code of Federal Regulations, Sections 10.30, 10.33, and 10.35.

Besides accepting public comments and petitions, FDA also schedules public meetings and hearings to discuss and explain its proposals. These usually are held with industry representatives or consumer groups, but anyone interested may attend and, with advance notice, may comment on a proposal. Meetings often are held in the Washington, D.C., area, but sometimes are set in other areas across the country. Meetings for the public to present views are announced in the *Federal Register*.

Questions about the comment, petition or hearing process should go to the FDA Dockets Management Branch, (301) 443-7542. Hours are 9 a.m. to 4 p.m., Eastern time, Monday through Friday.

Filing a Freedom of Information Request

Copies of comments on any given issue may be obtained through a Freedom of Information Act (FOIA) request to FDA. The request is best made by letter, specifying exactly what material is sought. Requesters usually should be specific about what comments they want, instead of asking for "all comments" received on a certain proposal, which in some cases can run thousands of pages. (Indexes of comments are available by FOIA request as well.)

FOIA requests should include an address and phone number and be sent to:

Food and Drug Administration
Freedom of Information Staff (HFI-35)
5600 Fishers Lane
Rockville, MD 20857

Requests also can be faxed to (301) 443-1726. For more information, call (301) 443-6310.

Chapter 25

Reporting Problem Products to the Food and Drug Administration

Have you had a problem with a food, drug, cosmetic, medical device, radiation-emitting electronic product, or veterinary drug? Did it cause you an injury or was it unsanitary or improperly labeled? Perform a public service and report the problem to the Food and Drug Administration.

FDA welcomes reports from the public alerting it to problems with products that it regulates. The reports help FDA ensure that products on the market are safe, effective, and properly manufactured, stored and labeled.

Each report is evaluated to determine how serious the problem is and what follow-up is needed. Depending on the seriousness of the problem, FDA will either investigate it immediately or during the next inspection of the facility responsible for the product.

What to Report

Before you report a product that you suspect caused an illness or injury, ask yourself the following:

- Did you use the product for other than its intended use?
- Did you fail to follow carefully the instructions for the product?
- Was the product old or outdated?
- Do you have an allergy or other medical condition that might have something to do with the suspected harmful effect?

FDA Backgrounder, November 1991, updated October 16, 1996.

If you answer yes to any of these questions, it's unlikely that reporting the problem to FDA will be of any benefit. Nevertheless, you should, of course, get proper medical care for your injury, if necessary. Otherwise, report the following:

Food

Report any product, including seafood and dairy products (but not meat or poultry, which is regulated by the U.S. Department of Agriculture), if it is unsafe, decomposed, filthy, or defective; contains foreign substances or particles, such as hair or insects; is not properly labeled; is processed or stored under unsanitary conditions; weighs less than its labeled weight; or has caused injury or illness.

Drugs

Report products whose appearance is unusual examples are a capsule that is cloudy or contains crystals when it should be clear; a package that has a part or parts of its tamper-evident safeguards missing or broken; a capsule or pill that is chipped, broken or off-color; or any product that is contaminated with foreign matter, such as hair or mold. Also, report any drug that has caused an injury or illness.

Cosmetics

Report products that contain filthy or harmful substances, are decomposed or spoiled, or have caused an injury.

Medical Devices

Report products that do not perform according to claims and instructions, have false or misleading labels, are labeled as sterile but have broken seals, or have caused an injury.

Radiation-Emitting Electronic Products (Such as Microwave Ovens or Video Display Terminals)

Report incidents in which an injury either has occurred or may occur from products that give off radiation.

Veterinary Drugs and Feed

Report the same problems with animal feed (including pet food) and veterinary drugs that would be reported for human foods or drugs.

Where to Report

Complaints may be made by telephone or in writing. Contact the FDA office nearest you by checking the blue pages of you telephone directory under U.S. Government, Department of Health and Human Services, Food and Drug Administration. You may contact FDA's headquarters by writing:

Food and Drug Administration
5600 Fishers Lane (HFC-160)
Rockville, MD 20857

Or phone FDA's emergency number (staffed at all times): (301) 443-1240.

How to Report

Report what happened as soon as possible after you've encountered the problem. Give names, addresses and telephone numbers of persons who were injured or made ill. Be sure to include your name, address, and phone number. Also provide the name and address of the doctor or hospital providing emergency medical treatment.

State clearly what the problem appears to be. Describe the product as completely as possible, particularly any codes or identifying marks that appear on the label or container (usually these are stamped or embossed on the lids of canned products.) Give the name and address of the store where the product was purchased and the date of purchase.

Keep any opened or unopened containers or packages of the product (don't open packages if you haven't already done so). You should also report the problem to the manufacturer or distributor shown on the label and to the store where you purchased the product.

Limits of Authority

FDA does not regulate prices of products or sales practices of stores. FDA cannot control the selection of food or sanitation in schools, prisons, or other institutions. FDA cannot enforce terms of guarantees, warranties or coupons, nor can it require stores or manufacturers to give refunds or disclose product recipes or formulas. Your local Better Business Bureau of Consumer Affairs may be able to help with some of these problems.

What to Report to Other Agencies

Complaints about the following should be made to the agencies listed. Consult your local telephone directory or public library for specific information.

- Meat and poultry products: U.S. Department of Agriculture

- Sanitation in restaurants and cafeteria: Local or State health departments.

- Unsolicited products in the mail: U.S. Postal Service

- Accidental poisonings: Poison control centers or hospitals.

- Pesticides, air, and water pollution: U.S. Environmental Protection Agency.

- Hazardous household products (including appliances, toys and chemicals): Consumer Product Safety Commission.

- Exposure to hazardous materials in the workplace: Occupational Safety and Health Administration of the U.S. Department of Labor.

- Advertising and warranties: Federal Trade Commission (except advertising for prescription drugs, which is regulated by FDA).

- Dispensing and sales practices of pharmacies: State Board of Pharmacy.

- Medical practice: State Board of Healing Arts

Once you've reported a problem to FDA, investigators will follow up according to agency procedures.

Chapter 26

How to Order Food and Drug Administration Materials

FDA has available the following free brochures on the new food label. For one copy only, write to: FDA (HFE-88), 5600 Fishers Lane, Rockville, Maryland 20847 (USA). To receive two to 25 copies, write to FDA (HFI-40) at the same address. Or, FAX your order request to +1 (301)-443-9057.

Please indicate publication numbers on all requests:

- *An Introduction to the New Food Label* (FDA 94-2271) by FDA and the USDA. An overview of food labeling changes with a poster of the "Nutrition Facts" panel.

- *How the New Food Label can Help you Plan a Healthy Diet* (FDA 94- 2273) by FDA and USDA. An overview written at the 5th grade reading level.

- *How to Read the New Food Label* (FDA 93-2260) by FDA and the American Heart Association. An introduction to food labeling changes, particularly those that apply to heart disease prevention.

- *Come Leer la Nueva Etiqueta de Los Alimentos* (FDA 93-2260S) by FDA and the American Heart Association. A Spanish version of *How to Read the New Food Label*.

US FDA/Center for Food Safety and Applied Nutrition, April 30, 1995

- *Using the New Food Label to Choose Healthier Foods* (FDA 94-2276) by FDA and the American Association of Retired Persons. A large-type brochure.

- Also available is *Focus on Food Labeling—An FDA Consumer Special Report*, containing the magazine articles Main Messages as well as four others. Copies are $5.00 each from the Government Printing Office at: Superintendent of Documents, P.O. Box 371954, Pittsburgh, Pennsylvania 15250-7594; reference stock number 017-012-00360-5.

- *FDA Consumer Magazine*—10 issues per year.

There's new information every day on how to get healthy and stay healthy. *FDA Consumer* brings that information to you. The latest findings on diet and nutrition. Reports on new medicine—their benefits and side effects. Important topics like sodium, osteoporosis, generic drugs, and children's vaccinations. *FDA Consumer* will help you understand all the latest research and what it means to you. There's health advice of special concern to women, the elderly, and parents. And you'll know the information is up-to-date and authoritative because *FDA Consumer* is the official magazine of the U.S. Food and Drug Administration, the consumer protection agency responsible for food, drugs, medical devices, and other products that enter your life every day. In fact, each issue of *FDA Consumer* brings you reports from FDA's own investigators, taking you behind the scenes to show how FDA works to protect you from unsafe or worthless products.

To obtain a subscription to *FDA Consumer* at a cost of $15.00 per year domestic US or $18.75 per year foreign mail to: New Orders, Superintendent of Documents, P.O. Box 371954, Pittsburgh, Pennsylvania 15250-7954 USA. Or fax using VISA or MC to: +1 (202)-512-2233.

Chapter 27

A Food and Drug Administration Guide to Choosing Medical Treatments

Medical treatments come in many shapes and sizes. There are "home remedies" shared among families and friends. There are prescription medicines, available only from a pharmacist, and only when ordered by a physician. There are over-the-counter drugs that you can buy-almost anywhere-without a doctor's order. Of growing interest and attention in recent years are so-called alternative treatments, not yet approved for sale because they are still undergoing scientific research to see if they really are safe and effective. And, of course, there are those "miracle" products sold through "back-of-the-magazine" ads and TV infomercials.

How can you tell which of these may really help treat your medical condition and which will only make you worse off—financially, physically, or both?

Many advocates of unproven treatments and cures contend that people have the right to try whatever may offer them hope, even if others believe the remedy is worthless. This argument is especially compelling for people with AIDS or other life-threatening diseases with no known cure.

Clinical Trials

Before gaining Food and Drug Administration marketing approval, new drugs, biologics, and medical devices must be proven safe and effective by controlled clinical trials.

FDA Consumer, 97-1223, June 1995.

In a clinical trial, results observed in patients getting the treatment are compared with the results in similar patients receiving a different treatment or placebo (inactive) treatment. Preferably, neither patients nor researchers know who is receiving the therapy under study.

To FDA, it doesn't matter whether the product or treatment is labeled alternative or falls under the auspices of mainstream American medical practice. (Mainstream American medicine essentially includes the practices and products the majority of medical doctors in this country follow and use.) It must meet the agency's safety and effectiveness criteria before being allowed on the market.

In addition, just because something is undergoing a clinical trial doesn't mean it works or FDA considers it to be a proven therapy, says Donald Pohl, of FDA's Office of AIDS and Special Health Issues. "You can't jump to that conclusion," he says. A trial can fail to prove that the product is effective, he explains. And that's not just true for alternative products. Even when the major drug companies sponsor clinical trials for mainstream products, only a small fraction are proven safe and effective.

Many people with serious illnesses are unable to find a cure, or even temporary relief, from the available mainstream treatments that have been rigorously studied and proven safe and effective. For many conditions, such as arthritis or even cancer, what's effective for one patient may not help another.

Real Alternatives

"It is best not to abandon conventional therapy when there is a known response in the effectiveness of that therapy" says Joseph Jacobs, M.D., former director of the National Institutes of Health's Office of Alternative Medicine, which was established in October 1992. As an example he cites childhood leukemia, which has an 80 percent cure rate with conventional therapy.

But what if conventional therapy holds little promise?

Many physicians believe it is not unreasonable for someone in the last stages of an incurable cancer to try something unproven. But, for example, if a woman with an early stage of breast cancer wanted to try shark cartilage (an unproven treatment that may inhibit the growth of cancer tumors, currently undergoing clinical trials), those same doctors would probably say, "Don't do it," because there are so many effective conventional treatments.

Jacobs warns that, "If an alternative practitioner does not want to work with a regular doctor, then he's suspect."

Alternative medicine is often described as any medical practice or intervention that:

- lacks sufficient documentation of its safety and effectiveness against specific diseases and conditions
- is not generally taught in U.S. medical schools
- is not generally reimbursable by health insurance providers.

According to a study in the Jan. 28, 1993, New England Journal of Medicine, 1 in 3 patients used alternative therapy in 1990. More than 80 percent of those who use alternative therapies used conventional medicine at the same time, but did not tell their doctors about the alternative treatments. The study's authors concluded this lack of communication between doctors and patients "is not in the best interest of the patients, since the use of unconventional therapy, especially if it is totally unsupervised, may be harmful." The study concluded that medical doctors should ask their patients about any use of unconventional treatment as part of a medical history.

Many doctors are interested in learning more about alternative therapies, according to Brian Berman, M.D., a family practitioner with the University of Maryland School of Medicine in Baltimore. Berman says his own interest began when "I found that I wasn't getting all the results that I would have liked with conventional medicine, especially in patients with chronic diseases.

"What I've found at the University of Maryland is a healthy skepticism among my colleagues, but a real willingness to collaborate. We have a lot of people from different departments who are saying, let's see how we can develop scientifically rigorous studies that are also sensitive to the particular therapies that we're working with."

Anyone who wants to be treated with an alternative therapy should try to do so through participation in a clinical trial. Clinical trials are regulated by FDA and provide safeguards to protect patients, such as monitoring of adverse reactions. In fact, FDA is interested in assisting investigators who want to study alternative therapies under carefully controlled clinical trials. Some of the alternative therapies currently under study with grants from NIH include:

- acupuncture to treat depression, attention-deficit hyperactivity disorder, osteoarthritis, and postoperative dental pain
- hypnosis for chronic low back pain and accelerated fracture healing
- Ayurvedic herbals for Parkinson's disease. (Ayurvedic medicine is a holistic system based on the belief that herbals, massage,

and other stress relievers help the body make its own natural drugs.)

- biofeedback for diabetes, low back pain, and face and mouth pain caused by jaw disorders. (Biofeedback is the conscious control of biological functions, such as those of the heart and blood vessels, normally controlled involuntarily.)

- electric currents to treat tumors

- imagery for asthma and breast cancer. (With imagery, patients are guided to see themselves in a different physical, emotional or spiritual state. For example, patients might be guided to imagine themselves in a state of vibrant health and the disease organisms as weak and destructible.)

While these alternative therapies are the subject of scientifically valid research, it's important to remember that at this time their safety and effectiveness

Avoiding Fraud

FDA defines health fraud as the promotion, advertisement, distribution, or sale of articles, intended for human or animal use, that are represented as being effective to diagnose, prevent, cure, treat, or mitigate disease (or other conditions), or provide a beneficial effect on health, but which have not been scientifically proven safe and effective for such purposes. Such practices may be deliberately deceptive, or done without adequate knowledge or understanding of the article.

Health fraud costs Americans an estimated $30 billion a year. However, the costs are not just economic, according to John Renner, M.D., Kansas City-based champion of quality health care for the elderly. "The hidden costs—death, disability—are unbelievable," he says.

To combat health fraud, FDA established its National Health Fraud Unit in 1988. The unit works with the National Association of Attorneys General and the Association of Food and Drug Officials to coordinate federal, state and local regulatory actions against specific health frauds.

Regulatory actions may be necessary in many cases because products that have not been shown to be safe and effective pose potential hazards for consumers both directly and indirectly. The agency's priorities for regulatory action depend on the situation; direct risks to health come first.

Unproven products cause direct health hazards when their use results in injuries or adverse reactions. For example, a medical device called the InnerQuest Brain Wave Synchronizer was promoted to alter brain waves and relieve stress. It consisted of an audio cassette and eyeglasses that emitted sounds and flashing lights. It caused epileptic seizures in some users. As a result of a court order requested by FDA, 78 cartons of the devices, valued at $200,000, were seized by U.S. marshals and destroyed in June 1993.

Indirectly harmful products are those that do not themselves cause injury, but may lead people to delay or reject proven remedies, possibly worsening their condition. For example, if cancer patients reject proven drug therapies in favor of unproven ones and the unproven ones turn out not to work, their disease may advance beyond the point where proven therapies can help.

"What you see out there is the promotion of products claiming to cure or prevent AIDS, multiple sclerosis, cancer, and a list of other diseases that goes on and on," says Joel Aronson, director of FDA's Health Fraud Staff, in the agency's Center for Drug Evaluation and Research. For example, he says, several skin cream products promise to prevent transmission of HIV (the virus that causes AIDS) and herpes viruses. They are promoted especially to healthcare workers. Many of the creams contain antibacterial ingredients but, "there is no substantiation at all on whether or not (the skin creams) work" against HIV, says Aronson. FDA has warned the manufacturers of these creams to stop the misleading promotions.

People at Risk

Teenagers and the elderly are two prime targets for health fraud promoters.

Teenagers concerned about their appearance and susceptible to peer pressure may fall for such products as fraudulent diet pills, breast developers, and muscle-building pills.

Older Americans may be especially vulnerable to health fraud because approximately 80 percent of them have at least one chronic health problem, according to Renner. Many of these problems, such as arthritis, have no cure and, for some people, no effective treatment. He says their pain and disability lead to despair, making them excellent targets for deception.

Arthritis

Although there is no cure for arthritis, the symptoms may come and go with no explanation. According to the Arthritis Foundation,

"You may think a new remedy worked because you took it when your symptoms were going away."

Some commonly touted unproven treatments for arthritis are harmful, according to the foundation, including snake venom and DMSO (dimethyl sulfoxide), an industrial solvent similar to turpentine. FDA has approved a sterile form of DMSO called Rimso-50, which is administered directly into the bladder for treatment of rare bladder condition called interstitial cystitis. However, the DMSO sold to arthritis sufferers may contain bacterial toxins. DMSO is readily absorbed through the skin into the bloodstream, and these toxins enter the bloodstream along with it. It can be especially dangerous if used as an enema, as some of its promoters recommend.

Treatments the foundation considers harmless but ineffective include copper bracelets, mineral springs, and spas.

Cancer and AIDS

Cancer treatment is complicated because in some types of cancer there are no symptoms, and in other types symptoms may disappear by themselves, at least temporarily. Use of an unconventional treatment coinciding with remission (lessening of symptoms) could be simply coincidental. There's no way of knowing, without a controlled clinical trial, what effect the treatment had on the outcome. The danger comes when this false security causes patients to forgo approved treatment that has shown real benefit.

Some unapproved cancer treatments not only have no proven benefits, they have actually been proven dangerous. These include Laetrile, which may cause cyanide poisoning and has been found ineffective in clinical trials, and coffee enemas, which, when used excessively, have killed patients.

Ozone generators, which produce a toxic form of oxygen gas, have been touted as being able to cure AIDS. To date this is still unproven, and FDA considers ozone to be an unapproved drug and these generators to be unapproved medical devices. At least three deaths have been connected to the use of these generators. Four British citizens were indicted in 1991 for selling fraudulent ozone generators in the United States. Two of the defendants fled to Great Britain, but the other two pleaded guilty and served time in U.S. federal prisons.

The bottom line in deciding whether a certain treatment you've read or heard about might be right for you: Talk to your doctor. And keep in mind the old adage: If it sounds too good to be true, it probably is.

Approaching Alternative Therapies

The NIH Office of Alternative Medicine recommends the following before getting involved in any alternative therapy:

- Obtain objective information about the therapy. Besides talking with the person promoting the approach, speak with people who have gone through the treatment—preferably both those who were treated recently and those treated in the past. Ask about the advantages and disadvantages, risks, side effects, costs, results, and over what time span results can be expected.

- Inquire about the training and experience of the person administering the treatment (for example, certification).

- Consider the costs. Alternative treatments may not be reimbursable by health insurance.

- Discuss all treatments with your primary care provider, who needs this information in order to have a complete picture of your treatment plan.

For everyone—consumers, physicians and other health-care providers, and government regulators—FDA has the same advice when it comes to weeding out the hopeless from the hopeful: Be open-minded, but don't fall into the abyss of accepting anything at all. For there are—as there have been for centuries—countless products that are nothing more than fraud.

Resources

Whether looking for an alternative therapy or checking the legitimacy of something you've heard about, some of the best sources are advocacy groups, including local patient support groups. Those groups include:

American Cancer Society
1599 Clifton Road, N.E.
Atlanta, GA 30329
(404) 320-3333, (1-800) ACS-2345

Arthritis Foundation
P.O. Box 19000
Atlanta, GA 30326
(1-800) 283-7800

National Multiple Sclerosis Society
733 Third Ave.
New York, NY 10017-3288
(212) 986-3240, (1-800) 344-4867

HIV/AIDS Treatment Information Service
P.O. Box 6303
Rockville, MD 20849-6303.
(1-800) 448-0440, TDD/Deaf Access: (1-800) 243-7012

Federal government resources on health fraud and alternative medicine are:

FDA (HFE-88)
Rockville, MD 20857
(1-800) 532-4440

Office of Alternative Medicine
NIH Information Center
6120 Executive Blvd., EPS
Suite 450
Rockville, MD 20852
(301) 402-2466

U.S. Postal Inspection Service
(monitors products purchased by mail)
Contact your local post office.

Federal Trade Commission
(regarding false advertising)
Room 421
6th St. and Pennsylvania Ave., N.W.
Washington, DC 20580
(202) 326-2222

Other agencies that may have information and offer assistance include local Better Business Bureaus, state and municipal consumer affairs offices, and state attorneys general offices.

Chapter 28

Food and Drug Administration and Medical Devices

FDA has just marked the 20th anniversary of the Medical Device Amendments to the Food, Drug, and Cosmetic Act.

Until 20 years ago, FDA was ill-equipped to protect Americans from dangerous or useless medical devices, because the agency had to prove a device was unsafe or ineffective before it could take action to remove the device from the market. In 1976, the landmark Medical Device Amendments were signed into law by President Gerald Ford. The law requires manufacturers of most medical devices—particularly moderate- or high-risk devices—to provide FDA with safety and effectiveness data before marketing.

FDA's Center for Devices and Radiological Health is charged with implementing the device law. The center has many functions, including working with FDA's field force to inspect device manufacturing plants; keeping track of problems with devices already in use and taking prompt action to correct them; and helping manufacturers produce better products by conducting laboratory research on the ways companies test their products and on specific device safety problems.

One of the most visible and important functions of the center is to review devices for safety and effectiveness before they are marketed. The center clears for marketing everything from contact lenses and artificial joints to x-ray machines. More than 550 categories of low-risk medical devices, including surgical gloves and therapeutic massagers, are exempted from pre-market approval.

FDA Consumer, December 6, 1996.

Challenged to speed product approvals without compromising consumer safety, the center has made some changes in the way it does business. (See "Inside FDA: Agency Changes Include Medical Device Review" in the November 1996 issue of *FDA Consumer.*)

In the following interview, center director D. Bruce Burlington, M.D., talks about what the medical device program has accomplished and what remains to be done.

Q. Twenty years have passed since enactment of the landmark Medical Device Amendments of 1976. Are Americans better cared for as a result of the amendments ?

A. I think the American people are significantly better off for having the medical device law. Today, Americans can really rely on devices. When a medical device is used in a doctor's office or hospital, patients can be confident that the operator knows how to use the device well and that it will work for them.

Americans can count on devices because of the system of pre- and post-market oversight made possible by the 1976 amendments. To ensure that products are well-manufactured, FDA inspects companies to see that they are following good manufacturing practices, keeping appropriate records on the design and manufacture of products, and maintaining a system for handling complaints.

Before a product even goes to market a company must present data to FDA showing not only that it will be well-manufactured, but also that it is safe and effective—that it won't harm people and will deliver its expected benefits. And if a product causes unforeseen problems, there's a feedback loop, a requirement that manufacturers report any serious problems to FDA so rapid action, including a product recall if necessary, can be taken to protect people from a faulty device.

There is yet another vital benefit of our regulation of devices under the medical device law: information. The largest source of risk in using a medical device isn't the product itself, but the interface between the user and the device. It is especially important for doctors to know how and when to use the product. Serving as a reliable, unbiased evaluator of this information may be the most important service FDA can provide to health professionals.

Q. What are some of the most significant accomplishments of the center during your service as director to date?

A. Several breakthrough devices have been approved by the center. One of the most important is our recent approval of the use of implantable defibrillators to prevent sudden death in people who have had heart attacks. This was the first approval for this use in the world, and it should save thousands of lives each year. Also in the area of cardiology, we approved a coronary stent, a cage-like device that's permanently implanted in a diseased coronary artery to expand it and allow normal blood flow. This is really changing the way cardiologists are performing balloon angioplasty to open up clogged arteries feeding the heart, making the procedure available to many patients who before would have had to undergo major surgery.

To help detect cervical cancer more reliably, we've approved a device that scans all pap smears read as normal by the technologist and identifies suspicious ones for a second review.

Also, we've approved a new microwave device to treat symptoms of enlarged prostate, a condition affecting millions of men. This device gives patients an alternative to treatment with drugs or surgery.

Two newly approved devices can potentially help millions of women who suffer from urinary incontinence. One is a disposable balloon-type device that the patient inserts into her urethra, and the other is an adhesive-backed foam pad that's placed over the urinary opening.

Another approval that's been prominent in the news is the use of excimer lasers to treat certain cases of nearsightedness, giving many people an alternative to eyeglasses or contact lenses.

An additional major accomplishment has been the center's recent emphasis on clinical trials—controlled studies in humans—for evaluating the safety and effectiveness of new devices. For 20 years, we'd been concentrating primarily on assuring that devices were well-designed and well-made. It goes without saying that these things are still important. But we've come to realize that for some devices—probably less than 10 percent—we also need clinical data from human studies. This gives us information on how the device will perform in actual patients, and gives the physician information about which patients are likely to benefit from the device and under what conditions. In the long run, I think the focus on clinical trials may have a bigger impact on the public than anything else we're doing.

Q. Government agencies are often criticized for making decisions that don't reflect the interests of the public and the regulated industry. Has FDA taken steps to avoid this pitfall?

A. Yes. To help the agency make decisions on policy matters or on specific devices, we want input from the public and industry. For policy issues, we often have grass-roots meetings—we've had several in the last year—to get suggestions on how to approach an issue. When we have a particular device in front of us that may be ready for marketing, very often we will have an advisory committee meeting. Most meetings are open, and consumer protection groups and members of the public are welcome to attend and tell us what they expect.

Because I also work as an emergency room physician, I get an additional, hands-on perspective. I can see the devices in action and can learn from patients and other physicians what they expect from the devices and from government oversight. It helps me to know which issues are peripheral so I can focus on the issues that really make a difference.

After balancing everyone's input, and with the intent of the law foremost in mind, FDA is ultimately responsible for deciding whether to allow a product on the market and whether it's necessary to take action against a product already on the market. In the end, the government official charged with making the decision is accountable to the public, and he or she must "take the heat" if a decision is criticized.

Q. Some critics say FDA is too slow in approving medical devices. Is the criticism justified, and what is the agency doing to speed up Americans' access to safe, effective medical devices?

A. We should take seriously those critics who raise valid points, and use their negative appraisals to improve our performance. We at FDA have to understand that new products do bring real benefits, and that delaying availability of a safe, effective medical device can harm people just as much as approving a faulty product.

At the same time, we must bear in mind that our goal is not simply to get products to the market, but to get products that work and that we know how to use. So we can't lose sight of our consumer protection mission as we look at changing the way FDA does business.

A little over three years ago, when I came to the center. we had a mountain of work that had built up over the previous couple of years. We had been through a period of incredibly intense internal scrutiny and external review, and we responded to that review by modifying the way we operate.

We've substantially dug out from under the mountain. Abbreviated applications—applications for a device that's essentially the same as something already on the market—are reviewed on time, usually within 90 days. For more complicated applications, we still have some work to do. We're making real headway, though, towards a record of timeliness.

Some people question whether patients in other countries get access to new devices sooner than patients in the United States. When it comes to products that are really new—those that represent breakthrough technologies or are the first of their kind—we use a system of expedited review which allows these kinds of devices to go to the head of the queue and receive review very quickly.

Under this system, we've approved several significant new devices in the past few years before they were approved anywhere else in the world. These include a prenatal test for genetic abnormalities, an ultrasound system to speed the healing of bone fractures, a bone growth stimulator for treatment of old, unhealed fractures, and the use of an implanted heart defibrillator to prevent sudden cardiac arrest in patients who have suffered heart attacks.

Of course, we have little control over the time it takes for a company to develop its product and collect data on its safety and effectiveness. But the next step—the company's interaction with FDA—must be productive and efficient. Long, drawn-out decisions aren't necessarily better than prompt ones. We at FDA need to make timely decisions to provide a clear and predictable business climate so that industry can do its job and bring new products to market. But we can't make sacrifices in the quality of data.

Complete, well-prepared applications move through the system more quickly than others. Once we have the good science necessary to make a decision, we should go ahead and make it, to reach closure on the issue and move on. That culture of decisiveness is especially important when we're dealing with the device industry, in which a product's market life often is only a few years.

FDA is committed to doing the best we can with the budget provided. By looking to the experience of businesses across America, we can learn lessons about how to get our job done better and more cheaply. To make the most efficient use of FDA's resources, we're looking for ways to get the same results with fewer people. The agency has really pushed the envelope regarding abbreviated device applications. We're allowing many products that previously would have required a comprehensive application to now be reviewed under an abbreviated application, which is usually processed in only 90 days.

We're pilot-testing a program of third-party reviews, which asks, "Which part of the work does it make sense for the agency to turn over to external parties?" We may be able to reduce review times by allowing carefully selected outside groups to perform the first stage of review of devices that don't present a substantial risk to the American public.

Q. Is it realistic to think that device regulation could be standardized worldwide to lessen the burden on device manufacturers who want to market their products internationally?

A. Today, medical device manufacturers may have to develop different sets of data for each country in which they seek approval. We are working toward harmonizing standards among countries where we can.

People are much the same around the world, and many of their diseases and injuries are the same. We ought to be able to reach agreement worldwide on what constitutes a safe, well-manufactured product. But the issue of whether a product delivers a sufficient benefit is harder because there are different expectations of the regulatory systems in the United States and, for example, Europe.

The United States has the gold standard for what is expected from companies when they want to bring a product to market, a gold standard not just in terms of knowing how a product is made but also of knowing how it works and under what circumstances it works. In Europe, device regulation focuses on whether devices are well-designed and well-made—their mechanical performance characteristics. It doesn't focus of efficacy—on whether the device works on patients—like our system does. We're not prepared to take a step down to a lower standard, and other countries with different expectations of government aren't ready to line up with the American system. So we don't expect to see total harmonization soon, with one reviewing body getting the product to the world market.

Q. What are the biggest challenges you expect your center to face over the next decade?

A. We have many of the same challenges that people have across government. Given the realities of the federal budget, we have to figure out how to get our job done with tight resources. We have to determine what's most important about what we do, and, where possible, share the public health responsibility with industry, academia, and health-care providers. We've already begun that process through the pilot testing of third-party reviews.

Also, in the last few years there's been a shift from the one-on-one, individual doctor and patient model of health care toward a managed care model where patient care is administered by large organizations like HMOs. With cost-effectiveness considerations playing a much larger role in medical decision-making, health-care organizations will need information for "technology assessment"—information not only on whether a device works, but how it compares to other devices and other forms of treatment.

In some ways this will make FDA's job easier, because every company that wants to market a product will know that its data will not only have to pass review by the agency, but will also have to convince the managed-care organizations that its product really makes a difference.

But this raises questions about FDA's role in this new era. Are we going to continue to evaluate each new device essentially in isolation, simply asking whether the product works and is safe, leaving it to others to do the comparisons? Or will the agency jump into the technology assessment arena? More and more, I think we'll have to focus on how to evaluate products in the context of the whole health care picture.

—by Tamar Nordenberg

Chapter 29

Food and Drug Administration Review and Approval Times

The process of bringing a drug to market is lengthy and complex and begins with laboratory investigations of the drug's potential. For a drug that seems to hold promise, pre-clinical animal studies are typically conducted to see how it affects living systems. If the animal studies are successful, the sponsoring pharmaceutical firm designs and initiates clinical studies in which the drug is given to humans. At this point, FDA becomes directly involved for the first time.

Before any new drug can be tested on humans, the drug's sponsor must submit an investigational new drug application to FDA that summarizes the pre-clinical work, lays out a plan for how the drug will be tested on humans, and provides assurances that appropriate measures will be taken to protect them. Unless FDA decides that the proposed study is unsafe, clinical testing may begin 31 days after this application has been submitted to FDA. As the clinical trials progress through several phases aimed at establishing safety and efficacy, the manufacturer develops the processes that will be necessary to pro-duce large quantities of the drug that meet the quality standards for commercial marketing.

When all this has been done, the pharmaceutical firm submits a new drug application (NDA) that includes the information FDA needs to determine whether the drug is safe and effective for its intended use and whether the manufacturing process can ensure its quality. The first decision FDA must make is whether to accept the NDA or

GAO/T-PEMD-96-6, February 1996.

to refuse to file it because it does not meet minimum requirements. Once FDA has accepted an NDA, it decides whether to approve the drug on the basis of the information in the application and any supplemental information FDA has requested. FDA can approve the drug for marketing (in an "approval letter") or it may indicate (in an "approvable letter") that it can approve the drug if the sponsor resolves certain issues. Alternatively, FDA may withhold approval (through a "non-approvable letter" that specifies the reasons). Throughout the process, the sponsor remains an active participant by responding to FDA's inquiries and concerns. The sponsor has the option, however, of withdrawing the application at any time.

Results in Brief

We found a considerable reduction in approval time for NDAs. It took an average of 33 months for NDAs submitted in 1987 to be approved but only 19 months on average to approve NDAs submitted in 1992. Further, the reduction in time was observed for all NDAs and not just for those that had been approved. The overall decrease in approval times was achieved through gradual reductions in time for applications submitted in each successive year. The priority that FDA assigns to an NDA and the experience of its sponsor are the two factors that significantly affect the likelihood that the NDA will be decided on quickly. FDA assigns priority status to applications for drugs that are expected to provide therapeutic benefit to consumers beyond that of drugs already marketed. These NDAs take an average of 10 months less to be approved than do standard applications (those for which there is no perceived therapeutic benefit beyond that for available drugs). Applications from the most experienced sponsors take an average of 4 months less time to be approved than those from less experienced sponsors.

The data available on review time for FDA and the counterpart agency in the United Kingdom are limited, but show that times are not faster in the UK.

Our Analysis

As mentioned above, 905 NDAs were submitted to FDA in the years 1987-94. Of these, approximately 1 in 5 NDAs (17 percent) were for priority drugs. The other NDAs were for drugs that FDA considered to offer little therapeutic benefit beyond that already available to patients.

Because there has been so much discussion of how long it takes to obtain approval for an NDA, it can be easily missed that in fact many NDAs do not ultimately get approved. Table 29.1 shows the final status of those NDAs as of May 1995.

As can be seen from the table, a relatively large percentage of applications were not approved. Only 390 of the 700 NDAs submitted through 1992 had been approved by May 16, 1995. In other words, 44 percent of the applications submitted were for drugs that FDA did not find to be safe and effective or that sponsors chose not to pursue further. Truly innovative drugs (known as new molecular entities or NMEs) were approved at a higher rate than non-NMEs (64 percent to 52 percent), and priority drugs were approved more often than standard drugs (76 percent to 52 percent). This means that whether an NDA is or is not ultimately approved is as relevant a question as how long approval takes.

Table 29.1. Final Status for NDAs Submitted 1987-1994[a].

	Year of submission							
Final status	**1987**	**1988**	**1989**	**1990**	**1991**	**1992**	**1993**	**1994**
Approved	56%	58%	56%	54%	58%	52%	33%	5%
Withdrawn	21	26	22	25	11	18	11	6
Refused to file	7	3	3	3	12	9	11	13
Approvable	1	2	2	3	5	5	7	4
Not approvable	14	12	17	15	13	16	23	11
Pending	0	0	0	0	1	1	11	51

[a]Final status as of May 16, 1995. Percentages may not total 100 because of rounding. Percentages for 1993 and 1994 do not total 100 because NDAs found "unacceptable for filing" because user fees were not paid are not included in the table.

How Long Does the Review Process Take?

Table 29.2 shows for 1987-92 the average time (in months) from when NDAs were first submitted to when final decisions were made for both NDAs that were approved and those that were not. The table also distinguishes between all NDAs and those that were approved in three categories: new molecular entities, priority applications, and standard applications.

As can be seen from the table, the processing time for all eight NDA categories fell considerably (45 percent for all NDAs and 42 percent for approved applications). In addition, the reductions in time came for NDAs submitted throughout the period of our study. This finding is consistent with FDA's statements that review time has decreased in recent years. Closer examination of the individual NDAs shows that they differed considerably in how long it took before a final decision was made. Some NDAs were approved within a few months (the shortest was 2 months); others took years (the slowest was 96 months). Among applications that were not approved, the variation was similar. Some were withdrawn on the day they were submitted. The longest outstanding application was 92 months old.

This considerable variation raises the question of what differentiates one NDA from the next: Do some factors predict the time it will take to reach a final decision? When we tested potential explanatory variables, we found that the priority FDA assigned to an application and the sponsor's experience in submitting NDAs were statistically significant predictors of how long review and approval took. More specifically, controlling for the effects of the other explanatory variables in the model, our regression analysis found that priority NDA applications are approved 10 months faster than standard applications and that applications from the most experienced sponsors are approved 4 months faster than applications from less experienced sponsors.

Table 29.2. *Average Number of Months From Initial NDA Submission to Final Decision,1987-92.*

Type	Year of initial submission					
	1987	**1988**	**1989**	**1990**	**1991**	**1992**
All NDAs	33	31	24	23	21	18
Approved NDAs	33	30	25	25	21	19
All NMEs	31	32	21	21	25	20
Approved NMEs	33	26	23	23	23	21
All priority	29	29	16	23	17	17
Approved priority	23	23	16	22	18	16
All standard	34	32	26	23	21	18
Approved standard	35	32	28	27	22	20

Process Measures of Time

The interval between first submission and final decision indicates how long the public must wait for drugs after sponsors believe they have assembled all the evidence to support an approval decision. Alternative measures provide insight into what happens to an NDA before FDA approves it. One such measure is the extent to which FDA is "on time" in making decisions (using criteria established under the Prescription Drug User Fee Act). We examined both the degree to which FDA was on time and the factors that influenced whether it made its decisions on time.

Of all the decisions FDA made on the NDAs submitted between 1987 and 1993, 67 percent were on time. Simpler decisions (for example, refusals to file) were made on time more often than relatively complex decisions (for example, priority applications in which the first decision was an approval). Overall, the on-time percentage remained relatively stable, varying between a low of 62 percent for NDAs submitted in 1992 and a high of 72 percent for NDAs submitted in 1987.

Another process measure of review time is based on where responsibility lies for different parts of the process—with FDA, for the intervals during which it acts on an application, or with the sponsor, for the intervals during which FDA waits for the sponsor to provide additional information or to resubmit the application. Sponsors accounted for approximately 20 percent of the time in the NDA phase for applications that FDA approved. Importantly, the time for both sponsors and FDA diminished for NDAs submitted between 1987 and 1992.

Approval Times in the United Kingdom

The United Kingdom's equivalent of FDA is the Medicines Control Agency (MCA). MCA publishes information similar to that contained in FDA's statistical reports, including data on workload (number and type of submissions) and time (how long it takes to review applications). MCA's 1994-95 annual report indicates that the assessment of an application for a new active substance (the apparent equivalent of what FDA terms a new molecular entity) took an average of 56 working days. This figure stands in sharp contrast to FDA's reports that show an average approval time of 20 months for applications for NMEs approved in 1994. No doubt, the sharp contrast in these two averages is one factor creating the impression that approval times are much shorter in the United Kingdom than they are in this country.

However, closer examination of the data in MCA's annual report shows that they should be compared to our data on FDA with caution. In the United Kingdom, MCA's assessment is only the first step in the process of drug review and approval. All applications for new active substances are also referred to a government body called the Committee on the Safety of Medicines (CSM). CSM's expert subcommittees also assess the application and then send these assessments, along with those from MCA, to the full committee. CSM then makes a recommendation to the Licensing Authority, which is the government body that actually grants or denies the product license. Moreover, because the rate of rejection of applications or request for modifications or additional information is very high (99 percent for applications submitted 1987-89), many applications go through an appeals process that may involve additional work on the part of the applicant, reassessment by MCA or CSM, and the involvement of another body called the Medicines Commission. Thus, the total time until the license is actually granted is considerably longer than the period of initial assessment by MCA. In contrast, the time that FDA reports includes all the steps between an accepted NDA and the final decision on it.

When one examines total time for both processes, the United Kingdom does not appear to be dramatically faster than the United States. One recent study compared approval times for 11 drugs that were approved in both countries during the period 1986-92. The median time in the United States (about 23 months) was 15 percent longer than the median time in the United Kingdom (20 months) l3 The most recent data from MCA show that overall approval times are actually somewhat longer than that. These data indicate that MCA granted licenses for applications representing 32 new active substances during the 12-month period ending September 30, 1994. The median time for granting a license was 30 months and the average was 24 months. The fastest license was granted in about 4 months, the slowest in 62 months.

FDA's data for the calendar year ending December 31, 1994, indicate that the agency approved a total of 22 new molecular entities. The median approval time was 18 months, average approval time about 20 months. The fastest approval reported by FDA took about 6 months and the slowest about 40 months.

Thus, the most recent data show that approval times for NMEs are actually shorter in the United States. In addition, a broader perspective shows that approval processes in many industrialized nations may be converging. Approval times over the past 10 years for France,

Germany, Japan, the United Kingdom, and the United States all seem to be moving toward the 2-year point. The trend in the United States (which had lengthy times throughout the mid-1980s) has been toward more rapid times, whereas the process has been getting slower in some of the other (originally faster) countries.

Summary

In sum, the data we have presented show that NDAs are moving more quickly through the drug review and approval process and that the amount of time to obtain an approval is approximately the same in this country and in the United Kingdom. Whether the improvement in FDA time is because of actions that the agency or the pharmaceutical industry has taken or because of some other factors is an issue that was beyond the scope of our study. However, the consistency of all our results supports the conclusion that the reduction in time is real and not an artifact of how time is measured. Further, the magnitude of the reduction (more than 40 percent) and the relative similarity of review times internationally should both be considered in the ongoing discussions of whether it is necessary to change the NDA review process or the agency in order to speed the availability of drugs to patients.

Chapter 30

American's Food Safety
Team: A Look at the Line-up

So there's a bug in your Brie. Understandably, you feel like telling someone, since the label didn't say anything about bugs. But who can help? Is it a wild bug or a domestic one? Does it swim? Was the Brie homemade or imported? Did the others at your party also get a bug in their Brie or were you the only lucky one? Is eating bugs good for you? Who's in charge here?

Responsibility for monitoring and regulating the origin, composition, quality, safety weight, labeling, packing, marketing and distribution of the food you eat and drink is shared by local, state, national and international government agencies. On these pages are condensed descriptions of the principal ones involved and a brief explanation of their roles and relationships.

U.S. Department of Agriculture (USDA)

Through inspection and grading, the U.S. Department of Agriculture enforces standards for wholesomeness and quality of meat, poultry and eggs produced in the United States. USDA also is involved in nutrition research and in educating the public about how to choose and cook foods and how to manage healthy or restricted diets.

USDA food safety activities include inspecting poultry, eggs, and domestic and imported meat; inspecting livestock and production plants; and making quality (grading) inspections for grain, fruits,

FDA Consumer, July/August 1988.

vegetables, meat, poultry and dairy products (including Brie and other cheeses). USDA's education programs target family nutritional needs, food safety, and expanding scientific knowledge. The department supports education with grants in food and agricultural sciences and conducts its own and cooperative food research.

Bureau of Alcohol, Tobacco and Firearms (ATF)

ATF, an agency of the Department of the Treasury, is responsible for enforcing the laws that cover the production, distribution and labeling of alcoholic beverages, except wine beverage that contain less than 7 percent alcohol, which are the responsibility of FDA. ATF and FDA sometimes share responsibility in cases of adulteration, or when an alcoholic beverage contains food or color additives, pesticides or contaminants.

Centers for Disease Control (CDC)

A branch of the Department of Health and Human Services, CDC becomes involved as a protector of food safety, including responding to emergencies, when foodborne diseases are a factor. CDC surveys and studies environmental health problems. It directs and enforces quarantines, and it administers national programs for prevention and control of vector-born diseases (diseases transmitted by a host organism) and other preventable conditions.

Department of Justice

When the problem with a food is a violation of federal law, marshals from the Department of Justice are the agents who seize products. The Justice Department's attorneys take suspected violators of food safety laws to court.

Environmental Protection Agency (EPA)

Among its many duties, EPA regulates pesticides. It determines the safety of new pesticide products, sets tolerance levels for pesticide residues in foods, which FDA enforces, and it publishes directions for the safe use of pesticides.

EPA also establishes water quality standards, including the chemical content of drinking water. These standards are used by FDA as guides in its regulation of bottled water sold in interstate commerce for human use.

Federal Trade Commission (FTC)

FTC's Bureau of Consumer Protection has, among it duties, the regulation of advertising of foods.

Food and Drug Administration (FDA)

FDA, a part of the Department of Health and Human Services' Public Health Service, is responsible for ensuring the safety and wholesomeness of all foods sold in interstate commerce except for meat, poultry and eggs, all of which are under USDA jurisdiction.

FDA develops standards for the composition, quality, nutrition and safety of foods, including food and color additives. It does research to improve detection and prevention of food contamination. It collects and interprets data on nutrition, food additives and environmental factors, such as pesticides, that affect foods. FDA also sets standards for certain foods and enforces federal regulations on labeling, food and color additives, food sanitation and safety of foods.

FDA inspects food plants, imported food products, and feed mills that make feeds containing medications or nutritional supplements for animals destined as food for humans. FDA monitors recalls of unsafe or contaminated foods and can get illegally marketed foods seized.

National Marine Fisheries Service (NMFS)

A part of the Department of Commerce, NMFS is responsible for seafood quality and identification, fisheries management and development, habitat conservation, and aquaculture production. NMFS has a voluntary inspection program for fish products. Its guidelines closely match regulations for which FDA has enforcement authority.

State and Local Governments

State and local government agencies cooperate with the federal government to ensure the quality and safety of food produced within their jurisdictions. FDA and other federal agencies help states and local governments develop uniform food safety standards and regulations, and assist them with research and information.

States inspect restaurants, retail food establishments, dairies, grain mills, and other food establishments within their borders. In many instances, they can embargo illegal food products, which gives them authority over fish, including shellfish, taken from those waters.

FDA provides guidelines to the states for this regulation. Twenty-eight states have their own fish inspection programs.

FDA also provides guidelines for state and local governments for regulation of dairy products and restaurant foods.

The departments responsible for food safety and inspection functions vary by state and community. Some are divisions of other agencies such as state agriculture or health departments.

Foreign Governments. Governments of at least 40 nations are now partners with the United States in ensuring food safety through memoranda of understanding that cover some two dozen food products, including shellfish. International cooperation is expanding in areas of food product inspection, certification, quality assurance, education and training, product studies, and regulatory standards.

Chapter 31

Food Safety from Farm to Table

A New Interagency Strategy to Prevent Foodborne Disease

In his radio message on January 25, 1997, President Clinton announced a new initiative to improve the safety of the nation's food supply. The President announced he will request $43 million in his 1998 budget to fund a nationwide early warning system for foodborne illness, enhance seafood safety inspections, and expand food safety research, risk assessment, training, and education. President Clinton also directed the Secretary of Health and Human Services and of Agriculture, and the Administrator of the Environmental Protection Agency to work with consumers, producers, industry, states, universities, and the public to identify additional ways to reduce the incidence of foodborne illness and to ensure our food supply is the safest in the world.

The President directed Secretaries Shalala and Glickman, and Administrator Browner to report back to him with recommendations in 90 days. He instructed them to explore opportunities for public/private partnerships to improve food safety. And he asked that their recommendations include ways to improve surveillance, inspections, research, risk assessment, education, and coordination among local, state, and federal health authorities.

Food Safety Initiative Page, NCID Home Page, Updated: February 25, 1997

We need your advice. Your perspective is essential in providing the President with a report that identifies current needs in food safety, as well as assuring the future safety of our food supply and the health of consumers. We need the perspective and suggestions of all groups who are concerned about food safety and public health to make this a successful endeavor.

The goal of this initiative is to reduce, to the greatest extent possible, the incidence of foodborne illness. The thoughts in this draft focus on the public health principle that society should identify and take preventive measures to reduce the risk of illness, and that it should focus its efforts on those hazards that present the greatest risks.

The ideas in this draft represent our preliminary thoughts on this subject. A comprehensive food safety plan, describing actions and resources necessary to achieve the goals of reduced foodborne illness, will require extensive deliberation and in-depth discussion with all stakeholders in food safety, including consumers, state, tribal, and local public health officials, industry, and members of the scientific community. This draft is intended not as a prelude to government action, but an exploration of what might result from the upcoming seminars and conferences. While this initiative focuses on reducing the incidence of microbial foodborne illnesses, we recognize that chemical contaminants are also a cause of foodborne illness, but with chronic long term effects.

Background

The American food system provides consumers with an abundant supply of convenient, economical, high-quality, and safe food products. This system is built on the enterprise and innovative capacities of those who produce and market food in the United States, and it is driven by the high expectations of American consumers for the foods they purchase for their families.

Foodborne illness, however, still occurs in the United States. Over the last four years the Clinton Administration has developed and implemented major steps towards reinventing food regulation:

- In 1993, the Vice President's National Performance Review issued a blueprint for reinventing our nation's food safety system.

- The Food Safety and Inspection Service (FSIS) and the Food and Drug Administration (FDA) issued regulations that will require the meat, poultry, and seafood industries to follow Hazard

Analysis and Critical Control Points (HACCP) procedures. HACCP, which calls for food industries to implement preventive measures of their own design, will streamline regulation of these foods, increase the industries' responsibility for and control of their own safety-assurance actions, and generally bring regulation of meat, poultry, and seafood in line with state-of-the-art scientific procedures.

- Beginning in 1994, the Centers for Disease Control and Prevention (CDC) embarked upon a strategic program to detect, prevent, and control emerging infectious disease threats, some of which are foodborne, and has made significant progress toward this goal in each successive year.

- The Safe Drinking Water Act of 1996 includes responsible regulatory improvements to help states and water systems prevent drinking water contamination problems. Resources are provided for the first time for drinking water infrastructure that will help hundreds of communities protect their residents from harmful contaminants.

While these advances are significant, they may not be enough. New pathogens, new food products, huge increases in imported foods, the growing importance of food exports, and increasing antimicrobial resistance among foodborne pathogens present new challenges to the nation's food safety programs. The food safety system is in need of reform, especially reform that builds on the preventive principles embodied in HACCP.

History of the Food Safety Initiative

Achieving a significant reduction in the incidence of foodborne illnesses requires the cooperative efforts of public health and regulatory agencies at the federal, state, tribal and local levels, as well as all other parties responsible for and concerned about food safety and reducing the incidence of foodborne illness (i.e., consumers, industry, and academia). Partnerships—between public agencies and industry, federal agencies and state, tribal or local agencies, public agencies and academia, to name a few possibilities—will be invaluable in leveraging the resources focused on reducing the incidence of foodborne illness and enhancing communication.

Representatives of various government agencies have drafted a structure for the food safety initiative for your further deliberations. Ad hoc working groups, representing the varied perspectives of the FDA, CDC, the Department of Agriculture's Research, Education and Extension agencies, as well as the FSIS and Animal and Plant Health Inspection Service (APHIS), and the Environmental Protection Agency (EPA), have been meeting for several months to identify major food safety concerns and propose recommendations on what resources and activities are needed to have a significant impact on reducing the incidence of foodborne illness both in the short term and over the long term. The working groups worked from the premise that an effective food safety initiative must have several, interrelated components which, together, have far greater impact on reducing the incidence of foodborne illness than is possible to attain with any single component. Moreover, these elements must form the groundwork for the design and implementation of strategies to meet current needs, for continually evaluating the effectiveness of ongoing activities, and for identifying and implementing strategies to meet future needs. These elements include surveillance, coordination, risk assessment, research, inspections, and education.

This draft, which primarily defines short-term activities, describes the elements of a food safety initiative and tentatively identifies critical issues and the working groups' current thinking on preliminary recommendations. In some cases these recommendations have been included as part of the President's FY98 budget. However, no specific decision as to what will constitute the final food safety initiative, including how the strategic planning process is structured, have been made. Input from groups and individuals such as yourself, state, tribal and local agencies, consumers, industry, academia, and other stakeholders will be incorporated into the food safety initiative.

Foodborne Illness: A Significant Public Health Problem

Foodborne infections remain a major public health problem. The Council for Agricultural Science and Technology, a private non-profit organization, estimated in its 1994 report, Foodborne Pathogens: Risks and Consequences, that as many as 9,000 deaths and 6.5 to 33 million illnesses in the United States each year are food-related. Hospitalization costs alone for these illnesses are estimated at over $3 billion a year. Costs for lost productivity for 7 specific pathogens have been estimated to range between $6 billion and $9 billion. Total costs for all foodborne illnesses are likely to be much higher. These estimates do not take into account the total burden placed on society by the chronic, often life-long consequences caused by some foodborne pathogens.

Additional, important safety concerns are associated with the greater susceptibility to foodborne infections of several population groups. These include persons with lowered immunity due to HIV/AIDS, those on medications for cancer treatment or for organ transplantation, as well as pregnant women (and their fetuses), young children, and elderly persons. Patients taking antibiotics, or antacids, are also at greater risk of infection from some pathogens. Other groups who may be disproportionately affected include persons living in institutional settings, such as hospitals and nursing homes, and those with inadequate access to health care, such as homeless persons, migrant farm workers, and others of low socioeconomic status.

Sources of Foodborne Contamination

Sources of food contamination are almost as numerous and varied as the contaminants themselves. Bacteria and other infectious organisms are pervasive in the environment. *Salmonella enteritidis* enters eggs directly from the hen. Bacteria (occasionally pathogenic) inhabit the surfaces of fruits and vegetables in the field. Molds and their toxic byproducts can develop in grains during unusually wet or dry growing seasons, damage and stress during harvesting, or during improper storage. Seafood may become contaminated from agricultural and other runoff, as well as by sewage, microorganisms, and toxins present in marine environments. Many organisms that cause foodborne illness in humans can be part of the normal flora of the gastrointestinal tract of food-producing animals without any adverse effects to the animal. Milk, eggs, seafood, poultry, and meat from food-producing animals may become contaminated due to contaminated feed, misuse of veterinary drugs, or poor farming practices, including production and harvesting activities, or disposal of solid waste on land. Foods may become contaminated during processing due to malfunctioning or improperly sanitized equipment; misuse of cleaning materials; rodent and insect infestations; and improper storage. Foods may become contaminated in retail facilities and in the home through use of poor food handling practices.

Although many hazards threaten the safety of our food, certain foodborne hazards are of particular public health concern, and would be targeted for immediate attention by this initiative. Studies have shown that the following microbial pathogens are the predominant foodborne pathogens. They are: *Salmonella* species, *Campylobacter jejuni/coli*, *Escherichia coli* O157:H7 and other related strains; the parasites *Toxoplasma gondii* and *Cryptosporidium parvum*; and the Norwalk virus.

The microbial pathogens listed above, and discussed in greater detail below, may give rise to diseases that are far more serious than the uncomfortable but relatively temporary inconvenience of diarrhea and vomiting, which are the most common symptoms of so-called "food poisoning." Foodborne infections can result in very serious immediate consequences, such as spontaneous abortion, as well as long-lasting conditions such as reactive arthritis, Guillain-Barr, syndrome (the most common cause of acute paralysis in adults and children), and hemolytic uremic syndrome (HUS), which can lead to kidney failure and death, particularly in young children. The microbial pathogens described below are not listed in order of importance or severity.

Salmonella

Salmonella species cause diarrhea and systemic infections, which can be fatal in particularly susceptible persons, such as the immuno-compromised, the very young, and the elderly. An estimated 800,000 to 4 million infections occur each year in the United States, most of them as individual cases apparently unrelated to outbreaks. Animals used for food production are common carriers of *salmonella*e, which may subsequently contaminate foods such as meat, dairy products, and eggs. Foods often implicated in outbreaks include poultry and poultry products, meat and meat products, dairy products, egg products, seafood, and fresh produce. Between 128,000 and 640,000 of these infections are associated with *Salmonella enteritidis* (SE) in eggs. Over the past decade, more than 500 outbreaks have been attributed to SE with over 70 deaths. In 1994, an estimated 224,000 people became ill from consuming ice cream in one outbreak alone.

Campylobacter

The bacterium, *Campylobacter*, is the most frequently identified cause of acute infectious diarrhea in developed countries and is the most commonly isolated bacterial intestinal pathogen in the United States. It has been estimated that between 170,000 and 2.1 million cases of *campylobacter*iosis occur each year with an associated 120-360 deaths. *Campylobacter jejuni* and *Campylobacter coli* (2 closely related species) are commonly foodborne, and are the infectious agents most frequently described in association with Guillain-Barr, syndrome, perhaps as frequently as 1 in 1000 cases. Several prospective studies have implicated raw or undercooked chicken as major sources of *C. jejuni/coli* infections. Unpasteurized milk and untreated water have also caused outbreaks of disease.

Escherichia Coli O157:H7

Several strains of the bacterium *E. coli* cause a variety of diseases in humans and animals. *E. coli* O157:H7 is a type associated with a particularly severe form of human disease. *E. coli* O157:H7 causes hemorrhagic colitis, which begins with watery diarrhea and severe abdominal pain and rapidly progresses to passage of bloody stools, and has been associated with HUS. HUS is a life-threatening complication of hemorrhagic colitis characterized by acute kidney failure, and is particularly serious in young children. *E. coli* O157:H7 has its reservoir in cattle, but the dynamics of *E. coli* O157:H7 in food-producing animals are not well understood. It has been estimated that approximately 25,000 cases of foodborne illness can be attributed to *E. coli* O157:H7 each year with an estimated 6 deaths. *E. coli* O157:H7 outbreaks have recently been associated with ground beef, raw milk, lettuce, and minimally processed and fresh fruit juices. The most recent outbreak, in the Fall of 1996 in 3 western states and British Columbia, was associated with unpasteurized apple juice and sickened 66 people and caused the death of one child.

Toxoplasma Gondii

T. gondii is a parasitic protozoan. It has been estimated that 1.4 million cases of toxoplasmosis occur annually with an associated 310 deaths. Otherwise healthy adults who become infected usually have no symptoms, but may get diarrhea. Pregnant women who become infected during pregnancy may pass the disease to their fetuses. In infants infected before birth, fatal results are common. Should the infant survive, the effects of infection are typically severe. The disease can also be serious in persons with weakened immune systems and often is fatal to people with HIV/AIDS. *T. gondii* has been found in virtually all food animals. The two primary ways that humans become infected are consumption of raw or undercooked meat containing *T. gondii* or contact with cats that shed cysts in their feces during acute infection. Under some conditions, the consumption of unwashed fruits and vegetables may contribute to these infections.

Cryptosporidium Parvum

C. parvum is a parasitic protozoan. The most common consequence of infection in otherwise healthy people is profuse watery diarrhea lasting up to several weeks. Children are particularly susceptible. Cryptosporidiosis can be life-threatening among persons with weakened immune systems. The largest recorded outbreak of cryptosporidiosis was a waterborne outbreak that occurred in Milwaukee, Wisconsin in 1993, affecting over 400,000 people. More recently, a waterborne outbreak in Las Vegas resulted in at least 20 deaths attributed to Cryptosporidium. The first large outbreak of cryptosporidiosis from a contaminated food occurred in 1993. This outbreak was attributed to fresh-pressed apple cider. Cryptosporidium is found in feces of infected mammals and has been transmitted through contaminated water and food.

Norwalk Virus

Norwalk viruses are important causes of sporadic and epidemic gastrointestinal disease, that involve overwhelming, dehydrating diarrhea. An estimated 181,000 cases occur annually with no known associated deaths. In January 1995, a multi-state outbreak of viral gastroenteritis due to Norwalk virus was associated with the consumption of oysters. A 1993 Louisiana outbreak of Norwalk virus gastroenteritis, involved seventy ill people and was associated with the consumption of raw oysters. In 1992, another outbreak occurred which included 250 cases. Outbreaks of Norwalk virus intestinal disease have been linked to contaminated water and ice, salads, frosting, shellfish and person-to-person contact, although the most common food source is shellfish. Several such outbreaks are believed to have been caused by oysters contaminated by sewage dumped overboard by oyster harvesters and recreational boaters.

The Current System for Protecting Food

Ensuring the safety of food is one of the core functions of government. It is carried out by a system that, while generally successful in protecting the public, can be confusing for its complexity and diversity. Authority is divided among federal, state, and local governments; and the private sector also plays an important role. From the farm to the consumer's dinner table, the responsibilities can be summarized as:

- On the farm, food is regulated by state agencies supported principally by the EPA, which acts to ensure that pesticides are approved for safe use, by the FDA, which oversees use of drugs and feed in milk- and food-producing animals, and by APHIS, which is concerned with food-animal disease control. Federal responsibility also covers production and harvesting activities that discharge wastewater to surface and ground waters, and solid waste to land, all of which could contaminate growing and process waters or grazing land.

- Food processing for foods other than meat, poultry, and egg products (except shell eggs) is regulated by the FDA, whose inspectors are responsible for visiting about 53,000 plants periodically, with emphasis on the highest risk foods or processing techniques. FDA has fewer than 700 inspectors and analysts devoted to this activity. Meat, poultry, and all other egg products are regulated by FSIS, whose 8,000 inspectors are present in 6,500 slaughter and processing establishments to ensure that these products are safe, wholesome, and properly labeled. State and local governments also inspect food processors, with varying frequencies and under varying standards.

- Food being transported in interstate commerce is subject to federal and state regulation, although that area has received little attention in the past. USDA's FSIS and HHS's FDA have jointly published an Advanced Notice of Proposed Rulemaking (ANPR) on whether regulations are needed to govern the handling of meat, poultry, seafood, eggs, and other foods susceptible to harmful bacteria during transportation.

- The importation of food from foreign countries is overseen by FSIS for meat, poultry, and most egg products and FDA for all other foods. If an imported food is suspect, it can be tested for contamination and its entry into the United States denied.

- Restaurants, supermarkets, and institutional food services (such as schools and hospitals) are generally regulated by states and local health authorities, and FDA publishes the Food Code, which consists of model recommendations for safeguarding public health when food is offered to the consumer. Recommendations are developed by consensus of state government representatives at the

Conference for Food Protection. FSIS and FDA are working with states to update the Food Code in light of the changing retail and food service environment and emerging food safety issues, especially with regard to meat, poultry, egg products, and seafood. The Conference for Food Protection serves as one forum for fostering cooperation among federal, state and local governments in the oversight of food products and the conditions under which they are produced, processed, transported, stored, and handled through retail sale or food service to the consumer.

- National standards for drinking water are set by EPA, and enforced generally by local public water authorities; FDA establishes complementary standards for bottled water.

- Surveillance of foodborne illness is primarily the responsibility of state and local health departments and the CDC, which seek to identify cases of illness, determine their source, and control outbreaks. FDA or FSIS are called in when a link to a regulated food is suspected.

- In the home, consumers also have a responsibility for proper handling and storage of food, as consumer mishandling contributes to many cases of foodborne illness. As a result of this knowledge, FSIS promulgated safe handling labels for raw meat and poultry products.

- Other responsibilities related to food safety include research into the cause and transmission of foodborne illness, and education on treatment and prevention of foodborne illness. These responsibilities are carried out by the USDA, FDA, CDC, EPA, the National Institutes of Health, other federal components, and the states. Basic biomedical research on pathogenic organisms is conducted at the National Institutes of Health. The federal government also supports related research in universities. The private sector supports research within its own laboratories and in universities.

The Food Safety System Must be Prepared for the 21st Century

The system for identifying and preventing foodborne illnesses described above was largely created in the early years of this century.

It must be modernized. The current system is inadequate to properly identify, track, and prevent food-related illness and to prevent future cases from occurring. State and federal resources are not closely coordinated and duplication of effort is not uncommon. In 1981, FDA inspected food firms every 2-3 years, but can now visit those plants, on average, only once every 10 years. Our understanding of some disease causing organisms is so limited that our ability to protect the public health is seriously constrained. Food processors, restauranteurs, supermarket managers, and consumers often don't understand the threat from foodborne pathogens and the methods available to prevent and control them.

Immediate Actions to Improve Food Safety

There are many causes of foodborne illness, many points at which foods can become contaminated, and numerous factors that make some groups of people more susceptible than others. Needless to say, no single preventive measure will ensure the safety of all foods. However, a number of practical preventive steps can be taken immediately to reduce the incidence of many foodborne infections.

Any initiative designed to improve the safety of the food supply should focus on the hazards and foods that present the greatest risks to public health, should emphasize development and implementation of preventive controls of those risks, and should seek opportunities for such controls through a collaborative process with the responsible sectors of the food industry and all other stakeholders. This prevention-control concept is HACCP, a science-based, state-of-the-art process for building safety into the production, handling and storage of food. HACCP is being implemented by the meat, poultry, and seafood industries with FSIS and FDA regulatory oversight. The application of such preventive controls to other types of food may be important to protecting food in the years to come.

Under this initiative, the federal government, in concert with state and local governments would conduct research and risk assessments to determine how foodborne illnesses occur and can be prevented or controlled; improve surveillance and investigative efforts to locate and monitor illnesses caused by food; achieve more effective and efficient monitoring of the safety of the food supply through inspections of food processors; and reinvigorate education of all those involved in food preparation focusing on the use of safe practices. These issues, and our current thinking about them, are described below.

A New "Early Warning System" for Public Health Surveillance

Background

The primary goal of the American system of public health is to prevent disease before it occurs. While prevention of all disease may not be possible, stopping outbreaks of foodborne illness before they affect large numbers of people is a major goal. America needs a more effective early warning system that can catch outbreaks early, preventing illness and death. Such a system will also advance our understanding of foodborne illness and further our prevention efforts. In his January 25 radio address, the President announced a new national early warning system for foodborne illness that he is funding in his FY98 budget.

Preliminary Problem Identification

Surveillance and investigation of foodborne disease are powerful tools to detect new foodborne disease challenges, to determine what the specific food sources are, and to learn how best to keep the foods from becoming contaminated in the first place. Rapid detection of outbreaks is critical to stopping them before they affect many people. A key element in an early warning system is the ability to detect, compare, and communicate unusual patterns of illness and laboratory findings within and among states and among federal partners. Enhancing the capacity of states to monitor foodborne disease and to investigate and control outbreaks will lead to better general control measures and fewer illnesses. One way to achieve this is to expand the existing Active Foodborne Disease Surveillance Network (sentinel sites) to identify, investigate and control a broad spectrum of foodborne diseases. A second important way to enhance early warning is to increase the capacity of many states to deal with new foodborne challenges. These enhancements will help us identify outbreaks and other foodborne disease challenges early, and prevent illness and deaths.

Current Thinking

The federal government in cooperation with state and local health departments is proposing to take the following steps to establish a new national early warning system for, and enhance surveillance of, foodborne disease. These changes will result in an improved system for detecting and reporting foodborne illnesses and outbreaks that will enable public health agencies to rapidly put into place measures to control the spread of foodborne disease. This system will also collect critical data to recognize trends and target prevention strategies, including HACCP systems, and to evaluate the effectiveness and efficiency of prevention strategies already in place.

Enhance and Expand the Active Foodborne Disease Surveillance Program

CDC, FDA, and USDA currently support five food sentinel sites at state health departments to track cases of foodborne infections and to determine the sources of the most common ones. The existing sites should be strengthened, and the number of "enhanced" sites should be increased to 7 in FY 97, and to at least 8 in the following year. The sites and federal food safety agencies should be electronically linked together to create a powerful new network to detect, respond to, and prevent outbreaks of foodborne illness. Adding additional states will improve geographic and demographic representation, making this network more likely to detect diseases and outbreaks that are regional rather than national in distribution.

Enhance Early Detection of Foodborne Disease Nationwide

In addition to establishing enhanced food sentinel sites, an early warning system would require improved early detection of foodborne disease in additional states in FY 98 by providing resources for improved surveillance, investigation, control, and prevention of foodborne disease outbreaks. While sophisticated laboratory studies can identify causes of illness and show relationships among bacteria, laboratory methods are insufficient without investigators who can collect samples, interview people, and trace the source of contamination to find out why the illness occurred. New electronic tools need to be developed to enable rapid detection of outbreaks, and to enhance communication about outbreaks to appropriate agencies. CDC also should provide additional resources to states to increase their surveillance and response capacity for the serious long-term consequences of foodborne disease, such as hemolytic uremic syndrome.

Modernize Public Health Laboratories

CDC should provide resources and training to upgrade public health laboratory capabilities in the Active Surveillance sites and in other states so that they can rapidly identify a broad range of foodborne infections including new parasitic and viral pathogens, and can use new techniques of DNA "fingerprinting." CDC would work with states to develop, standardize, and transfer those methods. These new capacities would allow rapid identification of the cause of some outbreaks that currently go undiagnosed.

Create a National Electronic Network for "Fingerprint" Comparison

CDC should fund a new computer network and database system that would capture bacterial "fingerprints" in a national database, linking CDC, FDA, USDA, and states that have this new capacity as well as the federal laboratories into a new national network. This technology would, for example, permit rapid recognition that an *E. coli* O157:H7 bacterium cultured from a patient in Washington was indistinguishable from one isolated from another patient in California, which would suggest to public health investigators that a product distributed in both California and Washington may be contaminated with the organism.

In addition to identifying, investigating, and reporting cases of foodborne disease in humans, surveillance of contamination levels in foods, in animals used for food, and in their feed is important to control and prevent foodborne diseases, and to monitor the measures that reduce the risk of exposure. Therefore, to make the "early warning system" fully operational, and to translate its findings into long-term improvements in the safety of the food supply, additional surveillance activities would be required.

Increase National Surveillance for Antimicrobial Resistance of Foodborne Pathogens

CDC should expand surveillance for antimicrobial resistance in *Campylobacter*, *Salmonella*, and *E. coli* O157:H7 isolated in humans, and FDA and USDA should take similar steps for bacterial samples from food-producing animals and food products, in a way that permits these data to be compared. CDC, FDA and USDA should develop standard procedures for sharing necessary information, and for responding to increases in resistance, or other "red flag events" such as the discovery of an important new resistant bacterium.

Enhance Oversight of Animal Feeds and Feedstuffs for the Impact of Drugs and Other Therapies in Food Animal Populations and Pathogens

FDA may consider increasing monitoring of animal feed processing to determine the nature and extent of pathogen contamination and the impact of control strategies on pathogen reduction in animals.

Coordination

Background

At the federal level, there are four agencies charged with responding to outbreaks of foodborne illness (including waterborne illness): FDA and CDC at HHS, FSIS at USDA, and EPA. While CDC's primary responsibility is to work with state and local health departments to identify and investigate sporadic cases and outbreaks of illness, FDA, FSIS, and EPA have the additional responsibility of taking regulatory action against the suspect products, or those who contaminate the air, land, or waters used to produce the food product. Which regulatory agency gets involved depends on the type of food involved, with FSIS having primary jurisdiction over meat, poultry, and egg products, FDA over all other foods including shell eggs and EPA over water and pesticides. While each agency has clearly defined areas of responsibility, most outbreaks of foodborne illness involve more than one agency.

In addition, investigations of foodborne illness usually begin at the community or state level. These illnesses may cross jurisdictional boundaries and may be linked to foods or food ingredients that were processed or produced in another state or by international trading partners, necessitating the involvement of federal agencies. Federal involvement is also necessary when contaminated foods from the same sources may be in grocery stores, restaurants, and homes in other parts of the country. Companies responsible for affected products also have a critical role to play as many product recalls are voluntary.

In most outbreaks of foodborne illness, federal agencies work with state and local health authorities in their investigations and implementation of control measures through consultation, diagnostic assistance, and recommendations for control measures. In some instances on-site assistance is requested by the local and state authorities. For large or multi-state outbreaks, federal agencies play a critical coordination role to assure consistency of approach and implementation of needed control measures.

Preliminary Problem Identification

Although significant coordination already occurs among the federal and state agencies, the mere fact that more than one agency is involved in any one outbreak of foodborne illness can cause some confusion. Many times a joint effort is hindered by a lack of communication or a misunderstanding of each agency's role in a particular situation.

Current Thinking

Improved coordination among the federal agencies, between federal and state agencies, and among the various state agencies would enhance the level of public health protection, make the best use of interagency collaboration, and avoid duplication of effort.

Improve Federal/State Coordination in the Management of Response to Foodborne Illness

A Foodborne Outbreak Response Coordinating Group made up of representatives of the federal and state agencies charged with responding to outbreaks of foodborne illness should be created to coordinate the investigation and response to significant outbreaks of foodborne illness. The overall goal of this group should be to ensure that a coordinated and professional response, with all governmental resources pulling together, is undertaken to effectively investigate and respond to foodborne illness. The group should determine jointly each agency's responsibilities during the various phases of outbreak investigations, and who would play the role of spokesperson for each phase or component of an outbreak. In addition, the group should coordinate communications and decisions about appropriate actions during outbreaks and appropriate follow-up to prevent similar outbreaks. The coordinating group should also meet several times a year to review its work and the response to outbreaks.

Each participating agency could fund and enhance programs that provide opportunities to exchange employees, on a temporary basis, among federal agencies and between federal and state agencies. Such an exchange would facilitate coordination by sharing expertise and providing an opportunity to better understand the various roles each agency plays in an investigation of a foodborne illness.

Improve Federal/State Coordination in the Management and Response to Foodborne Illness

Better coordination between federal and state agencies and among the various state agencies would speed the identification and subsequent control of foodborne illness and the removal of the contaminated foods from the distribution chain.

In order to improve coordination, the federal agencies can sponsor a national meeting with state and local officials to develop recommendations on how to better coordinate the overall government response to foodborne illness.

For example, one specific issue that is discussed in FDA's FY98 budget is the occurrence of *Salmonella enteritidis* in layer hens and improved monitoring of the hens and liquid bulk egg products (before pasteurization) for contamination. The federal agencies should work to establish a federal/state cooperative program to solve this problem.

Enhance the Basic Infrastructure for Foodborne Illness Surveillance and Coordination at State Health Departments

The epidemiology offices and laboratories within state health departments are charged with the surveillance of infectious and non-infectious conditions, and, along with other state officials, with the investigation of outbreaks. They collect surveillance data from physicians, laboratories, local health departments and other sources. Yet, the resources available in many states for the surveillance and investigation of foodborne diseases are limited and decreasing, thereby limiting the states' effectiveness. As a result, outbreaks may go undetected or are never investigated.

This problem could be rectified by making sure that, given an assessment and cataloguing of available state resources, states are provided support for foodborne disease surveillance programs and assistance to better investigate outbreaks of foodborne illness.

Risk Assessment

Background

It is a basic public health tenet that public resources devoted to reducing risks should be in proportion to the toll they take on human health. Risk assessment is the tool best suited to set priorities among public health risks. Furthermore, risk assessment is a requirement for any science-based system of preventive controls. Indeed, risk assessments and evaluations of alternative risk management strategies are often carried out for major federal regulations. Pursuant to the USDA's Reorganization Act of 1994, USDA is required to conduct risk analyses for all major regulations. Such evaluations ensure that risk reduction strategies are cost effective and promote the maximum net benefit to society of efforts to reduce foodborne illness. Sound risk assessments, including bacterial, parasitic, and viral food contaminants, are also critical to World Trade Organization treaty negotiations, which require that U.S. food safety standards be based on scientifically valid measures derived through risk assessment.

Preliminary Problem Identification

Risk assessment's objective is to characterize the nature and size of the risk to human health associated with hazards, and to make clear the degree of scientific certainty of the data and the assumptions used to develop the estimates. Risk assessments require a substantial amount of specific information on the hazard and on the exposed population to provide meaningful information for those making risk management decisions. Even for chemical hazards, for which risk assessment methods have been most thoroughly developed, data gaps force the use of assumptions about exposure, hazard potency, and characteristics of the population at risk, and mathematical "models" of chemical action or of the way that the body deals with a chemical.

Risk assessment is far less developed for foodborne pathogens. Intensive commitment is necessary to develop critically needed data such as pathogen behavior in numerous foods under hundreds of conditions, and information about especially sensitive populations, such as children.

Current Thinking

This initiative's risk assessment activities would focus on developing better use of data and better models to inform surveillance plans, HACCP-based prevention strategies for process control systems and for food inspections, and research programs to fill critical food safety information gaps.

Establish a Risk Assessment Consortium

All federal agencies with risk management responsibilities should establish jointly a new consortium at which federal agencies can set collective priorities for risk assessment research and collective priorities and strategies for the further development and implementation of risk assessment and risk management. The consortium should be established at the Joint Institute for Food Safety and Applied Nutrition, a collaborative activity of FDA's Center for Food Safety and Applied Nutrition and the University of Maryland.

The consortium should focus federal research on developing data for risk assessments, focused and applied specifically to address the scientific, risk-based goal of preventive control that is the central principle of this food safety initiative.

Research supported and conducted through this initiative should cover several areas critical to developing our ability to conduct risk assessments for foodborne disease-causing organisms and to assess the effectiveness of control measures. Data and methods developed in response to the Safe Drinking Water Act Amendments of 1996, for example, will be relevant to food safety evaluations.

Develop Better Data and Modeling Techniques to Assess Exposure to Microbial and Chemical Contaminants, Including Animal Drug Residues, Through the Food Supply

Risk assessment of foodborne illness is dependent on accurately estimating the quantity of a toxin or pathogen ingested by the consumer (i.e., exposure assessment). This initiative would address the numerous data and modeling deficiencies in estimating exposure to microbial and chemical contaminants. Specifically, research should be conducted in: incidence and prevalence of microbial pathogens and chemical hazards in food; typical behaviors of commercial and home preparation operations; validation of dynamic exposure assessment models; intake data regarding food consumption patterns of the general population and sensitive subpopulations; and specific data on food vehicles of sporadic and epidemic disease. Research using biomarkers should be pursued. Biomarkers are surrogates that indicate that exposure has occurred or that some effect has occurred, particularly when actual evidence of exposure and effect are difficult or impossible to obtain.

Develop Dose-Response Assessment Models for Use in Risk Assessment

Research is needed to estimate the relationship between the quantity of a biological agent and the frequency and magnitude of adverse human health effects in a population. Dose-response assessments typically include estimates of the rates of infection, morbidity, and mortality. For bacterial hazards, the World Health Organization's Expert Consultation on the Application of Risk Analysis to Food Standards Issues (FAO/WHO, March 1995) refers to these steps as "hazard characterization."

Bioscience Research

Background

Currently, one of the most critical needs in food safety research is for techniques to more rapidly and accurately identify and characterize foodborne hazards. FDA, CDC, EPA, and the USDA's Research, Education, and Economics agencies (the Agricultural Research Service, the Cooperative State Research, Education, and Extension Service) conduct research related to pathogenic microorganisms and other contaminants that threaten the safety of food.

Preliminary Problem Identification

New pathogens, some of them foodborne, have emerged over the last 10 years. Many of these organisms can not be easily detected, or detected at all in foods. Other microorganisms, previously thought to be innocuous, have emerged as more virulent. Just because organisms are present at levels that can not be easily detected, however, does not mean that the organisms can not cause human illness. Newly recognized pathogens are causing serious disease outbreaks. Foodborne pathogens are increasingly overcoming time-tested controls, such as heating and refrigeration, and are developing new virulence and new ways to evade our immune defenses.

Current Thinking

Effective control of foodborne pathogens requires that prevention be targeted at high-risk foods and at high-risk points in their production and distribution. These interventions ideally are guided by risk assessment, for which all too often we have insufficient data. Research is needed to support HACCP implementation, to enable verification that critical control points in HACCP systems are working, and to target the data gaps that hamper risk assessment. Among the data gaps and information needs identified here are numerous opportunities for collaboration and resource leveraging among federal agencies, the private sector, and universities.

Improved Detection Methods

As stated above, many foodborne pathogens cannot be easily detected, or detected at all in foods. Methods need to be developed, validated, and implemented for rapid testing of very low levels of *Campylobacter*, *Salmonella*, Toxoplasma, Vibrio, *E. coli* O157:H7, Cyclospora, Cryptosporidium, Norwalk virus and naturally occurring toxins in food animals, in agricultural and aquaculture products, animal feeds, and processed food products. Some research efforts may initially focus on *Campylobacter*, because those foodborne infections are so prevalent and may lead to chronic diseases (Guillain-Barré syndrome); also methods to isolate and identify this pathogen are time-consuming and expensive. Research could be coordinated with EPA's efforts to develop better test methods and assessments of health effects from Cryptosporidium and other contaminants in drinking water. Improved methods are needed for identifying foodborne pathogens, including emerging pathogens, in clinical specimens and to subtype known foodborne pathogens.

Understanding Antimicrobial Resistance

Microorganisms can become resistant to antimicrobial agents and conditions that have been traditionally relied on to eliminate or prevent the growth of foodborne pathogens, but have become insufficient to prevent breakthrough of newly emerging pathogens. Research is needed to determine how microorganisms associated with foodborne disease become tolerant to various types of antimicrobials and to traditional food safety safeguards such as heat or cold, low pH, high salt, and disinfectants and to elucidate factors in animal and plant production systems and processing environments that influence the development of resistance. This research will lead to the identification of food production and processing practices that are likely to permit pathogen contamination or proliferation and will provide guidance in the modification of traditional techniques or the development of new techniques to prevent or control pathogen growth.

Understanding Antibiotic Drug Resistance

Pathogens in food-producing animals may become resistant to drugs partially due to improper use of the drugs, particularly antibiotic drugs, in those animals. One possible way to deal with this problem might be to adjust the required period of drug withdrawal prior

403

to slaughter. For example, studies should be conducted to explore possible changes to "withdrawal time" requirements that could reduce transfer of resistant pathogens with minimal disruption to industry production practices. In addition, industry in collaboration with federal agencies could determine the basis for the ability of microorganisms to rapidly adapt to changing environments and, together, develop animal production and treatment mechanisms to minimize this adaptive ability.

Prevention Techniques: Pathogen Control, Reduction, and Elimination

Contaminants are introduced into the food supply at numerous points along the way from farm to store. Food animals may carry pathogens, but remain healthy themselves, complicating controls at the point of slaughter. Animal feed and drinking water can be "hidden" but significant sources of contamination. Possible research recommendations to address these problems for *Salmonella, Campylobacter,* Toxoplasma, Vibrio, *E. coli* O157:H7, Cyclospora, Cryptosporidium, and Norwalk virus in all food products are the following (to be carried out in conjunction with universities and the private sector):

- Develop drugs and other therapies to prevent initial colonization.

- Develop new methods to reduce or eliminate contaminants from animals and plants before slaughter or harvest.

- Develop new disinfection methods and equipment and systems modifications for processing and production plants, and wholesale and retail outlets.

- Develop new methods of surface decontamination of fresh fruits, vegetables, meat, poultry.

- Develop heat-based and/or other disinfection methods for seafood, meat, eggs, produce, and animal feeds.

Food Handling, Distribution, and Storage

Food production and processing often occur thousands of miles apart. Transportation systems for live animals, fresh produce, and packaged foods offer many opportunities for contamination, such as heat, cold, and other stresses that make animals and plants more susceptible to infection, and cross-contamination from the vehicle itself. Possible research recommendations include the following:

- Investigate immune system "biomarkers" of stress that might indicate predisposition to infection during transport.

- Develop in- or on-package sensors of storage conditions to alert consumers of products not stored safely.

Inspections

Background

Inspection of commercial food processors is an integral part of the food safety assurance system. Inspections are carried out by federal, state and local authorities, with state and local officials focusing primarily on restaurants, supermarkets and other retail establishments. At the federal level, consistent with legal mandates, FSIS has carcass-by-carcass inspection in meat, poultry, and slaughter plants while they are operating, and continuous inspection in meat, poultry, and egg-product processing plants—in all, about 8,000 inspectors for 6,500 domestic plants and for all imported meat, poultry, and egg products. FDA does periodic, random inspections of all other food processing plants—less than 700 inspectors and analysts for 53,000 U.S. plants and for all other imported foods.

Preliminary Problem Identification

At FDA, the number of inspections has decreased steadily since 1981, when 21,000 inspections were conducted, so that today resources exist to carry out only about 5,000 inspections per year. The result is that an FDA-regulated plant gets inspected by FDA, on the average, only once every 10 years. FDA also relies upon the states to conduct some inspections under contract, but that number has dropped from 12,000 in 1985 to 5,000 now. Moreover, the inspectional coverage of imported foods has dropped as well, as the same number of import inspectors are now inspecting almost twice as many imports as just five years ago. Certainly FDA is finding greater problems, e.g., the number of products recalled for life-threatening microbial contamination has increased almost 5-fold since 1988 and inspectors are finding more hazardous conditions in the plants they inspect. FSIS is faced with a similar challenge of continually providing the most effective inspection program with limited resources and growing threats to food safety.

Current Thinking

Scientists and other food safety experts have concluded that the most effective and efficient mechanism for assuring that food processors identify and control hazards that could threaten food is the application of the HACCP concept of built-in preventive controls. FDA has begun to implement HACCP for the seafood industry, and FSIS for the meat and poultry industries; FSIS intends to publish an ANPR requesting comments on HACCP systems for egg processing plants, and FDA plans to work with the food industry, as it has in a pilot program over the last 2 years. To ensure that HACCP is properly implemented, and to ensure more efficient and effective monitoring of the safety of the food supply, the following preliminary recommendations are being made.

Enhance Development of HACCP Procedures

FDA is considering whether and how to implement HACCP throughout the non-meat/poultry food industry for all appropriate food commodities. It is recognized that staged implementation, by commodity, might be necessary because of resource limitations. To ensure that HACCP is being properly implemented, FDA should conduct inspections and provide necessary training and outreach activities. FSIS will continue development of a HACCP-based inspection system. FSIS plans to conduct a public meeting and then subsequent field trials to gather data to support future decisions on designing new inspection procedures in a HACCP environment.

Upgrade FDA's Food Inspection Program

FDA has included implementation of seafood HACCP in its FY98 budget request. If HACCP is to be an effective program for ensuring that food processors have modern, state-of-the-art food safety procedures in effect, FDA must improve its inspection capabilities, so that the highest risk food plants (such as seafood) are inspected at least once per year. To maximize the joint federal/state role in inspections, development of new partnerships with the states may be considered, that focus on coordinating the inspection coverage and preventing duplication of effort.

FSIS and FDA may consider expanding and re-focusing existing cooperative agreements under which plants producing both meat and non-meat foods are inspected solely by FSIS inspectors, who have been trained in FDA inspectional standards. FSIS inspectors are already in these plants; their presence could be better utilized to maximize use of federal resources.

FSIS and FDA are considering whether and how to regulate the transportation of meat, poultry, seafood, eggs and other foods in order to safeguard the public from pathogenic microorganisms, as reflected in the ANPR published on November 22, 1996.

Enhance Federal/State Inspection Partnerships

Additional federal/state partnerships can ensure improved coordination between the federal food safety agencies and state regulators for the training of state inspectors in federal food safety standards, as well as provide the states with equipment and technology for the rapid sharing of inspection results and for a national database for the monitoring of all food inspections. This information sharing would help both federal and state regulators make inspections more effective and efficient.

FDA may consider establishing a process for certifying private laboratories that would be authorized to test samples of food products for contaminants. This may embody a similar process currently being discussed by a coalition of industry, private laboratories, professional associations, and accrediting bodies with input from federal agencies. Such private parties would provide a service to food firms wishing to demonstrate that their products meet applicable federal standards.

Enhance Inspectional Coverage of Imported Food, to Address the Problem of Rising Imports and FDA's Inability to Provide Adequate Inspections of Them

FDA should develop more Mutual Recognition Agreements (MRAs) with foreign countries, under which both countries agree to inspect each other's food exporting firms under equivalent procedures for ensuring safety. Once such MRAs are in place, FDA could better focus its import inspections on foods coming from countries with the least reliable safety standards.

Education

Background

Educating people about steps they must take to prevent and control foodborne illness is a vital link in the food preparation chain.

Educational efforts have already been made at the federal level. For example, FDA has a website which offers information on many food safety issues, has established a 24-hour seafood hotline, and has published brochures on such topics as food safety advice for persons with AIDS and posters on such topics as listeria in soft cheese. USDA has taken similar steps through its Cooperative Extension network, its Meat and Poultry Hotline, and by requiring safe handling instruction labels for meat and poultry products.

Preliminary Problem Identification

Despite these efforts, and the work that states, consumer groups and the food industry have done in this area, foodborne illness still occurs from a lack of knowledge of the risks involved at all stages of food preparation. For instance, choices consumers make about how they handle food prepared at home and whether they eat food that increases the risk of foodborne illness can have a significant impact on the incidence of foodborne illness. Studies show, for example, that 53% of the public eat food with raw eggs, 23% eat undercooked hamburger, 17% eat raw clams and oysters, and 26% do not wash their cutting boards after using them for raw meat or poultry.

Foodborne illnesses have also been traced to commercial food establishments. For example, many food establishments do not know that the pooling and undercooking of eggs can increase the risk of *Salmonella enteritidis*. Currently, a much higher percentage of those who receive their food in an institutional environment are victimized by the more serious consequences of foodborne illness. For example, during 1988 to 1992, *Salmonella* caused 69% of the 796 bacterial foodborne disease outbreaks; 60% of these *Salmonella* outbreaks were caused by S. *enteritidis*. S. *enteritidis* also resulted in more deaths than any other pathogen with 85% of these deaths occurring among residents of nursing homes.

Producers of animals used in human foods production and veterinarians treating such animals also need education in food safety practice. Drugs used to treat these animals are not always used appropriately, and can be purchased over the counter by non-veterinarians and misused, resulting in harmful residues in meat and milk, decreased effectiveness of these drugs, and increased antimicrobial resistance.

Finally, those responsible for the transportation of food are often unaware of unsafe practices that result in the contamination and mishandling of food during shipment.

Current Thinking

Understanding and practicing proper food handling procedures from farm to table would significantly reduce foodborne illness.

Improve Consumer Education

An alliance including industry and consumer groups should mount a comprehensive food safety awareness campaign for consumers, highly focused on messages and tactics targeted to the general public and to special populations such as high-risk consumers. The campaign should be centered around an easily recognized symbol or catch phrase and should include a national print and broadcast media campaign and incorporate food safety messages into school curricula. An emphasis should be placed on multilingual activities to ensure the widest coverage.

Innovative methods for sharing information related to food handling behaviors should be developed in order to reach larger audiences. As part of this effort, a National Food Safety Education Alliance of industry, consumer, trade, state and local food protection agencies, and academic organizations focused on changing unsafe food handling practices should be convened. Research should be conducted to determine effective methods of providing information and evaluation of educational programs. A national clearinghouse should be established to provide consumers and food safety educators with food safety information.

Improve Retail, Food Service, and Institutional Education

A highly focused campaign should be developed to change food workers' unsafe food preparation behaviors. A multilingual approach should be developed. An alliance of federal, state, and local health agencies, as well as private parties, should be formed to develop education efforts on food safety issues. Activities of the alliance should include educating retail food service workers about the safe handling perishable food product provisions in the 1997 Food Code.

In addition, guidelines should be developed by USDA and the states for retail and food service operations which process meat and poultry products to train state level inspectors to identify hazards at the retail level. Efforts should also be undertaken to educate the retail, food service and institutional industries in order to increase the use of HACCP principles.

Improve Veterinary and Producer Education

Development and implementation of a program could be considered to educate producers of animals for human food consumption, veterinarians, state and local regulators about proper drug use and the incorporation of HACCP principles into industry quality assurance programs. The program could entail regularly scheduled training sessions, including satellite teleconferences, educational symposia, and presentations at producer and practitioner meetings. Guidelines and educational materials could also be developed and disseminated through a national clearinghouse to food producers and the veterinary medical community.

Improve Industry Education in the Transportation Area

Government agencies could form an alliance to develop educational materials and train food transportation vehicle owners and operators and food processing establishments on hazards associated with the transportation of food products, particularly hazards associated with temperature controls, prior cargoes, and sanitation methods. Training and education for state and local health and transportation authorities could also be conducted so they can apply this information during inspections of food processing facilities and transportation vehicles in their jurisdiction.

A Strategic Plan for Reducing Foodborne Illness Over the Long Term

Background

The broad issues of a sustainable safe food system include, among other issues, improving the infrastructure for rapid identification and response to outbreaks, improving coordination among all food safety participants in numerous aspects of prevention and response, and developing a strategic, long-range research agenda. Stakeholders include food producers and manufacturers, consumers, academic institutions, representatives from the food service sector, including retail, restaurant, and institutional food service settings, veterinary and medical professionals, and federal, state, and local public health and agricultural officials.

Preliminary Problem Identification

Making the necessary improvements in the food safety system will not be easy. Because so many lines of authority must be crossed, so many new working relationships established, and so many fundamental changes in infrastructure made, the current system must be "reinvented." For example, the federal government needs to develop a long-term, coordinated research agenda to truly address research needs to support a fundamentally improved food safety system, and strategies for developing such an agenda would need to be developed through such a planning process. Extensive dialogue will be required among the many stakeholders in various regions of the country to agree upon priorities, strategies for achieving change, and a process for achieving change.

Current Thinking

A significant activity proposed as part of this food safety initiative is the creation of a process that facilitates the participation of all stakeholders in discussing the issues and setting an agenda for consideration of fundamental change in the food safety system. A contract could be established with an independent organization to bring together all major stakeholders for discussion of fundamental changes to the present food safety system. A major purpose of this strategic planning exercise would be to identify changes that should be made to the present organizational and procedural structure that would bring about permanent improvements in efficiency and coordination. Dialogue groups could be established to develop a strategic plan. Opportunities for input could include symposia held in geographically dispersed sites to encourage stakeholder participation.

Documents developed from the deliberations and recommendations of these symposia could be the focus of further discussion during a series of open meetings. The product of this series of dialogues, symposia, and hearings could form a report, which would provide the outline necessary for targeting needed structural changes in the federal/state food safety system.

Chapter 32

What to Do if You Have a Problem with Food Products

Problems:

A. Your hot dog has a strip of plastic inside.

B. The canned chili contains a metal washer.

C. You think a restaurant dinner made you ill.

D. A sugar-coated roach was in your box of cereal.

What Can You Do?

- For help with meat, poultry and egg products (examples A and B): Call the toll-free USDA Meat and Poultry Hotline at 1 (800) 535-4555.

- For help with restaurant food problems (example C): Call the Health Department in your city, county or state.

- For help with non-meat food products (example D): For complaints about food products which do not contain meat or poultry—such as cereal—call or write to the Food and Drug Administration (FDA). Check your local phone book under U.S. Government, Health and Human Services, to find an FDA office in your area. The FDA's Seafood Hotline is at 1 (800) 332-4010.

USDA Food Safety and Inspection Service Home Page, May 1996.

In order for the USDA to investigate a problem with meat, poultry or egg products, you must have:

1. the original container or packaging;
2. the foreign object (the plastic strip or metal washer, for example); and
3. any uneaten portion of the food (refrigerate or freeze it).

Information you should be ready to tell the Hotline on the phone includes:

1. your name, address and phone number;
2. the brand name, product name and manufacturer of the product;
3. the size and package type;
4. can or package codes (not UPC bar codes) and dates;
5. establishment number (EST) usually found in the circle or shield near the "USDA passed and inspected" phrase;
6. name and location of store and date you purchased the product.
7. You can complain to the store or the product's manufacturer if you don't choose to make a formal complaint to the USDA.

If You Think You are Ill, See a Physician

1. If an injury or illness allegedly resulted from use of a meat or poultry product, you will also need to tell the Hotline staff about the type, symptoms, time of occurrence and name of attending health professional (if applicable).

2. If you can't reach the Hotline staff, or if an injury or illness allegedly resulted from restaurant food, call your local the Health Department.

3. If an injury or illness allegedly resulted from non-meat food products, call or write to the FDA.

The bottom line: If you sense there's a problem with any food product, don't consume it. "When in doubt, throw it out."

For Further Information Contact:

FSIS Food Safety Education and Communications Staff
Meat and Poultry Hotline
Phone: 1-800-535-4555

Part Five

National Institutes of Health

Chapter 33

National Institutes of Health Almanac

Introduction

Begun as a one-room Laboratory of Hygiene in 1887, the National Institutes of Health today is one of the world's foremost biomedical research centers. An agency of the Department of Health and Human Services, the NIH is the Federal focal point for health research.

NIH is the steward of biomedical and behavioral research for the Nation. Its mission is science in pursuit of fundamental knowledge about the nature and behavior of living systems and the application of that knowledge to extend healthy life and reduce the burdens of illness and disability. The goals of the agency are as follows: 1) foster fundamental creative discoveries, innovative research strategies, and their applications as a basis to advance significantly the Nation's capacity to protect and improve health; 2) develop, maintain, and renew scientific human and physical resources that will assure the Nation's capability to prevent disease; 3) expand the knowledge base in biomedical and associated sciences in order to enhance the Nation's economic well-being and ensure a continued high return on the public investment in research; 4) exemplify and promote the highest level of scientific integrity, public accountability, and social responsibility in the conduct of science.

In realizing these goals, the NIH provides leadership and direction to programs designed to improve the health of the Nation by conducting

Excerpted from NIH Publication No. 96-5, September 1996.

and supporting research: in the causes, diagnosis, prevention, and cure of human diseases; in the processes of human growth and development; in the biological effects of environmental contaminants; in the understanding of mental, addictive and physical disorders; in directing programs for the collection, dissemination, and exchange of information in medicine and health, including the development and support of medical libraries and the training of medical librarians and other health information specialists.

The Organization

Office of the Director

The director of NIH gives overall leadership to NIH activities and maintains close liaison with the DHHS assistant secretary for health in matters relating to medical research, research training, health professions education and training, manpower resources, and biomedical communications.

The NIH director also maintains close communications with other constituents of DHHS in order to provide more effective program relationships.

To fulfill these responsibilities and obligations, the director is assisted by a professional executive and administrative staff.

A deputy director shares in the overall direction of the activities of the National Institutes of Health.

A deputy director for intramural research deals with the scientific policy problems of the research institutes and divisions and represents them in the overall policy councils of NIH. An associate director for intramural affairs and an assistant director for intramural planning aid in maintaining overall direction of all intramural research.

A deputy director for extramural research—in collaboration with an associate director for extramural affairs—directs the development and coordination of NIH policies and procedures for awarding funds in support of medical research and provides policy guidance for the Division of Research Grants, which administers and processes grant applications.

An associate director for disease prevention supervises medical technology assessment and transfer from the laboratory to the clinical setting. This assessment is provided through the Consensus Development Conference, under the Office of Medical Applications of Research.

The associate director for AIDS research formulates scientific policy and recommends allocation of resources for AIDS research at NIH.

An associate director for clinical care is adviser to the director on maters and policies pertaining to clinical research conducted or supported by NIH.

An associate director for research services is responsible for the management of technical and selected administrative services to all NIH components and provides national leadership in research safety policy and methodology. Four primary units function under the associate director—the Divisions of Engineering Services; Safety; Space Management; and Technical Services.

An associate director for science policy and legislation assesses the growth of medical research nationally and applies these findings to future program planning; evaluating external factors and trends affecting NIH activities, and evaluating legislative development relevant to NIH programs and policies. The associate director functions through two Divisions—Program Analysis and Legislative Analysis.

An associate director for administration guides NIH management procedures and activities; advises on, develops and implements policies, procedures and methods for budget, contracts and grants management, financial analysis, accounting, auditing, and personnel management functions. The ADA functions through seven divisions: Financial Management; Management Policy; Management Survey and Review; Personnel Management; Procurement; Logistics; and Contracts and Grants.

An associate director for communications is primary policy adviser on communications activities, including scientific and public information. The office is also responsible for overall direction, planning, and coordination of NIH information activities, and directs information liaison with DHHS and constituent agencies.

The Office of Recombinant DNA Activities (ORDA) was established in 1974 as a result of nationwide concerns over the safety of research involving the manipulation of genetic material. First located in the National Institute of General Medical Sciences, ORDA was transferred to the National Institute of Allergy and Infectious Diseases in September 1979, and in 1988, to the Office of the Director, NIH. ORDA is responsible for administering the Recombinant DNA Advisory Committee, and for ensuring compliance with the "NIH Guidelines for Research Involving Recombinant DNA Molecules." To this end, ORDA serves as a national focal point for information and for providing advice to organizations including biosafety committees, Federal agencies, state and local governments, and the biotechnology industry.

An associate director for research on women's health is responsible for ensuring that NIH-supported research focuses on issues pertinent

419

to women's health, assuring that women are included in biomedical and behavioral research, and enhancing opportunities for women in biomedical careers. The associate director serves as director of the Office of Research on Women's Health and as codirector of the Women's Health Initiative.

National Cancer Institute

Mission

NCI's overall mission is to conduct and support research, training, health information dissemination, and other programs with respect to the cause, diagnosis, prevention, and treatment of cancer and the continuing care of cancer patients and the families of cancer patients.

The National Cancer Program consists of 1) an expanded, intensified, and coordinated cancer research program encompassing the research programs conducted and supported by the institute, and the related research programs of the other national research institutes, including an expanded and intensified research program for the prevention of cancer caused by occupational or environmental exposure to carcinogens, and 2) the other programs and activities of the institute.

The National Cancer Institute also conducts control research for the prevention, detection, diagnosis, and treatment of cancer and for the rehabilitation and continuing care needs of patients respecting cancer. All cancer prevention and control activities focus on reducing cancer incidence, morbidity, and mortality through an orderly sequence of research on interventions and their impact in defined populations to the broad application of the research results through demonstration and education programs. NCI also supports:

- information and education programs to collect, identify, analyze and disseminate to cancer patients and their families, physicians and other health professionals, and the general public, information on cancer research, diagnosis, prevention and treatment (including nutrition programs for cancer patients and the relationship between nutrition and cancer).

- national cancer research and demonstration centers which conduct basic and clinical research into training in. and demonstration of advanced diagnostic prevention and treatment methods.

420

Other mission activities include:

- collaboration with voluntary organizations and other institutions and societies engaged in cancer research and cancer education activities. Encouraging and coordinating cancer research by industrial concerns showing particular capability for such research.

- Support of cancer research outside the United States to benefit the American people, and training of American scientists abroad and foreign scientists in the U.S.

- Operation of an International Cancer Research Data Bank to collect, catalog, store and disseminate the results of cancer research undertaken in any country for the use of any person in cancer research worldwide.

- Support for appropriate programs of education and training (including continuing education and laboratory and clinical research training). Authority to acquire, construct, improve, repair, operate, and maintain laboratories, other research facilities, equipment, and such other real or personal property as is determined necessary.

- Authority to make grants for construction or renovation of facilities, in consultation with the advisory council for the institute.

Research Programs

The NCI research programs take place in three settings: the laboratory, the clinic, and the community. In the laboratory, research is pursued on the biology of cancer, the fundamental properties of cancer-causing agents and processes, and the body's defense against and response to cancer. In the clinic, patient-oriented research is carried out concerning prevention, detection, diagnosis, treatment, and rehabilitation. In the community, research is carried out on the causes, risks, predispositions, incidence, and behavioral aspects of cancer, The components of this research triad interact. For example, populationor community-based research on the effects of exposure to a potential cancer-causing agent links to the laboratory where an understanding of the agent's effect on the cell can be explored. Through these linkages. NCI-funded research has identified a sexually transmitted papillomavirus as a primary cause of cervical cancer and subsequently explained why only certain viral subtypes are cancer-causing; and NCI-funded research has established the relationship between asbestos and mesotheliomas, between reproductive variables such as late menopause and breast cancer, and between dietary factors and a variety of cancers.

Likewise, community-based research on family clusters of cancers can lead to the isolation of the specific genes responsible for inherited cancer syndromes. The identification of specific genetic pathways in cells studied in the laboratory then can be used to predict the course of a patient's disease and his or her response to therapeutic interventions, or to find ways to detect these cancers very early in their development.

Research Areas

There are four fundamental cancer research areasin effect four basic goals of research: an understanding of cancer biology; identifying who is at risk for cancer and why; developing interventions to prevent, detect, diagnose, and treat cancer, and to enhance survivorship from cancer; and bringing research discoveries to the public and to practice.

Cancer Biology

The most remarkable progress in the last 25 years has been in knowledge of cancer biology. Researchers are finally beginning to understand what is required to turn a normal cell into a cancer cell. Cancer arises when a single cell changes so that it divides continuously, released from the controls that constrain the replication of normal cells. This transformation is due to changes in the function and activity of genes—segments of DNA containing the information that directs a cell to make a particular protein product.

Of the 100,000 genes found in the human genome, only the altered activities of a small number of genes are responsible for transforming a normal, well-behaved cell—be it in the breast, brain, blood, colon, prostate or other organ—into a cancer cell. Identifying these "cancer genes" defines the central scientific hunt in cancer biology. Their identification provides an unprecedented window into the nature of cancer. These genes normally function to instruct cells to produce accelerators that drive cells to proliferate, brakes that control proliferation, or mechanisms that underlie the repair of DNA damage or the elimination of damaged cells. Some individuals inherit an altered form of a cancer gene. These individuals carry a very high lifetime risk of developing cancer because fewer subsequent changes in DNA are required to take place in one of the trillions of cells in our bodies to transform that cell into a cancer cell.

DNA changes are the fundamental cause of all cancers. These changes can occur due to chemicals, viruses, radiation, and mistakes made each day in the course of duplicating the 3 billion units in our DNA when a cell divides. DNA, the molecule of life, is very vulnerable to damage, but each cell has the remarkable ability to recognize damage and correct it. The changes in DNA required to produce cancer result from the imbalance between damage and the cell's ability to repair the damage. When a normal cell recognizes damage to its DNA, it stops the process of growth and division called the cell cycle. A normal cell either repairs the damage or, if it fails, undergoes programmed cell death (apoptosis). In the development of cancer, checkpoint controls are lost and the cell continues to divide, transmitting its damaged DNA to its descendants. It is for this reason that cancer is beginning to be seen as a problem of genetic instability.

No one genetic alteration, however, is enough to make a normal, healthy cell a cancer cell. Rather, an accumulation of changes during the lifetime of a cell in a relatively small number of genes is required. This understanding allows us to begin to define the development and evolution of cancer from predisposition to precancer to cancer. Each cancer is ultimately defined by its particular pattern of altered and normal gene activity. This pattern determines the cancer's rate of growth, tendency to spread, responsiveness to hormones and therapies, and defines the ability of a person's immune system to recognize and respond to a cancer. These patterns will define what each cancer is and how many different cancers there are. By defining these molecular patterns, researchers are beginning to be able to describe what distinguishes each cancer from its normal counterpart. Advances in the ability to detect, diagnose, and treat each cancer will most likely be found in these differences.

Cancer Risk

Research on cancer risk quantifies the risk of developing cancer in various populations and strives to identify the factors responsible for these risks. Research in this area is critical to linking knowledge of biological processes to the detection, management, and ultimately, prevention of cancer. Studying people who are at high risk of cancer is particularly important, because it may be possible to identify more readily the factors influencing risk and to assess means for prevention and risk reduction. Behavioral scientists also contribute to understanding risk by studying how people perceive cancer-related risks and by learning how to motivate health professionals and high-risk persons to practice cancer risk reduction strategies.

Epidemiology is the principal discipline used to study cancer patterns in the population and the determinants of cancer risk. Epidemiologists have uncovered distinct cancer patterns among various population groups. For example, African American men have the highest prostate cancer risk of any group in the world, while men in Asian countries have a relatively low risk. Similarly, women in most Asian countries have the lowest rates of breast cancer, while those in the West have the highest. Interestingly, when Asian women migrate to the United States, their breast cancer risk rises over several generations until it matches that found in U.S. white women. These striking variations among populations have proven particularly useful in targeting further epidemiologic research into the causes of cancer. These studies underlie the commitment of the NCI to address the burden of cancer in all population groups in the United States to assure that all benefit from our research.

The epidemiologic approach has been successful in identifying many factors that increase cancer risk, some of which are environmental and lifestyle-related, while others are part of a person's genetic makeup. With the exception of a few genetic conditions, however, it is still not possible to predict with any degree of certainty that a person having one or more of these factors will develop cancer. This uncertainty is related to the need for a number of alterations to accumulate in the genetic material (DNA) of a single cell for that cell to be transformed into a malignant state.

The single most important exposure that increases cancer risk is the use of tobacco products, particularly cigarette smoking. Smoking is believed to contribute to more than 30 percent of all cancer deaths. In addition, certain aspects of the diet, particularly diets lacking in fruits and vegetables or high in fats, appear to be important contributors to cancer risk. An excess risk of cancer also has been linked to alcohol consumption, radiation (e.g., ultraviolet- and x-rays), certain occupational exposures (e.g., asbestos), environmental pollution (e.g., arsenic), some pharmaceutical agents (e.g., estrogenic drugs), certain viral infections (e.g., human immunodeficiency virus, and human papilloma virus [HPV]), and hormonal factors. In addition, epidemiology plays a key role in revealing inherited cancer predisposition syndromes, as are seen in women who inherit alterations in the BRCA1 gene.

With recent major advances in molecular biology, a strategy called molecular epidemiology has emerged, combining the strengths of epidemiology with sensitive laboratory probes and providing new insights into genetic susceptibility and gene-environment interactions. This kind of interdisciplinary approach promises to elucidate the risk profiles and biologic mechanisms involved in cancer etiology, making it possible to predict cancer risk with greater certainty.

Cancer Interventions

Ultimately, the purpose of understanding tumor biology and identifying cancer risk is to uncover effective ways to intervene in the cancer process. Important advances in both areas are leading to new strategies to prevent, detect, diagnose, and treat cancer.

Our ability to prevent cancer depends on identifying and removing (or at least reversing the effects of) specific risk factors. Clearly, the most important of these is tobacco use. The NCI has strongly supported recent initiatives to avert the initiation of tobacco use among children and teenagers and continues to develop a variety of approaches to cessation among those already addicted. The effect of dietary modification and administration of preventive agents to forestall the occurrence of cancer in high-risk populations is under study. The testing of tamoxifen as a breast cancer preventive in women at high risk for breast cancer is one approach. It should be quite clear, however, that major improvements in chemoprevention will depend on a better understanding of the fundamental mechanisms of carcinogenesis—the process by which normal cells are induced to become malignant.

Researchers have learned to see inside the body of a living human being with a precision that could not have been anticipated by a previous generation of physicians. Computed tomography, magnetic resonance imaging, and ultrasonography simply did not exist as useful clinical tools 25 years ago. Their development depended on first learning how the body interacts with x-rays, magnetic fields, and sound waves, and then figuring out how to create images from these interactions. These technologies permit doctors to locate internal tumors with unprecedented accuracy and to biopsy internal organs without the need for major surgical procedures. There is every reason to believe that further improvement in their powers of resolution will enhance the ability to detect small tumors even earlier than is possible with currently available method such as x-ray mammography. Invasive procedures, such as colonoscopy and bronchoscopy, are on the verge of giving way to "virtual" procedures involving the imaging of these internal structures without any actual invasion of the body by tubes or scopes.

The diagnosis of cancer depends on the microscopic appearance of tissue samples taken from growths or other suspicious lesions in the body. Advances in biological knowledge have improved our ability to subclassify cancers into accurate categories. For example, a better understanding of normal immune system development and biology has led directly to molecular techniques for classifying, for the first time, immune system tumors (lymphomas). More precise classification of cancers is important because it will lead to more precise prediction of clinical outcome for patients and to the discovery of more effective therapies. The experience with lymphoma serves as a model for what will very likely occur in a variety of malignancies. Tumor diagnosis and classification will be revolutionized in the coming years by application of emerging knowledge in molecular genetics. The past quarter century has seen major progress in the ability to treat certain cancers. In addition to well-publicized improvements in the cure rates for many uncommon tumors, such as Hodgkin's disease, certain lymphomas, testicular cancer, and a variety of childhood cancers, adding chemotherapy to surgery and/or radiation has increased the cure rates for patients with breast and colorectal cancer. High-dose chemotherapy with stem-cell rescue is effective in the leukemias and is undergoing definitive testing in breast cancer.

The application of molecular biology to the drug discovery process has ushered in the era of biological therapy by permitting the large-scale production of so-called "recombinant" proteins. Following directly from this approach, the availability of interferon-alpha has markedly improved the outlook for patients with a rare form of leukemia. Both interferon and interleukin-2 provide improved tumor shrinkage for some patients with kidney cancer. The availability of bone marrow stimulatory factors has enhanced the quality of supportive care by mitigating the toxicity of chemotherapy to the blood elements. Over the past 15 years, the formidable problem of treatment-related nausea and vomiting has been markedly lessened by the development of truly effective drugs that reduce this side effect.

NCI is committed to research to improve the quality of life for those who develop cancer. As treatment becomes increasingly effective in the coming years, the emergence of certain problems associated with surviving cancer will continue to be seen. These are of two general types. The first are the challenges to an optimal quality of life posed by the effects of cancer treatment itself.

Although most acute side effects of treatment are rapidly reversible, some, such as the loss of a body part, have a lasting impact. The widespread use of techniques such as breast reconstruction, conservative surgery, and customized limb prostheses have greatly improved the emotional and functional outlook for survivors of breast and bone cancer. The knowledge, gained in a landmark clinical trial, that chemotherapy followed by radiation treatment is as effective as total removal of the voicebox for cancer of the larynx has made preservation of natural speech possible for many patients with this condition. The recent FDA approval of effective drugs for protecting against the cardiac toxicity of the anthracycline antibiotics and the kidney toxicity of cisplatin can be expected to reduce the overall incidence of two particularly troublesome chronic effects of chemotherapy.

The second general problem is the propensity of many cancer survivors to develop second cancers at the same or other body sites. In some cases, this is a treatment effect; many current therapies that effectively treat the patient's primary cancer unfortunately also promote the development of second cancers in a small fraction of people who receive them. So, for example, women who have received radiation therapy to the chest for the treatment of Hodgkin's disease are at increased risk for developing breast cancer; and certain chemotherapy regimens are associated with the late appearance of acute leukemia in some patients who survive for years after the treatment. Sometimes, however, the development of a second cancer stems from influences having nothing to do with the therapy. Patients who survive a first cancer of the lung or oral cavity, for example, have a high incidence of subsequent tumors at those sites, probably because of the long lasting carcinogenic influences of tobacco. Inherited risk may also play a role. Some breast, ovarian, and colorectal cancer patients have a genetic predisposition to those cancers and are likely to develop other primary cancers. The solution to these persistent problems clearly is to discover more targeted and less toxic treatments and to develop better surveillance and prevention strategies for people whose risk is elevated for reasons unrelated to treatment.

Psychosocial and behavioral research has fundamental contributions to make to all aspects of cancer survivorship, both in improving the quality of life for cancer patients as well as those at increased risk of developing cancer. Psychosocial research investigates how cancer affects quality of life and finds ways to address survivors' needs so they can meet the everyday demands of life and return to a productive lifestyle. NCI is committed to such research to complement its cancer prevention, detection, and treatment research programs. This research will assume even greater importance as genetic advances pose difficult prevention and treatment choices.

Cancer Control

Cancer control research bridges the gap between laboratory, clinical and population-based research, and health care by focusing on how to bring our discoveries to the practice of cancer prevention, detection, treatment, and rehabilitation. Effective application is a challenge well-illustrated by the fact that significant smoking rate reductions have taken over 30 years to achieve since the first Surgeon General's report that showed conclusively the causal link between smoking and cancer.

The science of cancer control is necessarily multidisciplinary and involves behavioral research, epidemiology, health services research, and communication. A crosscutting theme is to identify the environmental, genetic, physiological, and psychosocial determinants of health, in order to achieve the adoption of new behaviors that can reduce the risk of cancer or improve the prognosis for persons with cancer.

Behavioral research is central to cancer control. A large proportion of cancer is caused or linked to behaviors such as smoking or diet. Through behavioral research, the behavior of individuals and health care professionals can be modified to include the adoption or promotion of healthy practices, such as smoking cessation, adoption of a low-fat, high-fiber, balanced diet, and practicing cancer screening regimens. The development and rigorous evaluation of smoking cessation interventions is urgently needed to assist the 45 million Americans who currently smoke, particularly those who smoke heavily. Research is under way to integrate effective pharmacotherapies with self-help approaches that address both the addictive and behavioral aspects of smoking. Of equal concern is developing strategies to prevent smoking among adolescents. To this end, behavioral scientists are trying to understand why African American adolescents are avoiding tobacco while white youths have been more resistant to messages about the harms of tobacco.

An important aspect of cancer control research is finding those factors that facilitate adoption of recommended regimens. This requires understanding the population in need. Regimens must be sensitive to the economic, cultural, ethnic and social forces acting upon populations. For example, to increase the adoption of Pap smears, which can prevent needless deaths from cervical cancer, the practices and customs of individuals, their communities, and health care professionals must be understood, and interventions tailored appropriately.

Cancer control research often begins by studying the patterns of cancer in populations through epidemiological studies or through the NCI surveillance system that monitors cancer incidence, mortality, and survival. Evaluating cancer patterns provides insight into who is developing cancer and what factors may have contributed to their disease. Researchers examine not only the changing burden of cancer, but also the public's and health profession's knowledge, attitudes, and practices related to cancer prevention, early detection, treatment, and rehabilitation. All of this information is essential for designing and evaluating interventions that may reduce the cancer burden. For example, surveillance data have shown clearly that there are survival differences between African American and white populations. Research is under way to identify the factors underlying these differences.

Effective and widespread communication plays a critical part in applying the knowledge gained in biology, epidemiology, and intervention research. The NCI supports research on cancer communication as well as innovative programs to provide information on cancer to the public and to the Nation's health professionals. Our scientific journal, the Journal of the National Cancer Institute, is one of the premier cancer journals in the world. Although designed primarily to facilitate communication between scientists and clinicians, the journal is often cited in the popular press and therefore is an important channel for public information. The NCI also supports communications between scientists, physicians, and the public through its nationwide Cancer Information Service (1-800-4-CANCER) and the PDQ computer-based cancer and clinical trials information system. These communication systems provide Americans—patients, the public, and physicians—with the most current information possible on cancer treatments and on effective prevention, early detection, and supportive care technologies.

New challenges for cancer control research abound. The evolving health care system poses the challenge of how to introduce cancer discoveries in these settings, and especially important, to find ways that cancer research can be directly integrated into health care through clinical studies. Developing cost-effective cancer interventions is essential and is an important part of cancer-related health services research. Discoveries in genetics and clinical science pose special challenges for cancer control. For example, with the advent of more precise and individual-specific ways of assessing the risk of developing cancer, researchers are faced with an array of new challenges in living with and understanding risk, and with tailoring prevention, detection, and treatment to individual needs.

Indeed, each research advance brings its own challenges which must be met to realize the promise of research.

National Eye Institute

Mission

Conducts, fosters, and supports basic and applied research, including clinical trials, related to the cause, natural history, prevention, diagnosis, and treatment of disorders of the eye and visual system, and in related fields (including visual impairment and its rehabilitation) through:

- Research performed in its own laboratories and clinics;

- A program of research grants, individual and institutional research training awards, career development awards, core grants, and contracts to public and private research institutions and organizations;

- Cooperation and collaboration with professional, commercial, voluntary, and philanthropic organizations concerned with vision research and training, disease prevention and health promotion, and the special health problems of the visually impaired and disabled and blind;

- Collection and dissemination of information on ongoing research and findings in these areas;

- Cooperation and collaboration with domestic and international organizations in worldwide prevention of blindness programs and projects.

Major Programs

The NEI's extramural research activities are organized into seven areas: retinal diseases; corneal diseases; lens and cataract; glaucoma strabismus, amblyopia, and visual processing; low vision and its rehabilitation; and collaborative clinical research.

Retinal Diseases

NEI-supported investigations include studies of the development, molecular and cell biology, molecular genetics, and metabolism of the photoreceptor cells and their dependence on the underlying retinal pigment epithelium; the mechanism of the retina's response to light and the initial processing of information that is transmitted to the visual centers of the brain; the pathogenesis of diabetic retinopathy; the fundamental causes of and etiologic factors responsible for uveitis; the molecular genetic mechanisms responsible for producing retinoblastoma and ocular melanoma; the characterization at the molecular level of the genes responsible for retinitis pigmentosa, age-related macular degeneration, and related disorders; and, the cellular and molecular events that accompany retinal detachment.

Corneal Diseases

NEI-supported projects include studies of the regulation of genes that express proteins unique to corneal tissue; the details of the macromolecular and supramolecular assembly of extracellular corneal matrices; the characterization of cytokines and cell surface receptors which interact with corneal cells, pathogens, and blood-borne cells; the creation and use of transgenic animals to study corneal diseases; the mechanisms that maintain corneal hydration and transparency; the physiologic basis for immune privilege in the cornea; corneal wound healing; the biomechanics of the cornea; the cellular and molecular mechanisms by which corneal transplants are rejected; and, the role of specific viral genes in the establishment, maintenance, and reactivation of corneal herpetic infections.

Lens and Cataract

NEI-supported research includes studies of the development and aging of the normal lens of the eye; the identification, at the cellular and molecular level, of those components that maintain the transparency and proper shape of the lens; the control of lens cell division; the delineation of the structural and regulatory sequences of crystallin and noncrystallin lens genes; the impact of oxidative insult on the lens; and, the role of aldose reductase in human cataractogenesis.

Glaucoma

NEI-supported projects involve studies of the gene expression and regulation of the extracellular matrix proteins of the trabecular meshwork; the identification and characterization of genes that are involved in the development of glaucoma; the basic mechanisms that control aqueous humor dynamics; the design of better pharmacologic agents to modulate aqueous humor secretion and outflow; and the roles of growth factors, potential cytoprotective substances, and other nutritive factors for maintenance of outflow structures and the optic nerve.

Strabismus, Amblyopia, and Visual Processing

The NEI supports a broad range of studies concerned with the function of the neural pathways from the eye to the brain, the central processing of visual information, visual perception, optical properties of the eye, functioning of the pupil, and control of the ocular muscles. A large number of congenital, developmental, and degenerative abnormalities affect the visual sensorimotor system, but two disorders are of primary concern: strabismus and amblyopia. These are frequent causes of visual impairment among children which may persist for life. Additional emphasis is placed on and support provided for research on optic neuropathies, eye movement disorders, and the development of myopia.

Low Vision

The NEI supports research in low vision and rehabilitation of people with visual impairments. Examples include projects aimed at improving the methods of specifying, measuring, and categorizing loss of visual function; devising strategies to help visually impaired people maximize the use of their residual vision; systematically evaluating new and existing visual aids; developing an adequate epidemiological base for blindness, partial loss of sight and visual anomalies; and studying the optical, electronic, and other rehabilatative needs of people with visual impairments.

Collaborative Clinical Research

Funding includes a number of clinical trials and other epidemiologic research projects encompassing single-center randomized clinical trials, multicenter randomized clinical trials, natural history studies, and risk factor analyses using case-control and prospective cohort methods. These projects have the goal of improving the understanding, prevention, and management of visual system diseases and disorders including, for example, diabetic retinopathy, age-related macular degeneration, corneal diseases, cataract, glaucoma, and optic nerve atrophy, the leading causes of blindness in the United States.

432

National Heart, Lung, and Blood Institute

Mission

The National Heart, Lung, and Blood Institute (NHLBI):

- Provides leadership for a national program in diseases of the heart, blood vessels, lungs, and blood; sleep disorders; and blood resources management.

- Plans, conducts, fosters, and supports an integrated and co-ordinated program of basic research, clinical investigations and trials, observational studies, demonstration and education projects related to the causes, prevention, diagnosis, and treatment of heart, blood vessel, lung, blood diseases, and sleep disorders conducted in its own laboratories and by scientific institutions and individuals supported by research grants and contracts.

- Conducts research on clinical use of blood and all aspects of the management of blood resources.

- Supports research training and career development of new and established researchers in fundamental sciences and clinical disciplines to enable them to conduct basic and clinical research related to heart, blood vessel, lung, and blood diseases; sleep disorders; and blood resources through individual and institutional research training awards and career development awards.

- Coordinates with other research institutes and all Federal health programs relevant activities in the above areas, including the related causes of stroke.

- Conducts educational activities, including development and dissemination of materials for health professionals and the public in the above areas, with emphasis on prevention.

- Maintains continuing relationships with institutions and professional associations, and with international, national, state, and local officials as well as voluntary agencies and organizations working in the above areas.

433

NHLBI Programs

Heart and vascular diseases affect at least 50 million people and continue as the leading cause of death in the United States. Important progress in the reduction of morbidity and mortality from these diseases has been achieved since 1963, when coronary heart disease mortality was at its peak.

The NHLBI uses research grants, program project grants, specialized center grants, cooperative agreements, research contracts, research career development awards, and institutional and individual national research service awards to support research and research training. The four program divisions and one center of the NHLBI offer support in the following areas.

Division of Heart and Vascular Diseases

The Division of Heart and Vascular Diseases plans and directs a program of fundamental and clinical research in heart and vascular diseases. AIDS-associated cardiovascular disorders are also included. The division provides training and career development for research in these areas; specific programs foster career development for minority students and scientists. Among these programs are minority institutional research training awards, minority school faculty development award, research development award for minority faculty, and short-term training for minority students program.

The division is divided into two program areas: heart research and vascular research. The heart program area oversees research in arrhythmias, bioengineering, ischemic heart disease, congenital and infectious diseases, heart failure, and interventional cardiology. The vascular program supports research in molecular genetics and medicine, atherosclerosis, hypertension; vascular biology, vascular medicine, and cardiovascular homeostasis and bionutrition.

Arteriosclerosis, coronary heart disease, and hypertension are among the major areas of emphasis within the division's research program. Examples of newly supported projects include:

• angiogenesis in breast cancer

• etiology of excess cardiovascular disease in diabetes mellitus

• gene-nutrient interactions in the pathogenesis of congenital heart defects

• innovative ventricular assist systems.

Quality-of-life endpoints have become important measures in clinical trials. The division initiated a multicenter, randomized clinical trial to test the efficacy of interventions that provide social support and ameliorate depression in post-MI patients in FY 1995. Coronary heart disease death and reinfarction are the primary endpoints. Secondary outcomes include health-related quality of life and adherence to medical and lifestyle change regimens.

Another clinical trial recently begun will compare the impact on total mortality of a strategy of attempting to maintain sinus rhythm with antiarrhythmic drugs to a strategy of merely controlling the heart rate. Important secondary endpoints will include quality of life and cost of therapies.

Several trials have suggested that beta-blockers improve ventricular function in congestive heart failure and may also reduce mortality. While a reasonable theoretical basis and suggestive clinical studies exist, the concept that beta-blockers reduce mortality in congestive heart failure patients remains unproven. The division has initiated a clinical trial to determine whether the addition of a beta-blocking agent to standard therapy reduces the total mortality of patients with moderate to severe congestive heart failure.

In FY 1995 the division supported Specialized Centers of Research on the genetic determinants of high blood pressure and ischemic heart disease in blacks. Solicitations of applications were issued for research on elucidation of mechanisms responsible for myocardial dysfunction, specifically, those involved in the transition from cardiac hypertrophy to overt heart failure; and for research on atherosclerotic lesions using human tissues.

Division of Epidemiology and Clinical Applications

In FY 1995 the division continued to give special attention to minority health issues. Obesity prevention in young Native Americans, CHD risk factors in middle-age black adults, and hypertension care among inner city minorities are a few examples. A study associated with atherosclerosis in larger arteries was extended to include the effect of hypertension on smaller arteries in the eyes and brains of blacks and whites.

A clinical trial to determine whether the combined incidence of nonfatal myocardial infarction (MI) and fatal CHD differs between hypertensives receiving alternative antihypertensive pharmacological treatment was initiated. A subset of hypercholesterolemic patients will be studied to determine whether reducing serum cholesterol levels with a lipid-lowering drug decreases the incidence of nonfatal MI and fatal CHD. The effects of selected diet patterns on blood pressure will be examined in another group of patients.

Behavioral studies are an important component of clinical trials and have been included in several intervention projects. A few examples supported by the division include:

- multicenter study to examine the effect of community-wide education on reducing the time from onset of cardiac symptoms to receipt of medical care.

- behavioral interventions in primary care to encourage sedentary patients to increase their physical activity.

- clinical trial to study the effects of psychosocial support on morbidity and mortality in patients recently hospitalized with acute MI.

- Multicenter clinical trials are being conducted to study the effects of various medical treatments for cardiac problems.

Some issues being investigated are:

- impact of implantable cardioverter defibrillators on survival of coronary bypass patients.

- effects on mortality of beta-blockers to standard therapy for chronic congestive heart failure.

- effect on mortality of two strategies of antiarrhythmic drug therapy in patients with atrial fibrillation.

Other projects supported by the division include:

- efforts directed toward genetic and nongenetic determinants of CHD and cardiovascular risk factors in population-based studies of twins and families.

- a pilot project comparing the effectiveness of an implantable cardiac defibrillator with conventional drug therapy in reducing mortality in patients who have been resuscitated from sudden cardiac death.

- a pilot study evaluating the effects of specific dosages of various drugs or drug combinations on several biochemical markers for atherosclerotic CVD in patients with peripheral arterial disease.

Office of Prevention, Education, and Control

OPEC, located in the NHLBI Office of the Director, is the institute's technology transfer arm, relaying the results of heart, lung, and blood research to health care professionals, their patients, and the public. Its function is to disseminate and translate up-to-date research findings that will help practitioners be more effective, and provide scientific knowledge to patients and the public that will enable them to make "healthy decisions."

The institute has targeted six areas for educationai emphasis with OPEC. They include: high blood pressure; cholesterol; asthma; heart attack alert; sleep disorders; and obesity. Three of these (high blood pressure, cholesterol, and obesity) address major modifiable risk factors for CVD.

The National High Blood Pressure Education Program (NHBPEP) was established in 1972 with a goal of reducing death and disability related to high blood pressure through professional, patient, and public education. Strategies to achieve this goal include stimulating education and information programs to increase public awareness about the disease, promoting activities encouraging detection of the disease especially for underserved groups, encouraging hypertensive patients to seek medical care and follow their doctor's advice, providing education programs and materials for health professionals, and providing technical support to community health programs so they may carry these activities to their geographic areas.

Since its creation, the NHBPEP has released five joint national committee (JNC) reports on the detection, evaluation, and treatment of high blood pressure. Each report has been based on the latest scientific research related to hypertension control and reflects the state-of-the-art regarding hypertension management.

The fifth JNC report, issued in 1992, includes and updates earlier recommendations for both pharmacologic and nonpharmacologic therapies for high blood pressure.

NHBPEP also released the Hypertension and Chronic Renal Failure Report, which gives an overview of this mounting public health problem; a Report on High Blood Pressure in Pregnancy, which affects about 10 percent of all pregnancies; and a new Report on Primary Prevention of Hypertension.

The National Cholesterol Education Program (NCEP) was launched in 1985. Its goal is to reduce illness and death from coronary heart disease in the United States by lowering the prevalence of high blood cholesterol. Through its educational efforts directed at the public, patients, and health professionals, the NCEP aims to raise awareness and understanding about high blood cholesterol as a risk factor for coronary heart disease and the benefits of lowering high blood cholesterol as a means of preventing coronary heart disease. Success of program efforts is demonstrated by the results of cholesterol awareness surveys conducted in 1983, 1986, and 1990 that show dramatic improvements in cholesterol-related knowledge, attitudes, and practices among physicians and the public.

In 1992 the NCEP convened a new adult treatment panel to update the existing guidelines for detecting and treating high blood cholesterol in adults. The panel's report was completed in June 1993. The NCEP published the report of the children and adolescents panel and developed booklets to help parents and children adopt heart healthy eating patterns. The program endorsed the expert panel recommendations for heart healthy eating by the general population to lower average cholesterol levels, and it developed methods to improve the accuracy of cholesterol measurement. In its educational activities, the NCEP is pursuing a dual strategy to encourage blood cholesterol reduction by high-risk individuals and by the general population.

The National Asthma Education Program (NAEP) was initiated in March 1989 to raise awareness of asthma as a serious, chronic disease and to promote more effective management of asthma through professional and patient education. The NAEP released two expert panel reports on asthma, International Guidelines on Diagnosis and Management of Asthma and Asthma and Pregnancy Report, in 1992. The international guidelines were developed by asthma experts from several countries and will be translated and distributed throughout the world.

The NAEP initiated activities to help health professionals and patients implement the recommendations of the expert panel's report on diagnosis and management of asthma. Examples include developing a speaker's kit for use by health care professionals in workshops or training sessions on dissemination of panel recommendations, preparing and asthma management kit to aid health professionals working with patients on disease control, producing a pamphlet for patients emphasizing that asthma can be controlled, and distributing information to schools that will enable the staff to develop skill related to asthma management and control.

The National Heart Attack Alert Program (NHAAP) was initiated in June 1991 to reduce morbidity and mortality from acute myocardial infarction (AMI) and sudden death through the education of physicians, nurses. emergency medical service personnel, and other health professionals about the importance of rapid identification and treatment of individuals with heart attack, symptoms and signs. To date, the program has developed recommendations for emergency department management of individuals with characteristic signs of AMI. In addition, it has prepared background papers on 911 emergency telephone systems: acquisition of emergency medical services systems, including staff and equipment; emergency medical dispatching procedures; and factors associated with patient/bystander delays in seeking care.

The NHLBI Obesity Education Initiative (OEI) was launched in 1991 to educate the public and health professional about the risk factors associated with obesity. Obesity is not only an independent risk factor for CVD, but also a contributor to high blood pressure and high blood cholesterol and is related to sleep apnea. The program is using both high risk and population based strategies to educate those groups about the relationship of overweight with heart disease and impaired lung function. The first targets persons with adverse health effects and medical complications associated with obesity. An expert panel will convene to address issues such as identification, evaluation, and treatment of obesity. A strategy development workshop was held in September 1992 to plan the population-based effort for the general public as well as special subgroups.

All of OPEC's education programs work in partnership with a wide range of organizations—governmental, professional, voluntary, community, private, industry, and educational—that have focused their activities on NHLBI-related health information and education. OPEC collaborates with these organizations to help achieve its program goals, disseminate educational materials, and obtain feedback for new program development. Mass media are used to achieve program goals.

Division of Lung Diseases

Lung diseases are among the leading causes of death and disability in the United States. Excluding cancer, it accounts for 224,000 deaths annually, and is a contributing cause to perhaps an equal number of additional deaths.

More than 25 million persons suffer from chronic bronchitis, emphysema, asthma or other obstructive or interstitial lung diseases. In 1993, pulmonary diseases accounted for 27 percent of all hospitalizations of children under 15 years of age.

The division plans and directs research in lung diseases, encompassing basic and targeted research, clinical trials and demonstration trials, national pulmonary SCORs, technological development, and application of findings. The division assesses the national need for research in the causes, prevention, diagnosis, and treatment of lung diseases; in technological development; and for manpower training in these areas.

Minority training is an important priority within the division. The Minority National Research Service Award, the Minority School Faculty Development Award, the Research Development Award for Minority Faculty. and the Short-Term Research Training for Minority Students Award are among the research career and training programs it supports.

The NHBLI established six centers for gene therapy in FY 1993. Presently, the centers are focusing mainly on cystic fibrosis (CF) research but include other areas associated with gene therapy for heart, lung, and blood diseases. Basic, preclinical, and clinical studies are directed toward developing safe, efficient, and efficacious vehicles for delivering genes to appropriate target cells. Basic science and clinical findings are identifying new directions needed to generate improved gene transfer vectors, to manage the inflammatory and immune consequences of vector transfer, and to develop alternative vector systems.

Asthma research is an important area of support for the division. In FY 1995, major focus was directed towards:

- gene mapping studies to locate and identify genes important to asthma. Discoveries in this field will facilitate the development of new modes of treatment and will lead to an understanding of causal interactions between the genes and environmental factors that are relevant in asthma.

- development and evaluation of innovative approaches to ensure optimal disease management and prevention in the elementary school setting.

- clinical trial to investigate long-term effects of two short-acting, beta-agonist treatment regimens. As part of the research effort, an inexpensive and easily reproducible method for testing the accuracy and precision of peak flow meters was developed for use in monitoring asthma.

- clinical trial to examine the effectiveness and side effects of two long-acting, beta-agonist treatment regimens The long-term effects of three different asthma medications will be examined in a 5-year, multicenter clinical trial conducted among 1,000 children.

440

- collaborative study with the NICHI to determine the effects of asthma and its treatment on pregnancy and the effects of pregnancy on asthma.

The division is very active in public education programs that increase awareness of asthma and its public health consequences that promote study of the association between asthma and the environment, and that reduce asthma morbidity and mortality throughout the world. In collaboration with the World Health Organization, it recently published a report entitled Global Strategy for Asthma Management and Prevention. Presently, it is preparing a report on the diagnosis and management of asthma in the elderly.

Smoking-related diseases are a major cause of mortality and morbidity in the United States. The division has an ongoing randomized trial that examines the effect of inhaled corticosteroids on the natural history of lung function in continuing smokers.

The division supports efforts associated with acquired immunodeficiency syndrome (AIDS) and tuberculosis (TB) research. Specific programs include:

- clinical study of cardiopulmonary complications of HIV infection in infants and children.

- several programs to address pathobiology of Pneumocystis carinii, basic cell biology of pulmonary manifestations of AIDS.

- development of lung-specific drug delivery systems for enhanced TB treatment, and behavioral interventions for control of TB.

Several new programs were begun in FY 1995. Included among them are:

- prospective randomized clinical trial to assess novel treatment methods in patients at risk for developing adult respiratory distress syndrome.

- epidemiological study to investigate causes and environmental and genetic risk factors for sarcoidosis.

- a study of causes of noninfectious pneumonia, an often fatal complication of bone marrow transplantation.

- multi-institutional collaboration to create a molecular profile of bronchopulmonary dysplasia that will provide insight into the condition and offer directions for developing new reagents for clinical interventions.

Division of Blood Diseases and Resources

Blood diseases, including both acute and chronic disorders, resulted in 271,000 deaths in 1994: 262,000 of them were due to thrombotic disorders and 9,000 were due to diseases of the red blood cells and bleeding disorders.

The division develops, administers, and coordinates programs that will reduce morbidity and mortality caused by blood diseases and lead to their primary prevention. These programs include hemophilia, Cooley's anemia, sickle cell disease, and disorders of hemostasis and thrombosis. The division also has a major responsibility to ensure the adequacy and safety of the Nation's blood supply. A full range of activities, including studies of transmission of disease through transfusion, development of methods to inactivate viruses in donated blood, improvement of blood donor screening procedures, research to reduce human error in transfusion medicine, and studies of emerging diseases that may be transmitted by blood transfusion, are used to achieve this goal.

The division's overall responsibilities are met by an integrated and coordinated program of grants, contracts, training and career development awards, and academic awards. Special emphasis is given to training and career development programs targeting minority students, faculty members, and investigators at minority schools.

Stem cell biology was an area of major focus in FY 1995. Advances in characterization and purification of hematopoietic stem cells enabled investigators to begin to examine different sources of the cells and to pursue strategies designed to hasten the translation of basic research into clinical application. Among the areas studied were:

- hematopoictic growth factors and cytokines.

- stem cell transplantation.

- aplastic anemias and other nonneoplastic disorders of the bone marrow.

- pathophysiology of bone marrow in AIDS and related hematologic disorders.

The new SCORs in hematopoietic stem cell biology were initiated to develop improved treatments for both inherited and acquired hematologic disorders found in blood cell production and other blood diseases.

Thalassemia is another research area within the division. On going studies examine:

- genetics, pathophysiology, prevention, diagnosis, and treatment of the disease.

- development of pharmacologic agents that enhance fetal hemoglobin production or rehydrate red blood cells.

- gene therapy.

- development of animal models.

Sickle cell research is another high priority area and is supported through Comprehensive Sickle Cell Centers. A mutidisciplinary approach is directed towards membrane function, red cell rheology, and adherence of red cells to vascular endothelium.

Unrelated-donor marrow transplantation and pathogenesis, prevention, diagnosis, and treatment of complications of transplantation are current areas of investigation. Special attention is directed to studies of transplantation of stem cells from marrow, peripheral, and cord blood.

The division to has been very active in disseminating its research findings to the medical community through workshops, meetings, and consensus development conferences. Topics have included plasma transfusion, platelet transfusion therapy, diagnosis of deep-vein thrombosis, impact of routine HIV antibody testing of blood and plasma donors on public health, infectious disease testing for blood transfusions, stem cell therapy, and immune function in sickle cell disease.

National Center for Sleep Disorders Research

The National Center on Sleep Disorders Research (NCSDR) plans, directs, and supports a program of basic, clinical, and applied research; health education; and prevention-related research in sleep and sleep disorders. It maintains surveillance over developments in its program areas; assesses the national need for research on the causes, diagnosis, treatment, and prevention of sleep disorders; and coordinates sleep research activities across the Federal Government.

Since its inception, the NCSDR has initiated several activities. A study that involves existing epidemiological cohorts is being conducted to determine if sleep apnea is an independent or contributing risk factor for the development of cardiovascular and cerebrovascular disease. The center, in collaboration with NICHD, established the Back to Sleep campaign to reduce the risk of SIDS. In FY 1995, the NCSDR coordinated and released a NIH-wide program announcement in Basic and Clinical Research on Sleep and Wakefulness.

In collaboration with the National Aeronautics and Space Administration (NASA) the center supports research on sleep and microgravity as part of the Neurolab Project. A new initiative for a sleep academic award was approved and will soon be released. The NCSDR collaborated and coordinated a number of NIH-and Government-wide activities including an NIH Workshop on Molecular Biology and Genetic Approaches to Sleep Control, and joint activities with the National Sleep Foundation and the Department of Transportation on the Drive Alert Arrive Alive Program.

The center works closely with the NHLBI Office of Prevention, Education, and Control on the sleep education program which includes conducting some focus group research. A number of professional and public/patient education publications were released along with the start of a Sleep Apnea Mass Media Campaign. The center recently published a summary of the report of the Stately Development Workshop on Sleep Education. NIAID Research Program Investigators at universities, hospitals, and private research institutions throughout the country receive support through grants and contracts administered by the Division of Microbiology and Infectious Diseases; Division of Allergy, Immunology, and Transplantation; and Division of Acquired Immunodeficiency Syndrome.

Division of Intramural Research

The 16 Bethesda-based laboratories and branches conduct clinical research on the normal and pathophysiologic functioning of the cardiac, pulmonary, blood and endocrine systems and basic research on normal and abnormal cell behavior at the molecular level. A brief synopsis of current research follows.

The Cardiology Branch focuses on the processes involved in microvascular medicated myocardial ischemia, the genetic basis and clinical treatment of hypertrophic cardiomyopathy, and molecular and cellular mechanisms of angiogenesis and restenosis.

The Hematology Branch conducts research on the pathogenesis of hematological diseases at the molecular and cellular levels and on the development of novel therapeautic strategies, including gene therapy. Other activities include research on the pathogenesis and treatment of aplastic anemia and B19 parvovirus-induced disease.

Vasoactive substances regulating blood pressure and hypertension, the molecular events leading to vascular hypertrophy and hyperplasia, and studies of pheochromocytoma are the principal interests of the Hypertension-Endocrine Branch.

The Molecular Disease Branch is concerned with elucidating the molecular mechanisms involved in lipid transport and metabolism in normal individuals and patients with disorders of lipid metabolism and atherosclerosis. The branch also conducts clinical studies on the effects of drugs and diet.

The principal goal of the Molecular Hematology Branch is to develop the understanding and technology necessary to carry out human gene therapy. Targeted diseases include genetic and cardiovascular disease and cancer. Mechanisms and regulation of gene expression are also studied.

Research in the Pulmonary/Critical Care Medicine Branch is directed toward understanding basic mechanisms of inflammatory and immune processes in the pathogenesis of the human lung. Techniques from cellular and molecular biology, with special emphasis on genetic strategies, have been applied in the treatment of cystic fibrosis.

The Laboratory of Animal Medicine and Surgery studies intracardiac flow dynamics with digital acquisition and analysis of color Doppler ultrasound imaging techniques.

The Laboratory of Biochemical Genetics studies the molecular mechanisms that regulate gene expression during embryonic development. Interests include homeobox genes and neuron-specific enhancer sequences.

The Laboratory of Biochemistry is concerned with the elucidation of various mechanisms of metabolic regulation. Special pathologic effects of oxidation, signal transduction, and protein chemistry.

The Laboratory of Biophysical Chemistry investigates physical and chemical properties of molecules in relation to their biochemical functions. Techniques used include nuclear magnetic resonance (NMR), mass spectrometry, and x-ray crystallography.

The goal of the Laboratory of Cardiac Energetics is a better understanding of the cellular processes involved in the performance of work in vivo by the heart. State-of-the-art noninvasive NMR and optical spectroscopy are used and include a 1-meter bore, 4.D tesla NMR for imaging and spectroscopic studies.

The Laboratory of Cell Biology investigates diverse problems on the molecular basis of cell motility, bioenergetics, heat-shock proteins, and protein structure through a variety of techniques from molecular biology to time-resolved fluorescence spectroscopy.

The Laboratory of Cell Signaling studies the mechanisms by which signal activated phospolipases like phospho-inositide-specific phospholipase C and phosphocholine-specific phospholipase D are modulated and the role these enzymes have in human disease.

Objectives of the Laboratory of Kidney and Electrolyte Metabolism are to understand renal function at the molecular and cellular levels. Areas of interest include epithelial transport, cellular osmoregulation, transport metabolism and hormonal regulation.

The Laboratory of Molecular Cardiology investigates the regulation, expression, and function of contractile proteins, invertebrate muscle and nonmuscle cells. The tools of molecular genetics, protein chemistry, and video-enhanced microscopy are used. Research in the pulmonary and molecular immunology section focuses on topics related to the T-cell activation process, with particular emphasis on the three classes of interleukin-2 receptors.

The Laboratory of Molecular Immunology does research in the T-cells activation process—studies with importance for immunodeficiency, cancer, and autoimmune diseases; the mast cells activation process—an important area for asthma and other allergic diseases and the mechanisms of drug-induced toxicities, with particular emphasis on the mechanisms of hepatitis resulting from inhalation anesthetics and nonsteroidal anti-inflammatory drugs.

National Institute of Allergy and Infectious Diseases

Mission

The National Institute of Allergy and Infectious Diseases conducts and supports research to study the causes of allergic, immunologic, and infectious diseases, and to develop better means of preventing, diagnosing, and treating these illnesses.

Encompassed in the institute mission are studies on the following:

• The immune system, its genetic control, maturation, characteristics and manipulation.

• Disorders and derangements of the immune system including asthma and other allergies, immunodeficiency states and autoimmunity.

• The role of the immune system in the pathogenesis of chronic diseases such as arthritis, chronic glomerulonephritis, and lupus erythematosus.

• The etiology, epidemiology, and pathogenesis of all types of infections (including those caused by viruses, mycoplasma, bacteria, fungi and parasites) involving a variety of organ systems.

• The diagnosis, treatment and prevention of all types of infections including research on antimicrobial, antifungal and antiviral therapy; and vaccines.

NIAID Research Program

Investigators at universities, hospitals and private research institutions throughout the country receive support through grants and contracts administered by the Division of Microbiology and Infectious Diseases; Division of Allergy, Immunology, and Transplantation; and Division of Acquired Immunodeficiency Syndrome.

Division of Microbiology and Infectious Diseases

Viral Diseases. Viruses are the major cause of infectious diseases requiring medical care in the United States. The cost in dollars or in days lost from work is estimated to be in the billions each year. Following an initial infection, which may occur without symptoms, many viruses persist in the body for life and may lead to serious medical problems, including immune complex diseases, degenerative diseases, cancer, heart disease, and ulcers.

NIAID supports basic studies of virus structure, replication, gene regulation and evolution as well as studies in animals and humans that investigate the viral epidemiology, pathogenesis and host immune response. This research program provides the foundation for the development of vaccines and antiviral therapies.

Respiratory infections are the major cause of acute illness in the U.S. NIAID supports the development and testing of new vaccines against virus-caused respiratory diseases such as influenza and respiratory syncytial and parainfluenza, which cause the majority of croup, bronchitis, and pneumonia in infants and children.

Viral hepatitis caused by hepatitis A, B, C, D, and E is another group of diseases with a major impact on health worldwide. In some parts of the world, hepatitis is the primary cause of liver cancer. Each year in the U.S., more than 600,000 new viral hepatitis infections occur which, when acute, can be debilitating and costly. Chronic disease resulting from infection with hepatitis B, C, and D is an even greater problem. Medical costs for chronic hepatitis are between $1 and $2 billion a year. NIAID-sponsored studies focus on virology, molecular biology, immunology, pathogenesis, development of antivirals, animal model development, vaccine development and clinical trials. Vaccines have now been licensed for hepatitis A and B.

Diarrheal diseases caused by viruses are particularly a problem among infants in developing countries. Experimental vaccines against rotaviruses—a major cause of infant diarrhea worldwide—have been extensively tested in children and infants.

Although there have been reports of possible viral associations in chronic fatigue syndrome (CFS), no specific causative role for any virus has been demonstrated. In order to explore the possible causes of CFS, the institute has funded CFS Cooperative Research Centers to provide a multidisciplinary approach to CFS research by conducting basic science and clinical investigations on CFS. NIAID also supports scientists who are studying the possible immune system dysfunction, reactivation of latent virus infections, exercise-induced fatigue in CFS patients, and the epidemiology of CFS.

Development of Antiviral Drugs. Because many drug sponsors do not have access to comprehensive antiviral screening facilities, NIAID has established screening facilities for the in vitro evaluation of an experimental compound's activity against the human herpes viruses—herpes simplex virus (HSV) I and 2, varicella zoster virus, cytomegalovirus (CMV), and Epstein-Barr virus—and the respiratory viruses—influenza types A and B, respiratory syncytial virus, parainfluenza, measles, and adenovirus. This service is available to any scientist with a potential antiviral compound and an inability to test it. NIAID supports drug evaluation studies, preclinically in animal models of human viral infections and in human clinical trials. Institute-supported investigators participating in the Collaborative Antiviral Study Group have tested drugs for herpes encephalitis, neonatal herpes and hantavirus. Other investigators have evaluated interferons for human papilloma infections such as genital warts.

Bacterial Diseases. In the last decade, several important bacterial diseases have emerged as new or recurring threats to the health of people in the U.S. and elsewhere, including Lyme disease and tuberculosis (TB).

Lyme disease, first recognized in the early 1980's in this country, is caused by a bacterium transmitted to humans by certain ticks. It has emerged as a significant problem in the northeast coastal areas, among others. NIAID spearheads NIH studies on Lyme disease, supporting research focusing on pathogenesis, improved therapies, better diagnostic tests, and vaccines.

Tuberculosis, a serious disease once thought to have been conquered in the U.S., is reemerging in certain American cities. TB has a staggering impact worldwide, since one-third of the world's population is infected with the TB bacterium. Although most people who are infected never develop active TB, those with weakened immune systems—especially those infected with HIV—are particularly vulnerable to active TB disease. Each year 8 million people worldwide develop active TB, and 3 million die.

With appropriate antibiotic therapy, TB usually can be cured. In recent years, however, drug-resistant cases of TB have increased dramatically. Particularly alarming is the increase in the number of persons with multidrug-resistant TB caused by bacterial strains resistant to two or more drugs. Even with treatment, the death rate for multidrugresistant TB patients is 40 to 60 percent.

As the lead institute responsible for research on TB, NIAID supports basic research into the biology of TB, the development of new tools to diagnose TB, the development of new drugs or ways to deliver standard drugs, clinical trials of anti-TB therapies, and the development of vaccines to prevent it.

NIAID also funds research on leprosy, or Hansen's disease, which is caused by a mycobacterium. Although treatable today, this disease affects between 15 and 20 million people worldwide, largely in subtropical climates. Research on atypical mycobacteria, which constitute a diverse and heterogeneous group of acid-fast bacilli that are widespread throughout the environment, is of increasing importance in light of the AIDS epidemic. Although these organisms rarely cause disease in healthy adults, they can cause serious opportunistic infections in people with impaired immune systems.

Cholera is a disease caused by the bacterium Vibrio cholera. Infection results in severe, dehydrating diarrhea that is particularly dangerous to infants and small children. In 1991 cholera reappeared in the Western hemisphere for the first time in 100 years. The epidemic has spread as far north as Mexico and is a threat to travelers to Central and South America.

In 1992 a new strain of V. cholera appeared in Asia and in the area of the Bay of Bengal. This new organism causes disease in adults as well as children. NIAID supports research aimed at understanding the pathogenesis of the disease, what constitutes protective immunity, and the development of effective vaccines.

Effective antimicrobial agents have significantly reduced the burden of bacterial infections, even though their usefulness is limited by increasing bacterial resistance to antibiotics and in those diseases with an onset and progression so rapid that effective treatment is difficult. NIAID supports the development and testing of bacterial vaccines for Hemophilus influenzae type b, Streptococcus pneumoniae, all causes of meningitis; pertussis (whooping cough); cholera; shigella; and typhoid fever.

Hospital-associated, or nosocomial, infections have emerged in recent years as a significant health problem and cause of increased morbidity and mortality. They directly contribute to rising health care costs. An estimated 2 million hospital-associated infections occur in the U.S. each year, at a cost of more than $3 billion.

Cram-negative sepsis following surgery or trauma remains the most serious threat to patients, with mortality rates ranging from 25 to 40 percent if sepsis occurs. NIAID supports studies on immune mechanisms—cellular and humoral—that protect healthy people against normal microbial flora commonly encountered every day. Another focus is the study of disturbances in resistance mechanisms in hospitalized or immunocompromised patients. Gramnegative bacteria from the gastrointestinal tract are the primary etiologic agents and many have become resistant to antibiotics.

Hospital acquisition and transmission of methicillin-resistant staphylococci, Candida, enterococci, and antibiotic-resistant gram-negative bacteria are important areas of investigation.

The interplay of bacterial toxins such as lipopolysaccharide and staphylococcal toxic shock toxin with host serum and cell components can result in fever, shock, and death. NIAID is investigating the underlying mechanisms of shock and its control and prevention.

Fungal Diseases. Severe, sometimes life-threatening systemic infections caused by fungal organisms have long been recognized in all age groups and in all parts of the U.S. Treatment requires prolonged administration of relatively toxic drugs and is sometimes ineffective, even in the otherwise healthy patient. Fungal infections are increasingly recognized as a major cause of morbidity and mortality in patients with impaired immune defenses. NIAID supports research on medically important fungi such as Coccidioides immitis, Histoplasma capsulatum, Blastomyces dermatitidis, Cryptococcus neoformans, Candida albicans, and Aspergillus fumigatus.

Antimicrobial Drug Development. As promising new antibacterial and antifungal agents are developed, they must be critically evaluated for safety and efficacy in humans. NIAID selects for trial licensed and unlicensed drugs that the pharmaceutical industry is unlikely to test further in humans, even though the drugs may show considerable clinical promise. Controlled, prospective, and multicentered studies are designed to compare efficacy, safety, duration, and costs with standard chemotherapeutic agents. Currently, the institute supports trials of new systemic antifungal agents, an improved treatment regimen for urinary tract infections in women, antibiotic prophylaxis of respiratory infections in children with cystic fibrosis, and together with NICHD, an antibiotic trial for vaginal infections in pregnant women.

Sexually Transmitted Diseases (STD). A dramatic increase in the number of new cases of STDs has occurred over the past 50 years in the United States. Gonorrhea, syphilis, genital herpes, genital warts, chlamydial infections, and pelvic inflammatory disease (PID) take an increasingly large toll emotionally, physically, and economically. Each year in the U.S. there are approximately 4 million new cases of chlamydia, 1 million new cases of gonorrhea and 1 million new cases of PID. Thirty million Americans are estimated to have genital herpes, and 24-40 million are thought to be infected with human papillomavirus (HPV), several types of which are associated with development of cervical cancer.

STDs often have long-term, devastating consequences—particularly for women and children. Infertility, ectopic pregnancy, cervical cancer, increased risk of infection with HIV, fetal death, low birth weight, and congenital infections resulting in permanent physical and mental damage to infants, can result from STDs. In 1990 economic costs associated with PID alone were estimated to exceed $4.2 billion.

Current research priorities and initiatives focus on vaccine development, the sequelae of STDs in women, behavioral research, HPV, genital ulcer disease, the development of rapid, inexpensive diagnostics, and the development of topical microbicides.

NIAID conducts and supports basic research necessary to develop vaccines against gonorrhea, chlamydial infections, and syphilis. Candidate vaccines for genital herpes are under study, and two phase I clinical trials as well as a phase II trial have been completed. Additional trials are under way.

Because of the severe and disproportionate impact of STDs on health of women and infants, NIAID seeks to develop and evaluate interventions to reduce the incidence and severity of complications of PID, such as infertility, ectopic (tubal) pregnancy, and chronic pelvic pain syndromes. Furthermore, because STDs are preventable causes of adverse outcomes of pregnancy such as fetal wastage, low birth weight, and congenital infections, this area is also a priority.

In recognition of the critical interplay between behavioral and biomedical risk factors for STDs, NIAID is developing a program in integrated, intervention-oriented behavioral research for the prevention and control of STDs.

Studies of the pathogenesis and natural history of HPV are important areas of research. The role of HPV in development of cervical dysplasia and malignancy, HPV's role in transmission of HIV, development of animal models of genital HPV infection, and improved methods for detection and management of HPV infection are among the research areas of interest to NIAID.

The expansion of research on the pathogenesis and natural history of genital ulcer disease and on the interrelationship between these diseases and HIV is of high priority. Research on chancroid, syphilis, and genital herpes is being emphasized.

Parasitic Diseases. Parasitic diseases, a major world health problem, affect billions of people and are responsible for millions of deaths annually. While their principal health and economic impact is felt primarily in poor and developing countries, many parasitic infections remain endemic within the United States and can present a threat to individuals with immature or compromised immune systems or in situations where normal sanitation procedures break down. In addition, increased foreign travel by U.S. citizens as well as immigration to the United States allows importation of so-called "exotic" parasites from other countries.

A variety of unicellular protozoa and multicenter helminths cause parasitic disease. Goals of NIAID-sponsored studies on the immunology of parasitic diseases include the development of effective vaccines against malaria, schistosomiasis, filariasis, and others; the intervention in the host response to prevent immunologically mediated disease processes; and the development or improvement of immunodiagnostic procedures. NIAID also supports basic research on the biochemistry and molecular biology of parasites to develop new chemotherapeutic agents or improve the efficacy of existing drugs. Development of drug resistance is a rapidly increasing problem, particularly in malaria. Application of modern biochemical and molecular technology to determine how resistance develops may reveal ways to reverse the phenomenon. NIAID supports Tropical Disease Research Units at domestic institutions to provide a stable environment for research on parasitic diseases. These programs apply relevant and innovative biomedical technology to develop new approaches to control parasitic diseases of particular interest to the institute, including malaria, schistosomiasis, filariasis, trypanosomiasis, and leishmaniasis.

Vaccine Development. Vaccines have virtually eliminated once common killers such as diphtheria, tetanus, and polio in the U.S. Nearly 25 major human diseases caused by infectious agents are preventable or controllable through vaccine use. Despite this success, both new and old infectious diseases continue to threaten the health of people around the world.

The aim of the NIAID vaccine program is to capitalize on the extraordinary advances in molecular biology and immunology in order to improve the safety, effectiveness, and efficiency of existing vaccines and enhance the development of new vaccines. This is also the goal of the children's vaccine initiative, a global project of which NIAID is an integral part.

As the lead PHS agency for vaccine research, NIAID coordinates a comprehensive program among scientists in government, industry, and academic settings. Vaccine research is conducted by NIAID scientists as well as by institute-supported investigators at research institutions, including seven Vaccine Treatment and Evaluation Units. The units conduct clinical trials of candidate vaccines to determine whether they are safe and immunogeniccapable of stimulating an immune response.

Research on HIV vaccines is supported by NIAID's Division of AIDS.

International Research

The institute's international research activities involve grants, contracts and intramural projects to promote scientific research on tropical and other diseases of great importance to the health of people in developing and developed countries of the world.

Immediate aims are to improve means for diagnosing, treating, and controlling these diseases with the ultimate goal of disease prevention. For example, the U.S.-Japan Cooperative Medical Science Program organized in 1965, provides an opportunity for American and Japanese scientists to cooperate in studying 10 disease-related areas of importance to the health of Asian people.

In September 1979, the International Collaboration in Infectious Diseases Research Program replaced the International Centers for Medical Research and Training which had been operational since 1960. Under the new program, research centers are established in tropical countries through multidisciplinary program project grants awarded to U.S. institutions. The program is designed to promote true collaboration and scientific exchange between U.S. scientists and their overseas counterparts. Attention is given to the six diseases of WHO's Special Programme for Research and Training in Tropical Diseases, although no disease of major health importance to a tropical country is excluded. In 1991 NIAID established Tropical Medicine Research Centers to provide overseas facilities for the study of tropical diseases within endemic areas.

Other international activities include the NIAID-USAID Regional Project on the Epidemiology and Control of Vector-borne Diseases in the Near East, carried out through Jordan, Morocco, Lebanon, Tunisia, and Israel to study leishmaniasis and hydatid disease. NIAID also coordinates studies on the immunology of infectious diseases as part of the Indo-US Science and Technology Initiative.

Division of Allergy, Immunology and Transplantation

This division focuses on the immune system as it functions in the maintenance of health and as it malfunctions in the production of disease. It encompasses basic and clinical research.

Basic research is supported in 1) immunobiology and immunochemistry and 2) immunogenetics and transplantation immunology. Clinical research is supported in asthma and allergic diseases, and immunologic diseases and immunopathology. NIAID's approach integrates the basic science disciplines with relevant clinical specialties.

Basic Immunology. The biology and chemistry of the immune system and its products are the concerns of this program area. Immunobiologic studies focus on the origin, maturation, and interactions of the immune system's major cells, lymphokines, and other substances produced by these and other cells that mediate immune reactions. Studies include the mechanisms responsible for the induction and regulation of the immune response. Immunochemical research encompasses the delineation of the chemical structure and function of antigens and antibodies; the chemical basis of immunologic specificity; the regulation of immunoglobulin synthesis; and the mechanisms of antigen-antibody reaction. Research projects in this area are designed to:

- Elucidate the critical immunologic functions of T cell receptors, cell-adhesion molecules, and cytokines and their receptors in various systems in the human body and in laboratory animals.

- Isolate and characterize human stem cells.

- Participate in the formulation of a repository of cell lines and gene probes for use in the study of mucosal immunity and digestive diseases.

- Elucidate the chemical nature and structure of small organic molecules that generate allergic and hypersensitive responses; and

- Investigate the interactions of selected immunotoxicants with the secretory immune subsystems of the gut and respiratory tract.

Genetics and Transplantation. The primary goals of genetics and transplantation research are to:

- Clarify the organization and mechanisms of expression of the genes on which immune function depends;

- Characterize protein products of genes, including histocompatibility antigens;

- Determine how these gene products condition the response to foreign antigens; and

- Develop regimens to modulate the immune response and facilitate engraftment of transplanted organs and tissues.

By supporting the acquisition, characterization and distribution of tissue typing reagents and the evaluation and improvement of tissue typing methodologies, the program facilitates the matching of donors and recipients for transplants. It also supports studies on the relationship of the human major histocompatibility complex (MHC) HLA antigens to disease susceptibility. Research projects in this area are designed to:

- Investigate the mechanisms and innovative use of immunosuppressive drugs;

- Develop new monoclonal antibodies directed against specific cells to prevent graft rejection;

- Further develop reagents for precise typing of MHC or tissue matching; and

- Delineate the development of the fetal and adult immune response, using in vitro systems.

Identification and Acquisition of Reagents. NIAID contracts serve as sources of standard reagents to identify cell surface antigens both within and outside of the major histocompatibility complex that play a role in immune response.

Some of these reagents are available for use in workshops or similar large-scale studies.

The institute also is a primary source of standard reagents for distribution and analyses for basic immunogenetic studies of murine transplantation antigens.

Transplantation. Program projects in transplantation immunology, located at major transplant centers, are currently funded by NIAID to facilitate the rapid translation of basic immunologic discoveries into clinical use. The centers carry out basic and clinical research pertinent to mechanisms of rejection, organ availability and preservation, and management of rejection.

National Cooperative Clinical Trial in Transplantation. NIAID established this trial to expedite the evaluation of new treatment modalities to prevent kidney graft rejection. Multicenter clinical trials to assess the potential efficacy of various therapies are conducted at eight kidney transplant units throughout the U.S.

Asthma, Allergy and Inflammation. More than 50 million Americans suffer from allergic diseases including asthma. NIAID supports studies encompassing the cause, pathogenesis, diagnosis, prevention, and treatment of allergic diseases. Various types of allergic problems under investigation include: immediate type hypersensitivity and its disorders, including asthma, allergic rhinitis, atopic dermatitis, urticaria and angioedema; allergic reactions and disorders caused by insect bites and stings, foods, airborne allergens, and infectious agents; manifestations of delayed hypersensitivity and contact dermatitis; and the mechanisms of drug reactions and chemical sensitization. Studies also include structure of the antibodies, particularly IgE, and the chemical mediators released by the interaction of antigen and antibody with target cells; the isolation and chemical characterization of the active fractions of allergenic agents; and the therapy and prevention of allergic disorders and hypersensitivity reactions by immunotherapy with specific antigens or drugs.

Asthma, Allergic and Immunologic Disease Cooperative Research Centers. A network of cooperative research centers represents an effort to integrate the basic concepts of immunology, genetics, biochemistry, and pharmacology into clinical investigations of patients with asthma, allergic and immunologic diseases. The program encourages collaboration between basic and clinical scientists, provides a research environment for such interactions, and implements clinical application of adequately tested research findings and procedures. It is believed that this will lead to an understanding of the pathophysiologic, biochemical, and immunologic mechanisms of these disorders.

National Cooperative Inner-City Asthma Study. NIAID established this study to assess the factors contributing to the increased morbidity and mortality from asthma among children residing in urban environments, and to develop and evaluate a comprehensive therapeutic, educational, and environmental intervention program designed around those factors identified as major contributors. Eight sites in seven cities nationwide are participating in this cooperative study.

Clinical Immunology. Investigations of underlying mechanisms of disease and applications of basic knowledge to the cause, prevention, and management of immunologic disorders are approached from either of two disciplines—clinical immunology or immunopathology. Studies of clinical immunology involve acquired and inherited diseases associated with dysfunctions of the immune system, whereas the immunopathology studies encompass genetics, cytology, biochemistry, pathology, and pharmacology of the immune system. Areas under investigation include:

- Immune deficiency diseases arising from primary defects in development or maturation of the immune responses;

- acquired immune deficiency disorders excluding AIDS;

- clinical manifestations mediated by products of lymphocytes;

- diseases associated with immune complexes and autoimmune phenomena; and

- immunotherapy of disease process, including the use of immunopotentiating and immunoregulatory substances.

DAIT supports program projects in mechanisms of immunologic diseases and autoimmunity aimed at increasing the understanding of pathophysiologic processes of immune-mediated diseases and the development of improved methods of diagnosis, treatment and prevention of disorders of the immune system.

Division of AIDS

The mission of the Division of AIDS is to increase basic knowledge of the pathogenesis, natural history, and transmission of HIV disease, and to promote progress in its detection, treatment, and prevention. DAIDS accomplishes this mission by planning, implementing, and evaluating programs in:

- fundamental basic and clinical research,

- discovery and development of therapies for HIV infection and its complications,

- discovery and development of vaccines and other preventive interventions, and

- training of researchers in these activities.

In accord with this mission, the division's efforts are organized around five broad scientific areas: 1) pathogenesis, 2) epidemiology and natural history, 3) therapeutics research and development, 4) vaccine and prevention research and development, and 5) pediatric disease.

HIV Pathogenesis. Research on the pathogenesis of HIV infection will advance the understanding of the biological causes of HIV-related disease and serve as a foundation for advancing treatment and prevention. Investigator-initiated research and the traditional research grant are the foundation of the division's activity in this area. Important research gaps are identified by division staff in concert with investigators and advisory committees. Other key NIAID resources for the study of pathogenesis include:

- longitudinal epidemiological studies of cohorts of individuals infected with, or at risk of infection with, HIV, and serially collected specimens stored in an DAIDS-supported repository;

- animal model research and development projects;

- the NIAID AIDS Reference and Reagent Repository, through which DAIDS acquires and distributes essential research reagents to scientists around the world; and

- the Centers For AIDS Research (CFARS), designed to support coordinated scientific and administrative activities that enhance the capacity for collaboration between basic and clinical research.

Epidemiology and Natural History. The division's goals in the area of epidemiology and natural history are to foster population-based research that will advance the understanding of the biology and clinical course of HIV infection and serve as a foundation for advancing treatment and prevention.

The division oversees several large longitudinal cohort studies that conduct multidisciplinary research involving specific populations of individuals infected with or at significant risk of infection with HIV. These include:

- Multicenter AIDS Cohort Study,
- San Francisco Men's Health Study, and
- Women's Inter-Agency HIV Study.

In addition to collecting clinical data obtained at serial examinations and interviews, all of these studies are linked to a DAIDS-supported repository that stores a variety of serially collected biological specimens from participants and subsequently retrieves them for use in experiments conducted by investigators around the world. These studies therefore represent a powerful investigative tool for basic and applied research in pathogenesis, diagnosis, behavior, treatment, and prevention.

Vaccine and Prevention Research and Development. Development and testing of vaccines and other biomedical interventions such as drugs and microbicides to prevent HIV disease is a key role of DAIDS-funded research.

NIAID's efforts in vaccine research and development are built on a strong foundation of investigator-initiated research in basic virology, immunology, and microbiology. In addition, the division uses a number of specific applied resources to advance its objectives. These include:

- National Cooperative Vaccine Development Groups (NCVDGs), in which research teams from industry, academia, and government collaborate to develop and test novel experimental HIV vaccine concepts;

459

- SIV Vaccine Evaluation Units, which conduct standardized and directly comparable evaluations of various SIV vaccine candidates;

- Chimpanzee Unit, which is used to prepare stocks of virus for use in chimpanzees and to evaluate candidate vaccine concepts and products in chimpanzees;

- the AIDS Vaccine Evaluation Group (AVEG), which conducts phase I and II clinical trials of candidate HIV vaccines;

- central immunology laboratory facilities in support of the activities of the NCVDGs, the SIV-VEUs, the Chimpanzee Unit, and the AVEG;

- HIV Variation Project, which investigates the rate and magnitude of genetic variation in HIV and related retroviruses and explores the impact of this variation on strategies to develop HIV vaccines;

- Cooperative Group for Investigations of AIDS Vaccine Adjuvants, which supports investigator-initiated research into the mechanisms of adjuvant action, develops new adjuvant formulations to stimulate immune responses and generate long-lasting immunity and immunological memory, and evaluates vaccine-adjuvant combinations in relevant animal models;

- HIV Vaccine Efficacy Trials Network (HIVNET), which consists of both domestic and international HIV/AIDS vaccine efficacy trials components to study candidate HIV vaccines in U.S. populations and internationally; and

- Collaborative Mucosal Immunity Groups (CMIG), which characterize the immune response to HIV in both infected individuals and uninfected vaccinated people and primates.

Researchers at HIVNET and PAVE sites plan to study cohorts of individuals at high risk for HIV infection in order to determine the feasibility of conducting vaccine efficacy trials within these populations.

Therapeutics Research and Development. The division's goal in therapeutics is to foster the discovery and development of interventions that will improve the quality and duration of life of HIV-infected individuals.

NIAID devotes substantial resources to the discovery stage of therapeutics research, attempting to focus resources on areas of promise that are receiving insufficient attention from the private sector.

The effort begins with a strong commitment to basic research in microbiology and pathogenesis. Upon this are built programs of targeted drug discovery with the National Cooperative Drug Discovery Groups (NCDDGs) for HIV and opportunistic infections (OIs) at the center. These consortia of academia, industry, and government investigators work collaboratively on focused "gap" areas of targeted drug discovery. Small portfolios of highly applied traditional investigator-initiated research round out this effort.

NIAID's preclinical development resources are limited in scope to those necessary to ensure that the national effort has the capability to carry out specific rate limiting developmental steps involving selected highly promising candidate agents that lack a private sponsor with sufficient resources or commitment. These "gapfilling" resources include capabilities for 1) chemical resynthesis; 2) analytical chemistry and quality control; 3) dosage form development and manufacturing; 4) small and large animal toxicology; and 5) in vitro screening and animal model efficacy studies.

In addition, the Special Program for Innovative Research on AIDS Treatment Strategies (SPIRATS) foster coordinated and interdependent basic and clinical research between state-of-the-art studies in HIV pathobiology and clinical evaluation of novel therapeutic strategies. NIAID conducts clinical trials of new therapeutics in three networks:

- AIDS Clinical Trials Group (ACTG)a large, multicenter clinical trials network;

- Terry Beirn Community Programs for Clinical Research on AIDS (CPCRA)—a community-based program designed to address questions of importance to primary care clinicians and extend opportunity for participation in trials to persons underrepresented in HIV research; and

- Division of AIDS Treatment Research Initiative (DATRI)—a program designed to rapidly address critical questions or innovative treatment approaches.

Pediatric Disease. DAIDS is working to identify and support the development of improved interventions to prevent and treat HIV infection and its sequelae in infants, children, and adolescents. DAIDS' goals in pediatric disease include: 1) preventing perinatal HIV transmission to infants and HIV transmission to adolescents and children; 2) developing technology for the early identification and diagnosis of

HIV-infected infants; and 3) developing and optimizing therapies for HIV and its sequelae in infants, children, and adolescents. Specific resources related to pediatric disease include:

- Women and Infants Transmission Study, a longitudinal cohort study of infected women and their children;

- the pediatric component of the AIDS Clinical Trials Group; and

- investigator-initiated research, both solicited and unsolicited, addressing issues of pediatric disease.

Division of Intramural Research

The institute's Division of Intramural Research (DIR) consists of 16 laboratories, of which 13 are on the Bethesda campus and at off-campus sites in Frederick and Rockville, Md., and 3 are located at the Rocky Mountain Laboratories in Hamilton, Mont. Scientists in these laboratories conduct basic and applied research in immunologic, allergic, and infectious diseases and related clinical disorders. Considerable effort is devoted toward vaccine development and the understanding of the immune system's ability to react to certain antigens.

The scope of laboratory investigations includes the disciplines of virology, parasitology, mycology, microbiology, biochemistry, immunology, immunopathology and immunogenetics. Additionally, the DIR supports a 52-bed inpatient service and an outpatient facility located in the Clinical Center on the NIH campus. Patients with a variety of diseases under study, including AIDS, vasculitis, immunodeficiencies, host defense defects, unusual fungal infections, asthma, allergies, various parasitic diseases and disorders of inflammation, are seen. Frequently these patients participate in new and exciting treatment or diagnostic procedures derived from ongoing laboratory research efforts.

Successful vaccines or therapies for infectious diseases derive from a myriad of research activities on the disease agent as well as interactions of the agent with the host. The human immunodeficiency virus associated with AIDS is a major challenge to DIR scientists and physicians. The development of suitable laboratory animal models is critical to developing therapeutic strategies and vaccines for AIDS.

DIR scientists are studying the immunopathogenesis of HIV infection as well as the immune response to the virus. Cytokines have been shown to induce the expression of HIV in latently or chronically infected cell lines, thus providing tools for understanding the mechanisms of the insidious progression of immunosuppression in HIV-infected individuals.

In addition, NIAID researchers are exploring the many components of HIV disease, including phases of immune system activation and suppression. In studying the dissemination of HIV to lymphoid tissues in the body such as the lymph nodes and spleen, the investigators have found that HIV is active within these tissues from the earliest stages of HIV infection. This finding provides a scientific rationale for early treatment when safer and more effective antiretroviral drugs become available. DIR investigators have conducted intensive studies of antiretroviral and immunomodulator therapies. Clinical trials of a number of therapies, including use of IL-2 to maintain CD4 levels, are under way.

NIAID intramural scientists are working to develop and test vaccines against a number of infectious agents such as viruses causing AIDS, hepatitis A, dengue fever, diarrhea in infants, and pneumonia and croup in infants and young children. Bacterial agents that cause sexually transmitted diseases such as chlamydia and gonorrhea, and Lyme disease are under active investigation. Approaches to the development of a vaccine against malaria are being explored. Promising new vaccine candidates are tested in the clinical setting for safety, immunogenicity, and if warranted, efficacy.

Basic immunologic studies are aimed at defining the components and mechanisms of action of the humoral and cellular responses. Receptors on T lymphocytes and peptides linked to the surface of antigen presenting cells are being defined. Information derived from these studies may allow the design of peptides that can inhibit specific immune responses and may have great importance in controlling the rejection associated with transplantation.

DIR researchers are carrying out intensive studies of the role of newly discovered cytokines in T-cell differentiation. Researchers have found that interleukin 12 (IL-12) plays a pivotal role in the induction of T-cell responses, which are important for the control of intracellular infections.

B lymphocytes, critical components of the immune response and responsible for antibody responses, are being dissected for studies of structure and function. Among the studies being conducted are those related to the control of B-cell immunoglobulin class switching. It has been shown, for instance, that IL-4 and INF-gamma reciprocally regulate IgGI and IgE responses in mouse systems. In addition, the role of TGF-beta in IgA class-switching has been clarified. These studies are important in the design of future vaccines that can enhance the production of certain forms of antibody.

Inflammation is an important aspect of immunity. One of the important mediators of inflammation is a series of nine proteins called the complement system. NIAID scientists identified a new protein present in large concentrations in plasma of humans. The new protein binds to the fourth protein of the complement cascade where it acts as an inhibitor of this important inflammation-producing system. The inhibitor also interacts with the kinin-generating and coagulation systems. Certain patients with unusual swelling disorders have an abnormality in the degradation of this protein, and thus the protein may be very important in certain swelling disorders.

The first evidence that an immunodeficiency can be treated with a naturally occurring product of lymphocytes was recently demonstrated by DIR scientists. Chronic granulomatous disease of childhood (CGD), a disease in which there is a defect in the ability of the scavenger cells of the immune system to produce hydrogen peroxide, renders the patient susceptible to certain infectious agents. A multicenter clinical trial of interferon gammain patients with CGD followed in vitro studies which demonstrated the effectiveness of interferon gamma in correcting the defect in phagocytes from these patients Interferon gamma was shown to significantly reduce the number of serious infections in CGD patients. These studies led to FDA approval of this drug for use in CGD.

Studies of the immune response to the causative agent of leishmaniasis have demonstrated that immunity to the parasite is not only to a specific antigen, but also to a certain immune cell. DIR scientists have shown that the outcome of leishmaniasis depends on whether the animal develops a THI response with T cells that produce IL-2 and IFN-gamma, or a TH2 response with T cells that produce IL-4 and IL-5. In the former case, granulomas develop that wall off and kill leishmania in the latter case, the infection is disseminated.

Studies of allergy are carried out by investigators working in basic immunology laboratories as well as by clinical and laboratory investigators working within the Asthma and Allergic Diseases Center. One effort has been the study of IgE antibody which mediates allergic responses by causing mast cells to release mediators of allergic responses. IL-4, produced by T cells, is essential for production of IgE in mice. Administration of IL-4 to mice prevented increases in IgE antibodies normally observed in immune responses to certain antigens. In other studies, DIR scientists have developed a "knockout" mouse that lacks receptors for IgE antibodies on the surface of mast cells. These mice will facilitate a better understanding of the role of IgE responses in the production of allergic symptoms.

Studies of the mechanisms of allergies have emphasized work on mast cells. Mast cells are the central cells of allergic responses because when activated by an allergen and IgE they release the mediators of allergy. New techniques have been developed in order to grow human mast cells in culture, an advancement that will enable more detailed investigations into their biology. An improved approach to the treatment of asthma has been devised by DIR researchers. The concept is based upon separating bronchodilators from agents that act to reverse specific processes in the pathogenesis of asthma. Specifically, patients are placed on symptomatic therapy in order to permit the more specific therapy to act. Inhaled cromolyn, systemic corticosteroids and immunotherapy are employed as specific agents while beta adrenergic agonists, theophylline, and atropine are symptomatic agents. This approach is gaining increased acceptance and should improve long-term treatment of asthma.

National Institute of Arthritis and Musculoskeletal and Skin Diseases

Mission

The National Institute of Arthritis and Musculoskeletal and Skin Diseases (NIAMS) was established in 1986. It conducts and supports basic, clinical, and epidemiological research and research training, and disseminates information on many of the most debilitating diseases affecting the Nation's health. Many of these diseases are chronic. They afflict millions of Americans causing tremendous human suffering and costing the U.S. billions of dollars in health care and lost productivity. These diseases include the many forms of arthritis and numerous diseases of the musculoskeletal system and of the skin.

The institute also conducts and supports basic research on the normal structure and function of joints, muscles, bones, and skin. Basic research involves a wide variety of scientific disciplines, including immunology, genetics, molecular biology, structural biology, biochemistry, physiology, virology, and pharmacology. Clinical research addresses rheumatology, orthopedics, dermatology, metabolic bone diseases, heritable disorders of bone and cartilage, inherited and inflammatory muscle diseases, and sports medicine.

NIAMS Programs

The NIAMS supports a multidisciplinary program of basic and clinical investigations, epidemiologic research, research centers, and research training for scientists within its own facilities as well as supporting grantees at universities and medical schools nationwide. It also supports the dissemination of research results and information through the National Arthritis and Musculoskeletal and Skin Diseases Information Clearinghouse and through the Osteoporosis and Related Bone Diseases National Resource Center.

The NIAMS Intramural Research Program conducts basic research in structural biology, biology of the immune system, biology of the skin, muscle biophysics, and development of bone and cartilage. It does clinical research on lupus, rheumatoid arthritis, genetic skin diseases, and inflammatory muscle diseases.

The Extramural Program supports research via grants and contracts in four branches: Arthritis; Musculoskeletal Diseases; Skin Diseases; and Muscle Biology. Support also is provided for the Epidemiology/Data Systems Program and the Centers Program. A wide array of basic and clinical research and research training in the fields of rheumatology, muscle biology, orthopedics, bone and mineral metabolism, and dermatology are being pursued through these programs.

Arthritis Branch. This program supports basic and clinical research on the normal function and components of connective tissue and the immune system and their dysregulation in rheumatic, genetic, and inherited diseases of connective tissue. The goals are increased understanding of the mechanisms involved in the initiation and development of rheumatic and degenerative diseases of the joints and the translation of these basic research findings to prevention, diagnosis, and treatment of disease.

The research supported by the program uses approaches emanating from immunology, pathology, physiology, behavioral medicine, and epidemiology. Some of the specific diseases being studied include rheumatoid arthritis, osteoarthritis, systemic lupus erythmatosus, scleroderma, fibromyalgia, juvenile rheumatic diseases, gout, ankylosing spondylitis and other spondyloarthropathies, and many other inherited and acquired connective tissue disorders. Specific areas under investigation include:

- Biochemistry, physical chemistry, and metabolism of normal cartilage and extracellular matrix components.

- Mechanisms of dysregulation of immune function in rheumatic diseases, including development of new immunotherapies,

- Basic and clinical research in rheumatic diseases, including fibromyalgia, with emphasis on the development of therapies to prevent disease onset,

- Basic and clinical studies in osteoarthritis,

- Research in arthritic manifestations of chronic Lyme disease, and

- Inherited connective tissue disorders, including the application of gene therapy approaches.

Epidemiology and Data Systems Programs. The epidemiology program provides an administrative core for efforts to encourage epidemiologic research in the fields of rheumatic, musculoskeletal and skin diseases. Epidemiologic studies of these diseases contribute knowledge related to the prevalence and economic and social burdens from these diseases, studying their natural history, identifying risk factors, and investigating disease etiologies.

The data systems program fosters systematic acquisition, storage, retrieval, and analysis of information concerning arthritis and skin diseases. Program effort is focused on assuring validity and comparability of data collected in separate institutions and integrating data resources with data needs.

Musculoskeletal Diseases Branch. This program supports studies of the skeleton and associated connective tissues. Broad areas of interest include skeletal development, metabolism, mechanical properties, and responses to injury. Research on osteoporosis, a disease afflicting many of the Nation's growing population of older people, is a major area of emphasis. Some other diseases and skeletal disorders under investigation are osteogenesis imperfecta, a genetic disorder that leads to fragile, easily fractured bones; Paget's disease of bone, which results in irregular bone formation and subsequent deformity; genetic disorders of bone growth and development, such as osteomalacia.

Other studies focus on the causes and treatment of acute and chronic injuries, including carpal tunnel syndrome, repetitive stress injury, and low back pain. The program supports development of technologies with the potential to improve treatment of skeletal disorders and facilitate the repair of trauma in the normal skeleton. These include drugs and nutritional interventions, joint replacement, bone and cartilage transplantation, and gene therapy. Sports medicine and musculoskeletal fitness are also areas of special research emphasis. Research areas support through this branch include:

- Bone diseases: Epidemiology and development of disease; environmental and genetic risk factors; treatment, prevention, and diagnosis.

- Bone biology: Mechanisms of bone resorption; hormone, growth factor, and cytokine effects on bone-resorbing and bone-forming cells; regulation of bone growth and development; interactions among proteins, minerals, and cells in bone; mechanisms of mineralization.

- Orthopedic research: Skeletal architecture and mechanical properties; mechanisms of fracture repair; biomaterials, orthopedic devices, joint replacement and repair; rehabilitation.

Muscle Biology Branch. This program supports research on skeletal muscle, its diseases and disorders, and its central role in human physiology and exercise. Topics include the molecular structure of muscle and the molecular mechanisms that produce force and motion. An aim is understanding the alterations in muscle resulting from increased exercise and, conversely, the atrophy that follows immobilization during injury or illness. Specific aims include understanding the molecular structure and assembly of muscle components, including those responsible for contraction and regulation of muscle action; the molecular basis of genetic muscle diseases, such as Duchenne/Becker muscular dystrophy, myotonic dystrophy, myotonias, and malignant hyperthermia; genetic processes of muscle development and assembly; musculoskeletal fitness, metabolism, and adaptive mechanisms; the role of growth factors and hormones; altered metabolism during aging; the effects of therapeutic drugs and abused substances on basic muscle processes; the cellular basis for impaired muscle function in disease; inflammatory muscle diseases and inflammation resulting from exercise or injury; molecular mechanisms of muscle repair and regeneration; and development of more satisfactory methods of treatment and recovery. Specific research covered by the branch include:

- Muscle physiology

- Structure and function of muscle and of individual muscle proteins

- Mechanisms of muscle contraction and force generation

- Muscle development and specialization
- Musculoskeletal fitness and adaptive biology, including exercise physiology
- Muscle diseases and disorders
- Sports medicine, muscle injury and repair.

Skin Diseases Branch. Research studies supported by this program are increasing understanding of the mechanisms underlying normal and abnormal skin function and development. Research investigations are conducted on the molecular structures of various skin cells, the immunologic functions of the skin in normal and disease conditions, and the development of diagnostic tests and effective therapies for an array of skin diseases that can cause discomfort, disfigurement, and/or chronic disability. The range of skin diseases include keratinizing disorders such as psoriasis and ichthyosis atopic dermatitis and other chronic inflammatory skin disorders blistering diseases such as epidermolysis bullosa and pemphigus and disorders of pigmentation such as vitiligo and disorders of the hair and nails. Basic science and disease areas in skin research include:

- Metabolic studies of skin
- Immunologically mediated skin disorders
- Disorders or keratinization, pigmentation, and hair growth
- Photobiology. photoallery, and phototoxic reactions
- Bullous diseases and the basement membrane of skin
- Acne and physiologic activity of sebaceous glands
- Skin manifestations of diffuse connective tissue disorders
- Heritable connective tissue diseases
- Skin manifestations of HIV infection and AIDS.

Centers Program. The NIAMS currently supports three types of research centers programs: Multipurpose Arthritis and Musculoskeletal Diseases Centers, Specialized Centers of Research, and Skin Diseases Research Centers.

The Multipurpose Arthritis and Musculoskeletal Diseases Centers were established in the National Arthritis Act of 1974. The purpose of these centers, located at 14 medical institutions and hospitals around the country, is to foster a multidisciplinary approach to the many problems or arthritis and musculoskeletal diseases and to develop capabilities for research in these areas. To this end, centers develop and carry out basic and/or clinical research studies. research in professional and patient education, and epidemiology and health services research.

Existing Specialized Centers of Research (SCORs) are targeted for rheumatoid arthritis, systemic lupus crythematosus, osteoarthritis, and osteoporosis. These centers aim to accelerate the pace of basic research on the causes of disease and to expedite transfer of advances in basic science into clinical applications and improved patient care.

NIAMS has six Skin Diseases Research Centers (SDRC), which promote collaborative efforts among scientists engaged in high quality research related to a common theme. By providing funding for core facilities, pilot and feasibilty studies, and program enrichment activities at the SDRC, the institute reinforces and amplifies investigations already ongoing.

Information and Education Efforts. The focus of most NIAMS information and education efforts is in the Office of Scientific and Health Communications. The efforts include the National Arthritis and Musculoskeletal and Skin Diseases Information Clearinghouse, which helps lay and professional audiences locate materials and information, and a campaign entitled "What Black Women Should Know About Lupus." A National Resource Center on Osteoporosis and Related Bone Diseases provides public information and develops educational efforts on prevention, diagnosis, and treatment.

Intramural Research Program

The NIAMS intramural program has six main components—the Arthritis and Rheumatism Branch, Laboratory of Physical Biology, Laboratory of Skin Biology, Laboratory of Structural Biology, Protein Expression Laboratory, and craniofacial development section—the first section within a planned Bone and Connective Tissue Biology Branch.

The Arthritis and Rheumatism Branch (ARB) conducts a variety of investigations-basic and clinical. The historical focus of the ARB has been the study of the autoimmune rheumatic diseases—particularly rheumatoid arthritis, systemic lupus erythematosus, and myositis. At present, studies in the laboratories and clinics also focus on genetic diseases affecting inflammation and the musculoskeletal system, the basic mechanisms of signaling in the cells of inflammation, animal models of disease, genetic-epidemiologic studies, the role of neuroendocrine-immune system interactions in disease, and a variety of novel approaches to the interruption of inflammation.

In the Laboratory of Physical Biology leading-edge physical and biological techniques are used to study biological systems. Efforts are devoted to studying the structure of muscle cells, the molecular structure and function of various muscle components, and the mechanism of muscle contraction. Significant effort also is directed at the study of target sizes of macromolecules by radiation inactivation. The mechanism of cell membrane assembly is being investigated by means of calorimetry.

The Laboratory of Skin Biology conducts basic and clinical research on the skin and skin diseases, with particular emphasis on the epidermis—the outermost layer of skin. Basic research includes study of the various structural proteins and enzymes, and their genes, that are specifically expressed in the epidermis; the processes by which these molecules are assembled to form a normal epidermis; and the processes of abnormal cornification (keratinization) that occur in a variety of genetic skin diseases. One section within the lab uses direct and indirect genetic approaches to identify the molecular bases of disorders of cornitication and malignant skin diseases. This section also assists in genetic analysis of a variety of hereditary diseases under study by other NIH investigators, including complex hereditary disorders such as arthritis.

The Laboratory of Structural Biology conducts research into the structural basis of the assembly and functioning of macromolecules (large biological molecules) and their complexes, such as viruses, cell membrane and cytoskeletal proteins, and proteins in the skin. There is particular interest in the mechanisms that control these processes. These investigations make extensive use of cryoelectron microscopy and three-dimensional image processing. The newest group in this laboratory, established in 1991, is devoted to x-ray crystallographic study of the high-resolution structure and function of biological macromolecules and multienzyme complexes, including the replication complex of bacteriophage T4, retroviral proteins, and host factors involved in HIV expression.

The Protein Expression Laboratory, formerly under the NIH Office of the Director, joined the NIAMS in 1996. This lab plans and conducts research on the expression, purification, and structural characterization of HIV and HIV-related proteins. Laboratory scientists also collaborate with NIH intramural researchers studying the structure and function of HIV and HIV-related proteins. The lab serves as a support and resource group for the expression and purification of these proteins

The craniofacial development section, established in 1996, conducts basic investigations at the molecular and cellular levels on the mechanisms of bone and cartilage formation as they relate to human genetic diseases such as achondroplasia, craniosynostosis, craniofacial dysostosis, and various other forms of skeletal dysplasias. Signal transduction pathways that determine and maintain cartilage and bone formation are of particular interest. Members of the lab will use relevant animal models combined with the power of molecular genetics to address fundamental questions in bone and cartilage development and extrapolate their findings to shed light on the cause and development of human skeletal diseases.

National Institute of Child Health and Human Development

Mission

The National Institute of Child Health and Human Development (NICHD) seeks to assure that every individual is born healthy, is born wanted, and has the opportunity to fulfill his or her potential for a healthy and productive life unhampered by disease or disability. In pursuit of this mission, the NICHD conducts and supports laboratory, clinical. and epidemiological research on the reproductive. Neurobiologic, developmental, and behavioral processes that determine and maintain the health of children, adults, families, and populations. The institute administers a multidisciplinary program of research, research training, and public information, nationally and within its own facilities, on reproductive biology and population issues on embryonic development as well as maternal, child and family health and on medical rehabilitation.

NICHD programs are based on the concepts that adult health and well-being are determined in large part by episodes early in life. that human development is continuous throughout life, and that the reproductive processes and the management of fertility are of major concern, not only to the individual, but to society. The institute holds the tenet that when disease, injury, or a chronic disorder intervenes in the developmental process, it is incumbent to restore or maximize individual potential and functional capacity.

The institute supports and conducts basic, clinical, and epidemiological research in the reproductive sciences to develop knowledge enabling men and women to regulate their fertility in ways that are safe, effective, and acceptable to various population groups, and to overcome problems of infertility. The purposes of institute-sponsored behavioral and social science research in the population field are to understand the causes and consequences of reproductive behavior and population change.

Research for mothers, children and families is designed to advance knowledge of pregnancy, fetal development, and birth to develop strategies to prevent infant and childhood mortality to identify and promote the prerequisites of optimal physical, mental and behavioral growth and development through infancy, childhood, and adolescence and to contribute to the prevention and amelioration of mental retardation and developmental disabilities. Much of this research focuses on the disciplines of cellular, molecular, and developmental biology to elucidate the mechanisms and interactions that guide a single fertilized egg cell through it development into a multicellular, highly organized adult organism.

Medical rehabilitation research is designed to develop improved techniques and technologies with respect to the rehabilitation of individuals with physical disabilities resulting from diseases, disorders, injuries, or birth defects. Research training is an area supported across all NICHD research programs, with the intent of adding to the cadre of trained professionals available to conduct research in areas of critical public health concern.

An overarching responsibility of the NICHD is to disseminate information emanating from institute research programs to researchers. practitioners and other health professionals, and to the general public.

Organization

The NICHD has six major components—the Center for Research for Mothers and Children, the Center for Population Research, and the National Center for Medical Rehabilitation Research, all extramural programs supporting research through grants and contracts the Division of Intramural Research the Division of Epidemiology, Statistics, and Preventive Research and the Division of Scientific Review.

Center for Research for Mothers and Children. The Center for Research for Mothers and Children (CRMC) supports research and research training in the biomedical and behavioral sciences. The work is designed to foster pregnancies and births that produce sound infants—infants who can grow to adulthood free of disease and disability. The CRMC has six branches.

The Endocrinology, Nutrition and Growth Branch supports research on the nutritional needs of pregnant women, fetuses, and children and on the interrelationships of nutrition, endocrinology, and growth and development. The branch also focuses on nutritional and hormonal aspects of growth and development, both the normal and abnormal biological development of the fetus and infant, and on the effects of perinatal conditions and events on development.

The Human Learning and Behavior Branch is concerned with the development of human behavior, from infancy, through childhood and adolescence, into early maturity. Studies are supported in developmental psychobiology, behavioral pediatrics, cognitive and communicative processes, social and affective development and health-related behaviors, as well as learning disabilities, dyslexia, language disorders, day care and unintentional injuries.

The Mental Retardation and Developmental Disabilities Branch focuses on the etiology, pathogenesis, epidemiology, diagnosis, treatment and prevention of mental retardation and related disabilities, examining the biomedical, behavioral and social processes involved. The branch also supports 14 Mental Retardation Research Centers where research is conducted on mental retardation and related aspects of human development.

The Developmental Biology, Genetics and Teratology Branch develops and supports research and research training in the etiology of congenital malformations. The branch also examines gene transfer, the genetic basis of human development, and the development of the immune system.

The Pregnancy and Perinatology Branch studies research related to pregnancy and maternal health, embryonic development, fetal growth, and infant well-being. The branch also supports research on high-risk pregnancies, low birth weight, premature birth, perinatal pharmacology and toxicology, sudden infant death syndrome, exercise during pregnancy, and the impact of conditions and/or treatments during pregnancy, such as antibiotics, analgesics, anesthetics, drug use and addiction, cigarette smoking, obesity and infections on the outcome of pregnancy.

The Pediatric, Adolescent and Maternal AIDS Branch develops and supports research on HIV infection and disease as it affects women of childbearing age, pregnant women, mothers, fetuses, infants, children, adolescents and families. Research efforts focus on the epidemiology, natural history, pathogenesis, behavioral aspects, treatment and prevention of HIV infection and disease.

The Center for Population Research. The Center for Population Research (CPR) conducts the Federal Government's central effort in population research. Through grants and contracts, the center supports:

- Fundamental biomedical research on reproductive processes influencing human fertility and infertility

- Development of better methods for regulating fertility;

- Evaluation of the safety and effectiveness of contraceptive methods now in use; and

- Behavioral and social science research on the reproductive behavior of individuals, and the causes and consequences of population change.

There are four branches in the CPR. The Reproductive Sciences Branch supports fundamental biomedical research and research training in reproductive biology and medicine relevant to problems of human fertility and infertility.

The Contraceptive Development Branch supports projects aimed at developing safe and effective methods for regulating fertility in both men and women. The Contraceptive and Reproductive Evaluation Branch funds a national research program focusing on the epidemiology of reproductive health including studies of contraceptive and noncontraceptive gynocological products, medical devices, and surgical procedures.

The Demographic and Behavioral Sciences Branch supports studies on the social, psychological, economic and environmental factors governing population change, relationship between individual, household, and social behavior and population change.

National Center for Medical Rehabilitation Research. The NCMRR funds research training and projects on restoring, replacing or enhancing the function of individuals with physical disabilities. Medical rehabilitation research is directed towards restoration or improvement of functional capability lost as a consequence of injury, disease, or congenital disorder.

The Applied Rehabilitation Medicine Research Branch supports research to develop and evaluate new physical medicine/rehabilitation techniques and methods in prosthetics, orthotics, bioengineering, and technology transfer.

The Basic Rehabilitation Medicine Research Branch supports research and training in the physical medicine/rehabilitation areas of replacement, recovery, and restoration of function in neural, muscular, cardiac, pulmonary, urinary, and other physiological systems.

The Division of Intramural Research. The intramural research program conducts fundamental and clinical research at the Clinical Center and laboratories at NIH.

A limited number of research patients are admitted to the program's clinical research projects under guidelines established by the director of the Clinical Center. Patients must be referred by a physician. The DIR is broadly concerned with the biological and neurobiological, medical and behavioral aspects of normal and abnormal human development. In addition to four major clinical research and training programs in the areas of genetics, endocrinology, and maternal-fetal medicine, a diversity of developmental models are under study in 11 fundamental research laboratories and branches.

Fundamental Research

In the laboratories of the scientific director, the section on viruses and cellular biology studies the molecular events which influence the fidelity of the genonme, facilitating both evolution and species stability. A major objective is to elucidate the mechanisms which determine whether DNA repair is error-free or -prone in bacteria and in primate cells. The dynamics of mutagenesis are also of interest.

The section on growth factors studies the biochemical and physiological actions of nerve growth factor, a peptide required for the development of the sympathetic and sensory nervous systems.

The Laboratory of Developmental Neurobiology studies cellular, membrane and molecular mechanisms that determine nervous system functions and that figure importantly in brain development and mental retardation.

The Laboratory of Molecular Genetics examines how genetic information is transferred and expressed during development in a variety of organisms from yeast to mammals.

The Laboratory of Developmental and Molecular Immunity conducts research into developmental and molecular biology of "natural" and immunization-induced immunity to bacterial and other antigens. Emphasis has been placed on the study of pathogenic mechanisms, immunoregulatory mechanisms of the host, and the development of vaccines directed against serious bacterial infections.

The Laboratory of Theoretical and Physical Biology applies mathematical, statistical, and computer-based techniques to the analysis of complex clinical, biological, and pharmacological problems.

The Laboratory of Mammalian Genes and Development studies fundamental questions of development, differentiation and oncogenesis. Gene regulation at specific stages of mouse development is studied.

The Laboratory of Molecular Growth Regulation focuses on the control of mammalian cell growth, gene regulations and immune system function. Its goal is to understand normal control mechanisms and disorders of growth control that are manifested as cellular immortalization, transformation, or senescence.

The Laboratory of Molecular Embryology investigates the mechanisms by which gene expression is stabilized in embryogenesis. The laboratory is concerned with understanding the molecular mechanisms by which stable states of gene activity are established and maintained. Attention has been focused on germ cell-specific class II and class III genes.

The Laboratory of Cellular and Molecular Neurophysiology studies how neurotransmitter receptors and ion channels regulate information processing in the central nervous system.

The Endocrinology and Reproduction Research Branch studies the secretion and cellular actions of peptide and protein hormones, with particular reference to hypothalamic-pituitary hormones and their receptor-mediated responses in endocrine and neural cells.

The Cell Biology and Metabolism Branch carries out research in the areas of cell, molecular, and receptor biology. The molecular mechanisms of iron metabolism, the biology of intracellular organelles and membrane traffic, the mechanisms which regulate the fate of newly synthesized membrane proteins, the genetic response to environmental stress, and the biology of receptors central to the immune system are of interest.

Clinical Research

The Laboratory of Comparative Ethology investigates cognitive, social and motivational development in humans and in nonhuman primates. Research focuses on early environmental influences on behavior, development, and on the complex relationships between the organism and its environment. Research undertaken with primates seeks to relate brain function to behavioral states.

The Developmental Endocrinology Branch conducts basic and clinical studies of endocrine disease with emphasis on adult and pediatric reproductive endocrinology. Fundamental research focuses on endocrine and reproductive processes and gynecologic disorders. A major objective is to translate research findings into practical bedside application.

The Human Genetics Branch interests range from studies on the etiology, diagnosis and treatment of genetic and developmental disorders of young people to very basic studies on eukaryotic gene expression utilizing recombinant DWA methodology. Current research projects concern lipid and carbohydrate metabolism, the mucopolysaccharidoses, heritable disorders of the bone and connective tissue, lysosomal storage diseases (e.g., cystinosis), temperature sensitive models of cellular differentiation, and heritable disorders of bone and connective tissue.

The Perinatal Research Branch, located in Washington, D.C., conducts clinical investigations of obstetric and neonatal conditions contributing to infant mortality. Emphasis is placed on antenatal diagnostic techniques, premature labor, and other causes of low birth weight.

Division of Epidemiology, Statistics, and Prevention Research

The division provides the institute with the skills of four disciplines: biostatistics, behavioral sciences, computer sciences, and epidemiology. The Biometry and Mathematical Statistics Branch provides statistical consulting and data analyses to support intramural and extramural investigators and conducts its own methodological research in biostatistics. It also participates as a statistical unit in studies and projects of NICHD).

The Epidemiology Branch studies determinants of high risk pregnancies and of infant mortality and childhood mortality including congenital malformations. Particular attention is give to determinants which lend themselves to interventions and prevention.

The Computer Sciences Branch serves as the division's central resource for systems analysis, design and programming expertise with emphasis on the development and implementation of analysis, statistical procedures and data processing procedures in epidemiology and biometry. It also houses the data coordination center for the NICHD study of early child care.

The Prevention Research Branch conducts biobehavioral research to promote healthful behaviors and to prevent or ameliorate disease during pregnancy, infancy, and childhood through adolescence. The focus is the development and evaluation of interventions in health care setting and school-based programs for children and adolescents.

Division of Scientific Review

The Division of Scientific Review is responsible for a broad range of functions related to the review of research and training grant applications and research contract proposals.

The division provides policy direction and coordination for the planning and conduct of initial scientific and technical merit review of applications for various types of grants, including program projects, centers, institutional training, career development and conferences. The division serves the same function for NICHD research and development contracts in the biomedical, clinical, and behavioral sciences.

National Institute of Dental Research

Mission

Established in 1948, the National Institute of Dental Research is the primary sponsor of oral, dental and craniofacial research and related training in the U.S. Its mission, to improve and promote oral health, is accomplished by conducting and coordinating research to establish the causes, develop better diagnostic methods and treatments, and ultimately find ways to prevent or substantially lower the risk of developing oral and craniofacial conditions; and by maintaining a cadre of trained scientists to conduct basic, clinical, and applied research.

Institute scientists and those affiliated with grant-supported NIDR programs have made great strides in improving the Nation's oral health through advances in diagnosis, treatment and prevention. NIDR has organized its efforts into three major components: the Division of Extramural Research, which provides grant and contract funds to the scientific community for research and research training; the Division of Intramural Research, centered in NIDR's laboratories and clinics in Bethesda, Md.; and the Division of Epidemiology and Oral Disease Prevention, which sponsors epidemiologic studies of oral diseases, engages in controlled clinical trials of potential preventive agents an regimens; and promotes their dissemination to the dental profession and the general public.

Together, NIDR's three organizational divisions conduct and support basic research in biochemistry, microbiology, immunology, physiology, anatomy, histology, cell and molecular biology, genetics, pathology, bioengineering, and the social and behavioral sciences.

NIDR also sponsors clinical, epidemiological and applied studies in the oral health sciences.

The institute promotes the timely transfer and adoption of research findings by the public, health professionals, and the research community. NIDR collaborates with other U.S. Government organizations within and outside the NIH, with health professional and voluntary associations and industry, and with health professional and voluntary associations and industry, and with investigators internationally in developing and implementing research programs of mutual interest.

Division of Extramural Research and Special Programs

NIDR is the primary sponsor of oral, craniofacial, and dental research and research training in the U.S. Through its extramural program, the institute provides funds for biomedical and behavioral research outside its intramural laboratories and clinics in Bethesda. Funds are made available in the form of grants, cooperative agreements and contracts which support scientists working in institutions throughout the United States and in foreign countries. These scientists carry out research ranging from laboratory studies on the basic causes of oral and dental diseases to clinical trials of new public health measures for treatment and prevention. Funds are also awarded to train new researchers in certain needed disciplines. In addition to the Office of the Director, which incorporates the Office of Policy and Coordination, and Research Training and Career Development, the extramural program consists of two components: 1) the Program Development Branch with seven parts: Caries, Nutrition and Fluoride; Periodontal Diseases; Craniofacial Development and Disorders; Biomaterials, Pulp Biology and Dental Implants; Oral Soft Tissue Diseases and AIDS; Behavioral, Pain, Oral Function and Epidemiology; and Salivary Glands Research and Oral Biology Centers and 2) the Program Operations Branch, including the Scientific Review, Grants Management, and Contracts Offices. Brief descriptions are presented in the following paragraphs.

The Caries, Nutrition and Fluoride Program supports research on the causes, early diagnosis, prevention and treatment of caries. High priority areas include total fluoride intake, fluoride metabolism and action, caries prevention and control, fluorosis, and fluoride retention in bone and its relationship to aging and bone diseases. In the area of nutrition, research is targeted to defining the role of nutrition in oral health and the influence of compromised oral/ craniofacial health on nutrition and general health.

The Periodontal Diseases Program supports research on the etiology, pathogenesis, prevention, diagnosis, and treatment of periodontal diseases. Areas of particular interest include microbial virulence factors involved in periodontal diseases, development of assays to identify periodontal pathogens, and the role of host immune response in both the prevention and pathogenesis of periodontal diseases. The program also supports research to identify behavioral, psychosocial, environmental, and genetic risk factors for periodontal diseases.

The Craniofacial Development and Disorders Program supports research in cellular and molecular biology, protein chemistry, and biomineralization to improve our understanding of the causes and treatment of congenital craniofacial anomalies such as cleft lip and palate, dentofacial malrelations, and ameliogenesis imperfecta. Areas of special interest include defining the human genes for craniofacial malformations, identifying factors that regulate craniofacial development, and testing orthodontic and surgical strategies for correcting malformations.

The Biomaterials, Pulp Biology and Dental Implants Program supports the development of biocompatible materials for preventing oral disease and restoring damaged tissues. The pulp biology component encourages research on the development and physiology of this soft tissue and its hard dentin covering, including studies on sensitivity and pulp inflammation. Implant research focuses on improving the implant tissue interface, developing improved implant materials, and supporting clinical trials.

The Oral Soft Tissue Diseases and AIDS Program fosters basic and clinical research on diseases that affect the soft tissues of the mouth, including viral, fungal and bacterial infections, and oral cancer. The AIDS component focuses on oral changes as diagnostic and prognostic indicators of human immunodeficiency virus infection and disease progression, salivary functions in HIV infection, and the role of saliva in preventing the oral transmission of HIV.

The Behavioral, Pain, Oral Function and Epidemiology Program supports research to identify the psychosocial and prevention factors that influence the onset and progression of oral diseases and disorders and how these conditions affect the quality of life. The pain component supports studies to enhance the understanding, management and prevention of chronic and acute orofacial pain conditions such as temporomandibular disorders and burning mouth syndrome. Other program interests include research and epidemiological studies on such areas as taste, smell, thermal and tactile sensitivity disorders, and on normal and impaired oral motor function.

The Salivary Glands Research and Oral Biology Centers Program focuses on improving knowledge of the development, structure, function, and diseases of the salivary glands and to determine the influence of salivary constituents on oral health.

NIDR also funded 28 center grants for $18 million, approximately 15 percent of the EP budget. The center awards supported noncategorical Research Centers in Oral Biology. Oral Health in Aging Centers, Periodontal Diseases Research Centers, Caries Research Centers, Materials Science Research Centers, Clinical Dental Research Core Centers, and Regional Research Centers for Minority Oral Health. These centers not only contribute new information to oral health sciences, but provide stimulating environments for collaborative efforts and training researchers and educators.

The Research Training and Career Development Program supports training and career development opportunities in all the program areas of oral health research.

Under the Program Operations Branch, the Scientific Review Office coordinates initial scientific peer review of a variety of large research grant applications such as centers and program projects, training and career development applications, small grants and conference grant applications, and coordinates and conducts project site visits and other review procedures. The Grants Management Office is responsible for all fiscal management activities associated with the review, negotiation, award, administration, and termination of grants. The Contracts Management Office has responsibility for all matters relating to solicitation, negotiation, award, and administration of research and development contracts.

Contracted Research Studies

NIDR's contracted research activities of the extramural and intramural research programs and the Epidemiology and Oral Disease Prevention Program fund studies to readily translate advances in the basic sciences to disease-oriented applied research as well as to provide support complementary to basic science investigations. Interagency agreements with other Federal agencies have also been utilized to provide support toward these NIDR goals.

Division of Intramural Research

NIDR's intramural research program conducts basic and clinical research directed toward increasing fundamental knowledge of oral diseases and related disorders. The latest techniques in biomedical science—particularly those of molecular biology, immunology and cell biology—are used. Areas under investigation include the biochemistry, structure, function and development of bone, teeth, salivary glands and connective tissues; the role of bacteria and viruses in oral disease; genetic disorders and tumors of the oral cavity: studies on the cause and treatment of acute and chronic pain; and the development of new and improved diagnostic methods. The intramural research program has approximately 300 employees and guest researchers in eight laboratories, a dental clinic and a pain research unit.

The Clinical Investigations and Patient Care Branch conducts research related to the diagnosis, prevention and management of oral and dental diseases. Primary efforts are directed at understanding regulation of events involved in salivary secretion. Other studies focus on xerostomia (dry mouth), establishing criteria for evaluating salivary gland status and developing treatment for hypofunctional glands.

The Bone Research Branch studies the development and structure of bones, teeth and cartilage. Emphasis is placed on acquired heritable disorders of the skeleton through research in bone and cartilage cell biology, skeletal tissue metabolism and matrix moleculesmajor components of most tissues and critical factors in oral tissue development, function and health.

The Neurobiology and Anesthesiology Branch has as its primary interests clinical and basic research on pain mechanisms, the development of new methods of assessing pain, and evaluating new approaches to pain control. Collaborative studies, including research on pain associated with cancer and diabetes, have been initiated with other institutes.

The Laboratory of Oral Medicine conducts basic and clinical research on viral infections, autoimmune disorders and endocrine diseases. Studies focus on development of transgenic mice to study genes and proteins of HIV and human immunodeficiency virus. Research is also aimed at cloning and sequencing autoantigens which play a role in triggering autoimmune diseases such as insulin-dependent diabetes mellitus.

The Laboratory of Developmental Biology investigates the roles and gene regulation of the extracellular matrix, a key component of connective tissue, and other cell interaction systems in embryonic development and related processes. Research focuses on such areas as normal and abnormal embryonic development of craniofacial and other tissues, cancer metastasis, and wound healing.

Research in the Laboratory of Cellular Development and Oncology is directed toward understanding the role of growth and regulatory factors in oncogenesis. Studies focus on molecular mechanisms responsible for conversion of normal cells to a malignant state.

Scientists in the Laboratory of Immunology conduct basic research on mechanisms of acute and chronic inflammatory diseases such as arthritis, periodontal disease and AIDS. Understanding the pathways of inflammation will enable investigators to devise methods to interrupt this process and ultimately halt the tissue destruction characteristic of these disorders.

Research in the Laboratory of Microbial Ecology is concerned with human infectious diseases and host immunity. Studies focus on efforts to define the disease-causing mechanisms of microbial organisms, to understand interactions between these organisms and their human host, and to develop methods to protect against disease.

Division of Epidemiology and Oral Disease Prevention

This division conducts research on the etiology, distribution, and epidemiology of a broad range of oral conditions and facilitates the rapid transfer and adoption of disease prevention and oral health promotion measures by the public and the profession. DEODP consists of three branches.

The Molecular Epidemiology and Disease Indicators Branch develops, evaluates, and refines various types of cost-effective genetic and biological markers and clinical indicators for use in epidemiologic studies of oral and craniofacial conditions as well as hundreds of systematic diseases that affect oral health. Oral markers and indicators will be used to predict or detect those at highest risk of developing oral and craniofacial conditions.

The Disease Prevention and Health Promotion Branch plans and conducts analytical, experimental and community intervention research to identify, develop, and evaluate methods for the control and prevention of orofacial diseases and conditions, especially in high-risk populations and among special care groups. The branch also plans and conducts research designed to promote oral health and encourages transfer of scientific knowledge of disease prevention and health promotion to appropriate target groups.

The Analytical Studies and Health Assessment Branch analyzes patterns of oral diseases and disorders and the need for and utilization of dental treatment and dental delivery systems.

National Institute of Diabetes and Digestive and Kidney Diseases

Mission

The National Institute of Diabetes and Digestive and Kidney Diseases conducts and supports research on many of the most serious diseases affecting the public health. The institute supports much of the clinical research on the diseases of internal medicine and related subspecialty fields as well as many basic science disciplines.

The institute's Division of Intramural Research encompasses the broad spectrum of metabolic diseases such as diabetes, inborn errors of metabolism, endocrine disorders, mineral metabolism, digestive diseases, nutrition, urology and renal disease, and hematology. Basic research studies include biochemistry nutrition pathology histochemistry chemistry physical, chemical, and molecular biology pharmacology and toxicology.

NIDDK extramural research is organized into four divisions: Diabetes, Endocrinology and Metabolic Diseases; Digestive Diseases and Nutrition; Kidney, Urologic and Hematologic Diseases; and Extramural Activities.

The institute supports basic and clinical research through investigator-initiated grants, program project and center grants, and career development and training awards. The institute also supports research and development projects and large-scale clinical trials through contracts.

NIDDK Programs

Division of Intramural Research. The Division of Intramural Research conducts research and training within the institute in 1993s laboratories and clinical facilities in Bethesda, Md., and at the Phoenix Epidemiology and Clinical Research Branch in Arizona.

The division has 10 branches and 12 laboratories, which cover a wide range of research areas. In addition, there is a section on veterinary sciences, a joint program between the NIDDK and the Cystic Fibrosis Foundation to do basic research and an institute-wide research training program in nutrition.

Eight branches are engaged primarily in basic and clinical research on diabetes, bone metabolism, endocrinology, hematology, digestive diseases, and genetics. The Phoenix Epidemiology and Clinical Research Branch develops and applies epidemiologic and biologic methods in field

485

studies throughout the world on selected populations at risk of developing specific diseases, especially diabetes and its complications. The 10th branch addresses mathematical modeling of biological problems. The laboratories are engaged in fundamental research related to the institute's mission (e.g., molecular biology, chemistry, mathematics, cell biology, toxicology, pharmacology, physics, biochemistry, neuroscience, and developmental biology). The laboratory animal science section provides research animal support and collaboration to the research programs of the institute.

Division of Diabetes, Endocrinology and Metabolic Diseases

The DEMD supports research and research training related to diabetes mellitus, endocrinology, and metabolic diseases including cystic fibrosis. In addition, DEMD leads the administration of the Trans-NIH Diabetes Program and coordinates federally supported diabetes-related activities. The division also administers the Trans-NIH Cystic Fibrosis Program.

Diabetes Programs Branch Diabetes Research Program. This program supports basic and clinical studies related to the etiology, pathogenesis, prevention, diagnosis, treatment, and cure of diabetes mellitus and its complications. The program also supports investigations related to pancreas and islet transplantation, automated insulin delivery systems, glucose sensors, the epidemiology of diabetes and its complications, and behavioral research related to diabetes.

Diabetes Centers Program. Two types of awards are made: Diabetes/Endocrinology Research Centers, exclusively oriented toward biomedical research goals, and the Diabetes Research and Training Centers (DRTC), which include training and information transfer components in addition to research. The DERCs and DRTCs integrate, coordinate, and foster interdisciplinary cooperation of investigators in diabetes and related endocrine and metabolic disorders. Both programs also provide limited funds for pilot and feasibility studies to encourage young investigators and new initiatives.

Clinical Trials Program. This program supports a multicenter randomized clinical trials on the treatment and prevention of insulin-dependent and non-insulin-dependent diabetes mellitus.

National Diabetes Data Group. The NDDG serves as the major Federal focus for the collection, analysis, and dissemination of data on diabetes and its complications.

WHO Collaborating Center for Diabetes. This center, sponsored by the Division of Diabetes, Endocrinology, and Metabolic Diseases, solicits and provides guidance in developing international research about diabetes through NIH research grants and contracts; promotes interchange of scientific and health information among WHO member countries; and provides expert advice and consultation to WHO and other international committees and agencies.

Endocrinology and Metabolic Diseases Programs Branch. Endocrinology Research Program. Basic and clinical studies of normal and abnormal functions of the pituitary, thyroid, parathyroid, and adrenal glands, as well as other components of the endocrine system are supported. Studies involve the mode of action of hormones, their biosynthesis, secretion, and metabolism as well as their binding to protein carriers, and interactions with other hormones and metabolites.

Hormone Distribution Program. This program makes available to the research community human and animal pituitary hormones, antisera against the hormones, and selected other hormonal and biological products. An important research resource for the scientific community, this program gives scientists access to hormones and antisera of known composition and potency, most of which are unavailable commercially.

Metabolic Diseases Research Program. This program funds investigator-initiated research into enzymatic mechanisms, biological transport, and membrane structure as they relate to the etiology, pathogenesis, and treatment for acquired or inborn errors of metabolism.

Cystic Fibrosis Research Program. This program supports investigator-initiated research and research center grants related to the genetic, metabolic, and nutritional aspects of CF and its complications.

Division of Digestive Diseases and Nutrition

This division supports research related to liver and biliary diseases, pancreatic diseases, gastrointestinal diseases, including neuroendocrinology, motility, immunology, and digestion in the GI tract, nutrient metabolism, obesity, eating disorders, and energy regulation. The division provides leadership in coordinating activities related to digestive diseases and nutrition throughout the NIH and with various other Federal agencies.

Digestive Diseases Branch Liver and Biliary Program. This program supports basic and clinical research into the normal function and the diseases of the liver and biliary tract. Areas of study include hepatic regeneration liver cell injury, fibrosis, and death basic and applied studies on liver transplantation metabolism of bile acids and bilirubin physiology of bile formation factors controlling cholesterol levels in bile gallbladder and bile duct function cholesterol and pigment gallstones inborn errors in bile acid metabolism chronic hepatitis that evolves from autoimmune, viral, or alcoholic disease and other liver diseases.

Pancreas Program. This program encourages research into the structure, function, and diseases (excluding cancer and cystic fibrosis) of the exocrine pancreas. Research efforts focus on hormonal and neural regulation of electrolyte, fluid, and enzyme secretion receptors for secretagogues stimulus-secretion coupling mechanisms gutislet-acinar interrelations organization and expression of pancreiltic genes protein synthesis and export tissue injury, repair, and regeneration physiology and pathology of trophic responses neural innervation transcapillary solute and fluid exchange pancreatic transplantation, storage, and preservation imaging of the pancreas pancreatic insufficiency acute and chronic pancreatitis and relevant experimental models and endocrine tumors.

Gastrointestinal Neuroendocrinology Program. This program supports both basic and clinical studies on normal and abnormal function of the enteric nervous system and the central nervous system elements that control the enteric nervous system. Research focuses on gastrointestinal hormones and peptides and studies on disease conditions associated with excessive or deficient secretions of neuropeptides.

Gastrointestinal Digestion Program. This program supports research on the process of food digestion in the gastrointestinal tract (GIT). Areas of research focus on the regulation of gene expression in the developing gastrointestinal tract the structure and function of the gut mucosa the cytoskeletal structure and contractility in brush border the growth and differentiation of gastrointestinal cells in normal and disease states intestinal transplantation. storage, and preservation and gastrointestinal tissue injury, repair, and regeneration.

Also supported are studies on gastrointestinal diseases such as maldigestion and malabsorption syndromes, celiac sprue, diarrhea, inflammatory bowel disease, gastric and duodenal ulcers, diseases of the salivary glands (excluding cystic fibrosis), and the effects of prostaglandins and other treatment modalities on the gastrointestinal tract and their possible role in the pathogenesis and treatment of digestive diseases.

Gastrointestinal Motility Program. This program supports research on the structure and function of gastrointestinal muscles, the biochemistry of contractile processes and mechanochemical energy conversion relations between metabolism and contractility in smooth muscle, extrinsic control of digestive tract motility, and the fluid mechanics of gastrointestinal flow. Areas of interest include the actions of drugs on gastrointestinal motility, intestinal obstruction, and diseases such as irritable bowel syndrome, colonic diverticular disease, swallowing disorders, and gastroesophageal reflux.

Gastrointestinal, Mucosal and Immunology Program. The research emphasis of this program focuses on intestinal immunity and inflammation. Areas of interest include: ontogeny and differentiation of gut-associated lymphoid tissue migratory pathways of intestinal lymphoid cells humoral antibody responses cell-mediated cytotoxic reactions and the role of cytotoxic effector cells in chronic intestinal inflammation genetic control of the immune response at mucosal surfaces immune response to enteric antigens in both intestinal extraintestinal sites granulomatous inflammation lymphokines and cellular immune regulation leukotrienes/ prostaglandin effects on intestinal immune responses T-cell mediated intestinal tissue injury the intestinal mast cell and its role in intestinal inflammation approaches to optimal mucosal immunoprophylaxis, including viral, bacterial, and parasitic diseases and diseases such as gluten sensitive enteropathy, inflammatory bowel disease, and gastritis.

Acquired Immunodeficiency Syndrome Program. This program encourages research into the characterization of intestinal injury, mechanism of maldigestion, and intestinal mucosal functions, as well as hepatic and biliary dysfunction in AIDS. In addition, studies are supported on mechanisms of nutrient dysfunction, nutritional management in the wasting syndrome and other aspects of malnutrition related to AIDS.

Digestive Diseases Centers Program. This program currently administers research core center grant awards. These awards provide a mechanism for integrating, coordinating, and fostering interdisciplinary cooperation between groups of established investigators who conduct programs of high-quality research that relate to a common theme in digestive disease research.

Clinical Trials Program. This program includes all prospective studies in digestive diseases and nutrition. Using 10 or more patients, studies compare two forms of treatment, one of which could be placebo or "standard" care.

Nutritional Sciences Branch Nutrient, Metabolism Program. This program supports basic and clinical studies related to the requirement, bioavailability, and metabolism of nutrients and other dietary components. Specific areas of research interest include the understanding of the physiological function and mechanism of action/ interaction of nutrients within the body the effects of environment, heredity, stress, drug use, toxicants, and physical activity on problems of nutrient imbalance and nutrient requirements in health and disease and specific metabolic considerations relating to alternative forms of nutrient delivery and use such as total parenteral nutrition.

The program also supports research to improve methods of assessing nutritional status in health and disease.

Obesity, Eating Disorders, and Energy Regulation Program. This program funds research on the biomedical and behavioral aspects of obesity, anorexia nervosa, bulimia, and other eating disorders.

The goals of such research are to establish a clear understanding of the etiology, prevention, and treatment of these multifaceted conditions. Areas of research interest focus on the factors that affect food choices, food intake, eating behavior, appetite, and satiety the effects of taste, smell, and gastric and humoral (including neurotransmitters) responses associated with dietary intake and subsequent behavior the physiological and metabolic consequences of weight loss or weight gain the effect of mild exercise on appetite and weight control and the individual variability in energy utilization and thermogenesis.

The program encourages investigations on the dietary determinants of the growth and control of adipocyte size and number the responsiveness of the adipocyte to various metabolic and pharmacologic stimuli the prevention of obesity and other eating disorders improved methods of assessing body composition examination of health risk factors associated with specific degrees of obesity or body composition and determining the effect of exercise on body composition. The program supports an obesity research core center, which serves as a resource for scientists studying various aspects of obesity.

Clinical Nutrition Research Units. The CNRU is an integrated array of research, educational, and service activities focused on human nutrition in health and disease. It serves as the focal point for an interdisciplinary approach to clinical nutrition research and for the stimulation of research in improved nutritional support of acutely and chronically ill persons, assessment of nutritional status, effects of disease states on nutrient needs, and effects of changes in nutritional status on disease.

Obesity/Nutrition Research Centers. The ONRCs encourage collaboration among researchers and a multidisciplinary approach to the treatment and prevention of obesity. They will help to capitalize on emerging research opportunities in obesity and to enhance the translation of research findings to the public.

US-Japan Malnutrition Panel. In 1965 President Lyndon B. Johnson and Japanese Prime Minister Eisaku Sato issued a joint communique, recognizing their mutual concern for the health and well-being of all the peoples of Asia. This effort led to the foundation of the U.S.-Japan Cooperative Medical Science Program, which operates within a bilateral government framework. The malnutrition panel was established in 1966 to foster and support investigator-initiated research to help alleviate the serious problem of malnutrition.

Current topics of importance to both the U.S. and Japan focus on consequences of changing dietary patterns on health, development of disease and disease prevention. Specific research areas addressing these topics include the nutritional significance of varying the polyunsaturated fatty acids in the diet, nutritional aspects of bone disease, endogenous mediators of nutritional metabolism, and improved methodologies applicable to nutritional assessment.

Special Programs Branch

Epidemiology and Digestive Diseases Data System. P.L. 99-158 authorized the establishment of this program for the collection, storage, analysis, retrieval, and dissemination of data derived from patient populations with digestive diseases and, where possible, data involving general populations to detect individuals with a risk of developing digestive diseases.

Liver Transplantation Database Project. The purpose of the 7-year project is to establish a liver transplantation database with data gathered from patients and donors from several transplant centers in the United States. To answer questions about transplantation, data are being collected from patients who are undergoing liver transplantation for various acute and chronic liver diseases and malignancies. The data relate to patients' conditions prior to operation, and in early and late postoperative periods and to donor livers and malignancies. The data will be evaluated and made available to investigators and clinicians.

Division of Kidney, Urologic and Hematologic Diseases

The division supports research on the physiology. pathophysiology. and diseases of the kidney, genitourinary tract, and the blood and blood-forming organs to improve or develop preventive, diagnostic, and treatment methods.

Kidney Research

Chronic Renal Diseases Program. This program supports basic and clinical studies related to the etiology, pathogenesis, prevention, diagnosis, and treatment of renal diseases that affect adults and children.

Areas of research focus on the primary and nonprimary glomerulopathies and renal disease resulting from various systemic diseases kidney disease of diabetes mellitus kidney disease of hypertension congenital and inherited renal diseases immune-related renal disease IgA nephropathy and tubulointerstitial nephritis.

End-Stage Renal Disease Program. This program focuses on the causes and physiology of uremia, and on hemo-dialysis, peritoneal dialysis, and renal transplantation. The program seeks to improve organ availability by supporting research on transplants across the ABO blood barrier, better cross-matching of donors with recipients, and innovative approaches to making organs available in all areas of the country.

Pediatric Nephrology Program. This program supports basic and clinical research on the causes, treatments, and prevention of kidney diseases of children. Research efforts focus on inherited and congenital renal diseases kidney disease of diabetes mellitus IgA nephropathy and kidney disease and hypertension, which starts in early childhood.

Renal Physiology/Cell Biology Program. This program supports research on the normal structure and function of the kidney including its biochemistry, metabolism, transport, and fluid-electrolyte dynamics. Research is targeted toward the metabolic and physiologic transport processes that regulate solute and water excretion, as are studies on the adverse effects of drugs, nephrotoxins, and environmental toxins in the kidney. Applying molecular and cellular techniques, the structure of genes and their regulations, growth factors and their signal transduction systems, transport and their genes are studied. The program also has an interest in studies on analgesic abuse and heavy metal nephropathy, as well as studies on certain causes of acute renal failure such as hypoxic renal cell injury.

Urology Research

Urology Program. This program supports basic and clinical research studies of the normal and abnormal development, structure, and function of the genitourinary tract and the affect of diseases and disorders such as diabetes mellitus, spinal cord injury, and multiple sclerosis on these organs.

An area of emphasis is research that will increase the knowledge of the etiology, diagnosis. pathophysiology, therapy. and prevention of the major pediatric and adult urological diseases and disorders.

Also emphasized is basic research and clinical applications of diagnostic and therapeutic modalities such as 1) shock-wave and laser lithotripsy. 2) urolithiasis inhibitors, 3) bladder substitution procedures and devices, and 4) prostate growth inhibitor and reduction therapies.

Women's Health Program. This program encourages and supports basic and clinical research on urological problems that disproportionately affect women. Areas include urinary incontinence, urinary tract infections, and interstitial cystitis.

Division-wide Research

HIV Program. The HIV program supports basic and clinical studies on renal and genitourinary tract structure and function and hematopoietic function in individuals with HIV infection. Studies on HIV infection focus on the effect of HIV therapies on marrow function and clinical course of dialysis and transplant patients, potential interactions of HIV infection and the immunosuppressive therapy used to prevent transplant rejection and effect on organ function.

Centers Program. The George M. O'Brien Kidney and Urologic Research Centers conduct interdisciplinary investigations that address the basic, clinical, and applied aspects of biomedical research in renal and genitourinary physiology and pathophysiology, nephrology, and urology.

The goal of the centers is to reduce mortality and morbidity of kidney and urologic diseases by providing a focus and means for clinical and basic science disciplines to develop the knowledge needed to improve diagnosis, treatment, and prevention.

Clinical Trials Program. This program develops cooperative clinical trials to prevent major chronic kidney, genitourinary, and hematologic diseases.

Epidemiology Program. This program supports the development of epidemiologic data and research related to major kidney, genitourinary, and hematologic diseases. Coordinated under this program are the U.S. Renal Data System the kidney and urologic disease interview and examination component of the third National Health and Nutrition Examination Survey, 1988-94 and management of the epidemiology grants portfolio.

Hematology Research

Hematology Program. This program supports basic and clinical studies of normal and disease states of the hematopoietic system, including sickle cell anemia, thalassemia, aplastic anemia, iron deficiency anemia, thrombocytopenia, hemolytic anemia, and purpura. Areas of interest include morphologic, physiologic, and biochemical aspects of the formation, mobilization, and release of blood cells erythrocyte metabolism and physiology, globin synthesis, ion transport, and enzymatic pathways iron metabolism and absorption erythropoietin and other hematopoietic growth factors, hemoglobin metabolism, structure, function, and genetic control porphyrins and prophyrias and metabolism and function of white blood cells and plasma serum proteins.

Office of the Director Advisory Boards

National Diabetes Advisory Board. The NDAB was established to review and evaluate the progress of the long-range plan to combat diabetes designed to accelerate research and to expand programs in diabetes control, health care, and education. The board is composed of members representing a variety of scientific, educational, health care, and public service disciplines. The board provides advice and recommendations to the Congress, the secretary of Health and Human Services, the directors of the NIDDK and the NIH, and the heads of other appropriate Federal agencies and maintains liaison with governmental and nongovernmental entities concerned with diabetes.

National Kidney and Urologic Diseases Advisory Board. The NKUDAB was established to formulate a long-range plan to combat kidney and urologic diseases. The plan has been designed to develop national programs in kidney and urologic diseases research, control, health care, and education. The board is composed of members representing a variety of scientific, educational, health care, and public service disciplines. The board reviews and evaluates the implementation of the plan, provides advice and recommendations to the Congress, the secretary of HHS, the directors of the NIDDK and the NIH, and heads of other appropriate Federal agencies and maintains liaison with governmental and nongovernmental entities concerned with kidney and urologic diseases research and control.

National Digestive Diseases Advisory Board. The NDDAB is authorized to review and evaluate the research, training, prevention, and control programs within the area of digestive diseases. The board is composed of members representing a variety of scientific, educational, health care, and public service disciplines.

The primary function of the board is to review and evaluate progress of the long range plan developed for digestive diseases update the plan to assure its continuing relevance provide advice and recommendations on plan implementation to the Congress, the secretary of HHS, the directors of the NIDDK and the NIH, and the heads of other Federal agencies and maintain liaison with advisory bodies of other Federal agencies involved in implementing the plan.

Information Clearinghouses

National Kidney and Urologic Diseases Information Clearinghouse. The clearinghouse serves as an information resource for professional and patient education in kidney and urologic diseases through direct response and referral. The clearinghouse collects patient and professional educational materials for the NKUDIC subfile of the Combined Health Information Database and works with educators and health professionals to develop and exchange educational material.

National Digestive Diseases Information Clearinghouse. The clearinghouse is a central point for the collection and dissemination of information and education materials about digestive diseases. The clearinghouse works closely with local and national digestive disease organizations, and professional groups, in developing fact sheets and establishing priority areas of disease information emphasis through the strategic long-range plan. The overall goal of the NDDIC is to increase knowledge and understanding about digestive diseases among patients, health professionals, and the public through the effective dissemination of information.

National Diabetes Information Clearinghouse. The NDIC functions as the central point for the collection and dissemination of information about educational materials, programs, and resources relevant to diabetes. The clearinghouse works closely with the Diabetes Research and Training Centers, local and national diabetes organizations, professional groups, state departments of health, and other Federal and state agencies. The overall goals of the NDIC are to increase knowledge and understanding about diabetes among patients, health professionals, and the public through the effective dissemination of information, and to function as a catalyst in assisting and enhancing the efforts of these various groups in the development and exchange of educational materials and diabetes information.

National Institute of Environmental Health Sciences, Research Triangle Park N.C.

Mission

Human health and disease result from three interactive elements: environmental exposures, individual susceptibility, and time. The NIEHS mission is to reduce the burden of human illness and dysfunction from environmental exposures by understanding each element and how they interrelate. NIEHS achieves its mission through multidisciplinary biomedical research programs, prevention and intervention efforts, and communication strategies that encompasses training, education, technology transfer, and community outreach.

The institute has initiated clinical programs that bring the results from the laboratory more quickly to the bedside, and has strengthened its programs in prevention to address the problems associated with environmental equity. NIEHS supports training in environmental toxicology, pathology, mutagenesis, epidemiology and biostatistics, with emphasis on attracting women and minorities. The institute also funds basic and applied research on the health effects of human exposure to potentially toxic or harmful environmental agents. In its research, NIEHS attempts to learn:

- The identification and characterization of potentially harmful environmental agents, particularly toxic chemicals

- How the substances affect human health, by studying their impact on a variety of biological systems

- What happens in these systems after exposure to hazardous agents

- What diseases are caused or aggravated by environmental factors

- The extent of exposure of various population groups, especially sensitive populations, to these agents and

- What effects these agents cause, by themselves and in combination with other environmental factors.

In rounding out these activities, NIEHS supports efforts to identify hazardous environmental agents before they are released into the environment. These include developing, testing, and validating biological assay systems to ascertain animal toxicity and to predict toxic effects which might occur in humans.

Program output is intended to aid those agencies and organizations, public and private, responsible for developing and instituting regulations, policies, and procedures to prevent and reduce the incidence of environmentally induced diseases.

Major Programs

Protecting the general health of Americans and preventing environmentally related diseases are recognized government responsibilities. The NIEHS through its research programs is providing a health science base for prevention and control activities. In doing this, the institute focuses not on specific body organs or diseases but on agents and processes—the ways and means through which man's health can be adversely affected by chemical and physical agents in the environment.

Population expansion and growth of technology have increased environmental contamination problems. New forms of energy production, expanded uses of plastics and aerosols, and greater development of the chemical industry pose the problem of releasing toxic chemicals into the environment. Recent experiences with asbestos, mercury, vinyl chloride, bischloromethyl ether, methyl butyl ketone, sulfuric acid mist, polychlorinated and polybrominated biphenyls, kepone, dioxins, methylisocyanate, and chlorophenol indicate these compounds are not theoretical threats but real causes of illness and death.

The institute consists of the Divisions of Intramural Research; Extramural Research and Training; and Toxicology Research and Testing.

The Division of Extramural Research and Training supports investigators at colleges, universities, and research foundations through individual research grants, program project grants and other support mechanisms. These research activities provide information essential to an understanding of the way in which human health is adversely affected by chemical, physical and other environmental factors. The breadth of the institute's mission n dictates a multidisciplinary approach to problem solving which involves major biological, chemical, and physical science disciplines.

The division develops priorities and funding levels to assure maximum utilization of available resources. It maintains an awareness of national research efforts and assesses the need for research and research training environmental health and provides advisory support to the institute in the development of the research grant policy. Through this division, the institute supports basic and applied research on the consequences of the exposure of humans to potentially toxic or harmful agents in the environment.

For administrative purposes, the research is divided into: 1) biological response to environmental agents 2) applied toxicological research and testing 3) biometry and risk estimation and 4) resource and manpower development. Research and training may span one, several, or all program areas.

Environmental Health Sciences Centers. These centers provide core support to facilitate multidisciplinarv research in environmental health problems. They fill critical needs in the national environmental health program that cannot be met by individual research grants or program project grants. Each center has a different thrust and problem orientation. Overall, they serve as national focal points and resources for research and manpower development in health problems related to air, water and food pollution occupational and industrial health and safety heavy metal toxicity agricultural chemical hazards and the relationships of environment to cancer, birth defects, behavioral anomalies, respiratory and cardiovascular diseases, and diseases of other organs.

Much of the research conducted by the centers, in addition to substantive contributions to preventive medicine has served to clarify the scope of environmental health problems and future needs in this field.

Marine and Freshwater Biomedical Sciences Centers. MFBS centers foster multidisciplinary research on marine and freshwater organisms in the study of mechanisms of toxicity of environmental agents, as models for human diseases and disorders resulting from exposure to environmental toxicants.

Research Manpower Development Programs. Research manpower development programs support pre- and postdoctoral training in toxicology, pathology, mutagenesis, and epidemiology and biostatistics as they pertain to the environment. Three mechanisms are used to fund training: 1) institutional awards for pre and postdoctoral trainees (training program) 2) individual awards for postdoctoral fellows only (fellowship awards), and 3) senior fellowship awards to support training for new research oriented physician-researchers to enhance the teaching of environmental and occupational medicine. The division uses the environmental/occupational medicine academic award for curriculum and institutional resource development.

The Superfund Basic Research Program is university-based basic research supported by NIEHS as part of the 1986 Superfund Amendments and Reauthorization Act. It combines basic research in the fields of ecology, engineering, and hydrogeology into a core program of biomedical research to provide a broader and more detailed body of scientific information to be used in decisionmaking related to the management of hazardous substances.

The Division of Intramural Research (DIR) plans and conducts basic, applied, and clinical research directed toward increasing fundamental knowledge of environmentally related diseases and disorders. Broad multidisciplinary research approaches are used including basic mechanistic studies at the cellular and molecular level applied toxicology testing, and clinical and epidemiology studies. Intramural scientists address such complex research issues as genetic susceptibility, receptor mediated pathobiology, differentiation and development, signal transduction, environmental regulation of cell proliferation and cell death, environmental carcinogenesis and mutagenesis, and environmental epidemiology.

These research endeavors, in turn, support specific biomedical and clinical program interests of the institute such as environmental contributions to aging and age-related diseases and conditions (e.g., neurodegenerative diseases like Alzheimer's and Parkinson's, osteoporosis, cancer of the breast, prostate, endometrium and lung), environmental factors and respiratory disease (e.g., asthma and respiratory fibrosis), environmental contribution to reproductive and developmental disorders (e.g. infertility, abnormal growth and development, reproductive senescence) and environmental factors and integrated organ systems (e.g. abnormal sexual development, hypersensitivity and immune suppression).

The DIR pursues its scientific goals principally through its laboratories and branches in three scientific programs: the Environmental Biology and Medicine Program, the Environmental Carcinogenesis Program, and the Environmental Toxicology Program. In addition, a number of interdisciplinary program projects, clinical studies and international collaborative research projects have been established to address high priority research areas.

National Institute of General Medical Sciences

Mission

NIGMS primarily supports basic biomedical research that is not targeted to specific diseases or disorders. Because scientific breakthroughs often originate from such untargeted studies, NIGMS-funded work has contributed substantially to the tremendous progress that biomedical research has made in recent years. The institute's training programs help provide the most critical element of good research: well-prepared scientists.

Each year, NIGMS-supported scientists make major advances in understanding fundamental life processes. In the course of answering basic research questions, these investigators also increase our knowledge about the mechanisms involved in certain diseases. Other grantees develop important new tools and techniques, many of which have applications in the biotechnology industry. In recognition of the significance of their work, a number of NIGMS grantees have received the Nobel Prize and other high scientific honors.

Three divisions: Cell Biology and Biophysics; Genetics and Developmental Biology; and Pharmacology, Physiology, and Biological Chemistry support research and research training in basic biomedical science fields. The institute also has a Division of Minority Opportunities in Research, which administers a number of programs that are designed to increase the number of minority biomedical scientists. Finally, NIGMS has a Division of Extramural Activities, which handles the grant-related functions of the Institute.

NIGMS was established in 1962. In fiscal year 1995, its budget was $905 million. The vast majority of this money funds grants to scientists at universities, medical schools, hospitals, and research institutions throughout the country. At any given time, NIGMS supports over 3,300 research grantsabout 14 percent of the grants funded by NIH as a whole. NIGMS also supports nearly half of the predoctoral trainees and about 30 percent of all the trainees who receive assistance from NIH.

The institute places great emphasis on the support of individual, investigator-initiated research grants. It funds a limited number of research center grants in selected fields, such as trauma and burn research and the pharmacological sciences (including anesthesiology), in which the interaction of basic and clinical researchers is critical for rapid scientific progress. In addition, NIGMS funds several research contracts that provide important resources for basic scientists.

NIGMS research training programs recognize the interdisciplinary nature of biomedical research today, and stress approaches to biological problems that cut across disciplinary and departmental lines. Such experience prepares trainees to pursue creative research careers in a wide variety of areas. Among the fields in which NIGMS has long offered institutional predoctoral training programs are the cellular, biochemical, and molecular sciences genetics the pharmacological sciences and systems and integrative biology. Another longstanding training activity, the Medical Scientist Training Program, provides investigators who can bridge the gap between basic and clinical research by supporting research training leading to the combined M.D.-Ph.D. degree. Several newer training programs were designed to capitalize on rapidly developing areas of science, including biotechnology, molecular biophysics, and the interface between the fields of chemistry and biology.

The institute supports postdoctoral research through individual fellowships in areas related to its scientific programs and institutional postdoctoral training in the fields of anesthesiology, clinical pharmacology, genetics (with an emphasis on medical genetics), and trauma and burn injury research.

NIGMS also has a Pharmacology Research Associate Program, in which postdoctoral scientists pursue research in NIH or Food and Drug Administration laboratories. It is intended for individuals with backgrounds in the basic or clinical sciences who wish to obtain advanced experience in an area of pharmacology, or for those who are already pharmacologists to gain experience in new fields.

Major NIGMS Programs

Division of Cell Biology and Biophysics. The Division of Cell Biology and Biophysics seeks greater understanding of the structure and function of cells, cellular components, and the biological macromolecules that make up these components. The long-range goal of the division is to find ways to prevent, treat, and cure diseases that result from disturbed or abnormal cellular activity. The division has two components: the Biophysics Branch and the Cell Biology Branch.

Biophysics Branch. This branch supports studies in the areas of biophysics and bioengineering, disciplines that use techniques derived from the physical sciences to examine the structures and properties of biological substances. Areas of emphasis in biophysical research include the determination of the structures of proteins and nucleic acids studies of the structural features that determine macromolecular conformation the structural analysis of macromolecular interactions and of ligandmacromolecular interactions the development of physical methodology for the analysis of molecular structure and the development and use of theoretical methods to investigate biological systems. Bioengineering research interests include the development and refinement of instruments needed to conduct research in the areas described above. These include nuclear magnetic resonance spectroscopy, mass spectroscopy, and other forms of spectroscopy x-ray and other scattering techniques microscopy and cell separation techniques. This area of research also includes the development of new bioanalytical methods and biomaterials.

Cell Biology Branch. This branch supports general studies on the molecular and biochemical activities of cells and subcellular components, as well as on the role of cellular dysfunction in disease. Emphasis is placed on research with applications to more than one cell type, model system, or disease state, as well as research that does not fall within the diseaseoriented mission of another NIH component. Representative studies include those on plasma and intracellular membranes, receptors, and signal transduction mechanisms the structure and function of the cytoskeleton cell motility the regulation of protein and membrane synthesis and the activation of cell growth subcellular organelles cell division and lipid biochemistry.

Division of Genetics and Developmental Biology

The Division of Genetics and Developmental Biology supports studies directed toward gaining a better understanding of the fundamental mechanisms of inheritance and development. These studies underlie the more targeted research projects supported by other NIH components. Most of the projects supported by the division make use of nonhuman model systems It is expected that the results of these studies will lead to the eventual diagnosis, prevention, therapy, and cure of human genetic and developmental disorders.

Among the areas under active investigation are the replication, repair, and recombination of DNA the regulation of gene expression RNA processing protein synthesis extrachromosomal inheritance population genetics and evolution developmental genetics cell growth and differentiation cell cycle control rearrangement of genetic elements neurogenetics and the genetics of behavior and chromosome organization and mechanics.

Along with its research and research training activities, the Division of Genetics and Developmental Biology supports the Human Genetic Mutant Cell Repository, a unique resource for scientists studying medical and human genetics. The repository establishes and stores well-characterized cultured cell lines representing metabolic and chromosomal disorders collected from patients and their families. These cells and DNA extracted from them, as well as somatic cell hybrids, are provided to qualified investigators at modest charge, thus permitting the researchers to study the molecular and cellular aspects of many rare genetic conditions using material that would otherwise be difficult to obtain.

Division of Minority Opportunities in Research

The Division of Minority Opportunities in Research administers research and research training programs aimed at increasing the number of minority biomedical scientists. Support is available at the high school, undergraduate, graduate, postdoctoral, and faculty levels.

The division has three components: the Minority Access to Research Careers (MARC) Branch; Minority Biomedical Research Support (MBRS) Branch; and Special Initiatives.

MARC Branch. The MARC branch supports research training at 4-year colleges, universities, and health professional schools with substantial enrollments of such minorities as African Americans, Hispanics, Native Americans, and Pacific Islanders.

The branch's goals are to increase the number and capabilities of minorities engaged in biomedical research and to strengthen science curricula and student research opportunities at minority institutions. MARC funds research training for honors undergraduates, predoctoral fellowships, faculty fellowships, and visiting scientist fellowships.

MBRS Branch. To increase the number of researchers who are members of minority groups that are underrepresented in the biomedical sciences, the MBRS branch awards grants to 2- or 4year colleges, universities, and health professional schools with substantial enrollments of minorities.

These grants support research by faculty members, strengthen the institutions' biomedical research capabilities, and provide opportunities for students to work as part of a research team.

Special Initiatives

The division develops and launches new research and research training programs and other initiatives for minority scientists. These include the Bridges to the Future Program (Bridges to the Baccalaureate Degree and Bridges to the Doctoral Degree), which is cosponsored by the NIH Office of Research on Minority Health.

The division is also responsible for organizing meetings and other activities that build networks among individuals and educational institutions to promote minority participation in sponsored research.

Division of Pharmacology, Physiology, and Biological Chemistry

The Division of Pharmacology, Physiology, and Biological Chemistry supports a broad spectrum of research and research training aimed at improving the molecular-level understanding of fundamental biological processes and discovering approaches to their control. Research supported by the division takes a multifaceted approach to problems in pharmacology, physiology, biochemistry, and biorelated chemistry that are either very basic in nature or that have implications for more than one disease area.

The goals of supported research include an improved understanding of drug action and mechanisms of anesthesia new methods and targets for drug discovery advances in natural products synthesis an enhanced understanding of biological catalysis a greater knowledge of metabolic regulation and fundamental physiological processes and the integration and application of basic physiological, pharmacological, and biochemical research to clinical issues in pharmacology, anesthesia, and trauma and burn injury.

Biochemistry and Biorelated Chemistry Branch. This branch supports basic research in areas of biochemistry, such as enzyme catalysis and regulation, bioenergetics and redox biochemistry, and glyco-conjugates. It also supports research in areas of biorelated chemistry, such as organic synthesis and methodology, as well as bioinorganic and medicinal chemistry.

Examples of biochemical investigations include studies of the chemical basis of the regulation and catalytic properties of enzymes, intermediary metabolism, the chemical and physical properties of the cellular systems for electron transport and energy transduction, and the biosynthesis and structure of carbohydrate-containing macromolecules.

Chemical investigation examples include the development of strategies for natural products synthesis, studies of the structure and function of small molecules, the chemistry of metal ions in biological systems, the development of novel medicinal agents or mimics of macromolecular function, and the creation of new synthetic methodologies.

The branch also supports studies in biotechnology. This work focuses on the development of biological catalysts, including living organisms, for the production of useful chemical compounds, medicinal or diagnostic agents, or probes of biological phenomena.

Pharmacological and Physiological Sciences Branch. This branch supports research in pharmacology, anesthesiology, and the physiological sciences. Studies range from the molecular to the organismal level, and can be clinical in nature. In the pharmacological sciences and anesthesiology, important areas being studied are the effects of drugs on the body and the body's effects on drugs. This includes investigations of the absorption, transport, distribution. metabolism, biotransformation, and excretion of drugs, as well as drug delivery strategies and determinants of bioavailability.

Understanding the mechanisms of drug interactions with receptors and signal transduction mechanisms is another major focus of this section. This includes studies of soluble and membrane-bound receptors and channels, secondary and tertiary messenger systems, mediator molecules, and their regulation and pharmacological manipulation. Examples of studies in the physiological sciences include basic and clinical investigations directed toward improving understanding of the total body response to injury, including biochemical and physiological changes induced by trauma.

Research supported in this section includes studies on the etiology of post-traumatic sepsis and the mechanisms of immunosuppression, wound healing, and hypermetabolism following injury. This section also supports research in basic molecular immunobiology, which focuses on using cells of the immune system to study fundamental cellular and molecular mechanisms.

Division of Extramural Activities

The Division of Extramural Activities is responsible for the grant-related activities of the institute, including the receipt, referral, and advisory council review of applications as well as grant funding and management. It maintains an overview of the institute's scientific and financial status and advises the NIGMS director and other key staff on policy matters and on the planning, development, and scientific administration of institute research and training programs. The division recommends budget allocations for the various NIGMS programs. It also acts as a liaison with other NIH components for activities relating to grant application assignments and foreign grants.

National Institute of Mental Health

Mission

Provides leadership at a national level on brain research, mental illness, and mental health. It plans, conducts, fosters, and supports an integrated and coordinated program of research, investigations, research training, and services research relating to the causes, prevention, diagnosis, and treatment of mental illnesses, and supports basic research in related scientific areas.

Provides grants-in-aid to public and private institutions and individuals in fields related to its areas of interest, including research project, program project, and research center grants.

Conducts a diversified program of intramural and collaborative research in its own laboratories and clinics.

Provides contracts for the funding of research and research support projects in areas related to the brain, mental illness, and mental health.

In many years of work with animals as well as human subjects, NIMH researchers have advanced understanding of the brain and vastly expanded the capability of mental health professionals to diagnose, treat, and prevent mental and brain disorders.

The institute also conducts information and educational activities, including the dissemination of information and educational materials on mental illness, for health professionals and the lay public, and maintains relationships with professional associations international,

national, and state and local officials and voluntary agencies and organizations working in the areas of mental health and mental illness.

NIMH Programs

Division of Clinical and Treatment Research. The Division of Clinical and Treatment Research (DCTR) is the largest of NIMH's extramural divisions. Scientists here carry out studies of mental disorders and their etiology, diagnosis, psychopathology, and treatment. From this research, clinical advances emerge to bring new hope to people with mental illness and their families. The division also supports research training, conferences, and workshops. DCTR has six branches. These are:

Schizophrenia Research Branch. Research sponsored by this branch centers on improving our understanding of the causes of schizophrenia, the severe disorder that NIMH has designated as its top research priority. Scientists searching for the underlying abnormalities responsible for schizophrenia derive important information from brain imaging and other advanced techniques that reveal the anatomical defects and disturbances of brain function occurring in the disease. They also use molecular genetic approaches to search for genes that may be involved in the disorder. In other research, investigators are exploring psychosocial factors that affect people with schizophrenia.

Clinical Treatment Research Branch. This branch provides support for a wide spectrum of research dealing with pharmacologic, biologic, and psychosocial treatment and rehabilitation of mental disorders in adults. Of particular interest is the development and evaluation of integrated psychosocial-biologic treatments. The branch supports treatment research focused on schizophrenia, tardive dyskinesia, depression, manic-depressive illness, panic disorder, obsessive-compulsive disorder, social phobia, general anxiety disorder, somatoform disorder, personality disorders, menstrual-related disorders, sleep disorders, and sexual disorders.

Mood, Anxiety, and Personality Disorders Research Branch. The mission of this branch is to foster research and research training that will help to alleviate the suffering of people who have depression, other mood disorders. anxiety disorders, eating disorders, or personality disorders. These conditions are the most common mental illnesses, and several of them are risk factors for suicide.

Child and Adolescent Disorders Research Branch. Research supported by this branch deals with the causes, diagnosis, treatment, and outcome of mental disorders in children and adolescents. The aim of these studies is to develop knowledge that can be used to help afflicted youngsters and their families. Conditions studied include attention deficit disorder, autism, affective disorders such as depression, anxiety disorders, conduct disorders, eating disorders, schizophrenia, and youth suicide.

Mental Disorders of the Aging Research Branch. This branch fosters a broad spectrum of research in the biomedical and behavioral sciences and in mental health services. The goal is to obtain much-needed information about the causes, prevention, and treatments of mental illnesses in the elderly, and to improve the rehabilitation of older people suffering from these disorders. Among the disorders under study are Alzheimer's disease and other dementias, depression, late-onset schizophrenia, and sleep disturbances.

Research Projects and Publications Branch. Working in concert with the other branches of DCTR, this branch has responsibility for the production, publication, and distribution of various scientific publications (such as the *Schizophrenia Bulletin*, the *Psychopharmacology Bulletin*, and the *Psychotherapy and Rehabilitation Bulletin*). Further, the branch coordinates data management, analysis, and reporting requirements of national clinical research studies.

Division of Neuroscience and Behavioral Science

The Division of Neuroscience and Behavioral Science (DNBS) supports behavioral, biomedical and neuroscience research and research training to develop and expand fundamental knowledge that can ultimately advance the diagnosis, treatment, and prevention of mental illnesses. DNBS is composed of the following four programs.

Behavioral, Cognitive and Social Processes Research Branch. Research supported by this branch concerns the cognitive, personality, emotional, and social processes involved in normal behavioral functioning and adaptation. This includes research on factors that increase vulnerability to maladaptive outcomes, as well as those that foster protection and resiliency. Branch goals include understanding genetic and experiential contributors to behavior the interrelations and interactions among social, pyschological, and biological processes and developmental changes and continuities across the lifespan. Experimental, correlational, and longitudinal designs are included, as are cross-cultural, behavioral-genetic, ethnographic, computational, and animal model approaches.

Behavioral and Integrative Neuroscience Research Branch. This branch supports research on brain mechanisms underlying cognition and behavior in functional organisms and through theoretical models, with a view to understanding how cognition/ behavior develops, how it is maintained, and how it is regulated. This knowledge is crucial for improved diagnosis and treatment of all disorders of cognition and behavior including mental illness.

Molecular and Cellular Neuroscience Research Branch. This branch supports research on the molecular and cellular basis of normal and abnormal brain function related to mental health and mental illness. Research areas supported include neurotrasmitter distribution and function, neuronal signal transduction, regulation of gene expression, neural development and its regulation, relationships of the nervous system to the endocrine and immune systems, and neuropharmacology and discovery of new psychotherapeutic agents.

Scientific Technology and Resources. Methodological and technological innovations not only permit new approaches to be taken to old questions, but also stimulate investigation by raising new questions. Such innovations have been responsible for quantum advances in all areas of science, including the brain and behavioral sciences. Because the breadth of brain and behavioral research extends from the molecular level to the behavioral level, the tools and approaches which have allowed progress in these areas are extremely varied: from novel ways to assess behavior to new systems for recording neural activity, to innovative methods for identifying gene expression.

Division of Epidemiology and Services Research

The Division of Epidemiology and Services Research (DESR) is the NIMH focal point for studies of the frequency of mental disorders and risk factors for their development prevention of mental disorders violence and traumatic stress and the support and development of mental health services researci1. Research topics include the organization, financing, delivery, and outcomes of services to those with mental disorders as well as research that attempts to enhance the quality of care delivered.

Services Research Branch. Research supported by this branch pertains to mental health care services provided in mental health care facilities, general health care facilities, and community settings. This includes studies on mental health services for children and adolescents, the elderly, and minority populations rural mental health services and research in other priority areas noted above.

Violence and Traumatic Stress Research Branch. Research supported by this branch centers on victims of interpersonal violence (including rape, sexual assault, child abuse, domestic violence, and criminal violence) victims of emergencies and catastrophic events (including disaster, combat, community violence, and accidents) perpetrators of interpersonal violence (including studies of the causes, prevention, and treatment of violent and aggressive behavior in children and adults) and issues of law and mental health (including studies of mentally disordered offenders and violent behavior among the mentally ill).

Epidemiology and Psychopathology Research Branch. Activities of this branch include identification and analysis of risk factors for mental disorders, determination of the rates of occurrence of mental disorders among adults and children (including minorities), development of standardized methods for assessment and classification of mental disorders, and sponsoring training in mental health epidemiology.

Prevention Research Branch. This branch supports research and research training in the prevention of mental disorders and related serious problems in high-risk populations and in the promotion of mental health. Included are theory-driven prevention trials of interventions that interrupt the development of dysfunctions and improve individual adaptive capabilities. Research directed at modifying known risk factors for mental disorders is supported, as are methodological studies especially relevant to preventive intervention research.

The branch also supports the NIMH Depression Awareness, Recognition, and Treatment (D/ART) program, a national professional and public education effort. To achieve its goal of alleviating unnecessary personal suffering and reducing the economic costs of depression, D/ART educates health and mental health professionals about the diagnosis and treatment of depressive disorders, informs the public about the symptoms and effective treatments for depression, and encourages depressed individuals to seek appropriate treatment.

Basic Prevention and Behavioral Medicine Research Branch. This branch supports research on 1) the basic behavioral, biological, genetic, and social factors and psychological processes that impact on physical health and the maintenance of emotional well-being and 2) on interventions to prevent, monitor, or enhance health-related behaviors and psychological states. Research supported by the branch encompasses a wide range of health-related studies on the biological, psychological, and psychosocial aspects of stress, immunology, sleep and its disorders, circadian rhythms, nutrition, eating behavior and disorders, reproductive function, sexual behavior, medical illnesses, exercise, and health-related attitudes and practices.

The major emphases of the branch's programs are to develop an understanding of the relationships among behavior and physical illness and emotional dysfunction and to identify ways of maximizing healthful behaviors and minimizing health-damaging behaviors. The branch s goal is to develop and integrate behavioral and biomedical science knowledge and techniques relevant to health and illness and to apply these techniques to prevention, diagnosis, intervention, and rehabilitation. Theory driven research is encouraged. Studies using either humans or animals are supported.

Division of Intramural Research Programs

NIMH Division of Intramural Research Programs (DIRP) plans and administers a comprehensive, long-term, multidisciplinary brain and behavioral research program dealing with the causes. diagnosis, treatment, and prevention of mental disorders, as well as the biological and psychosocial factors that determine normal and pathological human behavior. DIRP provides a national and international focus for mental health research.

Participating in DIRP activities are over 600 staff members, 50 percent of whom are investigators. Many foreign and domestic guest scientists also contribute to the research effort of DIRP. Work is conducted in laboratories at three main facilities located on the main campus of NIH in Bethesda, Md., at the Neuroscience Center at St. Elizabeth's Hospital (NSCSE) in the District of Columbia, and at the NIH Animal Center (NIHAC) in Poolesville, Md. Broad spectra of adult and childhood psychiatric disorders including schizophrenia and manic-depressive illness, are studied in patients at both the NIH and St. Elizabeth's facilities. In addition, hundreds of basic neuroscience projects examining many aspects of central nervous system structure and function are carried out at all three facilities.

Behavior, both normal and pathological, is studied through an interdisciplinary approach. A variety of methods is used to correlate changes in neuronal function with behavior and to identify and measure the neurochemical and neurophysiological substrates of behavior.

The regulation of central nervous system metabolism is examined at various levels to determine its role in relationship to health and disease. Relatively noninvasive brain imaging techniques such as positron emission tomography (PET). single photon emission tomography (SPECT), and functional magnetic resonance are used to study living subjects in various physiologic and pathologic states. Molecular studies focus on many aspects of synaptic neurotransmission, including the biosynthesis, release, reuptake, and metabolism of neurotransmitters. The effects of disease, dietary changes, hormones, and drugs on synaptic events constitute a major area of investigation within DIRP.

Clinical pharmacological studies designed to improve treatment of the mentally ill center on work with psychoactive and psychotherapeutic drugs. Included in these studies are efforts to identify biological events and clinical measures that can serve as predictors of therapeutic response to these drugs. Other work includes characterization of receptors for neurotransmitters and psychoactive substances whose mechanisms of action are unknown. Studies of the regulation and action of receptors at the cellular level constitute a major area of investigation.

Genetic studies include molecular genetic analyses of psychiatric and neurologic disorders, pharmacogenetic as well as epidemiologic and family studies. Data from these projects will aid in sorting out the important and complex interactions between biological systems (i.e., the central nervous system) and the environment that determine behavior.

DIRP comprises of 24 components, as follows: Research Services; Veterinary Medicine and Resources; Biological Psychiatry; Clinical Neurogenetics; Clinical Psychobiology; Child Psychiatry; Clinical Neuroendocrinology; Experimental Therapeutics; Clinical Neuroscience; Laboratory of Clinical Science; Laboratory of Psychology and Psychopathology; Laboratory of Developmental Psychology; Laboratory of Socio-Environmental Studies, Laboratory of Cerebral Metabolism; Laboratory of Neuropsychology; Laboratory of Cell Biology; Laboratory of General and Comparative Biochemistry; Laboratory of Molecular Biology; Laboratory of Neurochemistry; Laboratory of Neurophysiology; Clinical and Research Services Branch; Neuropsychiatry Branch; Clinical Brain Disorders Branch; Laboratory of Biochemical Genetics.

Division of Extramural Activities

The most important responsibility of the Division of Extramural Activities (DEA) is to oversee the review of grant applications. Its aim is to provide every applicant with expert and fair review of his or her application and thereby ensure that NIMH supports the research and other activities that offer the greatest promise of furthering knowledge relevant to mental health and mental illness. DEA also provides committee management services and oversees activities of the National Advisory Mental Health Council, the advisory body to NIMH. In these and other ways, DEA exercises leadership in developing, implementing, and coordinating NIMH extramural programs and policies.

DEA consists of the Office of the Director and three branches: Clinical Review; Neuroscience Review; and Behavioral and Applied Review. Each branch administers the initial review groups (IRGs) which provide scientific and technical review of applications for research and training grants, fellowships, and cooperative agreements, as well as concept review for research and development contracts. The branches of DEA monitor the review process to ensure quality and conformity to policy. They also interpret the IRGs' recommendations to the National Advisory Mental Health Council. DEA is responsible for management and logistics of the meetings of the council and for preparing a major portion of the director's report to the council. A member of DEA staff serves as executive secretary to the council.

The division takes steps to ensure that grant applications reviewed by the institute adhere to guidelines on ethical conduct of research and provide for the inclusion of women and minorities in studies on human populations. The division also promotes adherence to safeguards for human and animal research.

DEA also oversees the issuance of program announcements and requests for applications (RFAs) that let the research community know what kinds of studies NIMH is most interested in supporting. Ensuring that these announcements and RFAs are clearly written, programmatically accurate, and faithfully conform to relevant criteria is DEA's responsibility.

Another major responsibility of DEA is to monitor the progress occurring in scientific areas relevant to NIMH's mission. DEA tracks significant developments in various fields of mental health research and training that will have an impact on the quality, diversity, and volume of grant applications. These trends are analyzed in light of IRG structure, new program announcements, and patterns of funding. With this ongoing analysis, the division is able to be responsive to changes in the review needs of the institute and to contribute to the evolution of science related to mental health and mental illness.

Office on AIDS

The NIMH AIDS program supports extramural research, intramural research, research training programs, and research development activities.

Extramural Research Activities. The NIMH AIDS program involves research at the biological, psychological, and behavioral level, including natural history, descriptive investigations, and experimental studies. It focuses on 1) the central nervous system effects of human immunodeficiency virus (HIV) infection, specifically neuropsychological, neuropsychiatric, and neurological dysfunction; 2) brain-immune interactions; 3) clinical research on HIV-related mental disorders; 4) mental health services research on ESIV infection and the severely mentally ill: 5) behavior change and prevention of HIV infection; and 6) psychological and psychosocial impact of HIV infection.

Intramural Research. Intramural scientists have been conducting studies of a number of compounds that may prove effective in blocking infectivity by HIV. Other research areas include: clinical neuropsychiatric studies of AIDS patients; molecular biologic studies of the neurotropic impact of HIV on the brain; studies of cognitive dysfunction and dementia associated with AIDS; and the development of animal models to test novel antiviral drugs against HIV.

Research Training. NIMH has two program announcements for individual and institutional research training across all areas of NIMH AIDS research. These include awards to individual fellows and also institutional awards.

Research Development Activities. The program sponsors meetings to review work in progress in such areas as neuroscience, prevention. neuropsychology, and research training. Another activity is the development of reports to improve measurement and methodology in AIDS research and to stimulate the development of research applications.

Office of Prevention

This office coordinates and promotes institute research programs concerning the prevention of mental disorders and the promotion of mental health by developing, planning, executing, and assessing national programs to set institute goals and priorities. For example, the Office sponsors conferences and workshops that bring together prevention experts and Federal policy makers to improve and facilitate the development of prevention programs.

Office of Rural Mental Health Research

The ORMHR directs, plans, coordinates, and supports research activities and information dissemination on conditions unique to those living in rural areas, including research on the delivery of mental health services to such areas. Also coordinates related departmental research activities and related activities of public and nonprofit entities.

Office of the Associate Director for Special Populations

The associate director for special populations provides leadership, advice, and coordination in developing, and fostering implementation of NIMH programmatic and administrative policies to promote mental health concerns of racial/ethnic minorities and women initiates and advances plans, policies, and activities to improve health and mental health of the Nation's women and racial/ethnic minorities. The office uses program planning, research, research training and public educational activities to promote mental health and prevent mental illness among women and racial/ethnic minorities; provides leadership in establishment and maintenance of organizational linkages and collaborates on mental health concerns of women and racial/ ethnic minorities with components of HHS, other Federal agencies, professional organizations, and other health organizations and institutions; monitors progress of division level goals and programs which bear on racial/ethnic minority and women's issues; and provides leadership and program guidance for the Career Opportunities in Research Education and Training Program (COR), the Minority Institutions Research Development Program (MIRDP), and the Supplements for Underrepresented Minorities in Biomedical and Behavioral Research Program.

The COR Honors Undergraduate Program assists institutions with substantial enrollment of racial/ethnic minority students in training of greater numbers of scientists as teachers and researchers in disciplines related to research in mental health.

The MIRDP provides grants to institutions with substantial enrollment of persons from racial/ethnic minority groups for support of research projects, enhancement of existing research infrastructure, and for advanced training of faculty. These grants also provide support for graduate and undergraduate students to serve as research associates on MIRDP projects.

The Supplements for Underrepresented Minorities in Biomedical and Behavioral Research are administrative supplements to existing research grants for research and salary support for high school students, undergraduate students, graduate research assistants, and junior level investigators. The proposed research must be an integral part of the ongoing research of the parent grant supported by NIMH.

National Institute of Neurological Disorders and Stroke

Mission

Conducts, fosters, coordinates, and guides research on the causes, prevention, diagnosis, and treatment of the neurological disorders, and stroke, and supports basic research in related scientific areas.

Provides grants-in-aid to public and private institutions and individuals in fields related to its areas of interest, including research project, program project, and research center grants.

Operates a program of contracts for the funding of research and research support efforts in selected areas of institute need.

Provides individual and institutional fellowships to increase scientific expertise in neurological fields.

Conducts a diversified program of intramural and collaborative research in its own laboratories, branches, and clinics. Collects and disseminates research information related to neurological disorders.

Major Divisions. The institute is organized as six divisions: convulsive, developmental, and neuromuscular disorders; demyelinating, atrophic, and dementing disorders; fundamental neurosciences; stroke and trauma and a division of extramural activities for support and coordination. A division of intramural research conducts laboratory and clinical research in NIH laboratories.

Division of Convulsive, Developmental, and Neuromuscular Disorders

The division stimulates and supports wide ranging research on neurological illnesses, including disorders of early and adult life, epilepsy, neuromuscular disorders, and sleep.

The Development Neurology Branch supports research on the neurobiology of developmental disorders of children, including cerebral palsy and other motor disorders, mental retardation and learning disorders, autism and behavioral disorders, and birth defects and genetic disorders affecting the central nervous system. In addition, the branch supports research on neuromuscular disorders including the muscular dystrophies, myasthenia gravis, and the peripheral neuropathies.

The Epilepsy Branch encourages research to prevent epilepsy and improve its diagnosis and treatment. Research is supported on convulsive and other paroxysmal disorders of the nervous system, including narcolepsy and other disorders of sleep. The branch administers an extensive antiepileptic drug development and monitoring program.

Division of Stroke and Trauma

The division supports basic and clinical research on stroke, injury to the head and spinal cord, and cerebral ischemia. The Division also funds studies of chronic pain, tumors of the central nervous system, and nerve regeneration. Attention is given to new imaging techniques—positron emission tomography, magnetic resonance imaging, near-infrared spectroscopy, ultrasound, and computerized axial tomography—that allow precise, noninvasive anatomic and metabolic imaging of the brain, a major tool for studying the consequences of stroke and nervous system trauma.

Stroke research encompasses all aspects of cerebrovascular disorders. Of high priority are investigations into the causes and neurological consequences of stroke, cerebral edema, cerebral aneurysms, and arteriovenous malformations and the significance of the timing of treatment after a stroke has occurred. The division supports clinical trials that evaluate the efficacy of surgical and medical therapy in symptomatic as well as asymptomatic patients. Pilot studies are being conducted on procedures for stroke treatment and evaluation.

The division encourages research on injury to the head, spinal cord, and peripheral nerves. Major goals are to find ways to promote regeneration of damaged nerve tissue and to restore function after injury. Toward that end, the division supports studies of neural plasticity, trophic factors that promote nerve growth, control of mitogenesis, therapeutic drugs, and nerve tissue implants.

Tumor research focuses on how neoplasms of nervous and supporting tissue affect the structure and function of the nervous system. Treatment of tumors depends on understanding certain physiological processes, which are particular subjects of research. A key area under investigation is blood flow and its effect on delivery of therapeutic agents to the tumor.

Division-supported studies of pain emphasize the clinical aspects of headache, neck and back pain, and other chronic problems. Some studies focus on neuro surgical procedures for relieving pain. Others evaluate alternative pain treatments: acupuncture, electroanalgesia, spinal manipulation, psychotherapy, biofeedback, and hypnosis. Drugs currently being tested include narcotic drugs, nonsteroidal anti inflammatory analgesics, and polypeptide analgesics such as the enkephalins and endorphins. The division also encourages research on better ways to measure and assess clinical pain.

Division of Fundamental Neurosciences

This division places special emphasis on studies of the neurophysiology of cognitive processes, particularly those that can be studied at the neuronal level. Another area involves investigation of somatic-autonomic mechanisms of neuronal interaction. Research on nerve receptors, especially their isolation and purification, has made possible many important experimental and clinical studies. An area of increasing research activity involves the interrelationships between the nervous system and the immune system, neuroimmunomodulation.

Another major area of research interest is central nervous system plasticity—its ability to drop or modify old connections, form new ones, and reshape neural networks. Local circuits served by short-axon or axonless neurons have been thought of as comprising a "second" nervous system which might some day be made to modulate central nervous system activity.

An activity supported largely by research contracts is the development of neural prostheses—devices that use electrical stimulation to replace, modify, or extend function in neurologically impaired people. This research has yielded motor prostheses to restore hand and arm function in paralyzed individuals. Potential new prostheses presently being investigated include urinary bladder control implants based on microstimulation of the sacral spinal cord and a visual prosthesis for the blind, which utilizes microelectrodes in the visual cortex.

Division of Extramural Activities

The division provides administrative support and coordination for the institute's research grant, research training, and research contract activities. The division directs and carries out scientific and technical merit review of proposals for research contracts, program projects, clinical research centers, special research grants such as multi-institutional clinical trials, and career development and research training. Management services for research grants and contracts are provided.

The division coordinates training and career development of young investigators. Opportunities include institutional and individual training awards as well as support through research career development awards, awards for reentry into the neurological sciences, and an integrated clinical and research career development program for physicians that begins during residency.

Division of Intramural Research

The division conducts basic and clinical research in neurological and related disciplines. Notable achievements have included drug therapies for debilitating neurological diseases such as parkinsonism and new techniques to help scientists better understand how the brain and nervous system function. Major research advances in neurovirology, neurochemistry and neuroimmunology have also come from the division.

NINDS scientists continue to explore central nervous system disorders such as Creutzfeldt-Jakob disease that appear to be slow infections caused by transmissible virus-like agents. These agents are unique in some respects, but in others exhibit classical viral properties. Research focuses on delineating the agents' chemical, biological and genetic nature, and on learning the nature of disease pathogenesis.

Inherited disorders of lipid metabolism such as Gaucher's, Niemann-Pick, Fabry's, Krabbe's, and Tay-Sachs are studied. This work includes biochemical and diagnostic studies, carrier identification, and genetic counseling. Studies on the molecular basis of the diseases have reached a new frontier enzyme replacement therapy has been successfully developed for patients with Gaucher's. Gene replacement is also being explored for patients with this and other metabolic disorders.

Many research projects in computed tomography advance the clinical applications of the technique as well as provide scientists with a wealth of valuable research data. In other imaging work, studies with the PET scanner have shown a relationship between glucose uptake and brain tumor growth. This scanning technique allows scientists to obtain axial transverse or coronal images of the brain. It also provides dynamic functional data such as rates of glucose consumption in different parts of the brain measurements of the storage, degradation, and turnover of radioactively tagged metabolites. Functional magnetic resonance imaging is a new technique being used to study brain activity.

In the Neuroimmunology Branch, the role of immunological mechanisms as they may relate to the cause of diseases such as multiple sclerosis is being studied. Immunological and genetic factors are being examined in families with multiple affected members or in twins in which either one or both twins have multiple sclerosis. The role of HTLV-I and other retroviruses as the cause of demyelinating disease is being assessed. Finally, new approaches to the treatment of multiple sclerosis are being examined and MRI is being used as a tool to study the natural history of the disease and to assess the efficacy of experimental treatments.

In the Surgical Neurology Branch, NINDS scientists have undertaken intensive studies of brain tumors, pituitary tumors, neuronal implantation, gene therapy and immunotoxins for brain tumors, and selected aspects of cerebrovascular disease and epilepsy.

The Medical Neurology Branch's human motor control section focuses on how the brain controls voluntary movement and how these processes become deranged with different movement disorders. Recent advances have been made in understanding of focal dystonia and brain plasticity. The neuromuscular diseases section has made recent important observations on postpolio syndrome, neuromuscular disorders in AIDS, polymyositis, and neuropathies associated with paraproteinemia. The cognitive neuroscience section conducts innovative research on human cognitive processes such as planning, memory, and object recognition and investigates how these processes become impaired in the presence of neurological disease or trauma. A clinical neurogenetics unit has been formed.

The Epilepsy Research Branch investigates the pathophysiology of seizure disorders and cognitive function in individuals with epilepsy as well as the organization of language and memory function in normal controls, using positron emission tomography studies of cerebral blood flow, metabolism, and neurotransmitters intracerebral electrode recordings and magnetic resonance imaging. Animal and cellular models are used to study excitatory and inhibitory mechanisms, the neuropharmacology of antiepileptic drugs, and potential novel therapeutic compounds.

The Stroke Branch explores the mechanisms by which stroke risk factors operate and analyzes mechanisms of neuronal ischemic damage at physiologic and molecular levels. The goal of these studies is to improve the prevention and treatment of human cerebrovascular disease. A clinical stroke research program is integrated with the basic stroke research program.

A major goal of research in the Neuroepidemiology Branch is to understand factors influencing the occurrence of neurological disorders in population groups. Using epidemiological methods, the branch carries out research that may resolve clinical problems related to the cause, prevention, and treatment of nervous system diseases. The branch is currently involved in research on cerebral palsy, pediatric migraine, and progressive supranuclear palsy.

Clinical Neuroscience Branch research focuses on amine neurotransmitter mechanisms in the brain and peripheral autonomic nervous system, and on neurotransmitter function and metabolism in various neurological disorders. In addition, the section studies how neurotransmitters and other factors regulate the synthesis of neurotrophic factors, as well as systems in which neurotransmitters, in particular neuropeptides, can function as neurotrophic factors.

Exploring the design, conduct, and analysis of experimental or observational studies of the nervous system is the work of the Biometry and Field Studies Branch. Branch scientists develop new methods to meet the institute's needs for designing experiments and field studies, analyzing data, and devising statistical models of biological processes. The branch also acts as statistical coordinating center for several continuing or planned clinical trials and for longitudinal field studies involving U.S. and foreign scientists. In one cooperative international project, the goal is to determine whether electroencephalography can predict if a child who has had one seizure associated with fever will have another.

The Experimental Therapeutics Branch seeks to develop improved pharmacotherapies for neurologic diseases. At the molecular level, scientists are working to characterize central transmitter receptors and information transduction processes as well as to develop pharmaceutical approaches to the selective regulation of gene expression within the central nervous system. At the systems level, studies focus on basal ganglia function especially in relation to dopamine receptor mechanisms and the effect of drugs that influence motor behavior. At the clinical level, investigators attempt to elucidate pathophysiologic mechanisms and develop novel pharmaceutical interventions for neurodegenerative disorders that impair motor and cognitive function.

The Developmental and Metabolic Neurology Branch is concerned with inherited disorders of metabolism such as Gaucher's disease,

Niemann-Pick disease, Fabry's disease, and Tay-Sachs disease. Investigations include the identification of enzymatic and molecular defects, devising diagnostic and carrier detection methods for genetic counseling, and development of enzyme and gene replacement therapy for patients with these disorders. The branch is also involved in the development of transgenic animals that mimic human metabolic disorders. The pathogenesis of heritable disorders for which the metabolic basis is unknown such as type C Niemann-Pick disease, is also under investigation through "reverse genetics" including chromosomal mapping and identification of the mutated genes and the normal gene products.

The Neuroimaging Branch focuses it research on brain tumors, movement disorders, and stroke. The research tools used are: 1) positron emission tomography to assess the rate of glucose utilization in brain tumors and cerebral blood flow in ischemia and 2) magnetic resonance imaging (MRI) and spectroscopy (MRS) to assess diffusion and perfusion (MRI) and levels of various metabolites (MRS) in brain tumors and cerebral ischemia, and brain iron distribution in normal controls, as well as in patients affected by movement disorders (primarily Parkinson's disease and parkinsonism).

National Institute of Nursing Research

Mission

The National Institute of Nursing Research (NINR) supports research and research on the biological and behavioral aspects of critical health problems that confront the Nation. According to its mandate, the institute seeks to reduce the burden of illness and disability by understanding and easing the effects of acute and chronic illness, to improve health related quality of life by preventing or delaying the onset of disease or to improve clinical environments by testing interventions that influence patient health and reduce costs and demand for care. Particular emphasis is placed on subsets of the population who have special health problems and needs such as older people, women and minorities, and residents of rural areas. Research seeks to discover how cultural and ethnic identity affect behavior and differences in risk patterns and to determine the influence of socioeconomic status, geographic location, and other factors on health-related attitudes, decisions, and behaviors. NINR's intramural investigations center on managing symptoms of chronic illness such as the nutritional changes, myopathy, and fatigue that occur during treatment for HIV disease. Other studies, which focus on quality of life as an outcome of chronic illness, are being conducted in caregivers of persons with Alzheimer's disease and in persons with AIDS. NINR fosters collaborations with many other disciplines in areas of mutual interest such as long-term care for at-risk older people, genetic testing and counseling, behavioral aspects of tuberculosis, the special needs of women with physical disabilities, and environmental influences on risk factors related to chronic illness.

The institute also supports comprehensive research training and career development programs to prepare individuals with requisite interdisciplinary skills to conduct nursing research.

Major Programs

Extramural Research Programs. The NINR extramural program invites investigator-initiated applications containing innovative ideas and sound methodology in all aspects of nursing research consistent with the institute mission. A program priority is the integration of biological and behavioral research. Three dimensions — promoting health and preventing disease, managing the symptoms and disability of illness, and improving the environments in which care is delivered — cut across the following six areas.

- Research in chronic conditions, including arthritis, diabetes, and urinary incontinence, and in long-term care and caregiving.

- Research in health and risk behaviors, including studies of women's health developmental transitions such as adolescence and menopause and health and behavior research such as studies of smoking cessation.

- Research in cardiopulmonary health, including prevention and care of individuals with cardiac or respiratory conditions. This area also includes research in critical care, trauma, wound healing, and organ transplantation.

- Research in neurofunction and brain disorders, including pain management, sleep disorders, symptom management in persons with brain disorders such as Alzheimer's disease, and rehabilitation following brain and spinal cord injury. This also includes research on patient care in acute care settings.

- Research in immune and neoplastic diseases, including symptoms primarily associated with cancer and AIDS such as fatigue, nausea and vomiting, and cachexia. Prevention research on specific risk factors is also included.

- Research in reproductive and infant health, including prevention of premature labor, reduction of health-risk factors during pregnancy, delivery of prenatal care, care of neonates, infant growth and development, and fertility issues.

NINR's priority is to fund investigator-initiated research. To assure depth in certain scientific areas, however, the institute collaborated with the National Advisory Council for Nursing Research and nursing scientific community to develop the National Nursing Research Agenda. Initial areas for special focus in 1989-1994 were low birth weight: mothers and infants HIV infection: prevention and care long-term care for older patients symptom management of pain nursing informatics support for patient care and health promotion for children and adolescents. Areas identified for 1995-1999 are:

- Community based nursing models to examine nursing strategies designed to promote health and reduce risks of disease and disabilities from chronic conditions, particularly among rural, underserved, and minority populations.

- Effectiveness of nursing interventions in HIV/AIDS to evaluate biobehavioral nursing interventions to foster health promoting behaviors of individuals at risk for HIV/AIDS, and to ameliorate the effects of illness in those already infected.

- Cognitive impairmentdevelop and test biobehavioral and environmental approaches to remedy cognitive impairment and to examine prevention strategies that target those at risk.

- Living with chronic illness—test interventions that increase individual and family adaptation to chronic illness.

- Biobehavioral factors related to immunocompetence—identify biobehavioral factors and test interventions that promote immunocompetence.

Research Training and Career Development

This activity assures that there will be an adequate cadre of well-trained nurse scientists to meet future research needs. This is accomplished through national research service awards consisting of predoctoral and postdoctoral individual and institutional support, as well as senior fellowships for experienced investigators.

For career development, NINR offers a "Mentored Research Scientist Development Award—Nursing" which is available to doctorally prepared students who need a mentored research experience with an expert sponsor as a way to gain expertise in an area new to the candidate or would demonstrably enhance the candidate's scientific career.

Intramural Division

NINR's growing Division of Intramural Research develops and conducts clinical research that contributes to scientific knowledge for nursing practice and health care. It also provides research training opportunities for nurse scientists.

The Clinical Therapeutics Laboratory studies the biophysiologic and behavioral basis for and the effectiveness of clinical therapeutics relevant to nursing practice and health care. Ongoing investigations study the prevention, detection, and treatment of symptoms and side effects occurring during HIV infection and its treatment, such as fatigue, nutritional problems, and muscle weakness. Another series of CTL studies in aging individuals focus on treatment of another symptom, incontinence.

The Laboratory for the Study of Human Responses to Health and Illness studies quality of life and adaptation. Investigations focus on people's responses to illness and disability, as well as health promotion. Ongoing longitudinal investigations are conducted on the predictors of burdens and quality of life of caregivers of Alzheimer's disease patients, as well as the psychophysiologic predictors of quality of life of HIV-infected people. Another study is investigating how to more accurately measure and improve the functional status of people with chronic illnesses.

Investigators are in the process of developing protocols for a new Clinical Ethics Laboratory.

National Institute on Aging

Mission

In 1974 Congress authorized the establishment of the National Institute on Aging. The NIA is responsible for "conduct and support of biomedical, social, and behavioral research, training, health information dissemination, and other programs with respect to the aging process and diseases and other special problems and needs of the aged."

NIA is the lead agency in Federal efforts on Alzheimer's disease, housing the Office of Alzheimer's Disease Research (OADR). OADR promotes and encourages the advancement of Alzheimer's disease research programs supported by NIA and NIH, other Federal and state agencies, and private organizations.

Intramural Research

The bulk of the NIA intramural research program is conducted at the Gerontology Research Center in Baltimore, Md. The Laboratory of Neurosciences operates basic and clinical research programs from the Clinical Center at NIH. Via the NIH medical staff fellow, staff fellowship, a cooperative geriatric medicine fellowship with Johns Hopkins, intramural research training awards, and visiting programs, scientists at various stages of their careers gain sophisticated gerontology experience at the center. Over 300 postdoctoral investigators have been trained at the GRC since 1940.

The Longitudinal Studies Branch is responsible for the management and operation of the Baltimore Longitudinal Study of Aging (BLSA) and scientists in the branch conduct research using both historical and currently collected data. First, historical datasets in many areas are continuously developed to model group and individual patterns of aging. Second, new BLSA research is planned and implemented on the most promising findings. Examples include new research in prostate aging and disease, vision, hearing, strength, cerebrovascular aging, and age-associated changes in functional ability.

The BLSA is a primary and unique resource of the intramural program. Nearly 600 volunteer men, ranging in age from 20 to 96 years, come to the center every 2 years and undergo 2 1/2 days of extensive clinical, biochemical, and psychological tests. A women's program, initiated in 1978, has over 550 participants, helping scientists make important comparisons of sex differences across the life span.

Recently a cohort of women 45 to 55 years of age has been added to allow analysis of the perimenopausal period. A minority cohort is being added for studies relevant to hypertension.

Scientists in the Laboratory of Clinical Physiology conduct research emphasizing the physiological changes that occur throughout the entire adult life span. Studies include quantification of age changes, elucidation of mechanisms underlying these changes, and the relation between aging processes and specific disease states. There are specific programs to study endocrine and metabolic systems, especially growth and sex hormones, glucose and insulin homeostasis, bone and the immune system.

The Laboratory of Behavioral Sciences applies behavior analysis methodology to investigate mechanisms mediating the development of selected disorders of aging and to facilitate their prevention and remediation. Studies in the behavioral medicine section are concerned with interactions of stress and salt intake in blood pressure regulation and the development of hypertension. The focus is on effects of hypercapnic breathing on mechanisms of cell sodium regulation. In addition, behavioral nursing research is concerned with prevention of falls and hip fracture, and with relationships between incontinence, urinary tract infection, and hypertension. Studies in the behavioral physiology section are concerned with the effects of low and high ambient temperature on plasma volume, blood pressure, and other cardiovascular measures, and with the diurnal variation in cardiovascular response to thermoregulatory behavior.

The Laboratory of Personality and Cognition (LPC) conducts research on individual differences in psychosocial and intellectual functioning with aging and their influence on health and adaptation. LPC researchers are actively engaged in dispelling myths on aging, personality, and health, and have contributed new insights about the stresses faced by aging adults, the methods and strategies used by them to cope, and the effectiveness of their coping efforts. The LPC also conducts research on early markers of Alzheimer's disease as well as cognitive performance and aging, emphasizing the psychological mechanisms underlying age-related changes in memory, learning, and reasoning.

Researchers in the Laboratory of Cellular and Molecular Biology conduct studies at the cellular and molecular levels to assess basic mechanisms of aging that affect physiologic function. Included are studies on signal transduction, the interaction of cells with synthetic macromolecules, structural biology, stress responses, gene expression, oxygen radicals and mechanisms of neurodegeneration. Manipulations, such as diet, exercise, pharmacological/endocrinological and genetic interventions, are examined.

Laboratory of Biological Chemistry investigators conduct research in neurobiology in such areas as molecular neuropathology, mechanisms of cell death, neurotrophic factors, and molecular biomarkers of Alzheimer's disease. Other researchers focus on cell biology, including development of models to measure capacity of bone to regenerate, the study of aging cartilage and bone, mitochondrial defects, and the relation between cancer and aging.

The Laboratory of Molecular Genetics (LMG) is investigating the molecular basis for aging and age-dependent diseases, notably cancer. Studies are focused on DNA-related mechanisms such as genomic instability. DNA repair, DNA replication and transcription. The increased levels of DNA damage that have been observed with aging may be due to changes in DNA repair. A special interest is in the fine structure of DNA repair and the DNA repair processes in individual genes. Molecular mechanisms are being investigated and changes in the mechanisms with aging are studied.

The overall goals of the Laboratory of Cardiovascular Science are 1) to identify age-associated changes that occur within the cardiovascular system in humans and in animal models and to determine the mechanisms for these changes; 2) to study basic mechanisms of excitation-contraction coupling, of membrane transport and of energy-yielding oxidative pathways in cardiac muscle: 3) to determine mechanisms that govern normal and abnormal function of vascular smooth muscle and endothelial cells; 4) to study myocardial and vascular structure and function, gene expression, and responses to pharmacologic and gene therapy in disease models, and 5) to determine how age interacts with chronically altered cardiac and vascular disease states to determine the overall level of cardiovascular function.

In meeting these objectives, studies are performed in human volunteers, intact animals, isolated heart and vascular tissues and cells, subcellular organelles and molecules. The research program is conceptualized and implemented within three sections: cardiac function; energy metabolism and biogenetics; and membrane biology.

Investigators in the Laboratory of Neurosciences (LNS) study the function and structure of the central nervous system in relation to neurodegenerative and developmental disorders. Basic studies involve brain phospholipid metabolism during neuroplasticity and functional activation, and blood-brain barrier transport and drug delivery.

Studies in the cerebral metabolism section deal with research on animal models related to human aging and disease, as well as collaborative efforts with the brain aging and dementia section, which operates an eight bed patient care unit at the NIH Clinical Center. Physicians, pharmacologists, and physiologists work together on clinical brain imaging studies using positron emission tomography and magnetic resonance. Recent studies demonstrated that early metabolic deficits can be detected in brains of participants with a single memory disorder, presaging the later development of Alzheimer's dementia. Simulation PET studies have shown that metabolic deficits in Alzheimer's disease can be partially reversed with appropriate cognitive tests.

Epidemiology, Demography, and Biometry Program

This program collects and evaluates data on health and illness in the older population. The intramural scientific research carried out by EDBP staff is supplemented by research contracts, interagency agreements. and numerous working arrangements with Federal and non-Federal organizations. Basic information is generated on current and projected health and social status of older people.

A multicenter, prospective study of 14,000 older Americans entitled "Established Populations for Epidemiologic Studies of the Elderly" (EPESE) was initiated in 1980 to prospectively evaluate social, behavioral and environmental factors related to morbidity and mortality. A public use version of the EPESE baseline dataset for all four sites, as well as followup data from three sites, was made available to investigators in the U.S. The EPESE serves as a primary resource for a broad variety of epidemiologic studies of the elderly, including minorities.

The Women's Health and Aging Study was launched in 1991 as a comprehensive study of functional decline in older women with moderate to severe disability. The 5-year effort, being conducted under a contract awarded to Johns Hopkins University School of Medicine will closely follow about 1,000 women to evaluate changes in physical status over a 3-year study period. Other factors, such as mortality and use of long-term care, will be evaluated.

In 1991 the EDBP started the Honolulu-Asia Aging Study. A complex cross-national study, the research focuses on people already participating in the Honolulu Heart Program, an ongoing prospective study of cardiovascular diseases of American men ages 70 to 90 of Japanese ancestry. The aging study will use the heart program participants as a resource for research on dementia and to compare results with those generated by parallel studies in other Asian ancestry populations.

The Veterans Study of Memory in Aging was initiated in 1994 with Duke University to retrospectively study the association between closed head injury with Alzheimer's disease and other degenerative dementias. The project will study 3,000 U.S. Navy veterans who served 1994-45. Half of these men will have suffered closed head injury with loss of consciousness in 1944-45, and possibly at other times in their lives; the other half will have suffered no such head injury. Base upon results of cognitive screening, some of these men will be followed and about 140 of these men will eventually undergo an in person clinical examination for dementia. Subsequent analysis will indicate any associations.

Progressive loss of muscle mass, or sarcopenia, has been hypothesized to be a common pathway by which multiple diseases contribute to disability. EDBP is initiating a clinical research study, the

"Dynamics of Health, Aging and Body Composition" (HEALTH ABC) to characterize the extent of loss of muscle mass in older men and women, identify clinical conditions accelerating the loss of muscle, and examine the health impact of loss of muscle on strength, endurance, disability, and diseases common in old age. Approximately 3,000 men and women, ages 70-79, half of whom will be African American, will be enrolled at two clinical centers—the University of Tennessee, Memphis, and the University of Pittsburgh—and followed far 7 years for new onset of physical disability. The HEALTH ABC will provide invaluable information on optimal timing for interventions to prevent or reverse muscle loss and on high-risk groups most likely to benefit.

EDBP scientists performed a mortality followup study of a representative sample of persons dying over a 1 2-month period in Fairfield County, Conn. The study, known as the "Last Days of Life," allows for investigations into a number of important issues concerning the year prior to death in older persons.

Other areas of interest include disability and physical function; hip fracture and osteoporosis; heart disease; dementia; sleep disturbance; hearing and vision disorders; methodologic issues in aging research; and cross-cultural and international studies of aging and the diseases of aging.

Biology of Aging Program

The program supports biomedical studies through various NIH grant mechanisms and contracts. The program plans, implements, and supports fundamental molecular, cellular and genetic research on the mechanisms of aging. It also supports resource facilities that provide aged animals and cell cultures for use in aging research.

Animal Models. This program area funds research on the identification and development of animal models, both mammalian and lower organism, for use in aging research.

Biomarkers. This area supports research to identify and validate a panel of biomarkers of aging in a rodent model, with eventual application of these biomarkers to humans.

Cell Biology. This program area investigates aging at the cellular level and includes membranes and membrane receptors, growth factors, signal transduction, extracellular matrix, skin and cartilage, intercellular communication, and proteoglycan structure and function.

Differentiation. This area supports research on muscle biology and muscle regeneration, developmental genetics related to aging and age-dependent loss of differentiated cell function.

Endocrinology. The endocrinology program area supports basic research aimed at understanding the age-related changes in hormone production, metabolism, and action; reproductive aging; biology of menopause; age-related changes in control of prostate growth; and age-related changes in hormonal regulation of bone growth and bone cell function.

Genetics. This area supports research aimed at longevity assurance genes and sequence assurance genes, evolutionary genetics of aging and longevity, sexdependent biological influences on aging, and the role of somatic cell mutations in aging.

Immunology. This program area encourages research on age-related changes in the immune system including regulation of lymphocyte proliferation, regulation of immune specificity, response of the immune system to biochemical stimuli, autoimmune disease and other immunopathology, endocrine and neuroendocrine control of immune function, and interventions to retard and/or correct age-related decline in immune function.

Molecular Biology. This area funds studies on the generation and metabolism of free radicals, repair of free radical damage in DNA and lipids, erythrocyte senescence, mechanisms of programmed cell death, and mechanisms of life span extension by caloric restriction.

Molecular Genetics. This area supports research on regulation of cell proliferation in normal, aging, and transformed cells; senescence-related changes in cell cycledependent gene expression, the role of telomeres in cell senescence; and age-related changes in gene expression.

Nutrition and Metabolism. This program supports research on nutritional factors in age-related disease, changes in RDAs with age, roles of nutrition in immune function, roles of dietary factors in oxidative damage and antioxidant defenses, the role of nutrition in age-related changes in tissue function, and the age-related changes in the metabolism of nutrients.

Pathobiology. This area supports research on the molecular basis of Werner's syndrome, arthritis and other age-related diseases; age-related changes in mitochondrial function, molecular basis of age-related pathology; and age-related changes in response to biological stress, especially heat shock and acute phage responses.

531

Physiology. This area supports research on age-related changes in osteoblast and osteoclast function and bone matrix, the cardiovascular system, and electronic transport.

Protein Structure and Function. This area supports research on protein oxidation and turnover of damaged proteins, protein tertiary structure, glycation of proteins and the metabolism of glycated proteins, and the post-translational modification of proteins.

The Biology of Aging Program also includes the Office of Biological Resources and Resource Development and the Office of Nutrition. They coordinate NIA activities in the indicated areas and serve as liaison between NIA and other agencies.

Geriatrics Program

The program supports the development of clinical research on the special medical needs and problems of the growing aging population in the U.S.

The cardiovascular/pulmonary/renal program area develops and supports research on problems such as alterations in blood pressure regulation with age isolated systolic hypertension orthostatic hypotension aging changes in the microcirculation age-associated alterations in the composition of arteries and the effect of these alterations on cardiovascular function age-related change in quality, quantity, and function of the myocardium and the conduction system of the heart and changes with age in kidney and pulmonary function.

The centers program includes the support of the Claude Pepper Older American Independence Centers and the Teaching Nursing Home Program. Both support a broad spectrum of research relevant to health concerns of older people.

The endocrinology program area encourages and supports research aimed at providing an understanding of the age-related changes in endocrine function, including menopause, the mechanisms underlying these changes, and the impact of these changes on other physiologic systems.

The geriatric research and training program area supports clinical research on disorders that are concentrated predominately among older people or that are associated with increased morbidity and mortality in the elderly. In addition to these specific clinical problems, the program also addresses the lack of research on clinical problems in nursing homes and other sites of long-term care for the elderly. Another mission is to attract new investigators to the field of aging and to further the development of active investigators in clinical medicine and biomedical research.

The infectious diseases program area supports research on the relationship of physiologic changes associated with age or chronic disease to susceptibility to infections.

Other priorities include new strategies for evaluating vaccine efficacy in the elderly, potential prophylactic techniques for infections in the elderly, age-related changes in the effects of stresses such as chemotherapy, radiotherapy, and infection on granulopoiesis and lymphopoiesis, age-related changes in circulating levels of amyloid proteins and effects of amyloid deposition, and the interaction of aging and processes of carcinogenesis.

The mission of the musculoskeletal program area is to develop and support basic and clinical research on age-related changes in function of bone, muscle and cartilage. The program supports research on risk factors, prevention and treatment of falls, gait disorders and hip fractures in the elderly, as well as research on osteoarthritis, and urinary incontinence.

The nutrition, gastroenterology, and metabolism program area develops and supports basic and clinical research on effects of nutritional factors throughout the life span on longevity and age-associated morbidity assessment of nutritional status in the elderly effects of aging on nutrient digestion, absorption, and utilization and the contribution of nutritional status to the etiology and pathogenesis of diseases prevalent in the elderly.

The osteoporosis program supports basic and clinical research to identify age-associated processes which contribute to bone loss and osteoporosis markers and risk factors that are related to changes in bone mass, bone competence and the predisposition to falls and strategies based on modifying or reversing these processes. NIA especially emphasizes research on osteoporosis in advanced age, when the consequences, particularly those of hip fracture, become more severe and result in escalating morbidity and mortality.

Neuroscience and Neuropsychology of Aging

This program fosters and supports extramural and collaborative research and training to further the understanding of the neural and behavioral processes associated with the aging brain. Research on dementias of old age—in particular Alzheimer's disease—is one of the highest program priorities.

Neurobiology of Aging. The neurobiology of aging program area fosters research on age-related cellular and molecular changes in the structure or function of the nervous system. Studies of neuroimmunology, neurovirology, neuroendocrinology, neuropharmacology, sensory and motor processes, sleep, biorhythmicity, and neural plasticity are of particular interest.

Dementias of Aging. This program area supports research on basic, clinical, and epidemiological studies of Alzheimer's disease, including the incidence, prevalence, and risk factors for Alzheimer's and other dementias the development of new and improved cognitive and diagnostic screening methods and the treatment and management of dementing diseases.

Neuropsychology of Aging. The neuropsychology of aging office emphasizes research, including the use of animal models, and training on age-related changes in basic cognitive processes, learning and memory, as well as prosthetic devices and aids. The aim is to clarify the interdependence of brain function and behavioral capacity in aging.

Behavioral and Social Research

This program supports basic social and behavioral research through all award mechanisms on the aging process and the problems and needs of older people. It focuses on understanding how psychological and social aging interact with biological aging processes how older people relate to social institutions (e.g., the family, health care systems) and the antecedents and consequences of the dramatic changes in age composition of the population.

The goal of the program is to produce a scientific knowledge base whichby informing professional practice, public policy, and everyday lifecan maximize people's health, effective functioning, independence, and well-being in their middle and later years. In order to explain the wide diversity among older people, it encourages comparisons between males and females persons with differing racial, ethnic. and socioeconomic background and inhabitants of countries that vary in styles and standards of living.

Special attention is given to studies of the oldest old (those age 85 and over), one of the fastest growing segments of the population. Of special concern is the care of Alzheimer's disease patients and their families. Emphasis is also placed on many kinds of interventions that can prevent, postpone, or reverse such decrements of old age as chronic ill health, sense of incompetence, memory loss, functional disability, or withdrawal from active participation in social and economic roles.

The program is divided into three areas of research. It also supports development of datasets, methodologies, and other research resources, and it works with other agencies to coordinate the preparation of statistical data on aging.

Adult Psychological Development (APD) supports research concerned with behavioral and social mechanisms and processes influencing cognitive and intellectual functioning, personality, attitudes and interpersonal relationships over the adult life course. An emphasis is placed on research relevant to maintaining and improving well-being, independence, and effective functioning. Research is needed for seeking out the conditions under which age-related individual changes occur or do not occur, and for supplying information to use in the design of roles and environments that can utilize the special strengths of middle-age and older people and that can maintain and enhance their functioning. The two sections included are: cognitive functioning and aging and personality and social psychological aging.

Social Science Research on Aging (SSR) aims to understand the social and environmental conditions influencing health, well-being, and functioning of people in their middle and later years. Its two sections focus respectively on the dynamic processes linking health, behavior, and aging and on those linking social structures with behaviors, attitudes, health, and status of older people. Both sections are concerned with social and behavioral factors in health and functioning and with assessment and testing of planned and natural interventions for health promotion/disease prevention.

Special attention is given to research on aging and health care, especially such issues in long-term care as: family structures and relationships affecting provision of home care, and interventions to prevent the need for long-term care (e.g., injury prevention and control). Particular emphasis is placed on studies of long-term care of Alzheimer's disease patients and their families in line with the NIA initiative. This program also encompasses social science research on two other institute-wide initiatives: gender, health, and longevity, and minority health. The three sections included are: behavioral geriatrics research, health care organizations and older people in society.

Demography and Population Epidemiology (DPE) supports research and training on the dynamics and consequences of population aging, and aims to describe and understand the changing elderly population in terms of its social, demographic, economic, health, and functional characteristics, and the impact of these changes on society as a whole.

DPE also coordinates policy on aging-related statistical data within the NIA and across other institutes at NIH as well as with other relevant Federal agencies. The Office on Demography of Aging is located in the DPE/BSR, the focal point for coordinating demographic and economic research within NIA. The demography office is also the center of activity for the Federal forum of aging-related statistics, a group which serves a similar function in coordinating research governmentwide. DPE's three sections are: health and retirement economies, demography of aging, and population epidemiology.

National Institute on Alcohol Abuse and Alcoholism

Mission

The National Institute on Alcohol Abuse and Alcoholism (NIAAA) is responsible for research on the causes, consequences, treatment, and prevention of alcohol-related problems. NIAAA conducts and supports biomedical and behavioral research into the effects of alcohol on the human mind and body, prevention and treatment of alcohol abuse and alcoholism, and epidemiology of alcoholism and alcohol-related problems. In carrying out these responsibilities, the institute:

- Conducts and supports basic and biobehavioral research aimed at determining the causes of alcoholism, discovering how alcohol damages the organs of the body, and developing prevention and treatment strategies for application in the Nation's health care system;

- Serves as a national resource for the collection, analysis, and dissemination of scientific findings;

- Supports training and development of scientists for participation in alcohol research programs and activities;

- Conducts policy studies that have broad implications for alcohol problem prevention, treatment, and rehabilitation activities; and

- Conducts epidemiological studies as well as national and community surveys to assess the risks for and magnitude of alcohol-related problems among various population groups.

Programs and Activities

NIAAA supports research through a program of extramural grant support to scientists at leading U.S. research institutions, through interdisciplinary National Alcohol Research Centers Program grants, and through an active intramural research program on the NIH campus in Bethesda, Md. Additionally, NIAAA is involved in a number of important collaborations within NIH and the international community. Findings from these several research areas are made available and accessible through a wide variety of research dissemination activities.

Extramural Research

NIAAA's extramural research support is aimed at building a solid base of biomedical and behavioral knowledge for improved prevention and treatment of alcohol-related problems. Scientists from a variety of disciplines, including social and behavioral sciences, biology, and medicine participate in the extramural program. Current directions in extramural research span diverse areas such as genetic predisposition to alcoholism, patient-treatment matching studies, the neurosciences, alcohol and pregnancy research, the development of pharmacological interventions to treat alcohol abuse and alcoholism and its effects, and alcohol-related public health policies. Selected extramural program highlights are provided below.

Genetics. The legacy of alcoholism in families has prompted researchers to explore the genetic and environmental factors that contribute so heightened vulnerability to alcoholism and the genetic factors that appear to protect certain individuals from developing the disease. Among it research activities in genetics, NIAAA has a cooperative agreement for a multidisciplinary, collaborative study involving seven research institutions across the U.S. to determine how vulnerability to alcoholism is transmitted through families. This study, initiated in the fall of 1989, involves the detailed diagnostic evaluation and genetic typing of 2,400 individuals comprising several hundred families in which alcoholism may be inherited. The long-term objective of this research is to pinpoint genes that influence the susceptibility to alcoholism.

Alcohol and Pregnancy. NIAAA supports many laboratory studies of alcohol's effects on prenatal and postnatal development. In recent years studies to determine why and how alcohol adversely affects the developing fetus have uncovered a number of mechanisms that likely contribute in differing degrees to fetal alcohol syndrome. Alcohol may inhibit cell growth, migration, and differentiation by interfering with the signaling molecules that control these steps in development. Last year, NIAAA funded a new study of relationships between alcohol consumption levels and the prevalence of alcohol-related birth defects among several Native American communities at relatively high-risk of fetal alcohol syndrome.

The effects of low-level or moderate drinking on prenatal development are of considerable concern because this pattern of drinking is so prevalent. Because alcohol's effects on development lie on a dose dependent continuum, it is important to assess developmental patterns in children in relation to a wide range of prenatal exposure levels. NIAAA supports longitudinal studies of the relationship between maternal alcohol consumption during pregnancy and developmental outcomes in offspring. Neurobehavioral deficits are expressed in different forms according to age, and difficulties with social and academic functioning appear to be lifelong.

Medications Development. NIAAA is strongly committed to the development of pharmacological interventions to diminish the craving for alcohol, reduce risk of relapse, and safely detoxify dependent individuals undergoing treatment. Pharmacologic agents are at various stages of development ranging from preclinical research to clinical application for the treatment of alcoholism.

Naltrexone, an opioid antagonist, has recently been approved by FDA as a safe and effective adjunct to psychosocial treatment for alcoholism.

Since alcohol-seeking behavior is complex and involves several neurotransmitter systems and neurohormones, NIAAA is exploring a range of additional medications to modify drinking behavior. Serotonin uptake inhibitors have shown considerable promise in animal models and may assist alcoholics with collateral depression. Related topics of interest are medication compliance, differential effect of pharmacotherapies on subtypes of alcoholics, and effects of medications when combined with psychosocial interventions.

Neurosciences. NIAAA-funded research is exploring the numerous targets in the brain on which alcohol acts. New methodologies are now becoming available to measure how alcohol acts on neural circuits in the brain to alter behavior. Noninvasive, functional imaging technologies are being used in animal and human studies to identify the neural circuits involved in the reinforcing properties of alcohol leading to and maintaining addictive alcohol-seeking behaviors. In addition, important new assessments are being made of alcohol-linked behaviors in freely behaving animals performing behavioral tasks combined simultaneously with changes in neurotrasmitters and neuromodulators in specific brain circuits using in vivo techniques such as microdialysis, voltammetry, or electrophysiological recordings in multiple areas of the brain. Such studies will lead to the development of therapeutic agents to treat alcohol abuse and alcoholism.

Treatment. NIAAA continues to emphasize research to improve patient-treatment matching, i.e., assignment of patients to facilities, interventions, and treatment providers according to the patients psychological and behavioral characteristics and the nature of their alcohol dependence. One of the institute's primary initiatives is a cooperative grant focused on matching studies at multiple sites using large study populations. This large scale permits simultaneous testing of various treatment strategies, exploration of interactions between strategies, and standardization of techniques among the participating centers. In turn, these features will allow for more sophisticated analyses than were previously possible, and will enhance the generalizability of findings to applied treatment settings.

Community Prevention Trials. NIAAA supports an integrated group of community-based prevention trials, where the community serves as the unit of analysis. The focal problems to be prevented include alcohol-related trauma, underage drinking, and drinking and driving. All of the trials are testing the impact of environmentally oriented interventions (e.g., enhanced law enforcement, server training, and community coalitions). In addition, one project tests school- and community-activation procedures. Experimental and quasi-experimental designs are being utilized and two of the studies evaluate the effectiveness of naturally occurring interventions using the methodologies of natural experiments. Results from completed research indicate that community-based interventions can significantly reduce underage drinking as well as drinking and driving.

National Alcohol Research Centers Program. NIAAA administers 14 diverse Alcohol Research Centers nationwide through the institute's National Alcohol Research Center Grants Program. This program is interrelated with and complementary to all other research support mechanisms and scientific activities that investigate the causes, diagnosis, treatment, control, prevention, and consequences of alcohol abuse and alcoholism. The program provides long-term (typically 5 years) support for interdisciplinary research that focuses on particular aspects of alcohol abuse, alcoholism, or other alcohol-related problems. This program encourages outstanding scientists from many disciplines to provide a full range of expertise, approaches, and advanced technologies for developing knowledge in these areas.

A primary goal of any NIAAA-funded center is to become, through excellence in science research, a significant regional or national research resource. In addition, each center affords research training opportunities for persons from various disciplines and professions. Current areas of alcohol center focus are the genetic determinants of alcohol ingestion; epidemiology of alcohol problems; environmental approaches to prevention; effects of alcohol on cellular neurobiology; alcohol and the cell; etiology and treatment of alcohol dependence; alcohol and aging; genetic approaches to the neuropharmacology of alcohol, biobehavioral manifestations of adolescent alcohol abuse; genetics of neuroadaptation to ethanol; clinical and medical epidemiology; and etiology and pharmacological treatment of alcoholism.

Intramural Research

The overall goal of the NIAAA Intramural Research Program is to understand the mechanisms by which alcohol produces intoxication, dependence, and damage to vital body organs, and to develop tools to prevent and treat those biochemical and behavioral processes. Areas of study include identification and assessment of genetic and environmental risk factors for the development of alcoholism the effects of alcohol on the central nervous system, including how alcohol modifies brain activity and behavior metabolic and biochemical effects of alcohol on various organs and systems of the body noninvasive imaging of the brain structure and activity related to alcohol use development of animal models of alcoholism and the diagnosis, prevention, and treatment of alcoholism and associated disorders.

Studies on the effects of ethanol on cell membrane receptors, ion channels, and expression of genes coding for these important proteins are yielding intriguing insights into basic mechanisms of ethanol's action. Combined with studies on region specific effects of ethanol on the release of neurotransmitters, these investigations will elucidate how ethanol produces reward, dependence, tolerance, and brain damage. Behavioral studies on animals, using mainly mice and monkeys, combined with molecular genetics and behavioral manipulations during development, examine important protective and causal factors for alcohol abuse and dependence.

NIAAA utilizes a combination of clinical and basic research facilities which enables a coordinated interaction between basic research findings and clinical applications in pursuit of these goals. An inpatient ward and a large outpatient program are located in the NIH Clinical Center.

Genetics of Alcoholism. This research focuses on investigating the genetic determinants of the risk for alcoholism. Studies on impulsive and violent alcoholics show that there is a clinical subgroup of alcoholics with polydrug abuse and antisocial personality features who also display deficits in serotonin function. The goal of this research is to understand how natural variants of genes involved in serotonergic neurotransmission affect human behavior. Two approaches are used: molecular cloning and expression studies of genes involved in serotonin function, and intensive behavioral and neuropsychological studies of human families and animal strains with natural variants of serotonin genes.

In conducting this research NIAAA scientists examine a variety of populations to determine how genetics and environment interact in the development of alcoholism and concomitant psychopathologies including drug abuse, antisocial personality, anxiety, and mood disorders. Techniques include family transmission studies and genetic linkage analyses using selected candidate genes and a large number of polymorphic markers.

To identify genes for complex, heterogeneous psychiatric diseases, it is helpful to define genetic characteristics which could correlate more precisely with genotypes. Neurophysiologic differences in alcoholism may serve this purpose these differences include a diminished amplitude of a specific electrophysiological trait—called the P300 evoked potential—and the low voltage alpha component of the electroencephalogram. Approaches include family transmission studies and a genetic linkage study to map the genes determining the variants. Psychiatric interviews are conducted to correlate neurophysiological phenotype with clinical phenotype and behavior.

Alcohol and Essential Fatty Acids. NIAAA researchers are investigating the biological functions of essential fatty acids and the adverse effects of alcohol on these functions. A clinical study of alcoholics has indicated that there is a loss of essential polyunsaturated fatty acids in the tissues and blood cells of these patients. Such losses are believed to be related to the tissue damage that occurs in almost every organ system in alcoholics but particularly in the liver and brain. Alcohol is perhaps the only dietary constituent that is capable of depleting the omega-3 fatty acids from the brain, and this may lead to the degeneration of neural cells and a loss in brain and visual function. An interdisciplinary approach is taken in these studies.

Losses of organ polyunsaturated fats as a consequence of chronic alcohol abuse. the underlying metabolic mechanisms and modulating nutritional factors, and the consequences for membrane function as assessed by biochemical and biophysical means are an integral part of this work. Fluorescence spectroscopy and magnetic resonance imaging are the principal tools used to study the functions of polyunsaturated phospholipids in membranes. Mass spectrometry is used for sensitive analysis of fatty acid metabolites in humans. Studies are also being conducted on the lipid requirements of the nervous system during early development. and the full range of experimental and clinical approaches available in the laboratory are employed in this effort.

Molecular Mechanisms of Alcohol Action in the Brain. Recent NIAAA research studies have demonstrated that alcohol affects signal transduction systems involved in the regulation of nerve cell excitability and the transmission of information at synapses. Using newly developed physiological and molecular bioiogical techniques, institute scientists are working toward determining the molecular mechanisms of alcohol's interaction with these signal transduction systems. Scientists also will investigate the molecular alterations of neural function associated with alcohol tolerance, dependence, and withdrawal. This information, will significantly lead to our understanding of the molecular basis of alcohol dependence, and to development of new treatments and prevention strategies.

International Activities

The Office of Collaborative Research Activities initiates and fosters collaborative activities with other NIH institutes, government agencies, and other organizations interested in alcohol-related problems. These activities include cosponsorship of workshops and research projects as well as efforts to disseminate research findings. The office administers and manages an international program to further the institute's domestic goals.

Mutually beneficial collaborative research efforts have been developed with other countries and international organizations. Research information is exchanged on a regular basis with over 30 countries. This office also coordinates the institute's science education initiative. Special projects in collaboration with educators of K-12 students are in progress.

Among its many recent collaborative national and international activities, NIAAA has cosponsored projects with other institutes and organizations studying birth defects, liver disease, AIDS, women's health, minority health, aging. and health services research. NIAAA has supported scientific exchanges to increase the research capability of scientists in several foreign countries or to support collaborative research with grantees. The institute has responded to requests for joint research efforts, developed productive cooperative projects, or supported grantees to work with scientists in Finland, Poland, Mexico, Russia, the Czech Republic, Canada, Spain, and many other countries.

Research Dissemination

NIAAA maintains an active communication program aimed at sharing with health care practitioners, policy makers, others involved in managing alcohol-related programs about research findings with applicability to alcohol treatment and prevention efforts, and the general public. Our scientific communications vehicles include publications such as:

* Special reports to Congress on alcohol and health, triennial reports from the secretary of Health and Human Services to the Congress, which describe research findings and advances in the alcohol field;

* *Alcohol Health & Research World*, a quarterly professional journal available by subscription;

* *Alcohol Alert*, a publication designed to quickly disseminate research findings to health professionals: and

* Monographs on special topics or containing papers from NIAAA-sponsored workshops on critical research areas such as imaging and economics.

Research findings are also shared with the alcohol and general health care communities through two online database services supported by the institute. The first of these, the "Quick Facts" electronic bulletin board, provides access to alcohol-related epidemiologic data and facilitates communication among NIAAA staff and others interested in NIAAA programs and data.

Scientists, clinicians, and others interested in alcohol-related research also have direct access to NIAAA's comprehensive "Alcohol and Alcohol Problems Science Database" through Ovid Technologies, Inc.a commercial vendor. The database title is ETOH, named after EtOH, one of the chemical designations for ethyl alcohol. ETOH covers literature from the late 1960s to the present, contains over 93,000 bibliographic records, and covers all aspects of alcohol research: psychology, psychiatry, physiology, biochemistry, epidemiology, sociology, neuroscience, treatment, prevention, education, accidents and safety, criminal justice, legislation, employment, labor and industry, and public policy. The database also contains entries on books, monographs, government reports, dissertations, and conference papers.

Plans are under way to make ETOH available on the world wide web (WWW) institute home page. Currently, NIAAA's WWW features publications (many available as full text documents), news releases, grant and contract information, and other alcohol-related resources.

National Institute on Deafness and Other Communication Disorders

Mission

Conducts and supports research and research training with respect to disorders of hearing and other communication processes, including diseases affecting hearing, balance, smell, taste, voice, speech, and language through:

- Research performed in its own laboratories and clinics

- A program of research grants, individual and institutional research training awards, career development awards, center grants, and contracts to public and private research institutions and organizations

- Cooperation and collaboration with professional, commercial, voluntary, and philanthropic organizations concerned with research and training that is related to deafness and other communication disorders, disease prevention and health promotion, and the special biomedical and behavioral problems associated with people having communication impairments or disorders

- The support of efforts to create devices which substitute for lost and impaired sensory and communication functions

- Ongoing collection and dissemination of information to health professionals, patients, industry, and the public on research findings in these areas.

Major Programs

Research programs at NIDCD are intended to improve methods of prevention, diagnosis, treatment, and rehabilitation of clinical problems of deafness and other communication disorders.

Hearing

In recent years, the fields of cellular and molecular biology have furthered hearing research through the ability to clone genes for inner ear development and the assembly of human and animal cochlea-specific cDNA libraries. These advances offer researchers many new opportunities to study the characteristics of deafness, hereditary factors involved in hearing loss, and the genes that are critical for the development and maintenance of the human ear. Scientific advances have also been translated into cochlear implants, digital hearing aids, and tactile devices that provide information by stimulating the skin.

Great strides are being made in the study of the properties of auditory sensory cells, and of the characteristics of the response of the inner ear to sound. For many years, it was thought that sensory cells in the auditory and vestibular epithelia of birds and mammals were produced only during embryonic development. Thus, any loss of these cells as a result of drug treatment, noise trauma or aging was thought to result in permanent hearing deficits. However, recent research has shown that sensory cells in the vestibular epithelia of most vertebrates, including humans, can be regenerated.

Hearing impairment, a problem that crosses all ethnic and socioeconomic lines, is studied through NIDCD supported research. This research provides important information on otitis media, the most common cause of hearing loss in children, and presbycusis, hearing loss in the aging population.

Balance NIDCD supports research on balance and the vestibular system. These disorders afflict a large proportion of the population, particularly the elderly. The vestibular system, with its primary receptor organs located in the inner ear, is largely responsible for the maintenance of one's orientation in space, balance, posture and for visual fixation of objects during motion and regulation of locomotion and other volitional movements. Vestibular disorders can, therefore, yield symptoms of imbalance, vertigo (the illusion of motion), disorientation, instability, falling and visual blurring (particularly during motion). Major disorders affecting the vestibular system result from infection, trauma, impaired blood supply, impaired metabolic function and tumors.

In addition to its roles in the stabilization of gaze and balance, recent findings suggest that the vestibular system plays an important role in regulating blood pressure. This information holds potential clinical relevance to the understanding and management of orthostatic hypotension (lowered blood pressure related to a change in body posture).

The institute supports research to develop and refine tests of balance and vestibular disorders. Computer-controlled systems measuring the responses activated by stimulating specific parts of the vestibular sense organ are now available. Improved tests of vestibular disability will have important implications for planning programs of physical rehabilitation for patients with balance and vestibular disorders.

Smell and Taste

NIDCD investigators study the chemical senses of smell and taste to enhance understanding of how individuals communicate with their environment. For example, this research is providing insight into changing preferences and aversions for specific foods and flavors. Improved understanding of the interaction between chemoreception and food consumption will lead to improved nutrition from birth to old age.

Both the olfactory and gustatory systems offer special approaches for understanding fundamental mechanisms of plasticity. NIDCD scientists have found that smell and taste cells have the capacity to replace themselves throughout life. These are the only known mammalian sensory cells with this property.

Advances in the molecular and cellular biology, biophysics and biochemistry of the olfactory and gustatory systems are paving the way for improved diagnosis, prevention, and treatment of chemosensory disorders. The vertebrate olfactorv receptor neuron has become an important biologic model system in the area of molecular and cellular biology. The olfactory receptor gene family was recently described in mammals and may contain as many as 1,000 olfactory receptor genes. NIDCD scientists are presently characterizing genetic mechanisms of olfaction which will provide the opportunity to study the molecular pharmacology of the process of smell. In addition, the use of available biochemical and molecular probes will lead to a more complete characterization of the neurotransmitters throughout the gustatory system.

Voice, Speech and Language

Studies of voice and speech disorders are aimed at determining the nature, causes, treatment and prevention disorders such as stuttering, spasmodic dysphonia, and dysarthria. A recent study has demonstrated a new, effective treatment for one such disorder, spasmodic dysphonia—a hyperactivity of the muscles of the larynx which constricts the vocal folds and severely distorts speech. This treatment involves the injection of minute amounts of botulinum toxin into the laryngeal muscles. The toxin blocks the muscle stimulation and eliminates the hyperactivity, rendering a patient free of the symptoms for as long as 4 months.

Oral speech communication may not be a realistic option for individuals with severe dysarthria. Substantial progress has been made in the development of augmentative communication devices to facilitate the expressive communication of persons with severe communication disabilities. An investigation of conversational performance by augmentative communicative device users is in progress. Other funded research evaluates whether a low cost, laser activated keyboard for accessing personal computers is feasible. By providing access to computers, individuals with disabilities can immediately use personal computer software programs and speech synthesizers for augmentative communication.

Language research continues to expand our understanding of the role of each hemisphere of the brain in communication and language, of early specialization of the brain, and of the recovery process following brain damage. This research is intended to further understanding of the neural bases of language disorders. Research on acquisition, characterization and utilization of American Sign Language is expanding our knowledge of the language of people who are deaf.

National Institute on Drug Abuse

Mission

The National Institute on Drug Abuse (NIDA) provides national leadership for research on drug abuse and addiction. Through its extramural research program and its intramural research program at the Division of Intramural Research in Baltimore, NIDA supports studies on the biological, social, behavioral and neuroscientific bases of drug abuse as well as its causes, prevention, and treatment. In addition, NIDA supports research training, career development, public education and research dissemination in these areas. Through grants and contracts to investigators at research institutions around the country and overseas, NIDA supports research and training on:

- the neurobiological, behavioral, and social mechanisms underlying drug abuse and addiction

- specific biomedical and behavioral effects of drugs of abuse, including marijuana, heroin, and cocaine, on the body and brain

- effective prevention and treatment approaches, including a broad research program designed to develop new treatment medications and behavioral therapies for drug abuse

- the causes and consequences of drug abuse, including impact on society and morbidity and mortality in selected populations, e.g. ethnic minorities, youth, women

- investigation of the relationship of drug use to other problem behaviors, e.g., psychopathology, unemployment, violence

- biomedical, behavioral, and social factors associated with vulnerability/invulnerability to drug abuse and addiction

- the role of drug abuse as a factor contributing to the spread of HIV/AIDS, tuberculosis, and other diseases and the development of effective prevention/intervention strategies

- research on the mechanisms of pain and the search for a nonaddictive analgesic

- research on tobacco and nicotine addiction.

The intramural research program of NIDA's Division of Intramural Research (DIR), formerly the Addiction Research Center, located in Baltimore, Maryland, conducts interdisciplinary research on the causes, hazards, treatment, and prevention of drug abuse and addiction the behavioral mechanisms underlying the addictive process, and the addictive liability of new drugs. These studies range from basic molecular studies through laboratory work with animals, to clinical studies with human volunteers. The DIR uses the latest technologies, such as positron emission tomography to study the action of drugs in the human brain and transgenic techniques in which genetically altered mice are created to examine the role genes play in vulnerability to drug abuse. The DIR also serves as a national and international training center for researchers in the drug abuse field.

NIDA Programs

Division of Epidemiology and Prevention Research. The Division of Epidemiology and Prevention Research conducts research on the epidemiology, etiology, natural history and consequences of drug abuse and strategies to prevent drug abuse among general, special and underserved populations. Major research efforts focus on identifying risk and protective factors for drug abuse, and exploring the natural history of drug abuse and related comorbid conditions. The information obtained from these studies guides NIDA in determining its research priorities.

The division's programs address questions about what kind of drugs are being abused, to what extent and by whom. Activities range from support for surveys designed to monitor drug use trends among high school students, to developing networks of community researchers for the purpose of identifying new trends in patterns of drug use in the U.S., to conducting in-depth analyses of data which increase knowledge about the nature and extent of drug abuse, and to performing methodologic research to improve the measurement of drug abuse patterns.

The extramural community research program supports studies on the epidemiology and prevention of drug use and abuse-related consequences including HIV/AIDS, hepatitis B and C, and violence; the antecedents, determinants, correlates, and consequences of drug use and abuse and these conditions; the efficacy, effectiveness, and efficiency of community-based interventions in reducing these drug-abuse-related conditions; and innovative methodologies to improve community-based epidemiologic and prevention efficacy research.

The extramural epidemiologic research program funds research on the origins and patterns of drug use/abuse and the disease of addiction, including surveys among general and special populations; the identification and study of resiliency and risk factors for drug use and abuse; etiologic studies on drug use/abuse and the human developmental process; improved methodological studies and innovative statistical research designs; and international epidemiologic studies that focus on drug use, etiologic factors, and related concerns around the world.

The extramural prevention research program supports studies to develop and test strategies to prevent drug use, to prevent escalation from initial drug use to dependence among high risk individuals and groups, and to determine the efficacy of population-based, comprehensive multiple component interventions.

The division works with state, Federal, and international agencies and private organizations to encourage the sharing of drug abuse information and prevention models.

Division of Basic Research

Elucidating the basic behavioral and biomedical mechanisms underlying drug abuse, its causes, and its hazards is the goal of the Division of Basic Research. Research supported by the division helps form the foundation needed to make advances in the treatment and prevention of drug abuse. The division conducts research focusing on the behavioral processes underlying the use of abused substances, which includes studies of drugs' effects on human and animal behavior, as well as studies of social and other factors in drug abuse and addiction. NIDA-funded scientists also seek to understand how abused drugs influence performance, perception and cognitive functions such as learning and memory.

Because drugs affect the brain and its control over mood and behavior, a significant part of the division's research is connected to the broad field of neuroscience. With a clearer understanding of the brain's functions (e.g., the neurobiology of drug reinforcement), and how they are affected by illicit drugs, researchers hope to improve treatment for drug addiction and to prevent drug dependence. The division also supports studies on the motivational processes underlying drug use and relapse to drug use such as craving.

The division monitors a broad spectrum of neurobiological and other biomedical research including studies that seek to determine: the specific mechanisms mediating drugs' effects on the heart and other organs; the mechanisms of drug tolerance and dependence; the basic chemistry of drugs and their analogs; and the processes through which the body absorbs, metabolizes and excretes drugs. In addition, investigators funded by the division explore the effects of drugs on pregnancy and offspring and short- and long-term consequences of multiple drug use. The division also supports studies to determine the neurochemical and behavioral effects of newly developed drugs, with a special emphasis on finding nonaddicting analgesics. Other research develops methodologies for testing new compounds to determine their potential for abuse.

Division of Clinical and Services Research

The Division of Clinical and Services Research supports a program of research aimed at enhancing the understanding of the pathophysiology of drug abuse/addictive disorders, their complications including

AIDS, and their treatment, at the clinical level. The work of the division encompasses physiological/neurobiological, behavioral, medical, developmental, and services delivery approaches. In each of these areas the emphasis is on elucidation of mechanisms underlying the drug abuse/addictive disorders and their complications, the development, improvement and evaluation of treatments and access to quality and cost-effectiveness of care.

The Clinical Medicine Branch stimulates, plans and develops a national research program focusing upon the clinical health and developmental consequences of drug abuse/addictive disorders. The program encompasses studies of natural history of infectious (particularly HIV/AIDS and tuberculosis) and noninfectious complications of drug abuse/addictive disorders, effects of addiction on human development, efficacy of clinical interventions for complications of drug abuse/ addiction, and pathophysiology/pathogenesis of diseases associated with drug abuse disorders.

The Etiology and Clinical Neurobiology Branch conducts a national research program which focuses on the clinical neurobiology of drug abuse/addictive disorders. This program targets questions of how these disorders affect the structure, function and development of the human central nervous system, as well as how the structure and physiology of the human CNS and genetic factors affect susceptibility and development and course of drug abuse/addictive disorders.

In addition, the branch supports studies of the neurobiological mechanisms underlying both pharmacological and nonpharmacological treatments of drug abuse/addictive disorders. Investigations of neurobiological aspects of HIV infection/AIDS in patients with substance abuse/addictive disorders are also supported by this program. Approaches include functional and structural brain imaging, as well as other state-of-the-art techniques.

The Services Research Branch conducts a national research program addressing issues of financing and cost, organization, management and effectiveness of health services delivered to patients with drug abuse disorders, as well as health services delivered to such patients in relation to HIV/AIDS. Investigations are carried out at the client, program and system levels.

The Treatment Research Branch conducts a national research program concerned with developing. improving, and assessing behavioral and somatic treatments for drug abuse disorders, including treatments to reduce AIDS risk behaviors. Research on the treatment of patients with comorbid addictive and psychiatric disorders, investigations aimed at optimizing matching of patients to treatment modalities, and studies on diagnosis and classification of drug abuse disorders are also supported by the branch.

Medications Development Division

Finding new and better pharmacotherapies to treat drug addiction is the mission of the Medications Development Division. Its founding in 1990 strengthened NIDA's commitment to improving drug abuse treatment and preventing the spread of AIDS.

The division funds researchers at every step of the complex medication development process. By expanding NIDA's in-house pharmacological research capabilities, forging drug development agreements with pharmaceutical firms, and establishing a nationwide network of clinical research sites where new medications can be tested, the division is aggressively pursuing ways to enhance and quicken the medication development process.

The division continually searches for compounds that may be effective against drug use. By focusing on medications that have already achieved FDA approval, the division hopes to move rapidly to testing in humans—reducing the average 10 years it takes to get a new medication on the market.

Division of Intramural Research

NIDA's Division of Intramural Research, with a staff of more than 180, including 60 doctorate-level scientists, is one of the largest research facilities in the U.S. devoted to studying drug abuse and addiction.

Located in Baltimore, Md., the DIR provides an environment where NIDA scientists can collaborate within one facility on a variety of research projects crucial to understanding drug addiction.

Research conducted by intramural NIDA scientists in the DIR complements the many studies supported by NIDA awarded grants and contracts across the country and abroad. Areas under investigation include the causes, treatment, and prevention of drug abuse and addiction; the biochemical and behavioral mechanisms underlying the addictive process; the addictive potential of new drugs; and bases for selective individual vulnerabilities to abused drugs. Work ranges from basic molecular studies through laboratory work with animals to clinical studies with human volunteers. The center uses the latest research technologies, such as positron emission tomography, to study the action of drugs in the living human brain and transgenic techniques, in which genetically altered mice are created to examine the role genes play in vulnerability to drug abuse.

DIR researchers have played central roles in defining molecular sites for cocaine and opiate action and have used their insights to add to new therapeutic studies.

In addition to its research role, the DIR also serves as a training ground for researchers from across the world to receive training in its laboratories. Approximately 25 percent of all DIR personnel are trainees.

Special Programs

NIDA Training Programs. To ensure an adequate supply of professionals in the drug abuse field, NIDA's research training program includes individual fellowships and institutional training programs. NIDA's training emphasizes basic biomedical, clinical, behavioral, neuroscience, and epidemiological research in drug abuse.

In addition, NIDA instituted a Science Education Program in recognition of the need to improve science education and literacy in the U.S. The purpose of the program is to provide educators with tools that can be used to effectively interest students in science.

AIDS Program. Because transmission of HIV is linked directly and indirectly to drug abuse, NIDA's new Office on AIDS collects valuable information on ways of limiting behaviors associated with drug use that are likely to spread the disease. By devising strategies that drug abuse treatment and prevention practitioners can use to combat AIDS, NIDA is helping reduce the transmission of HIV among drug abusers, their sexual partners, and their children.

NIDA's AIDS program also focuses on sharing its research findings with researchers, at-risk groups, prevention and treatment practitioners, and the general public. As part of this effort, NIDA provides technical assistance to help communities form coalitions to increase awareness at the grassroots level of the association between AIDS and drug abuse. In addition, NIDA has developed several comprehensive, national public education campaigns to deliver mass media messages about the prevention of drug abuse and AIDS.

Research Program on Women and Gender Differences. In 1991, NIDA established the women's health issues group to provide leadership for research in the area of drug abuse in pregnant and parenting women and the effects of drug use and abuse on the offspring. In past research on drug abuse, research subjects, both humans and animals, have been almost exclusively male; as a result little data have been available on women. However, gender differences recently have gained attention in the field of drug abuse research. Preliminary data indicate that biological mechanisms involved in drug abuse-progression and initiation; antecedents and consequences; prevention and treatment-vary considerably between men and women. In response to this newly emerging field of research, NIDA in 1995 broadened its program to include research on drug use, abuse and addiction in women, regardless of age and reproductive status, and gender differences.

This institute-wide research program on women and gender differences includes the full range of NIDA supported research including basic research (both human and animal), epidemiology, etiology, antecedents and progression, consequences, prevention, intervention and treatment. Leadership is provided by the women's health coordinator and the women and gender research group, an advisory group with representation from each of NIDA's program branches.

Research Dissemination. As part of its overall mission to promote the use of research in reducing the problems of drug abuse in the U.S., NIDA carries out multifaceted activities to disseminate research results to researchers, prevention and treatment practitioners, other health care providers, policymakers, and the general public. NIDA's public information branch coordinates these activities, which disseminate the most up-to-date findings by NIDA-supported researchers and other leading investigators in the drug abuse field through print and audiovisual materials to diverse audiences.

Special Populations. Epidemiologic data show that drug abuse and HIV/AIDS have disproportionately severe consequences for minority populations. Minority group persons who abuse drugs are more likely to die and suffer from severe drug-related illnesses and are less likely to receive appropriate prevention and treatment services. More research is needed in order to develop a rigorous scientific knowledge base on minority populations and drug abuse that can support the formation of policy, prevention/intervention efforts, and a full range of treatment approaches (e.g., pharmacologic, clinical, behavioral) that are responsive and appropriate to each population's needs.

The Special Populations Office supports activities to encourage research on minority health issues related to drug abuse and is administratively responsible for some of the research training programs pertaining to minority and other populations. It also assesses and makes recommendations regarding research needs and strategies and monitors progress towards the achievement of these goals.

Division of Research Grants

Mission

Provides staff support to the Office of Extramural Research in the formulation of grant and award policies and procedures. Assigns applications to the components of the PHS, and to supporting NIH institutes, centers and divisions and initial review groups.

Provides for scientific review of NIH grant applications and advisory and consultative services relating to grant policy and management.

Collects, stores, retrieves, analyzes, and evaluates management and program data needed in the administration of extramural programs.

Disseminates information on extramural programs to the Congress, scientists, and general public.

Warren Grant Magnuson Clinical Center

Mission

The Warren Grant Magnuson Clinical Center (CC) provides hospital services to patients who participate in clinical research conducted at NIH. The CC strives to be a model for clinical research by assuring quality patient care, delivering excellent support services, and recruiting and maintaining expert staff. Authorized by Congress to provide patient care necessary to conduct biomedical research, the CC was specially designed to place patient care facilities close to research laboratories to promote the quick transfer of new findings of scientists to the treatment of patients. Institutes admit to their units and clinics only those patients (upon referral by personal physicians) who have the precise kind or stage of illness under investigation by scientist-clinicians.

CC departments are responsible for the hospital services, except for direct physician care, and conduct research in their own specialties.

In addition to biomedical research and patient care, the CC offers opportunities for advanced training to physicians, medical and nursing students, and members of the paramedical professions. This training includes a core curriculum in clinical research, a graduate and postgraduate program, a clinical electives program and many lecture series. Monthly clinical staff conferences present the results of the cooperative biomedical research carried out at the CC by scientists and clinicians of the institutes and CC departments.

Major Programs

Unlike most hospitals, the CC does not offer general diagnostic treatment services. In its beds and clinics are patients who consent to participate in one of the 1,000 studies (protocols) sponsored by 15 institutes conducting research on the NIH grounds. The 13-story, 350-bed hospital logs about 7,000 inpatient admissions each year. Another 68,000 outpatient visits are made annually. Nearly 1,400 healthy people serve each year as clinical research volunteers. Some 1,200 physicians and 700 nurses provide patient care.

Clinical Center departments specifically tailor their services to serve the unique needs of biomedical research and patient care at NIH.

Clinical Pathology provides laboratory services for CC patients, develops new test methods, conducts research in laboratory medicine, and offers subspecialty training programs in the subdisciplines of clinical pathology. Five services make up the department: clinical chemistry; hematology; immunology; microbiology; and phlebotomy. The department performs some 4 million tests per year for CC patients. Research focuses on lipoprotein disorders, mineral metabolism, thrombosis and hemostasis, identification of cell populations by flow cytometry and the identification of microorganisms causing human disease. Further, the department is developing tests using molecular biology in each of the four clinical services.

Critical Care Medicine. This department was established in November 1977 in response to a need for a modern facility to care for increasing numbers of critically ill patients. Critical care physicians, nurses, and technical staff working with highly advanced technology and equipment provide care for any CC patient with serious but reversible medical problems. The nine-bed unit performs clinical research in collaboration with other NIH institutes on AIDS, sepsis, and pulmonary biology in addition to providing care.

Diagnostic Radiology research focuses on rare diseases or those in which traditional imaging methods have presented major problems in diagnosis, detection, or followup. New areas of research in MRI (magnetic resonance imaging) have concentrated on developing "contrast" agents that improve image resolution and on defining and analyzing optimal strategies for rapid scanning. The ultrafast computerized tomography (CT) scanner can display diagnostic images of patients unable to hold still for more conventional scanners. This is especially valuable when treating infants, children, and extremely ill adults.

Nuclear Medicine provides a broad scope of diagnostic and therapeutic services for CC patients and engages in collaborative research with institute investigators on the safe application of radionuclides. Nearly 5,000 patient studies were conducted last year. A new, miniaturized, SPECT gamma camera for animal studies was produced by the physics group in collaboration with BEIP and institute investigators. This presentation was singled out for its excellence at the annual scientific meeting of the Society of Nuclear Medicine. Ongoing studies with NCI laboratories have further developed radiolabeled monoclonal antibodies for tumor diagnosis and therapy.

Positron emission tomography (PET) is a method of imaging the body's physiologic functions such as blood flow and metabolism. Patients receive a short, half-lived radiopharmaceutical containing a radioactive atom that is produced by a cyclotron. This substance, also called a radionuclide, emits positrons.

As the positrons encounter electrons in the body, they produce high-energy photons that can be traced by radiation detectors surrounding the body. By evaluating the concentrations, physicians can study blood flow or how the brain metabolizes glucose.

The PET department is organized as a scientific core concentrating on radiochemistry. Resources include two medical cyclotrons to produce the radionuclides six leadlined chemistry hoods where the radiopharmaceuticals are formulated laboratories for radiochemistry three PET tomographs and computer hardware and software for generating and analyzing the PET images.

Rehabilitation Medicine Department (RMD) has continued to provide comprehensive rehabilitation services to NIH research patients. Approximately 25,000 patients were seen by RMD staff in the medical, occupational therapy, physical therapy, speech-language pathology, recreation therapy, and biomechanics laboratory sections.

Recently, RMD developed new clinical programs to assess swallowing and tongue motion in children. These children had diagnoses of childhood dermatomyositis and Beckwith-Weidemann syndrome (BWS). A comprehensive musculoskeletal evaluation was devised to determine the degree of abnormalities in children with BWS and their unaffected siblings. This evaluation was designed to provide pediatricians with a screening tool to identify abnormalities frequently associated with BWS (hemihypertrophy, macroglossia, and scoliosis).

The ultrasound laboratory developed programs that will help provide real time imaging of the oral pharynx without exposure to radiation and will permit quantitation and sequencing of swallowing events in real-time.

The biometrics laboratory has developed simulation models that will be used to predict outcomes of therapeutic intervention prior to treatment.

Undergraduate and graduate-level training are provided routinely in RMD, including summer programs and student internships.

The Department of Transfusion Medicine (DTM) continues to provide safe blood and blood products for CC patients. This includes approximately 500 units of whole blood or red cells and approximately 1,800 units of platelets a month for treatment of patients undergoing surgery, bone marrow transplantation or therapy for such diseases as aplastic anemia, leukemia, or other malignant conditions. Projects include a core facility for providing hematopoietic cells for transplantation, immunotherapy, and gene therapy, expansion of molecular-level testing in the tissue typing (HLA) lab to meet all CC service needs, and establishment of stem cell infusion services in an outpatient transfusion clinic. The HLA lab was one of nine designated as a "lead laboratory" based on performance in an international cell exchange. It is the only lab in the world to be so designated for 6 consecutive years. The department's Blood Bank also acts as a reference center for transfusion problems referred by labs and hospitals throughout the country.

The department continues to investigate the relationship between blood transfusion and hepatitis. DTM staff expanded their studies of hepatitis C to look at blood donor risk factors and instituted clinical studies of the newly reported agent, hepatitis G. The apheresis activities included studies to stimulate the production of granulocytes and hematopoietic stem cells in normal donors in order to collect more effective transfusion components.

In 1990 the DTM was the site of the first human gene therapy experiments involving children with severe congenital immune deficiency disorders. Eight clinical research protocols are now being carried out in such diseases as breast cancer, AIDS, Fanconi anemia, Gaucher disease, and chronic granulomatous disease. Lymphocytes are harvested from donors and patients for potential cellular vaccines. Innovative cellular therapies complement the department's traditional role in transfusion therapy.

Hospital Epidemiology Service (HES) includes a physician, an epidemiologist, and five infection control specialists. HES has implemented a comprehensive infection control program that operates within the guidelines of several agencies: the Joint Commission on Accreditation of Healthcare Organizations, the Centers for Disease Control and Prevention (CDC), and the Occupational Safety and Health Administration. The HES seeks to prevent transmission of hospital infections by using ongoing educational programs, routine patient surveillance, investigations of outbreaks, isolation precautions, and employee health protocols.

Although tuberculosis historically has been a rare disease in the Clinical Center, with the recent implementation of protocols to study multidrug resistant tuberculosis and the issuance of revised guidelines from CDC, HES has focused on development of a comprehensive control plan to minimize transmission of tuberculosis. Similar to the hierarchy of controls used to control transmission of blood-borne pathogens, tuberculosis control has involved developing and implementing administrative (work practice) and engineering controls and using personal protective equipment.

Information Systems (ISD) consolidates the planning, development, and maintenance of CC computing activities. ISD manages the CC medical information system (MIS), a large, online computerized system that provides access to patient records and allows users to retrieve and add data. The department operates the computer center, providing round-the-clock service to patient units, clinical pathology, pharmacy, radiology, admissions, and other departments engaged in administrative, diagnostic, and therapeutic activities. In addition, ISD provides advice and support to CC departments about micro or minicomputers, or other computer hardware or software. MIS is used by over 4,000 physicians, nurses, and other hospital professionals. On a typical day, 1,200 different hospital staffers make 8,800 distinct accesses to the system write 5,300 orders and request nearly 20,000 online patient retrievals for 2,000 patients.

Pharmacy provides a 24-hour comprehensive service for patients. The clinical pharmacy service is staffed by pharmacists with advanced specialty training. They assist physicians in designing, monitoring, and evaluating patient drug regimens to assure proper, rational drug therapy. The clinical pharmacokinetic research lab monitors drug levels in patients and interprets patient response to drug therapy. The formulation, development, control, assay, dispensing, and clinical monitoring of investigational drugs make the CC's pharmacy program unique. Pharmacy manufactures nearly 1 million investigational drug units and registers and labels some 2 million units each year. The inpatient pharmacy mixes an average of 750 I.V. admixtures daily and dispenses close to 1 million unit doses of medicine yearly. The outpatient pharmacy fills approximately 400 prescriptions a day.

Other departments and offices supporting the research effort include anesthesiology; housekeeping and fabric care materials management; medical record; nursing; nutrition; outpatient; social work; spiritual ministry; and surgical services.

John E. Fogarty International Center for Advanced Study in the Health Sciences

Mission

The John E. Fogarty International Center for Advanced Study in the Health Sciences:

- supports international research and research training activities in targeted areas of emphasis;

- supports international scientific collaboration through international fellowships and scholarships, small grants, scientist exchanges, and conferences;

- identifies significant international research issues/opportunities and facilitates ICD interest and involvement;

- provides administrative services for recruitment of foreign scientists into the intramural research laboratories of the NIH;

- coordinates the activities of the NIH concerned with the health sciences internationally, and

- receives foreign visitors to NIH.

Major Programs

Grants. The FIC AIDS International and Training Research Program (ITRP) enables U.S. universities and other research institutions to provide HIV/AIDS-related training to scientists and health professionals from developing nations and to forge collaborative ties with research institutions in countries highly impacted by the AIDS virus.

In collaboration with NIEHS and CDC's National Institute of Occupational Safety and Health, the ITRP in Environmental and Occupational Health funds nonprofi t public or private institutions to support international training and research programs in general environmental and occupational health for foreign health scientists, clinicians, epidemiologists, toxicologists, engineers, industrial hygenists, chemists and allied health workers.

In cooperation with NICHD, the FIC International and Training Research Program in Population and Health funds U.S. nonprofit public or private institutions to support population-related sciences research.

The ITRP in Emerging Infectious Disease, developed in collaborations with NIAID, addresses the need for international training and biomedical and biobehavioral research in these disease areas.

FIC is also the U.S. Government's organizational focus for an interagency program to identify bioactive products from plant and marine sources while preserving the rich natural diversity of rain forests and oceans. Funded by NIH, the National Science Foundation, and the U.S. Agency for International Development, but administered by FIC, the International Cooperative Biodiversity Group Program promotes both economic growth and ecological conservation by demonstrating the value of biological resources from which natural pharmaceuticals are derived.

In cooperation with the NIH Office of Research on Minority Health, FIC has established a Minority International Research Training Program to provide international educational training and research opportunities to groups underrepresented in the scientific professions. Training grants are provided to U.S. colleges and universities, including consoritia with minority representation, to stimulate students to pursue scientific careers by enhancing their undergraduate and graduate training through international experiences. Awards are provided to faculty members to conduct independent research and to serve as mentors to students abroad.

A small grants program, called the Fogarty International Research Collaboration Awards, or FIRCA, is offered to U.S. institutions for collaboration between U.S. principal investigators on regular NIH research grants and scientists in Africa, Asia (except Hong Kong, Japan, Singapore, South Korea and Taiwan), Central and Eastern Europe, Latin America and the non-U.S. Caribbean, the Middle East, and Pacific Ocean islands (except Australia and New Zealand). The FIRCA provides funds for supplies and equipment necessary to the collaborative research project (for the foreign collaborator's laboratory only), and funds for travel for the U.S. principal investigator, the foreign researcher, and/or associates. A similar award; the HIV/AIDS and Related Illnesses Collaboration Award, provides small grants in support of cooperative research between NIH grant recipients and foreign institutions throughout the world.

Fellowships. Fellowship programs administered by the FIC enable foreign scientists to pursue their research interests in U.S. laboratories and, conversely, provide opportunities for U.S. researchers to work in foreign laboratories. The International Research Fellowship Program enables promising postdoctoral biomedical or behavioral scientists from developing and emerging nations to gain further research experience by working in the laboratory of a distinguished U.S. scientist on a problem of mutual interest.

The Senior International Fellowship Program is for U.S. researchers well recognized and established in their careers who wish to spend up to 12 months in a foreign laboratory pursuing a project of mutual interest to the fellow and the foreign host scientist.

Several foreign countries support fellowships that enable U.S. biomedical researchers who hold doctoral degrees to spend up to a year in a foreign research laboratory. The FIC is involved in the initial stages of these programs, but the funding and administration is by the foreign country. The FIC publicizes the availability of postdoctoral research fellowships from the Academy of Finland, the Health Research Board of Ireland, the Israeli Ministry of Health, the Japan Society for the Promotion of Science, the Japanese Science and Technology Agency, the Norwegian Council for Science and the Humanities, and the Swedish Medical Research Council. The FIC also arranges for receipt and technical merit review of applications and transmits the applications and reviewers' comments to the awarding country for final selection.

Additionally, FIC announces the availability of postdoctoral fellowships from the Alexander von Humboldt Foundation in the Federal Republic of Germany and from the National Science Council in Taipei, Taiwan.

Scholars-in-Residence. FIC contributes to advanced studies in the health sciences by capitalizing on worldwide intellectual resources, biomedical knowledge, research findings, and technological advances by bringing these to bear on the identification of health-related issues of international importance and by developing strategies that will have a worldwide impact on disease prevention.

The FIC Scholars-in-Residence Program provides the opportunity for a small number of eminent scientists to spend up to 12 months at the NIH interacting with intramural staff and conducting studies of international interest and importance in contemporary biomedicine and international health.

International Relations. The FIC serves as the coordinating link between NIH and other U.S. agencies, foreign governments and international organizations on international biomedical research matters. It is responsible for the administrative oversight of all intergovernmental agreements in which the NIH participates.

The center also fosters and facilitates international cooperation in biomedical research by disseminating information on foreign biomedical research activities to the NIH research institutes and informing foreign agencies and institutions about the international activities of the NIH preparing background materials for NIH senior staff participation in international meetings and discussions; providing advice to the director and deputy director, NIH, and to senior staff of the NIH research institutes on policies and procedures relating to international activities; assisting the institutes by obtaining clearances for awards requiring State Department approval and by interpreting DHHS and State Department procedures relating to international travel; serving as a channel for communications to and from U.S. embassies abroad and foreign embassies in Washington; and coordinating responses to inquiries on international issues.

The FIC ensures that NIH interests are represented as new opportunities for research collaboration in the life sciences areas through initiatives of the U.S. Government, foreign governments, multilateral and international organizations.

In its role as a WHO Collaborating Center for Research and Training in Biomedicine, the FIC provides research fellowships and grants, conducts studies, and sponsors workshops involving the NIH, WHO, PAHO and U.S. and foreign biomedical research organizations to identify and further strengthen the health of the U.S. population and contribute to the enhancement of health worldwide.

As the NIH focus of international activities, the FIC has both an integrative and admhlistrative role in activities supported by other PHS components and other Federal agencies. The FIC is the NIH representative in maintaining liaison with such international organizations as WHO, PAHO, the European Union, and the European Medical Research Councils.

The FIC director meets regularly with international representatives of the NIH ICD's to exchange information and views on NIH international activities and to discuss implementation of related policies and procedures.

International Services Branch. The ISB provides support to foreign scientists in the NIH visiting, special volunteer, and guest researcher programs.

For foreign scientists engaged in NIH intramural research, the ISB handles administrative and immigration matters ISB also provides via assistance to foreign special experts, exchange scientists, special volunteers, and visiting fellows engaged in research in the Center for Biologics Evaluation and Research, FDA.

Division of Computer Research and Technology

Mission

The Division of Computer Research and Technology incorporates the power of modern computers into biomedical programs and administrative procedures of NIH by focusing on three primary activities: conducting computational biosciences research developing computer systems and providing computer facilities. In fulfilling these responsibilities, the division:

- promotes the application of high performance computing and communication to biomedical problems, including image processing, structural biology, protein folding, database searching, gene linkage analysis, and computational chemistry, using the most advanced, massively parallel scalable computing

- applies computing technology to research problems involving macromolecular structure representation and modeling, and protein and DNA sequence analysis

- develops and provides computer networking facilities, and supports, guides, and assists other NIH components in local area networking

- provides professional programming services and computational and data processing facilities to meet NIH program needs

- conducts research in biomathematical theory and biophysical instrumentation to explain biological phenomena in terms of biochemistry and biophysics

- operates and maintains the NIH Computer Center and all centrally owned, shared-use computing resources; designs and develops software: and provides extensive personal support, training, and documentation for computer and network users

- develops computer-based systems for laboratory and clinical applications, and conducts computer science and engineering research and development

- consults and collaborates in computational, statistical, and mathematical aspects of data analysis: supports software systems to perform these analyses; and conducts independent research in statistics and mathematics with applications to biomedicine

- provides guidance and support to scientists and administrators throughout NIH in the effective use of personal computers, workstations, local area networks and associated automation technology

- serves as the central systems analysis, design and programming resource for data processing and database projects relating to scientific, technical, management, and administrative data

- serves as a scientific and technological resource for other parts of the PHS

- Applies mathematics, statistics, and computer sciences to biomedical problems such as signal processing, image processing, modeling physiological systems, and data analysis problems in laboratory experiments.

DCRT Programs

The office of the Director consists of the Office of Computational Biosciences and the Office of Computing Resources and Services, which provide leadership for the scientific (computational biology, computational chemistry) and administrative services of DCRT, respectively. The director and staff provide leadership with regard to NIH policy and programs involving computing networking and information systems, and provide liaison with the NIH Office of the Director, the ICDs, and numerous committees and user groups. The computational molecular biology section furnishes support, services, and training in sequence analysis and molecular modeling maintains and supports genetic/genomic databases and software and has introduced Gopher and Mosaic information services to NIH.

The Computational Bioscience and Engineering Laboratory (CBEL) provides high performance parallel supercomputing and image processing systems and leadership in the research, development, and biomedical application of massively parallel computers in a networked environment. CBEL collaborates with research investigators to model complex systems and analyze and interpret data, signals and images in computationally intensive task areas, including electron and light microscopy, x-ray crystallography and multidimensional nuclear magnetic resonance spectroscopy, molecular dynamics and quantum chemistry, drug design, protein folding, medical imaging, and radiation treatment planning.

The Laboratory of Structural Biology carries out biomolecular research using experimental approaches to directly measure forces between and within biomolecules as well as computational approaches to model and simulate biomolecular conformation and assembly. The MFS investigates the physical forces governing biomolecular function. The MGSS develops and implements computational methods on leading edge workstations and high performance parallel platforms, with the goal of increasing the realism of simulated molecular properties. The MGSS studies molecular motion and interaction using molecular mechanics and quantum mechanics based methods. The ABS develops and applies statistical-based methods to protein secondary structure prediction. structure-function prediction, and the classification of protein folds. The LSB develops computational methods for predicting the three-dimensional structures of proteins from primary sequences. The CMMS acts as a bridge between computational chemistry, providing software tools, guidance, and research collaboration.

The laboratory also develops computer programs and applications of general-purpose computers, workstations, supercomputers, and highly parallels computers for research in molecular and computational biology and chemistry.

The Physical Sciences Laboratory (PSL) brings to bear applications of mathematics and physics on a broad range of biomedical problems. Examples are the development of medical image processing methods, theories for using optical techniques in noninvasive diagnosis, studies of chemical reactions and diffusion in complex media, mathematical modeling of various aspects of cell and tissue physiology, and methods for describing macromolecular energetics.

PSL projects include an analysis of the detectibility and resolution of tumors by time-resolved optical spectrophotometry, development of a model to interpret data relating to calcium metabolism in the context of osteoporosis, and an investigation of structural transformations of clathrin-coated pits during receptor-mediated endocytosis. The laboratory serves as a general resource for collaborations involving physical sciences (e.g., crystallography, NMR spectroscopy) applied to problems of interest to medical researchers.

The Network Systems Branch provides leadership in developing and implementing networking and other communications technologies for the NIH campus and its outlying facilities, including connections with national and international data networks. The branch explores new technologies applicable to the NIH environment, provides continuous guidance and support for locally managed networks, and maintains liaisons with other DHHS components to improve the overall information dissemination infrastructure.

The Computing Facilities Branch (CFB) plans operates, and supports scientific and administrative computing resources for NIH-wide use and for use by other Federal Government agencies. CFB promotes awareness and efficient and effective use of computing resources by its customers: investigates new and emerging customer computing requirements; and conducts research and development to identify, evaluate, and adapt new computer architectures and technologies. Services are provided on several platforms.

Mainframe computer systems support large-scale administrative applications and massive data management requirements, including the NIH administrative database and the IMPAC and CRISP systems, as well as providing a variety of batch and interactive processing capabilities.

In addition, modern relational database management systems on the mainframes provide for client-server methods to access them. Scientific computing services are provided by a general purpose scientific computer system, supplemented by a vector supercomputer and a parallel supercomputer.

The Advanced Laboratory Workstation System offers network-based support and access to a distributed file system for users of scientific and engineering workstations. The branch provides round-the-clock oversight for these facilities and for a wide variety of Internet and World Wide Web services. CFB services are available to users 7 days a week, 24 hours a day via high-speed point-to-point and dial connections and via the Internet.

The Customer Services Branch (CSB) furnishes centralized, integrated computer support services to DCRT customers. As the primary interface to the NIH computing community, CSB performs its liaison role by consulting with customers to resolve computing problems and provide advice referring questions to appropriate experts within DCRT operating DCRT's computer training program and disseminating technical information, documentation, and certain software. The branch designs and develops methodologies for software change control, and it promotes NIH community awareness of DCRT services.

The Information Systems Branch (ISB) provides advice and assistance to research investigators, program officials, and administrators throughout NIH in planning and obtaining data processing and computation services. ISB serves as a central resource for systems analysis, design, and programming expertise for NIH management and data processing projects related to administrative, scientific, and technical data.

The branch develops and maintains specified central NIH administrative systems and general-purpose and information handling techniques for data management and information processing. ISB plans data processing and computation projects involving DCRT central facility computers as well as exchanges technical knowledge and operating expertise with other operations research, systems analysis, computer programming, and data processing organizations within and outside the NIH.

The Statistical Support Staff provides 1) a combination of research in mathematical statistics and computer information science with collaboration and service in all computational aspects of biomedical data analysis; 2) advice and consultation on the quantitative analysis of biomedical research data and use of the computer in such analysis, including interpreting output and developing statistical procedures when needed; 3) selection, maintenance and support of a large collection of mathematical/statistical computer systems for general use in the analysis of modeling of research data; and 4) training and teaching the effective use of these systems to biomedical researchers, administrators and other NIH users, including a rapid response to user queries.

National Library of Medicine

Mission

The National Library of Medicine, one of three national libraries, is the world's largest research library in a single scientific and professional field.

The library has a statutory mandate from Congress to apply its resources broadly to the advancement of medical and health-related sciences. It collects, organizes, and makes available biomedical information to investigators, educators, and practitioners, and carries out programs designed to strengthen existing and develop new medical library services in the U.S. It is the central resource for the existing national biomedical information system.

Major Programs

MEDLARS. The library's computer-based MEDLARS was established in January 1964 to achieve rapid bibliographic access to NLMs vast store of biomedical information. The principal objective of MEDLARS is to provide references to the biomedical literature for researchers, clinicians, and other health professionals. This is accomplished through: 1) preparation of citations for publication in Index Medicus, a comprehensive, subject-author index to articles from approximately 3,000 of the world's biomedical journals, and the NLM Current Catalog, a bibliographic listing of citations to publications cataloged by the Library; 2) compilation of other recurring bibliographies on specialized subjects of wide interest; and 3) provision of online search services through MEDLINE, TOXILINE, and other databases.

Agreements with foreign institutions provide MEDLARS services to an international community of health scientists.

Online Databases

In 1971 NLM initiated its MEDLINE service to provide an online bibliographic searching capability through terminals in libraries at medical schools, hospitals and research institutions throughout the country. By typing simple instructions on a terminal or personal computer connected by communications networks to the central computer, a physician or other health professional can retrieve almost instantaneously references to the most current indexed Journal articles in this area of interest. In addition to MEDLINE, other online databases deal with toxicology information, cataloging information, audiovisual materials, history of medicine, cancer literature, hospital and health care literature, medical ethics, and reproductive biology. Almost 150,000 institutions and individuals in the U.S. now have access to these databases.

Regional Medical Library Services

To provide more efficient dissemination of biomedical information, NLM has been developing a network arrangement through which MEDLARS and interlibrary loan services can be shared efficiently by medical libraries. The network consists of eight Regional Medical Libraries. Although NLM remains the heart of the network, more and more services are being provided directly by regional libraries.

Lister Hill National Center for Biomedical Communications

The center explores the use of computer, communication, and audiovisual technologies to improve the organization, dissemination, and utilization of biomedical information, and is the focus of the library's high performance computing and communications initiatives.

Toxicology Information Program

The general objectives of the program are to create computer-based toxicology data banks from scientific literature and from files of collaborating industrial, academic, and governmental agencies, and to establish toxicology information services for scientists.

National Center for Biotechnology Information

The NCBI, created in 1988, builds databases and information analysis/retrieval systems for genomic information and does research into advanced information-handling methods for biotechnology and related information.

National Information Center on Health Services Research and Health Care Technology

The goal of this program is to create information services that make the results of health services research readily available-including clinical guidelines, technology assessments, and health care technology.

Extramural Programs

The extramural grant and contract programs of NLM were originally authorized by the Medical Library Assistance Act of 1965 (P.L. 89-291) to provide better health information services through grant support to the Nation's medical libraries. The act, since extended by Congress, offers assistance for library resources, research in biomedical communications, biomedical publications, training for research careers in medical informatics, and Regional Medical Libraries. Research project grants in medical informatics are awarded under authority of title III, part A, sec. 301, of the PHS act.

National Center for Human Genome Research

Mission

The National Center for Human Genome Research (NCHGR) was established in 1989 to head the NIH's role in the Human Genome Project. The center's Division of Extramural Research funds research in chromosome mapping, DNA sequencing, database development, technology development for genome research, and studies of the ethical, legal, and social implications of genetics research in laboratories throughout the country.

In February 1993 NCHGR expanded its role on the NIH campus with the establishment of a Division of Intramural Research, focuses on applying genome technologies to finding human disease genes, developing DNA-based diagnostics and gene therapies. The division serves as a hub for NIH-wide human genetic research, enhancing the work of investigators in NIH institutes who are searching for specific genes and studying their function in health and disease.

Major Programs

Division of Extramural Research Mapping Technology Branch. This branch supports research with special emphasis on technology development to improve the resolution, information content, and utility of genomic maps. Specific areas of interest include new or improved methods to facilitate the efficient construction and annotation of genetic and physical maps strategies for identifying genes, coding regions, and other functional elements in genomic DNA and strategies for high-throughput mapping and sequencing of human cDNAs.

The Mapping Technology Branch is also the focal point in NCHGR for training, career development, and special programs. As such the branch plans and administers programs of individual pre- and post-doctoral fellowships, institutional training grants, career awards, minority awards, international exchanges, short courses, and chromosome-specific workshops and other meetings.

Mammalian Genetics Branch. The branch is responsible for the administration and support of research directed to the highly efficient construction of complete genetic and physical maps of individual mammalian chromosomes and entire mammalian genomes and to the sequencing of large (megabase) regions of mammalian DNA. The MGB supports research in genome informatics, including database research, development and maintenance of genome databases, and research into algorithms and techniques for genomic analysis.

This branch serves as the focal point in the NCHGR for policy development for the Genome Science and Technology Centers Program.

Sequencing Technology Branch. The Sequencing Technology Branch funds research to develop new methods, technologies, and instruments that will be the basis for fully integrated, innovative approaches to the rapid, low-cost determination of DNA sequence.

Areas of interest include both refinement and full automation of current approaches to DNA sequencing as well as novel approaches to achieve order-of-magnitude improvements in sequencing capability. The branch also supports research to develop maps and to determine the sequence of the genomic DNA of nonmammalian organisms. The branch promotes collaborative, multidisciplinary research aimed at closely integrating research at academic and industrial laboratories.

Ethical, Legal, and Social Implications (ELSI) Branch. This branch supports research to anticipate and resolve the ethical, legal and social issues arising from human genome research. Investigating these issues alongside the scientific research is a novel pursuit prompted by concern about the responsible use of information generated by human genetics research. This branch fosters public education and discussion of ELSI issues. The program has defined three priority areas of research: 1) clinical practices in the introduction of new genetic services, 2) access to and use of personal genetic information by parties outside the clinical setting, and 3) public and professional understanding of concepts and issues involving genetics.

Division of Intramural Research

NCHGR's Division of Intramural Research was established to serve as a hub where development of technology for the rapid isolation and analysis of disease genes will be carried out, together with research on DNA diagnostic technology and gene therapy. In the division's proposed basic research laboratories and clinical branches, highly experienced scientists and technicians, as well as post-doctoral fellows and other trainees, will develop and use the most advanced techniques to conduct research in medical genetics.

Research will include indentifying and understanding the molecular basis of human genetic disease and planning and carrying out clinical trials to test methods for the treatment and perhaps the cure of such diseases. Researchers in the division will collect and study families in which important diseases are inherited—a facet that will provide the nucleus for a physician training program in medical genetics—and translate basic science advances into effective, reliable, and costeffective DNA- and cytogenetic-based diagnostics.

The division will collaborate with other human genetics research efforts at NIH, complementing ongoing activities in human molecular genetics, structural biology, and gene therapy. It provides a core of support facilities as a resource for the NIH community.

These labs have expertise in genotyping and analyzing large families as a basis for genetic mapping, produce radiation reduced hybrid cell lines, perform chromosome microdissection, and support a physical mapping core to serve as a repository and distribution center for clones.

Since many common diseases appear to result from the interaction of more than one gene, as well as environmental factors, the intramural division will develop technologies to address the difficulties associated with analyzing multilocus diseases. As genetics increasingly becomes a part of everyday medicine, the division will play a major role in developing and participating in public education programs.

Technology Transfer Office. This program is responsible for the implementation of the Federal Technology Transfer Act of 1986 and serves as the focal point of pertinent legislation, rules and regulations and the administration of activities relating to collaborative agreements, inventions, patents, licensing and royalties and associated matters.

Laboratory of Genetic Disease Research. This unit studies genome organization and seeks to identify the causes of human genetic diseases. Using positional cloning techniques and model systems, investigators attempt to identify and characterize disease genes. This laboratory improves existing quantitative approaches to gene mapping, large-scale sequencing and lab automation technologies. Investigators in this lab determine the function of genes involved in human genetic diseases.

Laboratory of Cancer Genetics. While predisposition to some cancers is hereditary, many others result from genetic changes that occur throughout life. Using techniques of cytogenetics, chromosome microdissection and positional cloning, researchers in this laboratory seek to define the genetic changes in somatic cells that lead to cancer and the inherited mutations that predispose family members to cancer. Genes involved in the development of malignant characteristics in cancer cells, such as drug resistance and metastasis, is also studied.

Laboratory of Gene Transfer. This laboratory serves as the focal point at NIH for the development of human gene therapy techniques. Investigators develop vectors and other technologies to introduce cloned genes and DNAs into somatic cells to correct inherited diseases or the effects of acquired mutations in DNA.

Researchers explore gene therapy approaches in cultured cells and targeted introduction of genetic material into animal models. Transgenic animals that model human diseases are be developed for testing prototype gene therapy strategies.

Diagnostic Development Branch. One of the first clinical spinoffs of gene discovery is the development of DNA-based diagnostic techniques. Gene hunters in NCHGR's Laboratory of Genetic Disease Research are uncovering the genetic contributors to a number of inherited diseases. These efforts provide grist for the rapid translation of basic research findings into clinically applied technologies by researchers in the Diagnostic Development Branch. Branch scientists develop DNA-base and cytogenetic tools for diagnosis.

Medical Genetics Branch. This branch evaluates genetic disorders in a comprehensive clinic. Investigators examine patients and families affected by inherited disorders to identify and characterize novel genetic diseases. The Medical Genetics Branch also sponsors a physician training program in medical genetics, as well as a genetic counselor training program.

Clinical Gene Therapy Branch. Researchers in this branch apply developments in gene therapy to the treatment of human disease. Investigators work closely with those in the Laboratory of Human Gene Transfer and staff of the NIH Clinical Center. Researchers monitor and evaluate patients receiving experimental gene therapies.

In addition to the DIR's laboratories and branches, the division supports core resources in genetic mapping, quantitative analysis of genetic linkage data, molecular informatics, and technology development. The division also supports an education and outreach program, a visiting investigator program, and an ethics program to address questions surrounding participation of individuals and families in genetics research protocols as well as related issues.

National Center for Research Resources

Mission

NCRR conceives and develops a broad array of critical research technologies and resources and ensures their availability, thereby strengthening and enhancing biomedical research supported or performed by NIH.

The center, established on February 15, 1990, merged the Division of Research Resources—which provided extramural research resources to NIH-supported institutions, and the Division of Research Services—which provided resources to NIH intramural research programs.

Research resources and technologies provided by NCRR include General Clinical Research Centers—hospital inpatient and outpatient facilities staffed by specially trained medical personnel that host multicategorical clinical research studies; biomedical research technology resources-state-of-the-art computers, laboratories, and complex instrument systems that provide scientists with the latest tools from the physical sciences, mathematics, and engineering: animal resources—facilities such as the seven Regional Primate Research Centers and other valuable animal colonies at which laboratory models of human disease are developed and studied; and nonmammalian research models such as cell systems, lower organisms, and other biological materials critical to research on human diseases.

NCRR programs also provide funds for pilot research projects and unanticipated research opportunities, science education for minority students and teachers, and for enhancing the research capabilities of minority institutions that award doctorates in the health professions or health-related sciences. NCRR also offers the ICDs scientific library and translation services, and medical arts and photography.

Major Programs—Extramural

General Clinical Research Centers. NCRR's nationwide network of 75 General Clinical Research Centers offers a special environment for the study of research patients by medical scientists in their pursuit of improved diagnosis and treatment of human disease and disability. At clinical research centers, advances in basic sciences are translated into clinical tools used to diagnose, treat and prevent illness. Grants awarded through this program may be used for equipment, special laboratories, diet kitchens, salaries for highly trained staff (including nurses, dietitians, biostatisticians and other protessionals), and the hospitalization costs of research patients. Support for biostatistical as well as for data management and analysis also may be provided.

Regional Primate Research Centers. NCRR's seven regional Primate Research Centers provide unique research resources for biomedical and behavioral research using nonhuman primates as experimental animal models. Initial awards were made for construction of physical facilities at all seven centers. Operating awards are made each year following review of each center's proposed budget by NIH staff. The overall programs of each center also receive regular peer review from outside supporting agencies. Universities serve as host institutions for centers and provide academic environments of high standard for staff and visiting scientists.

Areas of emphasis include reproductive biology, infectious diseases. neurosciences, biobehavioral research, metabolic, nutritional and cardiovascular diseases, and environmental health and toxicology. Based on the availability of facilities and other resources, the centers maintain extensive collaborative programs for scientists from many institutions. Visiting scientist programs for investigators from the U.S. and abroad also are included within the centers.

Laboratory Animal Sciences. The Laboratory Animal Sciences Program funds research, research animal resources, and scientific training in the field of comparative medicine. Of particular interest is to develop new and improved animal models of human disease. To assist institutions in their efforts to meet animal care guidelines established by PHS and the requirements of the Animal Welfare Act, LASP supports projects to enhance the environmental conditions of laboratory animals and improve their health. The goal of LASP-supported training is to provide graduate veterinarians with the research skills and motivation to become career participants in biomedical and health research.

AIDS Animal Models. The Chimpanzee Biomedical Research Program was established in 1986 to provide a stable supply of healthy chimpanzees for biomedical investigations related to AIDS and hepatitis, and to perpetuate the chimpanzee population in the U.S.

The Specific-Pathogen-Free (SPF) Rhesus Monkey Breeding and Research Program was established in 1988 to create self-sustaining rhesus breeding colonies that are free from contamination with certain simian retroviruses and herpes B virus, and to make SPF animals available for PHS-supported research projects related to AIDS.

Biomedical Research Technology. A biomedical research technology resource combines expensive equipment, complex methodologies, and scarce expertise to help find solutions to important biomedical research problems. It serves investigators within a university, research institution, region, or the entire Nation. Biomedical research technology resource centers take many forms such as biomedical computer centers, biomedical engineering centers, and instrument-oriented centers for studying biomolecular and cellular structure and function.

Program funds support the technology resource allowing scientific collaborators to increase its usefulness in biomedical research. Thus, the resource adds a new dimension in special expertise and capability to the research potential of qualified investigators. Particular emphasis is placed on shared resources operating on a regional or national basis.

The program also funds grants for the development of new technologies and instrumentation for biomedical research.

Biomedical Research Support. The Biomedical Research Support Program includes three science education programs to improve science literacy and attract tomorrow's cadre of biomedical scientists. The Minority High School Student Research Apprentice Program (MHSSRAP), begun in 1980, provides summer "hands on" research experiences. The goal is to motivate minority students to pursue careers in health research or a health profession. The program includes teachers in elementary, middle and junior high schools, plus preservice teachers. The MHSSRAP is being phased out and replaced by the new competitive program "NCRR Minority Initiative: K-12 Teachers and High School Students."

The Science Education Partnership Award Program fosters alliances among educators, biomedical researchers, and local communities. Model programs further knowledge and excitement about the health sciences in young people (K-12) and the public.

The Science Teaching Enhancement Award Program is testing the feasibility of preparing science instructors (grades 6-12) to become master teachers. These individuals assume leadership roles in acting as liaisons between biomedical research scientists, their home institutions and science educators, school administrators, and others in the local school systems. The goal is to improve the quality of precollege science education.

The Institutional Development Award Program is a congressionally mandated effort to broaden the geographic distribution of NIH funding. The program helps investigators in designated states obtain long-range NIH research grant funding.

The unique Shared Instrumentation Grant Program provides funds for instruments costing $100,000 to $400,000. Groups of 10 or more NIH-supported investigators share NMR imagers, coupled hybrid mass spectrometers, scanning laser confocal microscopes, and the latest in gene sequencing equipment. This cost-effective program affords NIH grantees with tools for state-of the-art biomedical research.

Research Centers in Minority Institutions. Begun in 1985, the Research Centers in Minority Institutions Program is a congressionally mandated initiative. The program seeks to expand the national capability for research in health sciences by assisting, through grant support, predominantly minority institutions that offer doctorates in either the health professions or health-related sciences. The grants enhance the capacity of minority institutions to conduct biomedical and behavioral research by strengthening their research environments. Funds are typically used to hire additional research faculty in the biomedical and behavioral sciences, support training in specialized analytical methods, upgrade facilities, and purchase advanced scientific instruments.

Biomedical Models. The Biomedical Models Program develops and supports nonmammalian models such as lower vertebrates and invertebrates and nonanimal models such as cell systems, lower organisms, and nonbiological systems for biomedical research and provides biological materials that serve as important resources to the biomedical community. The program is enhancing and expanding utilization of nonmammalian models in biomedical research.

Major Programs—Intramural

Biomedical Engineering and Instrumentation. The Biomedical Engineering and Instrumentation Program supports intramural scientists in applications of engineering, mathematics, physics, and the physical sciences to the solution of problems in biology and medicine, through 1) collaborations involving measurement, imaging, mathematical and physical modeling, and design of specialized equipment, and 2) construction, modification, maintenance, repair, and lease of scientific equipment.

Veterinary Resources. The Veterinary Resources Program contributes to intramural research at NIH by procuring, housing, and maintaining laboratory animals at holding facilities in Bethesda and Poolesville. VRP provides technical consulting services to meet individual research needs in studies involving nonhuman primates, dogs, cats, rabbits, rodents, and livestock. Services and support available to intramural scientists include: disease diagnostics, animal model selection and development, genetic monitoring, germfree technology, behavior, nutrition, preoperative and postoperative care, cryopreservation, and surgery. VRP also manages the NIH Animal Genetic

Resource, which supplies scientists at NIH and around the world with a large selections of genetically defined small animal models.

Library Services. The NIH Library provides NIH with extensive research information resources and services. Housing approximately 80,000 monographs, 155,000 bound periodicals, and 2,600 current journal titles, the NIH Library is one of the country's largest biomedical libraries. It provides free access to a variety of databases including MEDLINE, AIDSLINE, PDQ, EMBASE, Biological Abstracts, Psychinfo, CANCERLIT, BIOETHICSLINE, and CHEMLINE. Several training courses are available on how to use these resources. The library also can translate foreign-language medical and scientific articles into English.

Medical Arts and Photography. The Medical Arts and Photography Branch provides NIH with complete visual communication services. MAPB designers, artists, photographers, video production specialists, etc., work with NIH personnel to produce effective visual presentations of biomedical research results. Services include design, graphics, video production, medical illustration, micro- and macrophotography, information and patient photography, and consulting.

Part Six

Appendices

Appendix A

Federal Government Health Information Resources

Office of **ADOLESCENT PREGNANCY** Programs
Department of Health and Human Services
200 Independence Avenue SW., Room 736E
Washington, DC 20201
(202) 245-7473

Services: The Adolescent Family Life (AFL) program seeks to discover new approaches to providing care services for pregnant adolescents and adolescent parents and emphasizes a primary prevention strategy based on reaching adolescents before they become sexually active. AFL encourages the active involvement of the adolescent's family in addressing issues related to adolescent pregnancy and promotes the postponement of teenage sexual activity. Adoption is promoted as a positive option to early parenting.

Division of Technical Information and Dissemination
Administration on **AGING**
Department of Health and Human Services
330 Independence Avenue SW., Room 4646
Washington, DC 20201
(202) 619 0641

Services: The Administration on Aging (AoA), created by the Older Americans Act (OAA) in 1965, is the only Federal agency devoted exclusively to the concerns and potential of older Americans. Help for the elderly under OAA is provided through programs administered by AoA, together with its

DHHS Publication, *Health Information Resources in the Federal Government*, Fifth Edition, 1990.

10 Regional Offices and 57 State and territorial units on aging, approximately 670 area agencies on aging, and Indian tribes. AoA's primary goals are to support a national network of State and area agencies on aging and Indian tribes in their efforts to reach out to older persons residing in communities across the Nation; develop and oversee a comprehensive and coordinated system of supportive services and opportunities to meet the social and human service needs of the elderly; and serve as an advocate on behalf of older people. AoA allocates funds to the State Agencies on Aging to administer and support a wide range of services and other activities, including services in the home, services and opportunities in the community, and services to individuals in long-term care institutions. AoA also supports improvements in quality of life and services for older people through research and training grants. Results of these studies are made available to professional organizations and the public.

Publications: *Aging Magazine.*

Public Information Office
National Institute on **AGING**
Department of Health and Human Services
Federal Building, Room 6C12
9000 Rockville Pike
Bethesda, MD 20892
(301) 496-1752

Services: The National Institute on Aging (NIA) was established in 1974 to conduct and support biomedical, social, and behavioral research and training related to the aging process and the diseases and other special problems and needs of the aged. NIA provides for the study of biomedical, psychological, social, educational, and economic aspects of aging through in-house research conducted at its Gerontology Research Center in Baltimore, MD, and through grant support of extramural and collaborative research programs at universities, hospitals, medical centers, and nonprofit institutions throughout the nation. NIA also provides support to institutions training scientists for research careers in aging. In addition, NIA sponsors the Alzheimer's Disease Education and Referral (ADEAR) Center, which provides in depth information of special interest to health and service professionals; patients, their families, and caregivers; and the general public. For more information, contact ADEAR,8737 Colesville Road, Silver Spring, MD 20910; (301)495-3311.

Publications: Free consumer materials are available on menopause, nutrition, arthritis, cancer, aging, Alzheimer's disease, constipation, crime, diabetes, exercise, hearing, high blood pressure, osteoporosis, medicines, senility, flu, urinary incontinence, skin care, and dental care. Some are translated into Chinese and Spanish. Professional materials are available on Alzheimer's disease and self-help groups. A publications list is available.

National Resource Center on Health Promotion and **AGING**
1909 K Street NW
5th Floor
Washington, DC 20049
(202) 728-4476

Services: The National Resource Center is designed to support State Units on Aging and others in the fields of aging and health in developing and implementing health promotion for older adults. The center offers training and technical assistance to State Units on Aging, maintains a health promotion library for professionals that can be accessed by telephone or letter, provides information on health promotion for minority populations, assists with program development, and provides information on State level programs. The center also provides resource lists and referrals to organizations that may be helpful in planning a health promotion campaign and offers individual consultation. In addition, a wide range of materials are available on health promotion topics, including exercise, nutrition, injury prevention, and medication use.

Database: The center maintains a database that is currently available only to staff members.

Service Limitations: The materials in the library are not available for loan, but may be viewed by appointment only.

Publications: *Health Promotion for Older Adults, Nutrition and Older Adults, Mental Health and Wellness and Older Adults, Healthy Aging: Model Health Promotion Programs for Minority Elders* (also in video), and *The National Resource Center on Health Promotion and Aging.* A publication list is available.

Serial publication: *Perspectives in Health Promotion and Aging,* (bimonthly).

National **AIDS** Information Clearinghouse
P.O. Box 6003, Mail Stop 1B
Rockville, MD 20850
(800) 458-5231

Services: The National AIDS Information Clearinghouse (NAIC) was established in 1987 by the Centers for Disease Control (CDC). Its purposes are to identify and respond to the needs of health professionals involved in the development and delivery of AIDS programs; ensure that the general public has access to information on AIDS; provide technical assistance to organizations involved in the fight against AIDS, particularly State health departments; assist in the development and assessment of resources; support all AIDS information delivery services of CDC, including the National AIDS hotline (800-342-AIDS; 800-344-SIDA-Spanish); and distribute single copies of selected publications. Requests for information from NAIC can be made either by mail or by phone.

Databases: Two databases form the core of information for NAIC: 1) the Resources Database, a directory of programs, projects and organizations providing AIDS-related services, and 2) the Educational Materials Database, containing information about specialized educational materials tailored to specific audiences and focusing on different aspects of AIDS.

The NAIC Resource Center is open to the public by appointment from 9 a.m. to 5 p.m., weekdays. The Resource Center contains copies of educational materials, videotapes, and reference works on AIDS and HIV infection.

Publications: NAIC distributes brochures, posters, and fact sheets about AIDS.

Office of Congressional and Public Affairs
Surgeon General of the **AIR FORCE**
Department of Defense
Bolling Air Force Base, Building 5681
Washington,DC 20332-6188
(202) 767-5046

Services: The Office of the Surgeon General of the Air Force develops and implements medical programs and policies that provide for the health care of active-duty and retired Air Force personnel and their dependents. The office will respond to inquiries about eligibility for and proper use of Air Force medical benefits, to include CHAMPUS (Civilian Health and Medical Program of the Uniformed Services) and the Dependent Dental Program. In most cases, however, this information is readily available at local Air Force medical treatment facilities. The Air Force Surgeon General manages an Air Force-wide health promotion program, which provides Air Force patients with education and counseling in preventive medicine techniques and the promotion of healthy lifestyles.

Communications and External Affairs
ALCOHOL, Drug Abuse, and Mental Health Administration
Parklawn Building, Room 13C-05 5600
Fishers Lane Rockville, MD 20857
(301)443-8956; (301) 443-3783 (general information)

Services: Inquiries on mental health, drug abuse, or alcohol can be directed to the Alcohol, Drug Abuse, and Mental Health Administration (ADAMHA). Requests for publications should be directed to the information offices of the components of ADAMHA: the National Institute on Alcohol Abuse and Alcoholism (NIAAA), the National Institute of Mental Health (NIMH), the Office for Substance Abuse Prevention (OSAP), and the Office for Treatment Improvement (OTI). In addition, requests for information and publications can be made to the National Clearinghouse for Alcohol and Drug Information (NCADI).

Serial publication: *ADAMHA News* (monthly).

Information Specialist
National Clearinghouse for
ALCOHOL AND DRUG INFORMATION
6000 Executive Boulevard P.O. Box 2345
Rockville, MD 20852
(301) 468-2600
(800) 729-6686 (Say No to Drugs)

Services: The National Clearinghouse for Alcohol and Drug Information (NCADI) was established in 1987, when the National Clearinghouse for Alcohol Information and the National Clearinghouse for Drug Abuse Information were combined. NCADI gathers and disseminates current knowledge on alcohol and drug-related subjects. Services include subject searches on an in-house automated database and response to inquiries for statistics and other information. NCADI also develops resource materials and operates the Regional Alcohol and Drug Awareness Resource (RADAR), a nationwide linkage of drug information centers.

Database: NCADI's online database, IDA (Information on Drugs and Alcohol), has two major components, a prevention materials resource and a traditional bibliographic resource. The bibliographic component is made up of journal articles, books, reports, proceedings, and conference papers and other primary source materials. The prevention materials component describes a variety of materials including, but not limited to, pamphlets, posters, videos, curricula, booklets, etc., which are reviewed for conformance with public health policy. Acquisitions are prevention and education oriented, and tend more to the psycho-social aspects of alcohol and other drug abuse rather than scientific and technical research. An effort is made not to duplicate existing databases. The database grows by 4,000 to 6,000 entries annually. All materials in IDA are housed in the NCADI library. IDA is accessed through the team of NCADI information specialists. The primary audiences requiring literature searches are educators, community and prevention planners, and policymakers.

Reference Services: A library is available and open to the public, Monday through Friday, 9:30 a.m. to 4:30 p.m. The collection contains information on all aspects of alcohol and other drug abuse including over 80 journals, newsletters, and major U.S. newspapers. Photocopying is available to patrons at $.10 per page.

Publications: Publications include *The Drug-Free Communities Series; Be Smart! Stay Smart! Don't Start!*, a prevention program for parents, teachers, and students age 8-12 as well as posters, pamphlets, resource lists, fact sheets, and directories. A free publications catalog is available.

Serial publication: *Prevention Pipeline* (bimonthly), available for $15.00 per year.

Office of Communications
National Institute of **ALLERGY** and Infectious Diseases
Department of Health and Human Services
Building 31, Room 7A-32
9000 Rockville Pike
Bethesda, MD 20892
(301) 496-5717

Services: The National Institute of Allergy and Infectious Diseases (NIAID) conducts and supports research on the prevention, diagnosis, and treatment of infectious, immunologic, and allergic diseases. NIAID is pursuing investigations in bacteriology, virology, mycology, immunology and parasitology. It has major responsibility for research on the immune system and on its disorders, including AIDS. NIAID is organized into an intramural research division and divisions that award grants and contracts to scientists in universities and private research institutions.

Publications: Free consumer materials are available on sinusitis, poison ivy allergy, mold allergy, pollen allergy, dust allergy, asthma, rabies, sexually transmitted diseases, influenza, toxoplasmosis, and the immune system. A publications list is also available.

Patient Administration Division
Office of the Surgeon General of the **ARMY**
HQDA (SGPS-PSA)
5109 Leesburg Pike
Falls Church, VA 22041-3258
(703) 756 0107

Services: Medical benefits programs for Army personnel and eligible civilians, including dependents, are developed and administered by the Office of the Surgeon General of the Army. The office responds to inquiries about eligibility for benefits.

Information Specialist
National **ARTHRITIS** and Musculoskeletal
and Skin Diseases Information Clearinghouse
9000 Rockville Pike, P.O. Box AMS
Bethesda, MD 20892
(301) 495-4484

Services: The National Arthritis and Musculoskeletal and Skin Diseases Information Clearinghouse (NAMSIC) is designed to help health professionals identify print and audiovisual educational materials concerning arthritis and musculoskeletal diseases, and to serve as an information exchange for individuals and organizations involved in public, professional, and patient education. Requests are answered by searching NAMSIC's database and other bibliographic sources and by making referrals to appropriate resources. Database: The database includes records for 6,300 documents published since 1975; about 1,000 records are added each year. The NAMSIC file is part of the Combined Health Information Database (CHID), publicly accessible online through BRS. Copies of materials found in the database are not provided by NAMSIC but may be reviewed there by appointment. Materials indexed include pamphlets, journal articles, and audiovisual materials. Personal information requests from patients are referred to appropriate organizations.

Publications: Bibliographies, reference sheets, and directories for professionals are available on such topics as arthritis, musculoskeletal diseases, rheumatic diseases, skin diseases, biofeedback, nutrition, pharmaceuticals, patient education, systemic lupus erythematosus, scleroderma, Lyme disease, gout, treatment centers, statistics, health care personnel, audiovisual materials, physical exercise, ankylosing spondylitis, radiology, surgery, and the handicapped. Also available are a publications list and irregular announcements of materials, resources, and services.

Serial publication: *Arthritis Clearinghouse Memo.*

Information Specialist
National Institute of **ARTHRITIS**
and Musculoskeletal and Skin Diseases
Building 31, Room 4C05
9000 Rockville Pike
Bethesda, MD 20892
(301) 496-8188

Services: The National Institute of Arthritis and Musculoskeletal and Skin Diseases (NIAMS) handles inquiries on arthritis, bone diseases, and skin diseases.

Service Limitations: Some requests for information are handled by the National Arthritis and Musculoskeletal and Skin Diseases Information Clearinghouse (NAMSIC).

Publications: Consumer publications are available on arthritis, epidermolysis bullosa, scoliosis, Paget's disease, psoriasis, vitiligo, and osteoporosis. Professional publications are available on arthritis and lupus erythematosus.

Information Services
National **AUDIOVISUAL** Center
National Archives and Records Administration
8700 Edgeworth Drive
Capitol Heights, MD 20743-3701
(301) 763-1896; (800) 638-1300
(301) 763-6025 (fax)

Services: The National Audiovisual Center (NAC) is the central source for purchasing or renting more than 8,000 federally produced audiovisual programs available to the public. Catalogs and referrals to free loan sources are provided free of charge. Several of the catalogs cover health-related topics, including such areas as alcohol and drug abuse, dentistry, emergency medical services, industrial safety, medicine, and nursing.

Database: NAC maintains a data file containing information on audiovisual materials produced by the Federal Government, which are available to the public.

Publications: NAC publishes subject area catalogs of available federally produced audiovisual materials such as films, videocassettes, slides, filmstrips, and audiotapes. Catalogs cover a variety of subject areas, including those related to health, and are issued and updated on an irregular basis.

Congressional and Public Affairs Staff
Center for **BIOLOGICS** Evaluation and Research
Food and Drug Administration (HFB-140)
5600 Fishers Lane (Park 1-58)
Rockville, MD 20857
(301) 443-7532

Services: The Center for Biologics Evaluation and Research answers inquiries on biologic products. These include vaccines, allergenics, blood, and blood products. The center also works with the Food and Drug Administration Consumer Affairs Officers, located in field offices, in answering inquiries on biologics.

Publications: Various publications are available, including guidelines and "Points to Consider" for clinical trials and manufacturing biologics.

Administrative Officer
Lister Hill Center for **BIOMEDICAL COMMUNICATIONS**
Department of Health and Human Services Building 30A
8600 Rockville Pike
Bethesda, MD 20894
(301) 496-4441

Services: The Lister Hill National Center for Biomedical Communications (LHNCBC) is the computer research and development division of the National Library of Medicine. LHNCBC projects develop and use new computer and information science methods to manage the vast and growing body of recorded knowledge in the life sciences. Research projects conducted and supported by the center concern technology applications as diverse as the development and evaluation of expert systems designed to support practitioner decision-making and the electronic representation of three dimensions of human anatomy for more accurate instruction in clinical education.

Publications: Reports issued by LHNCBC are available for sale by the National Technical Information Service. A publications list is available upon request from the Office of Inquiries and Publications Management, National Library of Medicine, 8600 Rockville Pike, Bethesda, MD 20894.

Reference Section
National Library Service for the **BLIND**
and Physically Handicapped
Library of Congress
1291 Taylor Street NW.
Washington, DC 20542
(202) 707-9287; (800) 424-8567

Services: The National Library Service for the Blind and Physically Handicapped (NLS), established by Congress in 1931, consists of a network of 56 regional and over 100 local libraries working in cooperation with the Library of Congress to provide free library service to anyone who is unable to read or use standard printed materials because of visual or physical impairment. NLS delivers books and magazines in recorded form or in Braille to eligible readers by postage-free mail and provides postage for their return. Specially designed phonographs and cassette players are also loaned free to persons borrowing "talking books." NLS also provides information on blindness, physical handicaps and library services to special groups on request. Persons interested in these services should contact the library serving their area. A list of local and regional libraries is available.

Publications: A bibliography of Braille and recorded materials on health topics will be sent on request.

Serial publications: *Braille Book Review* (bimonthly), *Talking Book Topics* (bimonthly), *Update* (quarterly), and *Musical Mainstream* (bimonthly).

CANCER Information Service
Office of Cancer Communications
National Cancer Institute
Building 31, Room 10A24
9000 Rockville Pike
Bethesda, MD 20892
(800) 4-CANCER; (808) 524-1234
(Hawaii-neighbor islands call collect) (301) 496-8664 (project officer)

Services: The Cancer Information Service (CIS) is the toll-free telephone inquiry system that supplies information about cancer and cancer-related resources to the general public and to cancer patients and their families. Callers are automatically put in touch with the office serving their area. Inquiries are handled by health educators and trained volunteers. Spanish-speaking staff members are available during daytime hours to callers from the following areas: California, Florida, Georgia, Illinois, northern New Jersey, New York, and Texas.

Publications: Free publications of the National Cancer Institute are available through CIS.

Public Inquiries Section
Office of **CANCER COMMUNICATIONS**
National Cancer Institute
Building 31, Room 10A24
9000 Rockville Pike
Bethesda, MD 20892
(301) 496-5583

Services: Requests for cancer information, posed by patients, the general public, and health professionals, are answered by the Public Inquiries Section of the National Cancer Institute's (NCI) Office of Cancer Communications (OCC). Responses include written response and distribution of NCI publications. Additionally, telephone inquiries are received through the Cancer Information Service national toll-free telephone number (800-4-CANCER). Referrals are made to other offices of NCI when appropriate.

Publications: Publications directed toward consumers include pamphlets, bibliographies, reprints, reports, and books with some titles prepared especially for minority populations. The pamphlet series, *What You Need to Know About Cancer*, provides information for cancer patients regarding symptoms, diagnosis, treatment, and rehabilitation of specific organ site cancers. Topics include breast cancer, radiation therapy, chemotherapy, cancer prevention including diet, skin cancer, DES exposure, dysplasia, Hodgkin's disease, leukemia, melanoma, Wilms' tumor, carcinogens, biopsies, and clinical trials. A list of NCI publications for patients and the public is available, as well as a list for health professionals.

Information
International **CANCER INFORMATION** Center
National Cancer Institute
9030 Old Georgetown Road Building 82
Bethesda, MD 20892
(301) 496-7403
(301) 480-8105 (fax)

Services: The International Cancer Information Center (ICIC) was established in 1984 to disseminate cancer research information useful in the prevention, diagnosis, and treatment of cancer to research scientists and clinicians around the world. ICIC includes an International Cancer Research Data Bank, which has been in operation since 1974. This information center disseminates the results of cancer research undertaken in any country for the use of cancer researchers and appropriate organizations or cancer centers in any country. The material in the data bank is highly technical.

Databases: ICIC's databases are PDQ and CANCERLINE. PDQ (Physician Data Query) provides physicians with data about prognosis, staging, and treatment options for 82 different types of cancer. It also includes information about active treatment protocols and the names of physicians who spend a major portion of their clinical practice involved in cancer treatment and groups that have organized programs of care for cancer patients. CANCERLINE's databases are: CANCERLIT—700,000 abstracts of published literature, papers, books, technical reports, monographs, and theses; and CLINPROT—over 7,000 summaries of investigational cancer therapy protocols. The databases are available through the National Library of Medicine's MEDLARS system and other selected databases.

Service Limitations: Inquiries from the public are usually referred to the Office of Cancer Communications, (301) 496-5583.

Serial Publications: *CANCERGRAMS*—current cancer research awareness bulletin with abstracts, *Oncology Overviews* (monthly)—retrospective abstract monographs, *Recent Reviews*—(annual volumes in three broad cancer subject areas—compilations of abstracts of major review articles), *Journal of the National Cancer Institute* (biweekly) primary source journal covering all areas of cancer research, cancer control, and prevention.

Reference Room
Clearinghouse on **CHILD ABUSE** and Neglect Information
P.O. Box 1182
Washington,DC 20013
(703) 821-2086

Services: The Clearinghouse on Child Abuse and Neglect Information serves as a major resource center for the acquisition and dissemination of child abuse and neglect materials. The clearinghouse is the information component for the National Center on Child Abuse and Neglect (NCCAN).

Database: At the core of the clearinghouse is a database consisting of child abuse and neglect documents. Literature searches of the database can be obtained from the clearinghouse as topical bibliographies or custom searches. The database is also directly available to the public through DIALOG. The clearinghouse strives to maintain a timely and comprehensive collection of materials. From its database and many other resources, the clearinghouse develops publications and services to meet the needs of its users.

Publications: Materials are available on topics including sexual abuse, child protection services, parenting, statistical data, program development, training manuals, treatment, prevention, and crisis intervention. A publications catalog is available free upon request.

Office of Research Reporting
National Institute of **CHILD HEALTH**
and Human Development
National Institutes of Health
Building 31, Room 2A-32
9000 Rockville Pike
Bethesda, MD 20892
(301) 496-5133

Services: The Institute of Child Health and Human Development (NICHD) conducts and supports basic and clinical research in maternal and child health and the population sciences. NICHD will respond to individual inquiries on related topics such as studies on reproductive biology and contraception; fertility and infertility; developmental biology and nutrition; mental retardation; pediatric, adolescent, and maternal AIDS; and developmental disabilities.

Publications: Consumer materials are available on anorexia nervosa, Cesarean childbirth, Down's syndrome, oral contraception, precocious puberty, premature birth, pregnancy, smoking and pregnancy, vasectomy, childhood hyperactivity, maternal health, and child health. Professional materials are available on sudden infant death syndrome, developmental disabilities, pregnancy, and genetics. A publications list is available. Publication distribution is limited to single copy requests.

Technical Information Specialist
Center for **CHRONIC DISEASE PREVENTION**
and Health Promotion
Centers for Disease Control
Building 1, SSB249, MS A34
1600 Clifton Road NE.
Atlanta, GA 30333
(404) 639-3492

Services: The Center for Chronic Disease Prevention and Health Promotion (CCDPHP), established in 1988, consists of the Division of Adolescent and School Health, the Division of Chronic Disease Control and Community Intervention, the Division of Diabetes Translation, the Division of Nutrition, the Division of Reproductive Health, the Office on Smoking and Health, and the Office of Surveillance and Analysis. CCDPHP's Office of the Director contains a Technical Information Services Branch, Editorial Services Branch, and Administrative Services Branch. CCDPHP plans, directs, and coordinates a national program for the prevention of premature mortality, morbidity, and disability due to chronic illnesses and conditions and promotes the overall health of the population.

Databases: CCDPHP maintains two databases: the Health Promotion and Education Database and the AIDS School Health Education Database.

These two databases are part of the federally sponsored Combined Health Information Database (CHID) that is available through BRS.

Publications: Serial publications: *Chronic Disease Notes* and *Reports and Diabetes Update.*

Public Affairs Specialist
CIVILIAN HEALTH and Medical Program
of the Uniformed Services (CHAMPUS)
Aurora, CO 80045-6900
(303) 361-3800

Services: The Civilian Health and Medical Program of the Uniformed Services (CHAMPUS) is a health benefits system of the uniformed services. Spouses and children of active duty members of the uniformed services, some former spouses, retirees and their family members, and spouses and children of deceased active duty members or deceased retirees have the benefit of coverage under CHAMPUS. Information about CHAMPUS eligibility, benefits, and exclusions is available from the Office of CHAMPUS or the health benefits advisor at any uniformed service medical facility.

Publications: CHAMPUS fact sheets and a handbook are available.

Office of Clinical Center Communications
Warren Grant Magnuson **CLINICAL CENTER**
National Institutes of Health
Building 10, Room 1C-255
9000 Rockville Pike
Bethesda, MD 20892
(301) 496-2563; (301) 496-4891 (patient referral)

Services: The Clinical Center, established in 1953 as the research hospital of the National Institutes of Health (NIH), is designed to bring patient care facilities close to research laboratories so new findings of basic and clinical scientists can be applied quickly to the treatment of patients. Patients are admitted upon referral by physicians to NIH clinical studies on cancer; allergy and infectious diseases; arthritis, diabetes, kidney, and digestive diseases; child health and human development; dental disorders: diseases of the eyes; heart, lung, and blood; neurological and communicative diseases and stroke; and mental and emotional illnesses. The center also serves as a training center for physicians and medical students.

Publications: Products for consumers include the Medicine for the Layman series, which consists of publications and videotapes based on lectures. Topics include allergies, arthritis, blood transfusions, the brain, cancer, depression, environmental health, epilepsy, heart disease, the lungs, and radiation therapy. All materials published by the center are free. Patient admission procedures are available to prospective patients.

Serial publications: *Clinical Electives for Medical and Dental Students* (annual), *Medical Staff Careers in Biomedical Research* (annual), T*raining for Fellowship Programs Catalog* (annual), *Summer Research Fellowship Program Catalog* (annual), and *Current Clinical Studies* (annual).

Director of Policy Analysis
Office of **CONSUMER AFFAIRS**
1009 Premier Building
Washington,DC 20201
(202) 634-4140

Services: The Office of Consumer Affairs (OCA), established in 1964 as the President's Committee on Consumer Interests, is responsible for providing the President and Federal agencies with advice and information regarding the interests of American consumers. OCA encourages and assists in developing new consumer programs, makes recommendations to improve Federal consumer programs, cooperates with State agencies and voluntary organizations in advancing consumer interests, promotes improved consumer education, recommends legislation and regulations to help consumers, and encourages the exchange of ideas among industry, government, and consumers.

Publications: *Consumer's Resource Handbook*, which provides information on how consumers can complain effectively and where to go for assistance, is available free from the Consumer Information Center, P.O. Box 100, Dept. 635H, Pueblo, CO 81009.

Serial publication: *Consumer News* (monthly newsletter).

CONSUMER INFORMATION Center
General Services Administration
Pueblo, CO 81009
(202) 501-1794 (information)

Services: The major function of the Consumer Information Center (CIC), founded in 1970, is to distribute Federal agency publications through its distribution center. CIC encourages agencies to develop and release useful consumer information on a wide variety of topics. CIC publishes a catalog of available materials and updates this listing quarterly and provides assistance to Government agencies for the development of pamphlets. Weekly news releases are sent to newspapers, consumer organizations, and agencies. CIC responds to mail orders for publications with a delivery time of about 3 weeks.

Service Limitations: There is a charge for many publications distributed by CIC, and a $1 handling fee is charged when ordering two or more free publications.

Publications: CIC distributes materials for consumers on such topics as children's health, food, drugs, medical services, exercise, weight control, and specific diseases and disorders.

Serial publications: *Consumer Information Catalog,* (quarterly) lists booklets distributed by CIC from over 30 Government agencies, and *New for Consumers* (monthly) highlights pamphlets available from the center.

Reference Department
National **CRIMINAL JUSTICE** Reference Service
National Institute of Justice
P.O. Box 6000
Rockville, MD 20850
(301) 251-5500; (800) 851-3420

Services: The National Criminal Justice Reference Service (NCJRS) was established in 1972 as a centralized information service for criminal justice practitioners and researchers. NCJRS provides reference services, collects publications for its collection, and provides other services, such as document loan, microfiche, and dissemination of publications. A computerized database includes abstracts of all materials entered into the NCJRS collection. A reading room is available (Second Floor, 1600 Research Boulevard, Rockville, MD). Health relevant areas covered by NCJRS include applications of behavioral and social sciences to the study of crime and criminal justice, stress, health care for confined populations, domestic relations, alcohol and drug information, rehabilitation and treatment, criminal behavior, and adult and juvenile offenders. NCJRS also operates the NIJ (National Institute of Justice) AIDS Clearinghouse, the only comprehensive clearinghouse for information and resources on AIDS as it impacts the criminal justice community. Database: The NCJRS online database of over 100,000 citations to documents on criminal justice issues is searchable by the public on DIALOG or by the specialists at NCJRS. All publications cited in the database are available at the NCJRS library.
Service Limitations: There is a charge for some services.
Serial publication: *NIJ Reports* (bimonthly journal)—free.

National Institute on **DEAFNESS**
and Other Communication Disorders
Building 31, Room 1B-62
National Institutes of Health
9000 Rockville Pike
Bethesda, Maryland 20892
(301) 496-7243 (voice); (301) 402-0252 (TDD)

Services: The National Institute on Deafness and Other Communication Disorders (NIDCD) became the 13th institute mandated by Congress within the National Institutes of Health in October 1988. NIDCD conducts and supports research and training with respect to disorders of hearing and other communication processes, including diseases affecting hearing, balance, voice, speech, language, touch, taste, and smell through research performed in its own laboratories. NIDCD also conducts a program of research grants, individual and institutional research awards, career development awards, center grants, and contracts to public and private research institutions and organizations. Other activities include conducting and supporting research and training through cooperation with professional, commercial, voluntary and philanthropic organizations concerned with deafness and other communication disorders; disease prevention and health promotion; and the special biomedical and behavioral problems associated with having communication impairments or disorders.

Publications: NIDCD offers an introductory brochure; pamphlets on hearing loss, stuttering, dizziness, speech and developmental language disorders, and aphasia; fact sheets; and *NIDCD Funding Mechanisms.*

DENTAL DISEASE Prevention Activity
Centers for Disease Control
1600 Clifton Road NE, Mail Stop E09
Atlanta, GA 30333
(404) 639-1830

Services: The Dental Disease Prevention Activity (DDPA) serves as a national resource for activities to prevent oral diseases and improve oral health. DDPA can provide information on fluoridation, infectious disease in dentistry, and dental sealants, as well as prevention of periodontal disease, baby bottle tooth decay, and oral effects of tobacco. DDPA also provides technical assistance to State and local health agencies and works with the professional dental community on issues related to the promotion of oral health.

Publications: Resource lists of educational materials on dental sealants and baby bottle tooth decay are available as are several publications on infectious disease in dentistry, the benefit of fluoridation, and community-based prevention strategies.

Program Analyst for Planning and Management
Division of Associated and **DENTAL HEALTH** Professions
Bureau of Health Professions
Health Resources and Services Administration
Parklawn Building, Room 8-101
5600 Fishers Lane
Rockville, MD 20857
(301) 443-6864

Services: The Division of Associated and Dental Health Professions serves as the Federal focus for the education, practice, service research, and the credentialing of personnel in the fields of dentistry, optometry, pharmacy, veterinary medicine, public health, health administration, and the allied health professions and occupations. The division supports and conducts studies and analytical activities to determine the present and projected requirements of the associated and dental health professions. The division also supports special educational initiatives related to health promotion and disease prevention, long-term care and geriatrics, dental care, and environmental health hazard control.

Publications: The division offers numerous publications of interest to personnel planners and administrators, including titles on allied health programs, allied health education and manpower, credentialing of health personnel, dental care, dental schools, dental manpower, environmental health, geriatric education, geriatric faculty health care administration, optometry, pharmacy education and manpower, public health manpower and education, and veterinary medicine manpower and education. Other titles include skill evaluation, dental insurance regulations, and the use of computers in dental practice. A publications list is available.

Information Officer
National Institute of **DENTAL RESEARCH**
National Institutes of Health
9000 Rockville Pike Building 31, Room 2C35
Bethesda, MD 20892
(301) 496-4261

Services: The National Institute of Dental Research (NIDR) was established in 1948 to improve the dental health of the people of the United States through research and education. Databases: The Research Data and Management Information Section maintains access to two computer-based information systems. NIDR ONLINE is an electronic bulletin board that contains full text of requests for applications, news for the dental research community, and news lists of NIDR publications. DENTALPROJ is a database containing abstracts of ongoing dental research supported by Government agencies and can be searched on the MEDLARS system using the same commands as Medline.

Publications: NIDR publishes a wide range of consumer-oriented pamphlets that are available free of charge upon request. Topics include dental health, fluoride treatment, canker sores, dry mouth, periodontal disease, dental sealants, and pain research. Posters and professional materials on school fluoride programs are also available.

Serial publication: *NIDR Research News* (irregular newsletter).

Director
Division of Consumer Affairs
Center for **DEVICES AND RADIOLOGICAL HEALTH**
Food and Drug Administration
1901 Chapman Avenue
Rockville, MD 20857
(301) 443-4190

Services: The Center for Devices and Radiological Health of the Division of Consumer Affairs (DCA) is responsible for analyzing factors affecting the safe and effective use of medical devices and radiation-emitting products by lay users and on patients and identifying those practices that promote health or adversely affect it. Trends relating to use of such devices are identified. In addition, DCA develops, implements, evaluates, and promotes education strategies and programs for patients and lay users of medical devices and radiation-emitting products to foster the safe and effective use of such devices. DCA also manages activities to study and evaluate education, training, and information such as labeling (instructions for device use) for patients and lay users of medical devices and radiation-emitting products to determine appropriateness, adequacy, and effectiveness. DCA answers consumer inquiries by telephone or mail on general issues relating to medical devices or radiation-emitting products. Devices range from such products as thermometers, hearing aids, contact lenses, condoms, magnetic resonance imaging devices, hemodialysis equipment, tampons, medical x rays, and pacemakers, to artificial hearts.

Publications: Publications cover topics such as pregnancy test kits, x rays, hearing aids, quack medical devices, IUDs, contact lenses, eyeglass lenses, ultraviolet radiation, and other general information on medical devices and radiological health products. Listings of *Federal Register* documents about medical devices and radiological health products are also available.

Information Office
National Institute of **DIABETES** and Digestive and Kidney Diseases
National Institutes of Health
9000 Rockville Pike, Building 31, Room 9A04
Bethesda, MD 20892
(301) 496-3583

Services: The Information Office of the National Institute of Diabetes and Digestive and Kidney Diseases (NIDDK), formerly the National Institute of Arthritis, Diabetes, and Digestive and Kidney Diseases, handles inquiries relating to diabetes, obesity, endocrine diseases, nutrition, digestive diseases, and kidney diseases. Requests for specific publications are handled by the National Digestive Diseases Information Clearinghouse, the National Diabetes Information Clearinghouse, and the National Kidney and Urologic Diseases Information Clearinghouse. Information requests on reimbursement programs for kidney dialysis are referred to the Health Care Financing Administration.

Publications: NIDDK distributes consumer publications on cystic fibrosis, human growth hormone, kidney stones, obesity, lithotripsy, and urinary tract infections. Publications for professionals cover cystic fibrosis, diabetes mellitus, digestive diseases, kidney diseases, and urology.

Serial publication: *NIDDK Research Advances* (annual).

Information Specialist
National **DIABETES INFORMATION** Clearinghouse
Box NDIC
9000 Rockville Pike
Bethesda, MD 20892
(301)468-2162

Services: National Diabetes Information Clearinghouse (NDIC), established in 1978, collects and disseminates information about patient education materials. NDIC maintains a meeting registry that includes regional, national, and international meetings, congresses, and symposia of interest to the diabetes community. NDIC distributes its own publications, as well as other diabetes-related materials. A library collection of approximately 5,000 items is open to the public, although materials do not circulate.

Database: NDIC maintains an automated database of patient and professional materials that is a component of the Combined Health Information Database (CHID). CHID is available to the public through BRS. Indexing is based on a thesaurus developed by NDIC.

Publications: Topical annotated bibliographies that provide ordering information are produced on such subjects as diet and nutrition, sports and exercise, and pregnancy. Other consumer materials are available on diabetes management, foot care, nutrition, dental care, insulin, self blood glucose monitoring, diabetes in older Americans, diabetes in young people, and eye care. Professional materials are available about all aspects of diabetes and its management including pregnancy, exercise, nutrition, diabetic retinopathy, and resources for patient education materials.

Serial publication: *Diabetes Dateline* (newsletter).

Program Specialist
National **DIFFUSION NETWORK**
555 New Jersey Avenue NW, Room 510
Washington, DC 20208-1525
(202) 357-6180 or (202) 357-6134

Services: The National Diffusion Network (NDN) makes educational programs available for adoption by schools, colleges, and other institutions by providing dissemination funds to programs considered to be exemplary. Persons known as facilitators, who serve as matchmakers between schools and NDN programs, are also funded by NDN. Many subject areas are represented among the 99 programs. Several are health-related, including programs for physical fitness and nutrition. A number of the programs are designed for handicapped persons. More than 26,000 program adoptions were completed in 1987-88.

Service Limitations: Services of NDN are oriented to teachers and educational administrators. Persons interested in more information are directed to contact one of the 53 State facilitators. A list of these facilitators is available from NDN.

Publications: A list of programs provided by NDN is available free. A catalog, *Educational Programs That Work*, provides summary data and a contact person for each program, and is available for a fee from Sopris West, Inc., 1120 Delaware Avenue, Longmost, CO 80501; (303) 651-2829.

Information Specialist
National **DIGESTIVE DISEASES** Information Clearinghouse
P.O. Box NDDIC
Bethesda, MD 20892
(301) 468-6344

Services: The National Digestive Diseases Information Clearinghouse (NDDIC) was established in 1980 to provide a central information resource on digestive health and the prevention and management of digestive diseases. It develops, identifies, and distributes educational materials; encourages production of needed materials; and responds to requests for information.

Database: NDDIC patient education materials are a part of the Combined Health Information Database (CHID), which is accessible through BRS.

Publications: Consumer materials are available on such topics as cirrhosis, diarrhea, gallstone disease, dyspepsia, heartburn, hiatal hernia, hepatitis B, ulcers, ulcerative colitis, irritable bowel syndrome, and Crohn's disease. Materials for professionals cover gallstones, biliary cirrhosis, Crohn's disease, endoscopy, neonatal hepatitis, liver transplantation, and digestive disease treatments. A directory of professional and lay digestive disease organizations and a glossary of digestive terms is also available.

Office of Public Affairs
President's Committee on Employment of
People with **DISABILITIES**
1111 20th Street NW., Suite 636
Vanguard Building
Washington, DC 20036-3470
(202) 653-5044

Services: The President's Committee on Employment of People with Disabilities, formerly the President's Committee on Employment of the Handicapped, was established in 1947. The committee strives to eliminate environmental and attitudinal barriers impeding the opportunities and progress of people with disabilities. Among its major activities is an ongoing public information campaign, which includes awards programs, print advertising campaigns, legislative liaisons reporting on disability legislation in the U.S. Government, exhibits, a speakers' bureau, and public service advertising. The committee is involved in National Disability Employment Awareness Month (October). The President's Committee has eight standing committees: Disabled Veterans; Employer; Disability and Employment Concerns; Employment Preparation; State Relations; Medical, Health, and Insurance; Labor; and Work Environment and Technology. Publications: Materials are available on employment of people with disabilities, independent living, the Rehabilitation Act (section 504), job accomodation, disabled veterans, and job placement. All publications are free and a publications list is available.

Serial publications: *Worklife* (quarterly magazine) and *Tips and Trends* (monthly newsletter).

Program Specialist
National Council on **DISABILITY**
800 Independence Avenue SW, Suite 814
Washington, DC 20591
(202) 267-3846 (voice); (202) 267-3232 (TDD)

Services: The National Council on Disability was established by Congress in 1973 and was transformed into an independent Federal agency in 1984. The 15 members appointed by the President and confirmed by Congress review all laws, programs, and policies of the Federal Government that affect individuals with disabilities. The council then makes recommendations to the President, Congress, and Federal agencies on these issues. In addition, the council is studying the availability of health insurance coverage for persons with disabilities and sponsors conferences for families caring for the disabled.

Publications: A report to the President, *The Education of Students with Disabilities: Where Do We Stand?*, is available.

Serial publication: *Focus* (quarterly newsletter).

Clearinghouse on **DISABILITY INFORMATION**
Office of Special Education and Rehabilitative Services
Switzer Building, Room 3132
330 C Street SW
Washington, DC 20202-2524
(202) 732-1241; (202) 732-1245; (202) 732-1723

Services: The Clearinghouse on Disability Information, formerly the Clearinghouse on the Handicapped, was created by the Rehabilitation Act of 1973. The clearinghouse responds to inquiries and researches information operations serving the handicapped field on the national, State, and local levels. It is especially strong in providing information in the areas of Federal funding for programs serving disabled people, Federal legislation affecting the handicapped community, and Federal programs benefiting people with handicapping conditions. The clearinghouse also refers inquirers to other appropriate sources of information.

Publications: Publications available from the Clearinghouse include OSERS *News in Print* (newsletter), *A Summary of Existing Legislation*

Affecting Persons with Disabilities, Educating Students with Learning Problems: A Shared Responsibility, and *Pocket Guide to Federal Help for Individuals with Disabilities.*

Director
National Institute on **DISABILITY AND REHABILITATION** Research
400 Maryland Avenue SW, Mail Stop 2305
Washington, DC 20202
(202) 732-1134

Services: The National Institute on Disability and Rehabilitation Research (formerly known as the National Institute of Handicapped Research) provides leadership and support for rehabilitation research. The institute's mission also encompasses the dissemination of information concerning developments in rehabilitation procedures, methods, and devices that can improve the lives of people of all ages with physical and mental handicaps, especially those who are severely disabled. The institute can provide statistical data on disabilities as well as information on research funding. Requests on specific topics are often referred to the National Rehabilitation Information Center.

Database: The institute maintains the Interagency Rehabilitation Research Information System, a database containing descriptions of recent and ongoing research projects involving rehabilitation. The database is accessible through BRS.

Publications: Professional publications include guides to funding mechanisms and grantee activities and compilations of statistical data. The institute also publishes Rehab Briefs, descriptions of research projects useful to practitioners.

Public Inquiries
Centers for **DISEASE CONTROL**
Management Analysis and Service Office
1600 Clifton Road NE, Mail Stop D25
Atlanta, GA 30333
(404) 639-3286; (404) 639-3534 (publications)

Services: Public Inquiries of the Centers for Disease Control (CDC) responds to inquiries from the general public and health care professionals on research conducted by CDC in the areas of environmental health, infectious diseases, health promotion and education, prevention services, and occupational safety and health. Callers and mail are referred to the appropriate CDC center, institute, or office and to other Federal, State, or private institutions. For inquiries concerning CDC's Center for Environmental Health and Injury Control, Center for Infectious Diseases, or Center for Prevention Services, the phone number and address listed above should be used. For inquiries concerning CDC's Center for Chronic Disease Prevention and Health Promotion, National Center for Health Statistics, National Institute for Occupational Safety and Health, Dental Disease Prevention Activity, Health Risk Appraisal Activity, Clearinghouse on Health Indexes, or Office on Smoking and Health, see separate listings appearing in this directory. Their appropriate addresses and phone numbers should be used when requesting information.

Serial publications: *Morbidity and Mortality Weekly Report (MMWR)* and *MMWR: Annual Summary — Information on Infectious Diseases in the United States.*

Director
Office of **DISEASE PREVENTION** and Health Promotion
Switzer Building, Room 2132
330 C Street SW
Washington, DC 20201
(202) 245-7611

Services: The mission of the Office of Disease Prevention and Health Promotion (ODPHP) is to provide leadership for disease prevention and health promotion among Americans. ODPHP undertakes this mandate through the formulation of national health goals and objectives; the coordination of Department of Health and Human Services activities in disease prevention, health promotion, preventive health services, and health information and education with respect to the appropriate use of health care; and the stimulation of public and private programs and strategies to enhance the health of the Nation. ODPHP is organized around four areas: prevention policy, clinical preventive services, nutrition policy, and health communication. ODPHP's Prevention Policy Staff manages the policy development and coordination function of the office. ODPHP oversaw the implementation and monitoring of the 1990 Health Objectives for the Nation and led the national project to develop health objectives for the year 2000. ODPHP's Clinical Preventive Services Staff promotes the appropriate use of immunizations, screening tests, patient counseling, and other prevention activities in clinical settings. The staff coordinated the U.S. Preventive Services Task Force's development of age- and sex-specific guidelines for preventive services. ODPHP acts as a catalyst for activities that strengthen the Department's capabilities and national leadership in nutrition research, nutrition monitoring, nutrition services and training, nutrition education, food safety and quality, and international nutrition. ODPHP promotes the effective communication of health information to the public and professionals regarding the behavioral determinants of disease, such as diet and exercise, and effective health promotion and disease prevention programs. ODPHP also operates the ODPHP National Health Information Center (ONHIC).

Publications: ODPHP offers publications in the area of Federal programs and policy, community and school health promotion programs, health promotion at the worksite, nutrition, and professional and consumer educational materials. A publications list is available from ONHIC. All ODPHP publications are ordered either from ONHIC or the U.S. Government Printing Office.

Legislative, Professional, and Consumer Affairs Branch
Center for **DRUG EVALUATION** and Research
Food and Drug Administration
5600 Fishers Lane (HFM8)
Rockville, MD 20857
(301) 295-8012

Services: The Center for Drug Evaluation and Research (CDER) responds to inquiries covering the entire spectrum of drug issues. The center develops CDER and agency responses to drug information requests under the provisions of the Food and Drug Administration's procedural regulations and established policies. Inquiries are received by telephone and mail; however, all Freedom of Information (FOI) requests should be via written correspondence to FOI Staff (HFI-35), 5600 Fishers Lane, Rockville, MD 20857.

Publications: Materials are available on pharmaceuticals, drug labeling, and consumer education.

Reference Specialist
HUD DRUG INFORMATION and Strategy Clearinghouse
P.O. Box 6424
Rockville, MD 20850
(301) 251-5154; (800) 245-2691

Services: The primary purpose of the HUD Drug Information and Strategy Clearinghouse is to promote strategies for eradicating drugs and drug trafficking from public housing. With a mandate from the 1988 Anti-Drug Abuse Act, the Department of Housing and Urban Development established the clearinghouse to provide housing officials, residents, and community leaders a source for information and assistance on drug abuse prevention and trafficking control techniques. Clearinghouse reference specialists also provide referrals, and copies of HUD regulations and legal opinions.

Database: The clearinghouse database consists of national and community program descriptions, publications, research, and news articles.

Publications: Resource lists are available.

Serial publication: *Home Front* (quarterly newsletter).

User Services Coordinator
ERIC Clearinghouse on Teacher **EDUCATION**
One Dupont Circle NW, Suite 610
Washington, DC 20036
(202) 293-2450

Services: The ERIC Clearinghouse on Teacher Education (ERIC/SP) acquires, evaluates, abstracts, and indexes journal and research literature in two subject areas: the preparation and development of education personnel and selected aspects of health education, physical education, recreation, and dance. The clearinghouse performs computer searches of the ERIC database on topics within the scope of the clearinghouse and sponsors workshops on searching the ERIC database. Documents are available in either microfiche or paper copy from the ERIC Document Reproduction Service.

Database: The ERIC database can be searched through either the clearinghouse or commercial database vendors that include DIALOG and BRS. Sources indexed for the ERIC database include research reports, program descriptions, curriculum guides, and journals.

Service Limitations: A fee is charged for selected services.

Publications: The clearinghouse produces monographs, bibliographies, and ERIC Digests.

Serial publications: *Resources in Education* (monthly abstract journal), *Current Index to Journals in Education* (monthly), and *Health, Physical Education, Recreation, and Dance Monograph Series* (irregular).

Office of **EMPLOYMENT** Projections
Bureau of Labor Statistics
Department of Labor
600 E Street NW, Room 9216
Washington, DC 20212
(202) 272-5282

Services: The Office of Employment Projections of the Bureau of Labor Statistics (BLS) develops long-term projections of industry and occupational employment for use in career counseling and educational planning. Employment projections are developed every 2 years, using an econometric model of the economy in the target year and staffing patterns projected from BLS survey data. Projections for the 1988-2000 period include approximately 35 health occupation and 8 health industry sectors.

Publications: Employment projections for the 1988-2000 period are published in the November *1989 Monthly Labor Review, Occupational Projections and Training Data* (BLS Bulletin 2350), and *Occupational Outlook Handbook, 1990-91 edition* (BLS Bulletin 2350). *Occupational Outlook Handbook* statements are also available in a set of 20 reprints, of which 4 are health-related. These statements describe the nature of the work, education and training requirements, job outlook, and earnings in approximately 240 occupations, including dentists, dental assistants, optometrists, physical therapists, radiologic technologists, and registered nurses.

Public Affairs Officer
National Institute of **ENVIRONMENTAL HEALTH** Sciences
P.O. Box 12233
Research Triangle Park, NC 27709
(919) 541-3345

Services: The National Institute of Environmental Health Sciences (NIEHS), established in 1966, supports and conducts basic research focusing on the interaction between humans and potentially toxic or harmful agents in their environment. The research concentrates on recognizing, identifying, and investigating environmental factors that may be harmful and quantifying those factors. NIEHS research also focuses on developing an understanding of the mechanisms of action of toxic agents on biological systems. Information based on research is transmitted to regulatory agencies, other Government agencies, Congress, the medical and research communities, industry, and the general public. NIEHS research is the basis of preventive programs for environment-related diseases and for action by regulatory agencies. Grants and awards are also made to research organizations.

Publications: Directories of NIEHS's research programs, monographs on topics such as chemical pollutants in the environment, and bibliographies are available.

Serial publication: *Environmental Health Perspective* (bimonthly journal).

Information Specialist
ENVIRONMENTAL PROTECTION Agency
Public Information Center, PM-211B
401 M Street SW
Washington, DC 20460
(202) 382-2080

Services: The Public Information Center of the Environmental Protection Agency (EPA) offers information about the agency, its programs, and activities. When appropriate, the center refers inquirers to the proper technical program or regional office. Public information materials on such topics as hazardous wastes, asbestos, air and water pollution, pesticides, and drinking water, which are produced by other EPA divisions, are distributed through the center. The Public Information Center is open to the public during normal working hours and responds to telephone and mail inquiries. EPA maintains a headquarters library and libraries in each of its 10 regional offices, which are open to the public. Documents may be used in the libraries, duplicated, or borrowed through interlibrary loan arrangements.

Publications: Materials are available on air pollution, pesticides, solid waste management, toxic substances, and water pollution. EPA publishes a wide selection of general publications that discuss the agency's programs and activities. Some of these materials are directed to children.

Information Officer
National **EYE** Institute
9000 Rockville Pike
Building 31, Room 6A-32
Bethesda, MD 20892
(301) 496-5248

Services: The National Eye Institute (NEI), established in 1968, has primary responsibility within the National Institutes of Health and the Federal Government for supporting and conducting research aimed at improving the prevention, diagnosis, and treatment of eye disorders. In addition, NEI encourages the application of research findings to clinical practice, heightens public awareness of eye and vision problems, and cooperates with voluntary organizations that engage in related activities.

Publications: Materials are available on glaucoma, cataracts, retinal detachment, macular degeneration, ocular histoplasmosis, retinitis pigmentosa, refractive errors, corneal diseases, and diabetic retinopathy. Information on NEI-supported research is also available.

Coordinator
FAMILY INFORMATION Center
National Agricultural Library, Room 304
Department of Agriculture
10301 Baltimore Boulevard
Beltsville, MD 20705
(301) 344-3719

Services: The Family Information Center provides information services to professionals concerned with family strengths, well-being, economics, and social environment and assists them in obtaining current literature regarding the family unit and its individual members. The center acquires print and audiovisual resources and develops resource lists, Pathfinders, and Special Reference Briefs. Document delivery services include lending books and audiovisuals through local or institutional libraries, providing photocopies of journal articles not easily found elsewhere, and helping determine which library owns a particular book, journal, or audiovisual. The center is part of the National Agricultural Library and is open to the public 8 a.m. to 4:30 p.m. eastern time, Monday through Friday.

Database: The center's database, AGRICOLA, is accessible through BRS and DIALOG.

Service Limitations: There is a fee for extended information and research Services.

Information Specialist
FAMILY LIFE Information Exchange
P.O. Box 30436
Bethesda, MD 20814
(301) 907-8198

Services: The Family Life Information Exchange (FLIE), formerly the National Clearinghouse for Family Planning Information, was established in 1978 to serve as a clearinghouse on family planning issues. In 1988 the name was changed and, as the Family Life Information Exchange, the focus has been broadened to include clearinghouses on adolescent pregnancy and adoption. FLIE collects materials related to these topics, distributes a number of DHHS publications, maintains a database with approximately 5,000 entries, and makes referrals to other information centers.

Publications: Topical bibliographies are compiled and disseminated to interested family planning professionals. Available publications include *Many Teens Are Saying No (English and Spanish), Adolescent Abstinence: A Guide for Family Planning Professionals, Your Contraceptive Choices: For Now, For Later,* and *Directory of Family Planning Grantees, Delegates,* and *Clinics.*

Serial publication: *Resource Memo.*

Associate Administrator for Communications
FAMILY SUPPORT Administration
370 L'Enfant Promenade SW., 6th Floor
Washington, DC 20447
(202) 2524518

Services: The Family Support Administration (FSA) was established to be responsible for programs that strengthen the American family, especially low-income families. Six major programs in FSA include Aid to Families with Dependent Children (AFDC), Job Opportunities/Basic Skills (JOBS) Training programs, Child Support Enforcement, Refugee and Entrant Assistance, Community Services Block Grant, and Low-Income Home Energy Assistance. AFDC recipients are automatically eligible for Medicaid. The Office of Refugee Resettlement provides funding for medical assistance to refugees. The State Legalization Impact Assistance Grant program provides medical assistance for eligible newly legalized aliens. The Community Services Block Grant program provides funding for community food and nutrition programs.

Publications: Assorted fact sheets and brochures dealing with the activities of the FSA components are available.

Information Specialist
Clearinghouse on **FAMILY VIOLENCE** Information
P.O. Box 1182
Washington, DC 20013
(703) 821-2086

Services: Established in 1987, the Clearinghouse on Family Violence Information provides information services to practitioners and researchers who work to prevent family violence and assist its victims. The clearinghouse maintains bibliographic databases of documents, audiovisuals, and national organizations. Services also include custom searches of databases and annotated bibliographies on frequently requested topics.

Publications: Available publications include *Child Abuse and Neglect and Family Violence, Audiovisual Catalog, Child Abuse and Neglect and Family Thesaurus, Family Violence, An Overview,* and *National Organizations Concerned With Family Violence Issues.* A number of bibliographies are also available, including database bibliographies.

Director
FEDERAL INFORMATION Center
General Services Administration
Washington, DC 20405

Services: The Federal Information Center (FIC) program was established in 1966 as a one-stop source of assistance for callers with inquiries about the Federal Government's agencies, programs, and services. The most current Government reference material and service directories are used in responding to inquiries. Residents of 72 metropolitan areas can dial an FIC on a local-call basis and residents of four States may dial an FIC via a toll-free telephone number. A complete list of FIC telephone numbers and addresses is available free from the Consumer Information Center, Pueblo, CO 81009. HR/0246

Office of Consumer Affairs
FOOD AND DRUG Administration
5600 Fishers Lane (HFE48)
Rockville, MD 20857
(301) 443-3170

Services: Charged with the responsibility of handling consumer inquiries for the Food and Drug Administration (FDA), the Office of Consumer Affairs (OCA) serves as a clearinghouse for FDA consumer publications. Approximately 70,000 requests are received each year, primarily in the areas of foods and cosmetics. Inquiries are referred to appropriate agency offices for reply, or are answered by OCA staff, utilizing data from agency offices or agency publications. Most inquiries are received by mail.

Publications: Consumer materials are available on foods, nutrition, sodium, Federal regulations, cosmetics, medical devices, drug labeling, pharmaceuticals, health fraud, radiological health, and Reye's syndrome.

Serial publication: *FDA Consumer* (monthly journal).

Coordinator
FOOD AND NUTRITION Information Center
Department of Agriculture
National Agricultural Library, Room 304
Beltsville, MD 20705
(301) 344-3719

Services: The Food and Nutrition Information Center (FNIC) was established to serve the information needs of persons interested in human nutrition, food service management, and food technology. FNIC acquires and lends books and audiovisual materials dealing with these areas of concern. The collection ranges from children's materials to the most sophisticated professional materials. Books and audiovisual materials may be borrowed from the library and a photoduplication service is available for journal articles. Eligible patrons may borrow directly from FNIC and others may obtain the sources through interlibrary loan. Individuals should check with the center regarding eligibility. The library is open to the public from 8 a.m. to 4:30 p.m., Monday through Friday. Requests for services may be made in person, by letter, or by telephone. There is a 24-hour answering service to monitor calls for requests during nonbusiness hours.

Database: FNIC uses the National Agricultural Library's database, AGRICOLA, for computerized literature searches.

Publications: Bibliographies and resource guides are available on such topics as sports, cardiovascular disease, dental health, older Americans, vegetarianism, cancer, diabetes, food composition, anorexia nervosa, bulimia, and various aspects of nutrition.

Information Specialist
Office of Public Awareness
FOOD SAFETY and Inspection Service
Department of Agriculture, Room 1165-S
14th and Independence SW
Washington, DC 20250
(202) 447-9351 (public inquiries)
(800) 535-4555 (meat and poultry hotline)
(202) 447-3333 (Metropolitan Washington, DC, hotline)

Services: Formerly the Food Safety and Quality Service, the Food Safety and Inspection Service (FSIS) was established in 1981 to administer the meat and poultry inspection program, which assures consumers that meat and poultry sold in the United States or shipped abroad is safe, wholesome, and truthfully labeled. FSIS inspects and analyzes domestic and imported meat, poultry, and meat and poultry food products; establishes standards and approves recipes and labels for processing meat and poultry products; and monitors the meat and poultry industries for violations of inspection laws.

Publications: FSIS produces a wide variety of pamphlets and other educational materials on such topics as food safety, food poisoning, labels on meat and poultry products, food additives, food labeling, sodium, herbs, and the food inspection program. A publications list is available.
Serial publication: *Food News for Consumers.*

Superintendent of Documents
U.S. **GOVERNMENT PRINTING** Office
Washington, DC 20402-9325
(202) 783-3238 (order and information desk)
(202) 275-3634 (for updates on publications)

Services: The U.S. Government Printing Office (GPO) was founded in 1861 for the production of U.S. Government documents. GPO was assigned the additional duties of sales and distribution in 1895. Yearly sales today exceed 40 million publications. More than 10,000 different titles may be printed during a single session of Congress. Publications prepared by Congress and the agencies and departments of the Federal Government are printed and distributed by GPO.
Database: The GPO Publications Reference File is used online at GPO and is searchable by the public on DIALOG. It is a complete listing of GPO materials. Searchable fields include subject, title, and author.
Service Limitations: Except for certain catalogs, GPO does not distribute any free publications. Payment is required in advance of shipment. However, single copies of many of its publications are available free from the issuing agencies.
Publications: The comprehensive listing of publications from GPO is the *Monthly Catalog of U.S. Government Publications*. It is divided by subject areas, a number of which are health-related. A series of free subject bibliographies list publications available in over 240 areas, including mental health, public health, medicine and medical science, and many other health areas. A free index of these bibliographies is also available.
Serial publication: *Health and Health-Related Publications*, a subject bibliography that lists new publications, is free.

Information Specialist
National Information Center for
Children and Youth with **HANDICAPS**
P.O. Box 1492
Washington, DC 20013
(703) 8934061; (800) 999-5599 (24-hour taped message)

Services: The National Information Center for Children and Youth with Handicaps (NICHCY), formerly the National Information Center for Handicapped Children and Youth, is a national information clearinghouse authorized by Congress under the Education of the Handicapped Act to assist parents, educators, caregivers, advocates, and others working to improve the lives of children and youth with disabilities. NICHCY has established a strong network with parent groups throughout the country. Services include personal responses to specific questions, referrals to other organizations/ sources of help, and technical assistance to parent and professional groups.

Publications: NICHCY develops and distributes fact sheets on specific disabilities, general information for parents, vocational/transitional issues, special education, and legal rights and advocacy, as well as information on parent support groups and public advocacy. Issue and briefing papers on current, relevant topics in the special education and disabilities field are also published. Information (pamphlets, booklets, and fact sheets) regarding pertinent disability issues obtained from other sources is available.

Serial publications: *News Digest and Transition Summary.*

Division of Public Information
National Institutes of **HEALTH**
Building 1, Room 344
9000 Rockville Pike
Bethesda, MD 20892
(301) 496-5787

Services: The Division of Public Information produces a variety of informational materials relating to the National Institutes of Health (NIH) as a whole. The division also responds to requests for information from the general public, the professional public, as well as media representatives. The division consists of the Editorial Operations Branch, the News Branch, and the Broadcast Services Branch. The Editorial Operations Branch produces publications covering all units, such as the NIH Almanac and the Scientific Directory and Annual Bibliography, as well as The NIH Record, an employee publication available to the public via paid subscription. The News Branch keeps abreast of trends in biomedical research, reviews NIH press releases, and produces "Search for Health" newspaper columns, and "News and Features," a photo-feature service for the media. The Broadcast Services Branch produces a weekly series of interviews featuring NIH physicians and scientists for use on radio, the 24-hour NIH Radio News Service (for radio stations), and other health information for radio and television. The Division of Public Information and its three branches will either respond to telephone or written requests or direct such requests to the proper NIH source. Materials produced by various NIH bureaus, institutes, and divisions, as found in the NIH Publications List, should be requested directly from the appropriate unit.

Serial publications: *NIH Almanac* (annual), *Scientific Directory and Annual Bibliography* (annual), *NIH Publications List* (annual), *NIH Brochure* (irregular), and *NIH Information Index* (irregular).

Executive Officer
Bureau of **HEALTH CARE DELIVERY** and Assistance
Health Resources and Services Administration
Parklawn Building, Room 715
5600 Fishers Lane
Rockville, MD 20857
(301) 443-2330

Services: The Bureau of Health Care Delivery and Assistance (BHCDA) serves as a national focus for efforts to ensure delivery of health care services to residents of medically underserved areas and to special groups. BHCDA assists States and local communities in providing health care to medically underserved populations through community health centers. Through project grants, funds are provided to help State, local, voluntary, public, and private entities meet the health needs of special populations such as migrant workers, the homeless, black lung disease victims, and high risk pregnant women. BHCDA provides direction for the Bureau of Prisons' medical program, the national Hansen's Disease Program, and the Federal Employee Occupational Health Program. BHCDA administers a health benefits program for designated Public Health Service beneficiaries. BHCDA also administers the National Health Service Corps (NHSC), which helps States and communities arrange for physicians, dentists, and other health care professionals to provide care in health manpower shortage areas (HMSAs). The NHSC Scholarship and Loan Repayment Programs help ensure the availability of trained health care providers to serve in HMSAs. Inquiries and publications requests are referred to the appropriate BHCDA office for response.

News and Information Branch
HEALTH CARE FINANCING Administration
200 Independence Avenue SW, Room 428-H
Washington, DC 20201
(202) 245-6145

Services: The Health Care Financing Administration (HCFA) administers Medicare, Medicaid, related quality assurance programs, and other programs. HCFA also makes certain that beneficiaries are aware of the services for which they are eligible, that services are accessible, and that they are provided in an effective manner. HCFA ensures that its policies and actions promote efficiency and quality within the total health care delivery system. Questions concerning Medicare or Medicaid can be asked at the above number or sent by mail to the agency. Questions are answered or referred to the appropriate office for response. Information on reimbursement programs for kidney dialysis are referred to the appropriate agency.

Publications: Consumer materials include descriptive brochures on the Medicare and Medicaid programs, available from local Social Security Offices.

Professional materials are available on Medicare and Medicaid program statistics, DRGs (diagnosis-related groups), health care financing, and medical care utilization.

Serial publication: *Health Care Financing Review* (quarterly journal).

Chief, Publications and Information Branch
Agency for **HEALTH CARE POLICY** and Research
Parklawn Building, Room 18-12
5600 Fishers Lane
Rockville, MD 20857
(301) 443-4100

Services: The Agency for Health Care Policy and Research (AHCPR) was established in 1968 as the National Center for Health Services Research. AHCPR is the primary source of Federal support for research on problems related to the quality and delivery of health services. ACHPR responds to the need for better data and information, new techniques, and innovative methods for improving health care delivery. AHCPR programs evaluate health services, assess technologies, and improve access to new scientific and technical information for research users. Research findings are disseminated through publications, conferences, and workshops.

Service Limitations: AHCPR research is targeted toward the needs of health care policy makers, including executive and legislative officials at Federal, State, and local levels, health care administrators, and others with responsibility for health care resource allocation.

Publications: Materials are available on medical treatment effectiveness, health care costs and utilizations, health care expenditures, health information systems, health technology assessment, and funding opportunities for grants and contracts. Single copies of publications are available free upon request from the AHCPR (send a self-addressed mailing label). An annotated publications list is also available.

Serial publication: *AHCPR Research Activities* (monthly) summarizes key research findings and the availability of new reports.

Office of **HEALTH FACILITIES**
5600 Fishers Lane
Parklawn Building, Room 11-03
Rockville, MD 20857
(301) 443-6560
(800) 638-0742 (Hill-Burton free hospital care information)
(800) 492-0359 (Hill-Burton information in Maryland)

Services: The Office of Health Facilities (OHF), formerly the Bureau of Health Facilities, was established in September 1978 to consolidate programs dealing with health facilities. The scope of activities of its three divisions includes administering insured and guaranteed loan programs for health facilities and monitoring health facilities to determine compliance with assurances made during application for Federal construction assistance. OHF also answers questions on the Hill-Burton free hospital care program and responds to patient inquiries on Hill-Burton facilities via the toll-free hotline. In addition, OHF supports the Bureau of Maternal and Child Health and Resources and the Health Resources and Services Administration.

Database: OHF maintains an in-house database that contains information on facilities obligated under the 20-year uncompensated care assurances (Hill-Burton) program. The data captured for facility obligations begun after January 1959 include location, name, type of facility, grant funds, and date obligation expires.

Publications: Publications are available on capital formation in health care facilities, cost containment in hospitals through energy conservation, guidelines for construction and equipment for hospital and medical facilities, criteria for design review and licensure surveys of solar systems in health care facilities, and energy issues in health. Also available are a guide on how to operate a Hill-Burton free care program and a directory of all facilities currently required to provide free care.

Chief Clearinghouse on **HEALTH INDEXES**
Office of Epidemiology and Health Promotion
National Center for Health Statistics
Centers for Disease Control
6525 Belcrest Road, Room 1070
Hyattsville, MD 20782
(301) 436-7035

Services: The Clearinghouse on Health Indexes provides information assistance in the development of health measures to health researchers, administrators, and planners. The clearinghouse definition of a health index is a measure that summarizes data from two or more components and purports to reflect the health status of an individual or defined group. Services provided to users include annotated bibliographies and reference and referral service. A library of 4,000 documents and journals is available to users by appointment.

Database: The clearinghouse is developing a share-ware PC-based version of its database, which will contain comprehensive information from 1973 to the present and core materials published earlier. Sources indexed by this database include journal articles, books, conference proceedings, Government publications, unpublished materials, speeches, and research in progress.

Serial publication: *Bibliography on Health Indexes* (quarterly).

Referral Specialist
Office of Disease Prevention and Health Promotion
National **HEALTH INFORMATION** Center
P.O. Box 1133
Washington, DC 20013-1133
(800) 336-4797; (301) 565-4167

Services: The Office of Disease Prevention and Health Promotion (ODPHP) National Health Information Center (ONHIC), formerly the National Health Information Clearinghouse, was established in 1979 to help the public and health professionals locate health information through identification of health information resources, an information and referral system, and publications. Utilizing a database that contains descriptions of health-related organizations, ONHIC staff refer inquiries to the most appropriate resources. Where appropriate, a direct answer is provided, primarily to requests for the names and addresses of organizations, publication ordering information, inquiries regarding ONHIC, or inquiries for which the staff has no database resource. A core collection of health reference materials, journals, newsletters, and educational materials is available for use by the public; advance arrangements are recommended.

Database: ONHIC's database of referral organizations is publicly accessible through DIRLINE, a database on the National Library of Medicine's MEDLARS system. The ONHIC component of DIRLINE contains descriptions of about 1,100 diverse health-related organizations. ONHIC'S DIRLINE records are labeled "HR" in the Secondary Source ID (SI) field. ONHIC staff do not diagnose, make direct referrals to health care professionals, answer questions about pharmaceutical side effects, or recommend treatment for medical conditions.

Publications: ONHIC offers a directory of selected health information resources in the Federal Government and provides resource guides on topics such as selected Federal information clearinghouses and information centers, national health observances, toll-free telephone numbers for health information, minority health, Spanish language health resources, and long-term care. ONHIC also distributes many of ODPHP's publications. A publications list is available.

Information Officer
Bureau of **HEALTH PROFESSIONS**
Health Resources and Services Administration
Parklawn Building, Room 8-05
5600 Fishers Lane
Rockville, MD 20857
(301) 443-3376
(800) 338-2832 (Vaccine Injury Compensation Program)

Services: The Bureau of Health Professions provides national leadership in supporting the development and use of the Nation's health personnel and serves as a focus for key health care practice issues such as quality assurance and medical malpractice. The bureau also administers the Vaccine Injury Compensation Program. The bureau supports health professions and nursing education in areas of high national priority, such as health care for minorities and the underserved, strengthened education concerning HIV/AIDS and substance abuse, and health care of the elderly. The bureau supports programs to foster interdisciplinary education and practice, to increase the supply of primary care practitioners, and to improve the distribution and utilization of health professionals. Financially needy students are assisted in pursuit of health careers. The bureau also collects and analyzes data and disseminates information on the characteristics and capacities of U.S. health training systems and assesses the Nation's health personnel work force, forecasting supply and requirements under a variety of utilization strategies.

Publications: Fact sheets on current health professions and nurse training authorities, reports to Congress on the status of health professions and nursing personnel, reports of studies, directories, and trend data on grants.

Office of Communications
HEALTH RESOURCES and Services Administration
Parklawn Building, Room 14-43
5600 Fishers Lane
Rockville, MD 20857
(301) 443-2086

Services: The mission of the Health Resources and Services Administration (HRSA) is to improve America's health care system and the health of the American people. The Office of Communications provides information on programs for the distribution, supply, use, quality, and cost-effectiveness of health resources, and on health services programs for certain segments of the population. Specific areas of concentration are health professions training, health services for Hansen's disease patients, community/migrant health centers, maternal and child health, migrant health, health facilities, and the National Health Service Corps. HRSA also administers programs concerned with health care for the homeless and Federal AIDS programs relating to pediatric AIDS service demonstrations, AIDS service demonstration projects, regional AIDS education and training centers, long-term and intermediate care facilities for AIDS patients, HIV services planning, and AIDS drug reimbursement. HRSA also administers programs relating to organ transplantation, Federal employee occupational health, rural health issues, and the National Practitioner Data Bank. Inquiries are answered directly or referred to the proper bureau or clearinghouse for response. Requests for publications should be directed to the issuing bureau, when known.

Publications: Informational materials, reports, bibliographies, studies, and guidelines are available along with a publications catalog.

Director
HEALTH RISK APPRAISAL Activity Center
for Chronic Disease Prevention and Health Promotion
Centers for Disease Control
Building 3, B43 1600 Clifton Road NE
Atlanta, GA 30333
(404) 639-3177

Services: The Centers for Disease Control's Center for Chronic Disease Prevention and Health Promotion provides health risk appraisal (HRA) general information and technical assistance in the use of HRAs through State and regional contacts. This office also maintains a computer bulletin board for health and safety professionals interested in HRA research and development. Current activities include the evaluation of HRA methods for community-based health promotion and the adoption of HRA methods for underserved populations. For those interested in using the current public-domain HRA computer software, a list of State and regional contacts is available.

Information
National **HEALTH SERVICE** Corps
Bureau of Health Care Delivery and Assistance
Parklawn Building, Room 7A-13
5600 Fishers Lane
Rockville, MD 20857
(301) 443-1400

Services: The National Health Service Corps (NHSC) was established in 1970 to recruit and place health professionals in health manpower shortage areas. Health professionals with service obligations under the NHSC Scholarship or Loan Repayment programs (administered by the Division of Health Services Scholarships) and volunteers are sent to communities with one primary care physician or fewer per 3,500 people. Information about NHSC's provision of a health practitioner for a community is available from this office.

Scientific and Technical Information Branch
National Center for **HEALTH STATISTICS**
Centers for Disease Control
6525 Belcrest Road, Room 1064
Hyattsville, MD 20782
(301) 436-8500

Services: Organized in 1960, the National Center for Health Statistics (NCHS) collects, analyzes, and disseminates data on health in the United States. Using surveys and registration systems, NCHS has developed data systems to collect statistics on births, deaths, marriages, and divorces in the United States; the extent and impact of illness and disability; determinants of health; health services; utilization of health care; health care costs and financing; and family growth and dissolution. Staff members respond to requests from professionals or consumers using publications, computer printouts, microdata tapes, and special tabulations.

Database: Much of the data collected and compiled by NCHS is part of the National Technical Information Service (NTIS) database, available online to the public through DIALOG and BRS.

Service Limitations: Requests for current statistical information on infectious diseases should be directed to the Centers for Disease Control rather than to NCHS.

Publications: Materials available include statistical data on health, nutrition, vital statistics, health care delivery, dental health, health resources utilization, health care personnel, families, contraception, and health care economics. A publications list, indexed by subject, is available upon request. Most NCHS publications must be purchased from the Government Printing Office. Findings from surveys conducted by NCHS are released in the *Vital and Health Statistics* series and the *Advanced Data* series.

Serial publications: *Vital Statistics of the United States* (annual report) and *Monthly Vital Statistics Report* (monthly).

Information Officer
National **HEART, LUNG, AND BLOOD** Institute
National Institutes of Health
Building 31, Room 4A-21
9000 Rockville Pike
Bethesda, MD 20892
(301) 496-4236

Services: The National Heart, Lung, and Blood Institute (NHLBI) was established in 1948 as the National Heart Institute. The primary responsibility of NHLBI is the scientific investigation of heart, blood vessel, lung, and blood diseases. NHLBI oversees research, demonstration, prevention, education, control, and training activities in these fields. NHLBI programs emphasize the prevention and control of heart, lung, and blood diseases and education concerning these diseases through more rapid transfer of knowledge into the mainstream of clinical medicine and personal health practices.

Service Limitations: Inquiries related to high blood pressure, cholesterol, smoking, asthma, and blood resources (blood banking, blood transfusion), as well as any information requests associated with cardiovascular disease prevention and heart-health promotion are handled by the NHLBI Education Programs Information Center.

Publications: Limited quantities of a variety of topical pamphlets and other publications are available free of charge upon request. NHLBI provides information on such topics as heart disease, the heart, arteriosclerosis, congestive heart failure, chronic obstructive pulmonary disease, angina, Raynaud's Disease, immune thrombocytopenic purpura, heart transplants, arrythmias, valvular heart disease, and sickle cell anemia. Professional materials are available on arteriosclerosis, lipid research, fetal hemoglobino pathies, cardiovascular diseases, coronary heart disease, asthma, and aplastic anemia. A publications list is available.

Information Specialist
National **HEART, LUNG, AND BLOOD** Institute
Education Programs Information Center
4733 Bethesda Avenue, Suite 530
Bethesda,MD 20814
(301) 951-3260

Services: The National Heart, Lung, and Blood Institute Education Programs Information Center was established in 1986 as a source of information and materials on cholesterol and smoking, two major risk factors for cardiovascular health. In 1987, it merged with the National High Blood Pressure Education Program. Two new programs, the National Blood Resource Education Program and the National Asthma Education Program, have also been added. Services include dissemination of public education materials, programmatic and scientific information for health professionals, materials on worksite health, and response to information requests. The center is a service of the National Heart, Lung and Blood Institute of the National Institutes of Health.

Databases: A cholesterol, high blood pressure, and smoking education database and a blood resource database are subfiles on the Combined Health Information Database (CHID), which is available on BRS Information Technologies.

Publications: Consumer materials are available on cholesterol, high blood pressure, smoking, asthma, chronic cough, heart disease, exercise, stroke, and blood resources. Professional materials are available on heart and lung health at the workplace, cholesterol, smoking programs, asthma, and blood resources.

Serial publications: *Infomemo*—provides program updates about cholesterol, high blood pressure, asthma, and smoking, and *Infoline*—describes the activities of the National Blood Resource Education Program.

National **HIGHWAY TRAFFIC SAFETY** Administration
Department of Transportation
400 Seventh Street SW, (NOA-40)
Washington, DC 20590
(202) 366-0123
(800) 424-9393 (hotline)

Services: The National Highway Traffic Safety Administration (NHTSA) was established in 1966 to reduce deaths, injuries, and economic losses resulting from motor vehicle crashes; improve highway safety by promoting both safer vehicles and safer driving practices; set and enforce Federal safety standards for all new motor vehicles; investigate alleged safety defects and order recalls where necessary; and conduct extensive research on improving vehicle safety. NHTSA also provides financial and technical assistance to State and local governments; awards grants to States for highway safety and to help combat drunk driving; works closely with private organizations to promote a broad range of driver and traffic safety programs, including programs to combat drunk driving; encourages use of safety belts and child safety seats; works to improve emergency medical services, driver licensing, traffic recordkeeping, and traffic law enforcement; investigates odometer fraud; sets bumper, fuel economy, and vehicle theft standards; and develops tests of crashworthiness of new cars. NHTSA maintains a toll-free hotline for consumer complaints on auto safety, reports of alleged defects, requests for auto safety recall information, and consumer publications on traffic and highway safety.

Publications: NHTSA publications include pamphlets, fact sheets, brochures, booklets, posters, and research notes on safety belt and child passenger safety seat use, drunk driving, and automobile safety; statistical reports on accidents and fatalities; and summary reports on compliance and auto manufacturer defect campaigns.

The National Resource Center
on **HOMELESSNESS** and Mental Illness
262 Delaware Avenue
Delmar, NY 12054
(800) 444-7415

Services: The National Resource Center on Homelessness and Mental Illness provides technical assistance and information concerning the service and housing needs of homeless mentally ill persons.

Database: The center maintains a comprehensive database of information on the homeless mentally ill population, prepares database searches in particular topic areas, and disseminates materials in the database that are not available from any other source.

Service Limitations: Ten cents per page for materials that must be photocopied; users in the Albany, NY, area may use materials on site. Database not currently accessible by outside users.

Publications: Three information packets are available, including *Case Management with Homeless Mentally Ill Persons, Financing Services for Homeless Mentally Ill Persons*, and *Training Staff and Volunteers Working with Homeless Mentally Ill Persons.*

Serial publication: *Access* (quarterly bulletin) provides information packets on discrete service issues and distributes an organizational referral list.

Reference Supervisor
HUD User (**HOUSING**)
P.O. Box 6091
Rockville, MD 20850
(301) 251-5154; (800) 245-2691

Services: HUD User is a computer-based information service designed to disseminate the results of research sponsored by the Department of Housing and Urban development. Services include personalized literature searches by reference staff of the computerized database, document delivery, and special products such as topical bibliographies and announcements of important future research.

Database: Health-related topics covered in the HUD User database, available through BRS, include housing safety, housing for the elderly and handicapped, and lead-based paint. HUD User is a service of the Office of Policy Development and Research, Department of Housing and Urban Development.

Service Limitations: There is a handling fee for all documents ordered from HUD User; please call before ordering.

Serial publication: *Recent Research Results* (bimonthly current awareness bulletin.

Office of Public Affairs
Office of **HUMAN DEVELOPMENT** Services
200 Independence Avenue SW, Room 348-F
Washington, DC 20201
(202) 245-2760

Services: The Office of Human Development Services (OHDS) administers human service programs, encourages the development of innovative service delivery strategies, and works to identify and eliminate barriers at all levels of government to the development of improved and more accessible social services. Questions are answered directly or referred to the appropriate OHDS agency, such as the Administration for Children, Youth, and Families, the Administration for Native Americans, or the Administration on Developmental Disability.

Publications: A brochure on OHDS is available.

Serial publication: *Children Today* (bimonthly magazine).

Information Specialist
State Planning and **HUMAN RESOURCE DEVELOPMENT** Branch
National Institute of Mental Health
5600 Fishers Lane, Room 7-103
Rockville, MD 20857
(301) 443-4735

Services: The State Planning and Human Resources Development Branch (SPHRDB) coordinates National Institute of Mental Health (NIMH) activities relating to mental health needs of persons in emergency conditions arising from crises in the physical environment. SPHRDB also analyzes and evaluates current research and developments; collaborates with other Public Health Service agencies, the Federal Emergency Management Agency, and other public and private agencies to administer crisis counseling programs in areas that have been declared disaster areas by the President of the United States; and develops and disseminates relevant educational materials.

Service Limitations: The services of SPHRDB are for use by mental health professionals and State and local agencies involved with emergency planning.

Publications: Publications offer guidelines for the prevention and control of stress among emergency workers and discuss appropriate services for victims of disasters. A publications list is available.

Project Share (**HUMAN SERVICES**)
P.O. Box 30666
Bethesda, MD 20824
(301) 907-6523; (800) 537-3788

Services: Established in 1976, Project Share provides reference and referral services designed to improve the management of human services by emphasizing the integration of those services at the delivery level to human services planners and managers. In addition, Project Share acquires and makes available documents containing current research and development activities, project descriptions, and accounts of the experiences of State and local governments in the planning and management of human services delivery. Turnaround time on requests is 3 days. Project Share is currently focused on the programmatic areas of the Family Support Administration.

Database: The database, which contains approximately 14,000 records, is updated quarterly and covers the years since 1972. Access to the collection is achieved using an automated retrieval system. Abstracts are included for each record, and indexing is done using a taxonomy. Sources indexed by the database include research reports, conference proceedings, papers, descriptions of ongoing and completed projects, operating manuals, and bibliographies.

Service Limitations: Fees are charged for publications and searches. Reduced membership plan rates are available upon request.

Publications: Professional materials are available on human services administration, teen pregnancy, program evaluation, elderly board and care, respite care, volunteerism, and domestic violence.

Communications Director
INDIAN HEALTH Service
Parklawn Building, Room 6-35
5600 Fishers Lane
Rockville, MD 20857
(301) 443-3593

Services: The Indian Health Service (IHS) provides comprehensive health services through IHS facilities, tribally contracted hospitals, health centers, school health centers, and health stations. Health services provided include medical, dental, and environmental health programs. Special program concentrations are in disease prevention and health promotion, alcoholism, substance abuse, suicide, accidents, maternal and child health, nutrition, and otitis media (inflammation of the middle ear).

Publications: Reports, directories, brochures, and pamphlets highlighting IHS activities are available.

National Commission to Prevent **INFANT MORTALITY**
Switzer Building, Room 2014
330 C Street SW
Washington, DC 20201
(202) 472-1364

Services: The National Commission to Prevent Infant Mortality was created by Congress (P.L. 990-660) and established on July 1, 1987. The commission consists of 16 members, including members of Congress, Cabinet heads, representatives from State governments, and members of the maternal and child health care community. The primary mission of the commission is to make universal access to early, comprehensive maternity and infant care accessible to all and to make children's health and well-being a national priority.

Database: ERIC, UD 026381, Death Before Life: The Tragedy of Infant Mortality.

Director
National **INJURY INFORMATION** Clearinghouse
U.S. Consumer Product Safety Commission
5401 Westbard Avenue, Room 625
Bethesda, MD 20892
(301) 492-6424

Services: The National Injury Information Clearinghouse, a division of the U.S. Consumer Product Safety Commission (CPSC), collects, investigates, analyzes, and disseminates injury data and information relating to the causes and prevention of death, injury, and illness associated with consumer products. The clearinghouse compiles data obtained from accident investigation reports, consumer complaints reported incidents, death certificates, news clips, and the CPSC-operated National Electronic Injury Surveillance System (NEISS). NEISS gathers data from a sample of hospitals that are statistically representative of emergency departments in the United States. From these data, estimates can be made of product-related injuries associated with consumer products. The clearinghouse responds to about 6,000 requests for information each year.

Service Limitations: Since September 1987, the fees for services include research time, computer time, number of computer lines printed, and review time. The Commission Secretary may waive or reduce fees when special circumstances warrant.

Publications: Publications include statistical analysis of data in the automated files and CPSC analysis of hazard and accident patterns.

Serial publication: *NEISS Data Highlights* (annual newsletter).

Deputy Director
Office of **INTERNATIONAL HEALTH**
Parklawn Building, Room 18-87
5600 Fishers Lane
Rockville, MD 20857
(301) 443-1774

Services: The Office of International Health (OIH) provides support to the Assistant Secretary for Health and the Secretary of the Department of Health and Human Services (DHHS) in developing policy and coordinating activities of the Public Health Service (PHS) agencies in the field of international health. OIH works closely with the World Health Organization and other international organizations. OIH oversees PHS participation in over 25 binational cooperative health agreements. Several desk officers serve as experts on various regions of the world. OIH will respond to questions regarding United States participation in international health agreements and programs.

Publications: OIH publications are available for purchase from the National Technical Information Service. A publications list is available from OIH. Professional materials are produced on health planning, health manpower, breastfeeding, communicable diseases, and international health.

Information Specialist
National **KIDNEY AND UROLOGIC DISEASES** Information Clearinghouse
Box NKUDIC
Bethesda, MD 20892
(301) 468-6345

Services: The National Kidney and Urologic Disease Information Clearinghouse (NKUDIC), sponsored by the National Institute of Diabetes and

Digestive and Kidney Diseases, is an information resource and referral organization. NKUDIC provides education and information on kidney and urologic diseases to patients, professionals, and the public. NKUDIC also makes referrals to other appropriate organizations.

Database: NKUDIC maintains the kidney and urologic diseases subfile of the Combined Health Information Database (CHID). Staff may also produce custom literature searches from CHID.

Service Limitations: Some publications require a fee to cover shipping and handling costs.

Publications: Available materials include brochures; bibliographies on diabetes, kidney disease, and audiovisual materials; and fact sheets entitled *Prevention and Treatment of Kidney Stones, Understanding Urinary Tract Infections,* and *Benign Prostatic Hyperplasia.*

Serial publication: *KU Notes* (bulletin).

Public Information Officer
National **LIBRARY OF MEDICINE**
Building 38, Room 2S-10
8600 Rockville Pike
Bethesda, MD 20894
(800) 272-4787 (general information)
(301) 496-6308 (library hours)
(301) 496-6095 (reference desk)
(800) 638-8480 (MEDLARS management)
(301) 496-6193 (MEDLARS management)

Services: In support of its mission to collect, preserve, and disseminate biomedical information, the National Library of Medicine (NLM) has assembled the largest collection of biomedical literature in the world. Included are over 4 million books, journals, technical reports, and other print and audiovisual materials in 40 biomedical fields, as well as the Nation's largest medical history collection. Services of NLM include computer-based literature retrieval services, interlibrary loan services, programs of grant support for medical libraries, communications research and training, toxicology information services, and publications. Medical reference questions should be directed to the NLM Reference Desk.

Databases: NLM has 30 specialized databases composing the Medical Literature Analysis and Retrieval System (MEDLARS) available through a nationwide network of 15,000 centers. Individuals with microcomputers and modems can have direct access through the software GRATEFUL MED, available for both IBM-PC and compatible machines and Apple Macintoshes. Fact sheets and pocket guides describing the databases are available. A MEDLARS management service desk at NLM is staffed to answer questions about the online system.

Publications: Numerous catalogs, guides, and indexes to specific NLM materials are available.

Serial publications: *Index Medicus*, (monthly), *NLM Current Catalog*, (quarterly), *NLM Audiovisuals Catalog* (quarterly), and *Bibliography of the History of Medicine* (annual for sale by the Government Printing Office.

Program Director
National Center for Education in
MATERNAL AND CHILD HEALTH
38th and R Streets NW.
Washington, DC 20057
(202) 625-8400

Services: The National Center for Education in Maternal and Child Health (NCEMCH) responds to information requests from consumers and professionals, provides technical assistance, and develops educational and reference materials. The NCEMCH Resource Center contains professional literature, patient education materials, curricula, audiovisuals, and information about organizations and programs. Major content areas include pregnancy and childbirth, child and adolescent health, nutrition, high-risk infants, chronic illness and disability, human genetics, women's health, and maternal and child health services and programs.

Publications: NCEMCH produces newsletters, bibliographies, booklets, brochures, resource guides and other educational materials, which are listed in a publications catalog. Most are free. The reference collection includes over 3,000 books and reports and 70 journal titles in the subject areas described above. NCEMCH operates 8:30 a.m. to 5 p.m. on weekdays, and the reference collection is open to the public by appointment.

Serial publication: *MCH Program Interchange*—published about 10 times a year, highlights a different topic in each issue.

Information Specialist
National Clearinghouse for **MATERNAL AND CHILD HEALTH**
38th and R Streets NW
Washington, DC 20057
(202) 625 8410

Services: The National Clearinghouse for Maternal and Child Health continues and expands the activities of the National Clearinghouse for Human Genetic Diseases. The clearinghouse is the centralized source of materials and information in the areas of human genetics and maternal and child health. The clearinghouse staff also responds to inquiries, disseminates approximately 500 publications, and produces fact sheets, topical bibliographies, and referral lists in the field.

Database: An inhouse online database of topics, agencies, and organizations related to human genetics and maternal and child health is being developed.

Publications: Clearinghouse publications cover such topics as breastfeeding, developmental disabilities, phenylketonuria (PKU), metabolic disorders, nutrition, prenatal care, perinatal care, and genetic diseases. Directories of clinical genetic service centers and Federal programs and voluntary and professional organizations in maternal and child health are also available.

Information Officer
Office of Research Reports
National Institute of General **MEDICAL SCIENCES**
Building 31, Room 4A-52
9000 Rockville Pike
Bethesda, MD 20892
(301) 496-7301

Services: The Office of Research Reports responds to inquiries relating to the institute's activities in basic biomedical research. Program areas include the cellular and molecular basis of disease, genetics, pharmacological sciences, biophysics and physiological sciences, and biomedical research and research training for minorities. Information on types of research and research training support available for institutions and individuals may be obtained from the office.

Publications: Consumer materials are available on genetics, basic research, and cell biology. Professional materials are available on research grants and training programs, basic research, genetics, and structural biology.

Public Inquiries
National Institute of **MENTAL HEALTH**
5600 Fishers Lane, Room I5C05
Rockville, MD 20857
(301) 443-4513

Services: Public Inquiries of the National Institute of Mental Health (NIMH) assumed many of the duties of the NIMH Science Communication Branch and the National Clearinghouse for Mental Health Information. The staff collects scientific, technical, and other information on mental illness and health from the staff and operating components of NIMH and outside sources; classifies, stores, and retrieves information; and answers general inquiries from the public within 2 weeks.

Publications: Public Inquiries distributes single copies of NIMH publications at no charge. There are several consumer publications in Spanish. A publications list is available.

Serial publications: *Caring About Kids* and *Plain Talk*—NIMH series of fliers and pamphlets.

Executive Director
President's Committee on **MENTAL RETARDATION**
Department of Health and Human Services
330 Independence Avenue SW, Room 5325
Washington, DC 20201
(202) 619-0634

Services: The President's Committee on Mental Retardation (PCMR) advises the President and the Secretary of the Department of Health and Human Services on appropriate ways to provide services for persons with mental retardation and on ways to prevent this type of disability. Areas of concern are full citizenship, prevention of biomedical and environmental causes of retardation, family and community support services, international activities, and public information. PCMR sponsors forums and conferences and prepares annual reports to the President.

Publications: Publications include annual reports, bibliographies, conference reports, and program descriptions on such topics as legal rights of the mentally retarded. A publications list is available.

Special Assistant
Office of **MINORITY HEALTH**
Department of Health and Human Services
Humphrey Building, Room 118F
200 Independence Avenue SW
Washington, DC 20201
(202) 245-0020

Services: Established in 1985, the Office of Minority Health (OMH) serves as the focal point for the implementation of the recommendations and findings from the Report of the Secretary's Task Force on Black and Minority Health. Community-based projects are being designed to reduce the more than 60,000 excess deaths each year among minority Americans. Major activities include conferences, grants for innovative community health strategies developed by minority coalitions, and research on risk factors affecting minority health.

Publications: The report mentioned above, in eight volumes, may be obtained from OMH.

Information Specialist
Office of **MINORITY HEALTH RESOURCE** Center
P.O. Box 37337
Washington, DC 20013
(800) 444-6472

Services: The Office of Minority Health Resource Center (OMH-RC) responds to information requests on minority health, locates sources of technical assistance through the Resource Persons Network, and provides referrals to relevant organizations. Activities concentrate on the minority health priority areas. Bilingual staff members are available to serve Spanish-speaking requestors.

Database: The automated Resource Persons Network and Materials database can locate materials and technical assistance.

Service Limitations: The database is not accessible by outside users.

Publications: Publications include the *Closing the Gap* series and the *Report of the Secretary's Task Force on Black and Minority Health*.

Health Care Operations
Office of the Director, **NAVAL MEDICINE**
Office of the Surgeon General of the Navy
Bureau of Medicine and Surgery
Washington, DC 20372-5120
(202) 653-1727

Services: The mission of the Director, Naval Medicine, is to provide the Chief of Naval Operations centralized, coordinated policy formulation, guidance, direction, and oversight, and professional and technical advice on all health care related programs; to ensure that adequate medical resources and trained personnel are available to meet Navy and Marine Corps contingency plans; and to ensure that the Navy's responsibility to safeguard and protect the health of Navy and Marine Corps personnel, their dependents, and other personnel, as authorized by law, is met. The office responds to inquiries about eligibility for benefits.

Service Limitations: Formal health information is provided only to Federal agencies and authorized beneficiaries.

Publications: Health information fact sheets, brochures, and booklets are designed and disseminated by several Medical Department commands, but these are for the use of authorized beneficiaries and are not available to the general public.

Head
Scientific Publications Section
Office of Scientific and Health Reports
National Institute of
NEUROLOGICAL DISORDERS AND STROKE
Building 31, Room 8A06
9000 Rockville Pike
Bethesda, MD 20892
(301) 496-5924

Services: The National Institute of Neurological Disorders and Stroke (NINDS) conducts and supports research and research training on the causes, prevention, diagnosis, and treatment of neurological disorders and stroke. NINDS awards grants for research projects, program projects, and center grants; provides training support to institutions and fellowships to individuals in the field of neurological and disorders and stroke; conducts intramural and collaborative research; and collects and disseminates research information.

Publications: Consumer materials are available on amyotrophic lateral sclerosis, aphasia, autism, cerebral palsy, dementias, epilepsy, Friedreich's ataxia, Huntington's disease, multiple sclerosis, muscular dystrophy, myasthenia gravis, neurofibromatosis, Parkinson's disease, shingles, spina bifida, spinal cord injury, torsion dystonia, stroke, head injury, Gaucher's disease, Nieman-Pick disease, Fabry's disease, Tay-Sachs disease, Farber's disease, metachrometic leukodystrophy, and lipid storage diseases. Professional materials are available on neurological disorders, stroke, epilepsy, Alzheimer's disease, and spinal cord injuries. A publications list is available.

Reference Librarian
Public Document Room
NUCLEAR REGULATORY Commission
2120 L Street NW, Lower Level
Washington, DC 20555
(202) 634-3273 (reference librarian)
(800) 638-8282 (hearing impaired)
(800) 492-8106 (Maryland residents only)

Services: The Public Document Room (PDR) of the Nuclear Regulatory Commission (NRC) is the headquarters and principal collection in a system of more than 130 local public document rooms. The PDR collection contains about 1,640,000 items and adds an average of 265 documents a day. Reports, meeting transcripts, existing and proposed regulations, copies of licenses, and official correspondence are available for inspection and reproduction by the public. The majority of the documents relate to design, construction, operation, and inspection of nuclear power plants and to the use, transport, and disposal of nuclear materials. Staff librarians will help users locate materials through indexes and a database of descriptive citations of documents added since October 1978. The local PDRs are generally located in public and university libraries. A national toll-free number, (800)638-8081, is maintained by the local PDR in Bethesda, Maryland, for assistance with questions about collection content, search strategies, and retrieval of information in the local PDRs. PDR headquarters provides a similar service.

Publications: *Citizen's Guide to U.S. Nuclear Regulatory Commission Information, Public Document Room User's Guide,* and *Public Document Room File Classification System* are all aids to finding information in the PDR system.

Administrator's Office
Human **NUTRITION INFORMATION** Service
Department of Agriculture
6505 Belcrest Road
Hyattsville, MD 20782
(301) 436-7725; (301) 436-5078 (electronic bulletin board)

Services: The Human Nutrition Information Service (HNIS) conducts applied research in food consumption, nutrition knowledge and attitudes, dietary survey methodology, food composition, and dietary guidance and nutrition education techniques. HNIS uses the research data to monitor the food and nutrient content of diets of the American population, assess dietary status and trends in food consumption, further understand the factors that influence consumer food choices, maintain the National Nutrient Data Bank of the nutrient content of foods, provide dietary guidance in food selection and preparation and in food money management, and develop materials and techniques to help increase nutrition knowledge and to improve food selection and management. HNIS conducts the Nationwide Food Consumption Survey, the Continuing Survey of Food Intakes by Individuals, and the Diet-Health Knowledge Survey. Within the Department of Agriculture, HMS coordinates the review and publication of Dietary Guidelines for Americans and develops information to help Americans put the guidelines into practice.

Publications: HNIS reports results of research on food consumption, food composition, and dietary guidance in both technical and popular publications, in forms that can be used by computers and by electronic bulletin board via telephone modem at (301) 436-5078. An HNIS publications list that includes ordering information is available to the public at the address above.

Office of Information
National Institute for **OCCUPATIONAL SAFETY** and Health
Centers for Disease Control
Building 1, Room 3106
1600 Clifton Road NE
Atlanta, GA 30333
(404) 639-3061

Services: The Office of Information serves as the point of contact relating to the policies of the National Institute for Occupational Safety and Health (NIOSH). The office answers questions of a nontechnical nature in the occupational safety and health field and provides single copies of NIOSH publications to visitors.

Database: The Registry of Toxic Effects of Chemical Substances (RTECS), formerly called the Toxic Substances List, is compiled annually and is searchable via the National Library of Medicine's MEDLARS system.

Service Limitations: Telephone or mail requests for publications and technical inquiries are referred to the Clearinghouse for Occupational Safety and Health.

Director of Information and Consumer Affairs
OCCUPATIONAL SAFETY AND HEALTH Administration
U.S. Department of Labor
200 Constitution Avenue NW, Room N-3647
Washington,DC 20210
(202) 523-8148

Services: Under the Occupational Safety and Health Act of 1970, the Occupational Safety and Health Administration (OSHA) was created to encourage employers and employees to reduce workplace hazards and implement new or improved safety and health programs; establish separate but dependent responsibilities and rights for employers and employees to achieve better safety and health conditions; maintain a reporting and record-keeping system to monitor job-related injuries and illnesses; develop mandatory job safety and health standards and enforce them; and provide for the development, analysis, evaluation, and approval of State occupational safety and health programs. The Act also provides six distinct provisions for protecting the safety and health of Federal workers on the job. OSHA also encourages a broad range of voluntary workplace improvement efforts, including consultation programs, training and education efforts, grants to increase safety and health compliance, and a variety of other similar programs.

Publications: Materials are available on occupational health, occupational safety, asbestos, back injuries, emergency response, hazard communication, Federal regulations, hearing, accidents, statistical data, and carcinogens. Some are available in Spanish. OSHA also has a number of audiovisual presentations. In addition, OSHA develops and distributes training programs on health and safety. Some materials are available from the National Technical Information Service or Government Printing Office. A print and audiovisual publication list is available upon request with a self-addressed mailing label.

Technical Information Branch
Clearinghouse for
OCCUPATIONAL SAFETY AND HEALTH INFORMATION
4676 Columbia Parkway, Mail Stop C-19
Cincinnati, OH 45226
(513) 533-8326
(800)35-NIOSH

Services: The Technical Information Branch (TIB), formerly the Clearinghouse for Occupational Safety and Health Information, established in

1976, is a merger of several technical information components that existed within the National Institute for Occupational Safety and Health (NIOSH). TIB provides technical information support for NIOSH research programs and provides information to others on request. Services include reference and referral, interlibrary loans, and information about NIOSH studies. The library consists of about 12,000 books and 1,100 periodicals in 2 library locations with no restrictions on their onsite use.

Database: NIOSHTIC is a current and retrospective database indexing materials dating back to the 1800s covering the field of occupational safety and health. The database contains approximately 170,000 citations and grows at a rate of about 9,000 citations per year. Updates are made monthly. Sources indexed by this database include journal articles, materials from the International Labor Organization's Clearinghouse for Occupational Safety and Health, the International Occupational Safety and Health Information Center database, and references from NIOSH Criteria Documents and Current Intelligence Bulletins. Abstracts are contained in each record. A thesaurus is used for indexing the documents. The database is available through DIALOG and Pergammon as Occupational Safety and Health (NIOSH). NIOSHTIC is available on CD-ROM.

Publications: Publications include a subject indexed catalog of NIOSH materials that gives information about availability. A new publications list is issued periodically. TIB disseminates all NIOSH numbered publications. Archived copies of all NIOSH publications can be obtained on microfiche or in hardcopy from the National Technical Information Service (NTIS).

Information Specialist
National Information Center for
ORPHAN DRUGS and Rare Diseases
P.O. Box 1133
Washington, DC 20013-1133
(800) 456-3505

Services: The National Information Center for Orphan Drugs and Rare Diseases (NICODARD), a component of the Office of Disease Prevention and Health Promotion (ODPHP) National Health Information Center (ONHIC), gathers and disseminates information and responds to inquiries from patients, health professionals, and the general public. Orphan drugs or products are those used to prevent or treat rare diseases. Rare diseases or conditions are defined as those with a prevalence in the United States of 200,000 cases or fewer. NICODARD information specialists respond to questions by using ONHIC's computer database, library, and referral system. ONHIC's database contains descriptions of many health-related organizations, including rare disease voluntary organizations. Information specialists determine which organization(s) can best answer the question, then refer the caller or forward the question to the organization(s) for direct response. Other questions are answered with information from the ONHIC library or other resources. NICODARD staff does not diagnose illness or provide medical advice. In addition to responding to inquiries, NICODARD gathers information to enhance the ONHIC database and library collection, refers inquiries to voluntary and other organizations, and gathers research data. NICODARD is sponsored by the Office of Orphan Products Development, Food and Drug Administration.

Director of Information
President's Council on **PHYSICAL FITNESS** and Sports
450 Fifth Street NW., Suite 7103
Washington, DC 20001
(202) 272-3430

Services: The President's Council on Physical Fitness and Sports (PCPFS) is an outgrowth of the President's Council on Youth Fitness, established in 1956. PCPFS conducts a public service advertising program, prepares educational materials, and cooperates with government and private groups to promote the development of physical fitness leadership, facilities, and programs. PCPFS also works with schools, clubs, recreation agencies, and major employers on program design and implementation; advises Federal agencies on the conduct of fitness-related programs; and offers a variety of testing, recognition, and incentive programs for individuals, institutions, and organizations.

Publications: Materials are available on exercise, school physical education programs, corporate fitness, and physical fitness for youth, adults, and senior citizens. Citations, including abstracts, come from 2,000 journals. A publications list is available.

Serial publications: *President's Council on Physical Fitness and Sports Newsletter* (bimonthly)—articles on conferences, exemplary physical fitness programs, information about free materials, sports competitions, and news from other organizations); and *Physical Fitness/Sports Medicine* (quarterly bibliography)—extracted from the MEDLARS database encompassing exercise physiology, sports injuries, physical conditioning, and medical aspects of exercise.

InformationSpecialist
POLICY INFORMATION Center
Department of Health and Human Services
HHH Building, Room 438-F
200 Independence Avenue SW
Washington, DC 20201
(202) 245-6445

Services: The Policy Information Center (PIC), formerly the Evaluation Documentation Center, provides a centralized repository of evaluations and short-term evaluative research and policy oriented projects conducted by the Department of Health and Human Services (DHHS); program inspections and audits conducted by the Office of Inspector General of DHHS; projects relevant to DHHS conducted by the Congressional Budget Office, General Accounting Office, and Office of Technology Assessment; and most recently, reports conducted by the Institute of Medicine and the National Research Council's Committee on National Statistics, both part of the National Academy of Sciences. PIC collects the information on a one-page description sheet that contains administrative data and an abstract for the DHHS-sponsored projects. The projects are monitored throughout the life of the study. Non-DHHS reports are entered at time of completion.

Database: All descriptions are stored in the computer-readable PIC database. PIC also maintains a library of final reports and executive summaries and makes these available to departmental personnel and others. Copies of final reports are available to the general public through the National Technical Information Service for a fee.

Serial publication: *Compendium of HHS Evaluations and Other Relevant Studies* (annual)—project descriptions of all in-process and completed studies entered into the PIC database.

Deputy Director
Office of **PREPAID HEALTH CARE**
Health Care Financing Administration
Wilbur J. Cohen Building, Room 4360
330 Independence Avenue SW
Washington, DC 20201
(202) 619-0815

Services: The Office of Prepaid Health Care (OPHC), an office of the Health Care Financing Administration (HCFA), includes all components of the former Office of Health Maintenance Organizations of the Public Health Service. OPHC serves as the departmental focal point to advance the managed care concept under Medicare and Medicaid and has regulatory authority over federally qualified health maintenance organizations (HMOs). Specific activities are carried out in the areas of Federal qualifications of HMOs and compliance with provisions of the Public Health Service Act dealing with federally qualified HMOs; granting and administration of Medicare contracts between HCFA and federally qualified HMOs, "competitive medical plans" (CMPs), and other types of managed care plans; and policy direction and technical assistance to HCFA regional offices and State agencies on Medicaid managed care issues. OPHC also serves as the focal point for directions in national health care policy related to managed care.

Publications: OPHC distributes materials on HMOs and competitive medical plans and maintains financial, enrollment, and service area information on such plans.

Project Director
National Clearinghouse for **PRIMARY CARE** Information
8201 Greensboro Drive, Suite 600
Mclean, VA 22102
(703) 821-8955

Services: Established in 1983, the National Clearinghouse for Primary Care Information (NCPCI) provides information services to support the planning, development, and delivery of ambulatory health care to urban and rural areas that have shortages of medical personnel and services. NCPCI distributes publications focusing on ambulatory care, financial management, primary health care, and health services administration that will be of special interest to professionals working in primary care centers funded by the Bureau of Health Care Delivery and Assistance.

Service Limitations: Although NCPCI will respond to requests from the general public, its primary audience is health care practitioners and administrators.

Publications: Materials are available on childhood injury prevention programs, health education, governing boards, financial management, sexually transmitted diseases, lead poisoning, administrative management, and clinical care. Bilingual medical phrase books, a directory of federally funded health centers, and an annotated bibliography are also available.

Information Specialist
Consumer **PRODUCT SAFETY** Commission
5401 Westbard Avenue, Room 332
Bethesda, MD 20892
(800) 638-2772 (Consumer Product Safety hot line-national)
(800) 638-8270 (hearing impaired—national)
(800) 492-8104 (hearing impaired—Maryland)

Services: The Consumer Product Safety Commission (CPSC) was established in 1972 to reduce injuries and deaths resulting from the use of consumer products. CPSC maintains the National Injury Information Clearinghouse, conducts investigations into incidents of alleged unsafe/defective products, and establishes product safety standards. CPSC assists consumers in evaluating the comparative safety of products, and conducts information and education programs to increase consumer awareness of dangerous products. CPSC operates the National Electronic Injury Surveillance System, which monitors a statistical sample of hospital emergency rooms for injuries associated with consumer products. CPSC maintains a free telephone hotline workdays 8:30 a.m. to 5 p.m. to provide information about recalls and about product safety. Hotline operators are on duty to receive reports on product-related accidents workdays 11:30 a.m. to 4:30 p.m.

Publications: CPSC publishes a variety of publications describing hazards associated with such products as children's toys and electrical products and suggesting ways to avoid these hazards. Descriptions of the laws and regulations CPSC administers are also available. To receive information and a publications list, consumers may write to CPSC, Washington, DC 20207.

Office of Communications
PUBLIC HEALTH Service
Department of Health and Human Services
200 Independence Avenue SW, Room 717-H
Washington, DC 20201
(202) 245-6867

Services: The Office of Communications of the Public Health Service (PHS) provides information on PHS, its components, and its programs. General inquiries from the public and questions regarding the policies of the Office of the Assistant Secretary for Health, which oversees PHS, are answered or referred to one of the seven PHS agencies.

RADIOPHARMACEUTICAL Internal Dose Information Center
Medical Sciences Division
P.O.Box 117
Oak Ridge Associated Universities
Oak Ridge, TN 37831-0117
(615) 576-3450

Services: The Radiopharmaceutical Internal Dose Information Center serves researchers at government agencies and nuclear medicine centers as well as private physicians having questions about internal radiation dose calculations, especially those involving radiopharmaceuticals. Information about the internal distribution of radioactive compounds is collected, interpreted, and correlated. The staff provides information to researchers who are developing new radiopharmaceuticals and answers requests for dose estimates. The center is often contacted when specialized knowledge of radiation dose calculation techniques is required and when an accidental intake of radioactive material occurs. The Department of Energy and the Food and Drug Administration sponsor the center.

Database: An inhouse database contains more than 34,000 bibliographic references concerning radiopharmaceutical kinetics, decay scheme data, calculation techniques, phantoms, and mathematical models.

Information Specialist
National **REHABILITATION INFORMATION** Center
8455 Colesville Road, Suite 935
Silver Spring,MD 20910
(301) 588-9284
(800) 34-NARIC

Services: The National Rehabilitation Information Center (NARIC), established in 1977, is a service of the National Institute on Disability and Rehabilitation, Department of Education. NARIC supplies publications on disability-related topics, prepares bibliographies tailored to specific requests, and assists in locating answers to questions. The NARIC collection includes materials relevant to the rehabilitation of all disability groups, as well as documents relevant to professional and administrative practices and concerns. The collection contains over 300 periodical titles and over 20,000 research reports, books, and audiovisual materials. The public can use the collection or order materials from NARIC.

Database: REHABDATA contains bibliographic information and abstracts for the entire NARIC collection, including materials produced from 1950 to the present. Direct access to the database is available through BRS. In addition, the REHABDATA thesaurus is a useful aid for database searching.

Service Limitations: There is a charge for photo duplication. Customized literature searches of the NARIC databases are available for nominal fees.

Publications: Materials include a periodical holdings list and subject catalog. NARIC also publishes a directory of rehabilitation librarians.

Serial publication: *NARIC Quarterly,* free newsletter.

Office of the Commissioner
REHABILITATION SERVICES Administration
Department of Education
Switzer Building, Room 3028
330 C Street SW
Washington, DC 20202
(202) 732-1282

Services: The Rehabilitation Services Administration (RSA) administers a number of programs authorized under the Rehabilitation Act of 1973, as amended. A major program is the basic State-Federal vocational rehabilitation (VR) program under which State VR agencies provide a wide variety of services to eligible physically and mentally handicapped individuals to enable them to become gainfully employed. Other State administered programs include independent living services, which offer support to handicapped individuals to enable them to function more independently in the home and community, and supported employment services, which provide intensive time-limited support to severely handicapped individuals at the workplace in coordination with ongoing services provided by other public or private community resources. In addition to the programs that offer direct services to individuals, RSA supports a number of programs and projects to strengthen and improve the rehabilitation services delivery system. Among these are the Client Assistance Program, projects with industry, the establishment of rehabilitation facilities, services to handicapped migratory and seasonal farmworkers, Native American services, and training grants to increase and upgrade the supply of rehabilitation personnel. RSA also supports a number of special projects that focus on strengthening and improving services for severely disabled people, including those handicapped by blindness, deafness, epilepsy, cerebral palsy, multiple sclerosis, and spinal cord injuries. The Helen Keller National Center for deaf-blind youth and adults is authorized to provide special services for the rehabilitation of persons who are both deaf and blind. RSA also administers the Randolph-Sheppard Act, under which blind persons are licensed to operate vending facilities on Federal and other property.

Publications: RSA distributes program information and a list of State vocational rehabilitation agencies.

Serial publication: *American Rehabilitation* (quarterly).

Information Officer
National Center for **RESEARCH RESOURCES**
National Institutes of Health
Building 12A, Room 4007
9000 Rockville Pike
Bethesda, MD 20892
(301) 496-5793
(301) 251-4970 (Research Resources Information Center)

Services: The National Center for Research Resources (NCRR), a component of the National Institutes of Health (NIH), comprises six extramural programs and four intramural programs/branches. The extramural programs fund development and support of biomedical research resources at institutions nationwide, generally health professional schools, colleges, and universities. The extramural programs include general clinical research centers, animal resources, biomedical research technology, biomedical research support, research centers in minority institutions, and biological models and materials resources. The intramural components, providing research resources for NIH intramural investigators, are the biomedical engineering and instrumentation program, library branch, medical arts and photography branch, and the veterinary resources program. The Research Resources Information Center, a contractor-operated service of NCRR, provides publications and answers questions covering the spectrum of biomedical science and technology. Inquiries pertaining to grants funded by extramural programs should be directed to the appropriate program at the following address:

5333 Westbard Avenue
Westwood Building
Bethesda, MD 20892

General Clinical Research Centers Programs
Director
(301) 496-6595
Room 10A03

Animal Resources Program
Director
(301) 496-5175
Room 857

Biomedical Research Technology Program
Director
(301) 496-5411
Room 8A15

Biomedical Research Support Program
Director
(301) 496-6743
Room 10A11

Research Centers in Minority Institutions
Director
301) 496-6341
Room 10A10

Biological Models and Materials Resources
Program Director
(301) 402-0630
Room 8A07

Inquiries pertaining to grants funded by intramural programs and branches should be directed to the appropriate program at the following address:

9000 Rockville Pike
Bethesda, MD 20892

Biomedical Engineering and
Instrumentation Program
Director
(301) 496-4741
Building 13, Room 3W-13

Library Branch
Chief
(301) 496-2447
Building 10, Room 1L-25G

Medical Arts and Photography Branch
Chief
(301) 496-2868
Building 10, Room B2L-316

Veterinary Resources Program
Director
(301) 496-2527
Building 14G, Room 102

For inquiries on biomedical science and technology contact:

Science Advisor
Research Resources Information Center
1601 Research Boulevard
Rockville, MD 20850
(301) 2514970

Publications: A variety of reports, resource directories, and reprints are available for consumers and health professionals

SCHIZOPHRENIA Research Branch
Division of Clinical Research
National Institute of Mental Health
Parklawn Building, Room 10C-16
5600 Fishers Lane
Rockville, MD 20857
(301) 443-4707

Services: The Schizophrenia Research Branch plans and supports programs of research, research training, and resource development in the classification, assessment, etiology, genetics, clinical course, and outcome, as well as pharmacologic, somatic, and psychosocial treatment and rehabilitation, of schizophrenia and related disorders. It reviews and evaluates research developments in the field and recommends new program directions. It collaborates with organizations within and outside the National Institute of Mental Health to stimulate work in the field through conferences and workshops. In a coordinated effort with the Office of Scientific Information, the branch disseminates research knowledge. It utilizes the full range of assistance and procurement instruments such as research grants, cooperative agreements, and contracts to develop and execute programmatic activities, including the collection, organization, and analysis of relevant data.

Service Limitations: The branch's information services are limited to **use by mental health professionals and researchers.**

Serial publications: *Schizophrenia Bulletin* (quarterly journal) and *Psychopharmacology Bulletin* (quarterly journal).

Reference Service
SCIENCE and Technology Division
Library of Congress
Adams Building, 5th Floor
101 Independence Avenue, LA5112
Washington, DC 20540
(202) 707-5664

Services: The Science and Technology Division provides reference services and serves as a focal point for the millions of books, journals, and technical reports on scientific and technological topics at the Library of Congress (LC). Direct reference services are provided to users by telephone, by mail, or in person. Bibliographic guides and research reports by division subject specialists and reference librarians provide indirect reference service. The division also has primary responsibility for recommending LC acquisitions in all fields of science and technology except technical agriculture and clinical medicine.

Publications: Various library guides on the use of the Science Reading Room, including How to Find Technical Reports in the Library of Congress, are available.

Serial publication: *LC Science Tracer Bullet* (informal series)—topics in the series include acupuncture, diabetes mellitus, anorexia nervosa/bulimia, AIDS, hypertension, birth defects, drug abuse, nuclear medicine, osteoporosis, Alzheimer's, electromagnetic fields (physiology and health effects), stress, noise pollution, and medicinal plants. Individual *Tracer Bullets* and a master list of the *Tracer Bullets* series are available free. HR/2001

Technical Information Center
Office on **SMOKING AND HEALTH**
Centers for Disease Control
Park Building, Room 1-16
5600 Fishers Lane
Rockville, MD 20857
(301) 443-1690

Services: The Office on Smoking and Health (OSH) offers bibliographic and reference services to researchers through its Technical Information Center (TIC). TIC publishes and distributes a number of titles in the field of smoking and health and possesses the computer capability, through its automated search and retrieval system, to generate comprehensive bibliographic printouts on topics of current interest in smoking and health. In addition to the bibliographic services offered, OSH has an Epidemiology Branch for the collection and analysis of numeric data sets which contain significant tobacco use information. This section also designs and conducts national surveys on smoking behavior, attitudes, knowledge, and beliefs among adult and teenagers on a periodic basis, and works with other individuals and organizations that are interested in incorporating smoking behavior as part of their survey research activities. Visitors may use the collection weekdays from 8:30 a.m. to 5 p.m. Advance arrangements for visits are suggested.

Database: The Smoking and Health Database contains almost 50,000 citations and abstracts. Sources indexed include journal articles, conference reports, and newsletters. Reference services are also provided by telephone. Copies of reference items are provided only in single copies, and only in cases where material cannot be obtained from other sources.

Publications: OSH offers consumer publications on smoking and teenagers, smoking and pregnancy, and smoking cessation. Materials for professionals cover cancer, heart disease, and lung disease associated with smoking.

Serial publications: *Smoking and Health Bulletin* (quarterly)—abstracts of current literature, *Bibliography of Smoking and Health* (annual), and *Health Consequences of Smoking* (the annual report of the Surgeon General).

Associate Commissioner
Office of Public Affairs
SOCIAL SECURITY Administration
West High Rise Building Room 4200
6401 Security Boulevard
Baltimore, MD 21235
(301) 965-1720

Services: The Office of Public Affairs of the Social Security Administration (SSA) provides public information materials about the Social Security and Supplemental Security Income (SSI) programs, as well as information on entitlement to Medicare. Inquiries concerning the Social Security and SSI programs can be directed to the Office of Public Affairs. Inquiries about the Medicare program should be directed to Health Care Financing Administration, Office of Beneficiary Services, Room 648, East High Rise Building, 6401 Security Boulevard, Baltimore, MD 21235. At the local level, inquiries can be made to any Social Security office.

Library collection: The collection holds 29,639 titles on topics including social sciences, health economics, law, personnel management, business and administrative management, and computer/information systems. The library is open 8:30 a.m. to 5 p.m. to Federal employees and open to the public by special arrangement.

Database: Custom searches for SSA personnel are provided.

Publications: Pamphlets on Social Security benefits, disability benefits, and supplemental security income are available. Medicare brochures can be obtained from the Health Care Financing Administration. Publications are free of charge.

Project Director
National **SUDDEN INFANT DEATH SYNDROME** Clearinghouse
8201 Greensboro Drive, Suite 600
McLean,VA 22102
(703) 821-8955

Services: The National Sudden Infant Death Syndrome Clearinghouse was established in 1980 to provide information and educational materials on sudden infant death syndrome (SIDS), apnea, and other related issues. Clearinghouse staff responds to information requests from professionals, families with SIDS-related deaths, and the general public by sending written materials and making referrals. The clearinghouse maintains a library of standard reference materials covering etiology, epidemiology, research, counseling, effects on families, training of emergency personnel, legal aspects, treatment, and prevention of SIDS. The clearinghouse staff also compiles annotated bibliographies on a variety of topics and maintains and updates mailing lists of State programs, groups, and individuals concerned with SIDS. In addition, the clearinghouse has fact sheets, catalogs, and bibliographies on areas of special interest to the community.

Database: The clearinghouse has an inhouse database of bibliographic references to professional and family-oriented print materials.

Publications: The clearinghouse distributes publications on SIDS to professionals, parents, and the public.

Serial publication: *Information Exchange* (quarterly newsletter)—promotes the exchange of information among SIDS groups nationwide.

National Second **SURGICAL OPINION** Program
Health Care Financing Administration
200 Independence Avenue SW
Washington, DC 20201
(202) 245-6183 (public information specialist)
(800) 638-6833; (800) 492-6603 (Maryland only)

Services: The National Second Surgical Opinion Program, established in 1978, is an information resource for people faced with the possibility of non-emergency surgery. The program sponsors the Government's toll-free telephone number to assist callers in locating a surgeon or other specialist. Written requests for information are answered within 14 days.

Publications: A pamphlet is available that poses questions a patient should ask and suggests ways to find a specialist to get a second opinion. Write Surgery, Department of Health and Human Services, Washington, DC 20201.

National **TECHNICAL INFORMATION** Service
Department of Commerce
5285 Port Royal Road
Springfield, VA 22161
(703) 487-4650

Services: The National Technical Information Service (NTIS) is the central source for the public sale of U.S. and foreign government-sponsored research and development and engineering report and other analysis prepared by Federal and local government agencies. NTIS provides access to both completed and ongoing research.

Database: The NTIS bibliographic database contains more than 1.4 million summaries of completed government research and development and engineering results. The searchable files begin with 1964. More than 60,000 information items are added annually. These consist of 55,000 technical reports, plus computerized datafiles, databases, software, proceedings, training guides, manuals, and other items. The bibliographic database is updated twice monthly and is available for lease. It is also available online from BRS, Datastar, DIALOG, Orbit, and STN, and on CDROM from Dialog, OCLC, and Silver Platter. Batch searching and SDI services are available through NERAC, Inc. Reports indexed in the N1IS bibliographic database can be ordered as paper copy or microfiche. Datafiles, databases, and software are available on magnetic tape and diskette. The Federal Research in Progress (FEDRIP) database provides access to ongoing federally funded research projects. FEDRIP is a compilation of input from nine Government agencies. The areas of health and medicine are most prominent for input from the National Institutes of Health, the Veterans Administration, and the National Institute for Occupational Safety and Health. FEDRIP is updated monthly and is available for lease or online from DIALOG.

Publications: A free copy of the NTIS Products and Services brochure (#PR-827) is available.

Serial publication: Abstract newsletters—weekly bulletins providing summaries of the most recent reports added to the NTIS collection in specific fields such as agriculture and food, biomedical technology and human factors engineering, environmental pollution and control, health planning, medicine, biology, and toxicology.

Program Manager for Health
Office of **TECHNOLOGY ASSESSMENT**
Congress of the United States
Washington, DC 20510
(202) 228-6590; (202) 2244996 (publications)

Services: The Office of Technology Assessment (OTA) assesses complex scientific and technological issues for the benefit of Congressional committees. Comprehensive analyses are conducted on issues such as energy, the environment, national security, transportation, and health. OTA provides reports, testimony, and workshops to clarify the range of policy options on an issue and the potential effects of adopting each option.

Publications: OTA publishes an annual report, press releases, a catalog of publications, research reports, and report summaries. The summaries are available to the public free of charge. Assessments in the health field have included such topics as the cost-effectiveness of medical technology, Federal immunization policy, physician reimbursement, medical information systems, adolescent health, rural health, child health, and priorities for tropical disease research, aging, genetic therapy, occupational health, medical devices, pharmaceuticals, health care costs, disabilities, environmental health, and unconventional cancer treatment. Research reports are for sale by the National Technical Information Service or the U.S. Government Printing Office. OTA can provide availability and price information. A publications list and an informational brochure are also available.

Communications and Inquiries
Department of **VETERANS** Affairs
810 Vermont Avenue NW
Washington, DC 20420
(202) 233-5081

Services: The Department of Veterans Affairs (VA) was established as the Veterans Administration in 1930 and elevated to cabinet level on March 15, 1989. The VA provides a wide range of veterans' benefits in such areas as health care, education, housing, disability pensions, and life insurance. Through its network of hospitals, clinics, and nursing homes, the VA provides a full range of medical, long-term care, and patient support services. Veterans with service-related illnesses or injuries receive priority for VA medical services, and special consideration is also given veterans who are in financial need, over 65 years old, or holders of the Congressional Medal of Honor. The VA is also involved in medical research and the training of health professionals. Training programs include undergraduate, graduate, and continuing education, a medical library, and assistance for health manpower training institutions. VA benefits are restricted to U.S. military veterans.

Publications: The VA publishes annual reports and booklets describing benefits and programs and produces audiovisual materials for medical staff training.

National Resource Center on
WORKSITE HEALTH PROMOTION
North Capitol Street NE, Suite 800
Washington, DC 20002
(202) 408-9320

Services: The National Resource Center for Worksite Health Promotion provides information about currently operating worksite health promotion programs in American corporations. The center also provides bibliographies of lowcost and free worksite health promotion materials available to businesses and develops lists of vendors offering health promotion services.

Database: The resource center's database contains information about currently operating selected worksite health promotion programs in American corporations.

Publications: *Wellness Programs for Older Workers and Retirees*, and *Worksite Wellness Media Reports* are available.

YOUTH DEVELOPMENT Information Center
National Agricultural Library
U.S. Department of Agriculture
Room 304, 10301 Baltimore Boulevard
Beltsville, MD 20705
(301) 344-3719

Services: The Youth Development Information Center provides information services to professionals who plan, develop, implement, and evaluate programs designed to meet the changing needs of America's youth. The center combines the technical and subject-matter expertise of the Cooperative Extension Service's nationwide educational network with the information specialists and resources of the world's foremost agricultural library. The center also assists educators and researchers working with youth in obtaining current literature regarding communication, educational design, youth development, youth program management, and volunteerism. In addition, the center acquires print and audiovisual resources and develops resource lists and bibliographies. Document delivery services include lending books and audiovisuals through local or institutional libraries; providing photocopies of journal articles not easily found elsewhere; and helping determine which library owns a particular book, journal, or audiovisual. The center is part of the National Agricultural Library, which is open to the public 8 a.m. to 4:30 p.m. Monday through Friday.

Database: AGRICOLA is accessible through BRS and DIALOG.

Service Limitations: There is a fee for extended information and research services.

Appendix B

Directory of State Health Departments

Alabama

State Department of Public Health
State Office Building
Montgomery, AL 36130-1701
Telephone: (205) 242-5052
Fax: (205) 240-3097

Alaska

State Department of Health and
Social Services
Division of Public Health
P. O. Box 110601
Juneau, AK 99811-0600
Telephone: (907) 465-3039
Fax: (907) 586-1977

Arizona

State Department of Health Ser-
vices
1740 West Adams St.
Phoenix, AZ 85007
Telephone: (602) 542-1024
Fax: (602) 542-1062

Arkansas

State Health Building
4815 W. Markham
Little Rock, AR 72205-3867
Telephone: (501) 661-2111
Fax: (501) 661-2601

California

State Department of Health Ser-
vices
714 P St., Office Building #8/1253
Sacramento, CA 95814
Telephone: (916) 657-1425
Fax: (916) 657-1156

Colorado

State Department of Public Health
Division of Consumer Protection
4210 East 11th Ave.
Denver, CO 80220
Telephone (303) 331-6752
Fax: (303) 320-1529

Connecticut

State Department of Health Services
150 Washington St.
Hartford, CT 06106
Telephone: (203) 566-2038
Fax: (203) 566-1710

Delaware

State Department of Health and Social Services
Division of Public Health
Cooper Memorial Building
Water and Federal Sts.
Dover, DE 19901
Telephone: (302) 739-4701
Fax: (302) 739-3008

District of Columbia

Department of Consumer and Regulatory Affairs
614 H St., NW
Washington, DC 20001
Telephone: (202) 727-7170 Fax: (202) 727-7842

Florida

State Department of Health and Rehabilitative Services
State Health Office
1317 Winewood Blvd.
Tallahasee, FL 32301
Telephone: (904) 487-2705
No Fax

Georgia

State Department of Human Resources
Division of Public Health
878 Peachtree St., NE
Atlanta, GA 30309
Telephone: (404) 894-7505
No Fax

Hawaii

State Department of Health
Kinau Hale Building
1250 Punchbowl St.
P. O. Box 3378
Honolulu, HI 96813
Telephone: (808) 548-6505
Fax: (808) 548-3263

Idaho

State Department of Health and Welfare
Division of Health
450 West State St.
Statehouse Mail
Boise, ID 83720-9990
Telephone: (208) 334-5946
Fax: (208) 334-5694

Illinois

State Department of Public Health
Office of Health Protection
535 West Jefferson
Springfield, IL 62761
Telephone: (217) 782-3984
Fax: (217) 524-6090

Indiana

State Board of Health
Bureau of Consumer Protection
1330 West Michigan St.
P. O. Box 1964
Indianapolis, IN 46206-19645
Telephone: (317) 633-0313
Fax: (317) 633-0776

Iowa

State Department of Public Health
Lucas State Office Building
Des Moines, IA 50319-0083
Telephone: (515) 281-5605
Fax: (515) 281-4958

Kansas

State Department of Health and Environment
Landon State Office Bldg.
900 S.W. Jackson St.
Topeka, KS 66612-1290
Telephone: (913) 296-0461
Fax: (913) 296-7119

Kentucky

Cabinet for Human Resources
275 East Main St.
Frankfort,KY 40621
Telephone: (502) 564-7130
Fax: (502) 564-6533

Louisiana

State Department of Health and Hospitals
Office of Public Health
325 Loyola Ave.
P. O. Box 60630
New Orleans, LA 70160
Telephone: (504) 568-5051
Fax: (504) 568-2609

Maine

State Department of Human Services
 Bureau of Health
State House Station 11
Augusta, ME 04333
Telephone: (207) 289-3201
No fax

Maryland

State Department of Health and Mental Hygiene
Office of Food Protection and Consumer Health Services
4201 Patterson Ave.
Baltimore, MD 21214-2299
Telephone: (410) 764-3579
Fax: (410) 764-3591

Massachusetts

Executive Office of Human Services
State Department of Public Health
150 Tremont Street
Boston, MA 02111
Telephone: (617) 727-0202
Fax: (617) 727-6496

Michigan

State Department of Public Health
3423 North Logan St.
P. O. Box 30195
Lansing, MI 48909
Telephone: (517) 335-8022
Fax: (517) 335-8298

Minnesota

State Health Department
State Dept. of Health Bldg.
717 Delaware St., SE
Minneapolis, MN 55440
Telephone: (612) 623-5460
Fax (612) 623-5067

Mississippi

State Board of Health
P. O. Box 1700
2423 North State St.
Jackson, MS 39215-1700
Telephone: (601) 960-7634
Fax: (601) 960-7948

Missouri

State Department of Health
1730 East Elm St.
P.O.Box 570
Jefferson City, MO 65102
(314) 751-6001
Fax: (314) 751-6010

Montana

State Department of Health and
Environmental Sciences
Food and Consumer Safety Bureau
W. F. Cogswell Bldg.
Capitol Station
Helena, MT 59620
Telephone: (406) 444-3671
Fax: (406) 444-2606

Nebraska

State Department of Health
301 Centennial Mall South
P. O. Box 95007
Lincoln, NB 68509
Telephone: (402) 471-2133
Fax: (402) 471-0383

Nevada

State Department of Human Resources
Health Division
505 East King St., Rm. 600
Carson City, NV 89710
Telephone: (702) 687-4740
Fax: (702) 687-3859

New Hampshire

State Department of Health and
Human Services
Divison of Public Health Services
Health and Welfare Bldg.
6 Hazen Drive
Concord, NH 03301-6527
Telephone: (603) 271-4501
Fax: (603) 271-2896

New Jersey

State Department of Health
Consumer Health Services
Health-Agriculture Bldg.
John Fitch Plaza
CN-369
Trenton,NJ 08625
Telephone: (609) 984-0794
Fax: (609) 292-3580

New Mexico

State Department of Health
1190 St. Francis Drive
Santa Fe, NM 87503
Telephone: (505) 827-2389
Fax: (505) 827-0097

New York

State Department of Health
Office of Public Health
Tower Building, Empire State Plaza
Albany,NY 12237-0001
Telephone: (518) 474-0180
Fax: (518) 474-7471

New York City Department of
Health
125 Worth St.
New York, NY 10013
Telephone: (212) 788-5261
Fax: (212) 571-1167

North Carolina

State Department of Environment
Health and Natural Resources
512 North Salisbury St.
P. O. Box 27687
Raleigh, NC 27611-7687
Telephone: (919) 733-4984
Fax: (919) 733-6801

North Dakota

State Department of Health and
Consolidated Laboratories
Division of Consumer Protection
2635 East Main Ave.
P. O. Box 937
Bismarck, ND 58502-0937
Telephone: (701) 221-6147
Fax: (701) 221-6145

Ohio

State Department of Health
246 North High St.
P. O. Box 118
Columbus, OH 43266-0118
Telephone: (614) 466-2253
Fax: (614) 644-8526

Oklahoma

State Department of Health
Consumer Protection Service
1000 Northeast Tenth St.
GCGD-0305
Oklahoma City, OK 73113-1299
Telephone: (404) 271-8056
Fax: (405) 271-7339

Oregon

State Department of Human Re-
sources
Health Division
1400 S.W. Fifth Ave.
P. O. Box 231
Portland, OR 97207
Telephone: (503) 229-5032
Fax: (503) 274-2524

Pennsylvania

State Department of Health
Health and Welfare Bldg.
7TH and Forster Sts.
P. O. Box 90
Harrisburg, PA 17108
Telephone: (717) 787-6436
Fax: (717) 783-3794

Rhode Island

State Department of Health
3 Capitol Hill
Providence, RI 02908-5097
Telephone: (401) 277-2231
Fax: (401) 277-6458

South Carolina

State Department of Health and
Environmental Control
Health Protection
J. Marion Sims Bldg.
2600 Bull St.
Columbia, SC 29101
Telephone: (803) 734-4880
Fax: (803) 734-4874

South Dakota

State Health Department
Division of Public Health
Joe Foss Bldg.
445 East Capitol Ave.
Pierre, SD 57501-3185
Telephone: (606) 773-3364
Fax: (605) 773-4840

Tennessee

State Department of Health and
Environment
Cordel Hull Bldg.
Nashville, TN 37247-0101
Telephone: (615) 741-3111
Fax: (615) 741-2491

Texas

State Department of Health
Bureau of Consumer Health Protection
1100 W. 49th
Austin, TX 78756-3189
Telephone: (512) 458-7537
Fax (512) 458-7622

Utah

State Department of Health
P. O. Box 16660
Salt Lake City, UT 84116
Telephone: (801) 538-6111
Fax: (801) 538-6694

Vermont

State Department of Health
60 Main St.
P. O. Box 709
Burlington, VT 05402
Telephone: (802) 863-7280
Fax: (802) 863-7425

Virginia

State Department of Health
1500 East Main St., Rm. 214
Richmond, VA 23218
Telephone: (804) 786-3561
No Fax

State Dept. of Agriculture and Consumer Services
1100 Bank St.
P. O. Box 1163
Richmond, VA 23209
Telephone: (804) 786-2042
Fax: (804) 371-2945

Washington

State Department of Health
Health Promotion/Chronic Disease
Prevention
M/S LL-14,
Olympia, WA 98504
Telephone: (206) 753-7521
Fax: (206) 586-5440

West Virginia

State Department of Health and
Human Resources
State Office Bldg., #3
1900 Kanawha Blvd., East
Charleston, WV 25305
Telephone: (304) 348-2971
No Fax

Wisconsin

State Department of Agriculture,
Trade, and Consumer Protection
801 West Badger Rd.
P. O. Box 8911
Madison, WI 53708
Telephone: (608) 266-7220
Fax: (608) 266-1300

Wyoming

State Department of Health and
Social Services
317 Hathaway Bldg.
Cheyenne, WY 82002-0710
Telephone: (307) 777-7656
Fax: (307) 777-7439

Appendix C

Public Health Information on the Internet

Centers for Disease Control and Prevention

Agency for Toxic Substances and Disease Registry
http://atsdr1.atsdr.cdc.gov:8080/

Centers for Disease Control and Prevention
http://www.cdc.gov

Epidemiology Program Office
http://www.cdc.gov/epo

Morbidity and Mortality Weekly Report
http://www.cdc.gov/epo/mmwr/mmrw.html

National Center for Chronic Disease Prevention
http://www.cdc.gov/nccdphp/

National Center for Environmental Health
http://ww.cdc.gov/nceh/ncehhome.htm

National Center for Health Statistics
http://www.cdc.gov/nchswww/nchshome.htm

National Center for HIV, Sexually Transmitted Diseases, and Tuberculosis
http://www.cdc.gov/nchstp/od/nchstp.html

National Center for Infectious Diseases
http://www.cdc.gov.ncidod/ncid.htm

National Institute for Occupational Safety and Health
http://www.cdc.gov/niosh/homepage.html

Department of Agriculture

Animal & Plant Health Inspection Service
http://www.aphis.usda.gov

Department of Agriculture
http://www.usda.gov

Food and Consumer Service
http://www.usda.gov/fcs/fcs.htm

Grain Inspection Packers & Stockyards Administration
http://www.usda.gov/gipsa

National Agricultural Library
http://www.nalusda.gov

Department of Health & Human Services

Administration for Children and Families
http://acf.dhhs.gov

Administration on Aging
http://www.aoa.dhhs.gov

Department of Health and Human Services
http://www.os.dhhs.gov

Health Resources and Services Administration
http://www.os.dhhs.gov/hrsa

Indian Health Service
http://www.tucson.ihs.gov

National Clearinghouse for Alcohol and Drug Information (Prevention Online)
http://www.health.org

National Health Information Center
http://nhic-nt.health.org

Office of Minority Health
http://www.os.dhhs.gov/progorg/ophs/omh

Secretary of Health and Human Services
http://phs.os.dhhs.gov/progorg/ospage.html

Food and Drug Administration

Center for Devices and Radiological Health
http://www.fda.gov/cdrh/index.html

Center for Drug Evaluation and Research
http://www.fda.gov.cder

Center for Food Safety and Applied Nutrition
http://vm.cfsan.fda.gov/list.html

FDA Consumer
http://www.fda.gov/fdac

Food & Drug Administration
http://www.fda.gov

MEDWATCH
http://www.fda.gov.medwatch/

National Institutes of Health

Magnuson, Warren Grant Clinical Center
http://www.cc.nih.gov

National Cancer Institute
http://nci.nih.gov

National Center for Human Genome Research
http://www.nchgr.nih.gov

National Center for Research Resources
http://www.ncrr.nih.gov

National Eye Institute
http://www.nei.nih.gov

National Heart, Lung, and Blood Institute
http://www.nhlbi.nih.gov

National Institute of Allergy and Infectious Diseases
http://www.niaid.nih.gov

National Institute of Arthritis and Musculoskeletal and Skin Diseases
http://www.nih.gov/niams

National Institute of Child Health and Human Development
http://www.nih.gov/nichd ,

National Institute of Diabetes and Digestive and Kidney Diseases
http://www.niddk.nih.gov

National Institute of Dental Research
http://www.nidr.nih.gov

National Institute of Environmental Health Sciences
http://www.niehs.nih.gov

National Institute of General Medical Sciences
http://www.nih.gov/nigms

National Institute of Mental Health
http://www.nimh.nih.gov/home.htm

National Institute of Neurological Disorders and Stroke
http://www.nih.gov/ninds

National Institute of Nursing Research
http://www.nih.gov/ninr

National Institute on Alcohol Abuse and Alcoholism
http://niaaa.nia.gov

National Institute on Drug Abuse
http://www.nida.nih.gov

National Institutes of Health
http://www.nih.gov

National Institutes of Health Research Grants Division
http://www.drg.nih.gov

National Library of Medicine
http://www.nlm.nih.gov

Other Selected Government Agencies and Independent Agencies

Consumer Information Center
http://www.pueblo.gsa.gov

Consumer Product Safety Commission
http://ww.cpsc.gov

Department of Veterans Affairs
http://www.va.gov

Environmental Protection Agency
http://www.epa.gov

Federal Emergency Management Agency
http://www.fema.gov

Federal Trade Commission
http://www.ftc.gov

General Accounting Office
http://www.gao.gov

General Services Administration
http://www.gsa.gov

Government Printing Office
http://www.access.gpo.gov

Health Care Financing Administration
http://www.hcfa.gov

Library of Congress: Links to State and Local Government Web Sites
http://lcweb.loc.gov/global/state/stategov.html

Occupational Safety and Health Administration
http://www.osha.gov

Persian Gulf Veterans' Illness
http://www.va.gov/health/environ/persgulf.htm

Social Security Administration
http://www.ssa.gov

Veterans Affairs Medical Center
http://pet.med.va.gov:8080

Index

Index

Index

NOTE: Page numbers followed by "n" represent footnotes; *italic* page numbers represent figures.

A

abortion rates, adolescents 30-31
abusive behavior prevention, Healthy
  People 2000 goal 184-85
Access 623
accidents and injuries
  cause of death 42-43, *78,* 87, *94*
  see also motor vehicles
Accreditation of Laboratory Animal
  Care, American Association for 295
ACIP *see* Immunization Practices,
  Advisory Committee on (ACIP)
Acquired Immunodeficiency Syn-
  drome, Division of 444, 447
ACS *see* American Cancer Society (ACS)
Active Foodborne Disease Surveil-
  lance Network 394
activity limitations
  causes *12*
  disorders and injuries 11
ADAMHA News 586
ademocarcinoma 145
Administrative Procedure Act 307

*Adolescent Abstinence: A Guide for
  Family Planning Professionals* 610
adolescent birth rates 168, 177
Adolescent Pregnancy Programs, Office of 583
adolescents
  AIDS 16-17
  birth rates 40
  fraud avoidance 359
  health education 61
  mortality rates 29-30
  pregnancy rates 30-31
  vaccines 246
  see also children; young adults
Advanced Data 621
Advanced Notice of Proposed
  Rulemaking (ANPR) 391, 407
*Advance Report of Final Mortality
  Statistics* 37
*The Advance Report of Final Mortal-
  ity Statistics, Monthly Vital Statistics Report (MVSR)* 79
*Advance Report of Final Natality Sta-
  tistics* 37
Aeronautics and Space Administration, National (NASA) 444
African-Americans
  cancer rates 119-63
  health status indicators 169-70

E

E. coli 222, 223, 389, 396, 403, 404
early detection
  chronic disease prevention 58-59,
  61
  food safety 394-97
Ebola virus 222
economic burden of chronic disease
  54-76
*Educating Students with Learning
  Problems: A Shared Responsibility*
  604
educational attainment, life expectancy 101
Educational Programs That Work 602
*The Education of Students with Dis-
  abilities: Where Do We Stand?* 603
education programs 59-61
  cancer 163
  food safety 407-10
  Healthy People 2000 goal 185
EIP *see* Emerging Infections Program
  (EIP)
Emerging Infections Program (EIP)
  236
emphysema
  cause of death *56*
  described 73
  research 439
endometrium cancer 144
enteritis, cause of death *56*
enterococci, resistant 237
environmental health, Healthy
  People 2000 goal 186
Environmental Health, National Center for (NCEH) 211-12
  internet address 657
Environmental Health Perspective 608
Environmental Health Sciences, National Institute of (NIEHS) 496-500,
  560
  Environmental Biology and Medi-
    cine Program 500
  Environmental Carcinogenesis Pro-
    gram 500
  Environmental Health Sciences
    Centers 498

Environmental Health Sciences,
National Institute of (NIEHS),
continued
  Environmental Toxicology Program
    500
  Extramural Research and Training,
    Division of 498
  internet address 660
  Intramural Research, Division of
    499-500
  Marine and Freshwater Biomedical
    Sciences Centers 499
  Public Affairs Officer 608
  Research Manpower Development
    Programs 499
  Superfund Basic Research Program
    499
Environmental Protection Agency
  (EPA) 168, 170, 175, 276, 279, 324,
  352, 380, 386, 391, 392, 397, 402,
  403
  internet address 661
  Public Information Center 608
EPA *see* Environmental Protection
  Agency (EPA)
epidemics 221-22
Epidemiology Program Office (EPO)
  217
  internet address 657
epilepsy
  described 73
  research 517
EPO *see* Epidemiology Program Office (EPO)
Epstein-Barr virus 448
ERIC Clearinghouse on Teacher Education 606-7
Escherichia coli (E. coli) 222, 223,
  389, 396, 403, 404
esophageal cancer 145
"Established Populations for Epidemiologic Studies of the Elderly"
  (EPESE) 529
ethnic factors
  AIDS (acquired immune deficiency
    syndrome) 32
  birth rates *38*, 39-41
  cancer patterns 119-63
  causes of death *72*, 77-83

Environmentally Induced Disorders Sourcebook

Basic Information about Diseases and Syndromes Linked to Exposure to Pollutants and Other Substances in Outdoor and Indoor Environments Such As Lead, Asbestos, Formaldehyde, Mercury, Emissions, Noise, and More

Edited by Allan R. Cook. 620 pages. 1997. 0-7808-0083-4. $75.

Fitness & Exercise Sourcebook

Basic Information on Fitness and Exercise, Including Fitness Activities for Specific Age Groups, Exercise for People with Specific Medical Conditions, How to Begin a Fitness Program in Running, Walking, Swimming, Cycling, and Other Athletic Activities, and Recent Research in Fitness and Exercise

Edited by Dan R. Harris. 663 pages. 1996. 0-7808-0186-5. $75.

Food & Animal Borne Diseases Sourcebook

Basic Information about Diseases That Can Be Spread to Humans through the Ingestion of Contaminated Food or Water or by Contact with Infected Animals and Insects, Such As Botulism, E. Coli, Hepatitis A, Trichinosis, Lyme Disease, and Rabies, along with Information Regarding Prevention and Treatment Methods, and a Special Section for International Travelers Describing Diseases Such as Cholera, Malaria, Travelers' Diarrhea, and Yellow Fever, and Offering Recommendations for Avoiding Illness

Edited by Karen Bellenir and Peter D. Dresser. 535 pages. 1995. 0-7808-0033-8. $75.

"A comprehensive collection of authoritative information." — *Emergency Medical Services, Oct '95*

"Targeting general readers and providing them with a single, comprehensive source of information on selected topics, this book continues, with the excellent caliber of its predecessors, to catalog topical information on health matters of general interest. Readable and thorough, this valuable resource is highly recommended for all libraries."
— *Academic Library Book Review, Summer '96*

Gastrointestinal Diseases & Disorders Sourcebook

Basic Information about Gastroesophageal Reflux Disease (Heartburn), Ulcers, Diverticulosis, Irritable Bowel Syndrome, Crohn's Disease, Ulcerative Colitis, Diarrhea, Constipation, Lactose Intolerance, Hemorrhoids, Hepatitis, Cirrhosis and Other Digestive Problems, Featuring Statistics, Descriptions of Symptoms, and Current Treatment Methods of Interest for Persons Living with Upper and Lower Gastrointestinal Maladies

Edited by Linda M. Ross. 413 pages. 1996. 0-7808-0078-8. $75.

". . . very readable form. The successful editorial work that brought this material together into a useful and understandable reference makes accessible to all readers information that can help them more effectively understand and obtain help for digestive tract problems." — *Choice, Feb '97*

Genetic Disorders Sourcebook

Basic Information about Heritable Diseases and Disorders Such As Down Syndrome, PKU, Hemophilia, Von Willebrand Disease, Gaucher Disease, Tay-Sachs Disease, and Sickle-Cell Disease, along with Information about Genetic Screening, Gene Therapy, Home Care, and Including Source Listings for Further Help and Information on More Than 300 Disorders

Edited by Karen Bellenir. 642 pages. 1996. 0-7808-0034-6. $75.

". . . geared toward the lay public. It would be well placed in all public libraries and in those hospital and medical libraries in which access to genetic references is limited."
— *Doody's Health Sciences Book Review, Oct '96*

"Provides essential medical information to both the general public and those diagnosed with a serious or fatal genetic disease or disorder."
— *Choice, Jan '97*

Head Trauma Sourcebook

Basic Information for the Layperson about Open-Head and Closed-Head Injuries, Treatment Advances, Recovery, and Rehabilitation, along with Reports on Current Research Initiatives

Edited by Karen Bellenir. 414 pages. 1997. 0-7808-0208-X. $75.

Health Insurance Sourcebook

Basic Information about Managed Care Organizations, Traditional Fee-for-Service Insurance, Insurance Portability and Pre-Existing Conditions Clauses, Medicare, Medicaid, Social Security, and Military Health Care, along with Information about Insurance Fraud

Edited by Wendy Wilcox. 530 pages. 1997. 0-7808-0222-5. $75.

Continues next page

Immune System Disorders Sourcebook

Basic Information about Lupus, Multiple Sclerosis, Guillain-Barré Syndrome, Chronic Granulomatous Disease, and More, along with Statistical and Demographic Data and Reports on Current Research Initiatives

Edited by Allan R. Cook. 608 pages. 1997. 0-7808-0209-8. $75.

Kidney & Urinary Tract Diseases &Disorders Sourcebook

Basic Information about Kidney Stones, Urinary Incontinence, Bladder Disease, End-Stage Renal Disease, Dialysis, and More, along with Statistical and Demographic Data and Reports on Current Research Initiatives

Edited by Linda M. Ross. 602 pages. 1997. 0-7808-0079-6. $75.

Learning Disabilities Sourcebook

Basic Information about Disorders Such As Autism, Dyslexia, Hyperactivity, and Attention Deficit Disorder, along with Statistical and Demographic Data and Reports on Current Research Initiatives

Edited by Linda M. Ross. 600 pages. 1998. 0-7808-0210-1. $75.

Men's Health Concerns Sourcebook

Basic Information about Topics of Special Interest to Men, Including Prostate Enlargement, Impotence and Other Sexual Dysfunctions, Vasectomies, Condoms, Snoring, Sleep Apnea, Hair Loss, and More

Edited by Allan R. Cook. 600 pages. 1998. 0-7808-0212-8. $75.

Mental Health Disorders Sourcebook

Basic Information about Schizophrenia, Depression, Bipolar Disorder, Panic Disorder, Obsessive-Compulsive Disorder, Phobias and Other Anxiety Disorders, Paranoia and Other Personality Disorders, Eating Disorders, and Sleep Disorders, along with Information about Treatment and Therapies

Edited by Karen Bellenir. 548 pages. 1995. 0-7808-0040-0. $75.

". . . provides information on a wide range of mental disorders, presented in nontechnical language."
— Exceptional Child Education Resources, Spring '96

"The text is well organized and adequately written for its target audience." — Choice, Jun '96

"The great strengths of the book are its readability and its inclusion of places to find more information. Especially recommended." — RQ, Winter '96

"Recommended for public and academic libraries."
— Reference Book Review, '96

". . . useful for public and academic libraries and consumer health collections."
— Medical Reference Services Quarterly, Spring '97

Ophthalmic Disorders Sourcebook

Basic Information about Glaucoma, Cataracts, Macular Degeneration, Strabismus, Refractive Disorders, and More, along with Statistical and Demographic Data and Reports on Current Research Initiatives

Edited by Linda M. Ross. 631 pages. 1996. 0-7808-0081-8. $75.

Oral Health Sourcebook

Basic Information about Diseases and Conditions Affecting Oral Health, Including Cavities, Gum Disease, Dry Mouth, Oral Cancers, Fever Blisters, Canker Sores, Oral Thrush, Bad Breath, Temporomandibular Disorders, and other Craniofacial Syndromes, along with Statistical Data on the Oral Health of Americans, Oral Hygiene, Emergency First Aid, Information on Treatment Procedures and Methods of Replacing Lost Teeth

Edited by Allan R. Cook. 560 pages. 1997. 0-7808-0082-6. $75.

Pain Sourcebook

Basic Information about Specific Forms of Acute and Chronic Pain, Including Headaches, Back Pain, Muscular Pain, Neuralgia, Surgical Pain, and Cancer Pain, along with Pain Relief Options Such As Analgesics, Narcotics, Nerve Blocks, Transcutaneous Nerve Stimulation, and Alternative Forms of Pain Control, Including Biofeedback, Imaging, Behavior Modification, and Relaxation Techniques

Edited by Allan R. Cook. 608 pages. 1997. 0-7808-0213-6. $75.

Pregnancy & Birth Sourcebook

Basic Information about Planning for Pregnancy, Fetal Growth and Development, Labor and Delivery, Postpartum and Perinatal Care, Pregnancy in Mothers with Special Concerns, and Disorders of Pregnancy, Including Genetic Counseling, Nutrition and Exercise, Obstetrical Tests, Pregnancy Discomfort, Multiple Births, Cesarean Sections, Medical Testing of Newborns, Breastfeeding, Gestational Diabetes, and Ectopic Pregnancy

Edited by Heather Aldred. 752 pages. 1997. 0-7808-0216-0. $75.